Eberhard Krüger and Wilfried Schilli, Editors
Oral and Maxillofacial Traumatology, Volume 1

Oral and Maxillofacial Traumatology

Edited by

Eberhard Krüger, M.D., D.M.D.

Professor and Head of Department of Oral and Maxillofacial Surgery,
University of Bonn, Federal Republic of Germany

and

Wilfried Schilli, M.D., D.M.D.

Professor and Head of Department of Oral and Maxillofacial Surgery,
University of Freiburg, Federal Republic of Germany

Volume 1

quintessence books

Quintessence Publishing Co., Inc., 1982
Chicago, Berlin, Rio de Janeiro and Tokyo

Composition and printing: Kupijai & Prochnow, Berlin
Binding: J. Godry, Berlin
Printed in Germany

ISBN: 0-931386-68-3

List of Contributors

Jacques A. Baart, D.D.S.
Department of Oral Surgery. Teaching Hospital, Free University Amsterdam, The Netherlands

Rudolf Fries, M.D.
Professor and Head of Department of Maxillofacial Surgery, General Hospital, Linz, Austria

Walter Hoffmann-Axthelm, M.D., D.M.D.
Professor Emeritus of History of Medicine and Dentistry, Free University of Berlin, now Freiburg i. Br., Federal Republic of Germany

Eberhard Krüger, M.D., D.M.D.
Professor and Head of Department of Oral and Maxillofacial Surgery, University of Bonn, Federal Republic of Germany

Willem A. M. van der Kwast, D.D.S.
Professor and Head of Department of Oral and Maxillofacial Surgery. Teaching Hospital, Free University Amsterdam, The Netherlands

Jürgen Lentrodt, M.D., D.M.D.
Professor and Head of Department of Maxillofacial Surgery, University of Düsseldorf, Federal Republic of Germany

Hans-Georg Luhr, M.D., D.M.D.
Professor and Head of Department of Maxillofacial Surgery, University of Göttingen, Federal Republic of Germany

Herbert Niederdellmann, M.D., D.M.D.
Professor, Department of Oral and Maxillofacial Surgery, University of Freiburg, Federal Republic of Germany

Berton A. Rahn, M.D., D.M.D.
Swiss Research Institute, Laboratory for Experimental Surgery, Davos, Switzerland

Bernhard Rottke, M.D., D.M.D.
Professor and Head of Department of Dental and Maxillofacial Radiology, University of Hamburg, Federal Republic of Germany

Wilfried Schilli, M.D., D.M.D.
Professor and Head of Department of Oral and Maxillofacial Surgery, University of Freiburg, Federal Republic of Germany

Norbert Schwenzer, M.D., D.M.D.
Professor and Head of Department of Maxillofacial Surgery, University of Tübingen, Federal Republic of Germany

Wolfgang Steinhilber, M.D., D.M.D.
Professor and Head of Department of Oral and Maxillofacial Surgery, Rudolf Virchow Hospital, Berlin, Federal Republic of Germany

Foreword

In view of the current increase in those injuries affecting predominantly the maxillofacial region, a comprehensive description of the traumatology of that section of the body is particularly desirable.
The pair of editors, together with the contributing authors–each of whom is an outstanding specialist in his field–have produced a work that is especially timely because of its extensive description of the technique of rigid internal fixation. Publication in the English language makes world-wide distribution possible. The book is suitable as a text for the oral and maxillofacial surgeon in training. Beyond that, it will be of great practical use to all those who are responsible for the care of patients with maxillofacial injuries in operating rooms on a day-to-day basis.

Hamburg, October 1981 Karl Schuchardt

Preface

Why a book about maxillofacial traumatology? The question can be answered relatively easily. This division of maxillofacial surgery has undergone such rapid development in the past decade that the available books cannot be contemporaneous any longer. That reason seemed to us to justify compilation of a new traumatology book. But a new book today soon may be out of date as well if, during the period in which it is being prepared, advances are made that cannot be included sufficiently in its contents.

This book is directed in the first instance to the maxillofacial surgeon active in the operating room. In addition to the long accepted conservative methods of fracture treatment, the surgical techniques, and especially rigid internal fixation, are discussed in detail. Functionally stable osteosynthesis of mandibular fractures with plates and lag screws, which makes intermaxillary fixation superfluous, has been developed in Europe to a perfectly routine method. Building on the experiences of surgery of the extremities, a system has been devised for the mandible that allows precise adjustments and exact fixation of the fragments with compression, thus permitting immediate functional stress. During the period in which this book was being written, acceptance was gained for stable osteosynthesis with miniplates for the management of midface fractures, so that here too, the need for intermaxillary fixation was obviated, a condition impossible until now with ordinary internal wire fixation. This most recent advance just made it into this book.

In addition to presentation of maxillofacial aspects, the associated topics of neurosurgery, ENT surgery and ophthalmology are taken up. The book is directed as well to dentists, surgeons, orthopedic surgeons, and anesthesiologists; in short, to practitioners of all the specialties dealing with traumatology.

Although most of the authors work in continental Europe, it is our purpose to make this book available to as many interested persons as possible in all nations; for this reason the work is published in the English language. Its international character is underlined through the use of the tooth numbering system of the F. D. I. throughout (see footnote, p. 173), and the use of abbreviations from World Medical Periodicals in the references. Non-English titles of references have been supplemented with English translations.

The scope of the material to be presented requires a 2-volume work. That design seemed more sensible to us than a rather clumsy, mammoth single volume.

Bonn and Freiburg, October 1981

Eberhard Krüger — Wilfried Schilli

Acknowledgements

The editors would like to record their gratitude to the contributing authors for the excellence of their work.

Mr. Walter A. Lerch prepared the drawings with great artistic sensitivity, which we would like to point out with special praise.

Mr. Henry M. Koehler of Chicago is owed the special thanks of all German-writing authors for his fundamental role in the translation of the manuscripts.

Finally, the editors would like to thank Mr. H. W. Haase, Mr. G. Kirsten and the staff of the Quintessence Publishing Co. for their willing cooperation and readiness to grant the editors' wishes for these volumes.

Bonn and Freiburg, October 1981

Eberhard Krüger Wilfried Schilli

Contents

Chapter 8

Mandibular Fractures

Chapter 1

The Treatment of Maxillofacial Fractures and Dislocations, in Historical Perspective

Walter Hoffmann-Axthelm

1. Antiquity

We will never know with certainty the time when an early *Homo sapiens* first adjusted a fracture intentionally or when he aligned a dislocation. Perhaps it occurred during the early Stone Age, that a broken extremity was splinted with wood or bamboo sticks or was embedded in clay that was allowed to harden. It is a long way from that point to the appropriate care of a facial fracture as we know it.

The early Egyptian *Smith* papyrus is one of the oldest surgical writings known. It was written in hieroglyphs in the middle of the 16th century B. C., at the beginning of the New Kingdom, a time when Egypt was developing into the leading power of the world. Its predominantly surgical content, however, reflects knowledge gathered a thousand years before, perhaps in the time of the pyramid builders of the Old Kingdom (2650-2150 B.C.). Among other things this work contains a careful and precise description of the alignment and support of the fractured nasal bone:

> "When you examine a man with a break of the column of his nose; his nose is broadened, his face is planar; the swelling on it (the fracture) rises high. He bleeds from his nostrils: Then you must say about this: a fracture of the column of the nose. An ailment that I will treat. Then you should cleanse (his nose) with two plugs of linen. Then you should place two plugs of linen moistened with oil or grease into his nostrils. Then you should lay him down on his bed until his swelling is drawn out. Then you should apply a pillow of linen to hold his nose together. Treat him thereafter with oil/grease, honey, fibers every day, until he is better."[1]

While we have here a treatment plan that is still valid (with a grain of salt), the anonymous author avoids treatment of infected fractures of the jaw:

> "If you examine a man with a fracture of his mandible, you should put your hand on it; and if you find the fracture, in that it becomes displaced under your fingers. Then you must say: one with a fracture in his mandible; and a wound has broken above it; the discharge(?) has stopped flowing(?); he has a fever as a result of it. An ailment that one cannot treat."[2]

This point of view, of giving up on cases held to be hopeless, was typical for ancient physicians, even the Greeks. A change in this attitude began only under the influence of Christianity.

In a manner that is still valid today, alignment of a dislocation of the mandible was described thus:

> "If you examine a man (with) a dislocation of his mandible, and you find his mouth opened, and he is unable to close his mouth, then you should place one of your fingers on (each) of both of his claw bones of his mandible on the inside of his mouth (and) both of your thumbs under his chin. Then you must let them (i.e., both claw bones) fall (back) so that they again lie in their correct places. Then you must say: one with a dislocation on his mandible. An ailment that I will treat. Then you should bandage him with bandages(?) (and) honey every day until he is well."

[1] Reference was not made to the texts of *Breasted* (1930) as is usual; rather, the more recent translation of *Westendorf* (1966) was used: *Westendorf* (1966) pp. 50f.; *Breasted* (1930) pp. 234f.

[2] *Westendorf* (1966) pp. 62f.; *Breasted* (1930) pp. 301f.

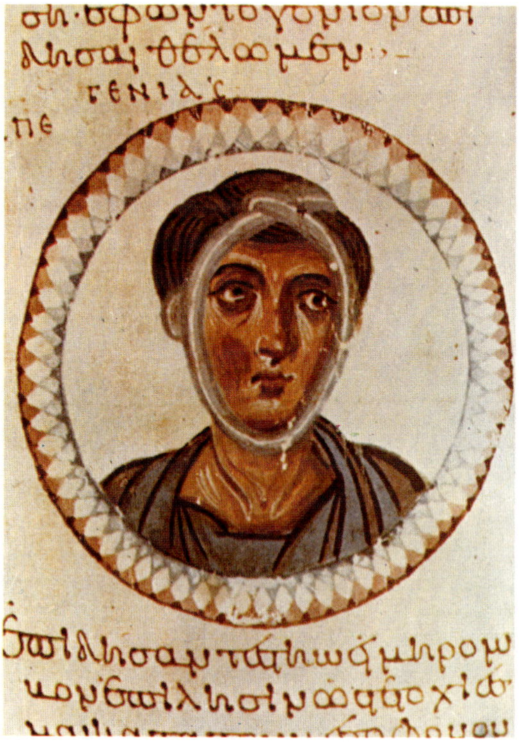

Fig. 1-1 *Soranos:* Jaw bandage (Florence, Codex Laurentianus pl. LXXIV, 7 fol. 232^{v}).

Here the ascending rami of the mandible with the associated condyles and articulation are described in an extraordinarily plastic way as claw bones.[3]

The comprehensive clay tablet medical literature of Mesopotamia, to the extent that we understand it today, does not include any mention at all of treatment of fractures.[4] Nevertheless, we find in the Code of *Hammurapi*, a stone-inscribed collection of the great Babylonian king (approximately 1792-1750 B.C.), the following:

> "If a physician set a broken bone for a man or cure his diseased bowels, the patient shall give five shekels of silver to the physician."

The first clear therapeutic guidelines are found at the turn of the fifth to the fourth century B.C. in the writings of the Hippocratic physicians. Here partial and complete fractures of the mandible ("like those of a stalk") are differentiated. The former is reduced

> "by making suitable lateral pressure with the fingers on the tongue side, and by counter-pressure from without. If the teeth at the point of injury are displaced or loosened, when the bone is adjusted fasten them to one another, not merely the two, but several, preferably with the gold wire, but failing that, with thread, till consolidation takes place" (*Hippocrates*).[5]

Then wax pads and linen wrappings should be used as a loose bandage, perhaps in the same manner as described by the Greek *Soranos* of Ephesos in his book "On Bandages" in the second century A.D. (Fig. 1-1). But the Hippocratics do not expect much from the effort, because the bandage must be repositioned again and again:

> "One should make frequent palpation on the

[3] *Westendorf* (1966) p. 63; *Breasted* (1930) pp. 303f. In case 22 we read about the claw-bone: "That is the end of its mandible. The claw-bone ends in his temple, like the claw-bird grasps for something." *Westendorf* (1966) p. 61; *Breasted* (1930) p.293

[4] Oral communication Prof. Dr. *Franz Köcher*, (1979) Berlin

[5] *Hippocrates*, On joints 32; Engl. transl. Vol. 3 pp. 257f.

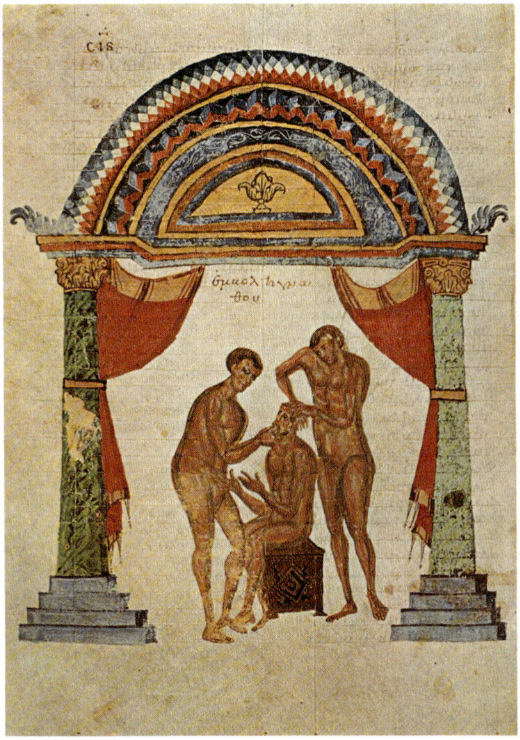

Fig. 1-2 *Apollonios* of Citium: "Setting a jaw" (Nicetas Codex).

tongue side, and hold the distorted part of the bone adjusted with the fingers for a long time. It would be best if one could do so throughout; but that is impossible."[6]

One may assume from this that the ligature described served only to splint the loosened teeth, but not the jaw.

For the care of a continuous fracture,

"which rarely happens, one should adjust it in the manner described. After adjustment you should fasten the teeth together as was described above, for this will contribute greatly to immobility, especially if one joins them up properly and fastens off the ends as they should be."

We can see from this that the author of this portion of the Corpus Hippocraticum, one of the oldest sections thereof and perhaps written by *Hippocrates* (approximately 460-375 B.C.) himself(?), was on the right path without, however, recognizing it completely.

"Next, one should take Carthagian leather; if the patient is more of a child, the outer layer is sufficient, but if he is more adult, use the skin itself. Cut a three-finger breadth, or as much as may be suitable, and, anointing the jaw with gum—for it is more agreeable than glue—fasten the end of the leather to the broken-off part of the jaw at a finger's breadth or rather more from the fracture. This is for the lower part; and let the strap have a slit in the line of the chin, so as to include the chin point. Another strap, similar or a little broader, the same interval from the fracture as the former one; and let it also be split for going round the ear."[7]

Still fully valid today is the Hippocratic criticism of the usual bandages, as they are applied by some practitioners without intelligence:

"But any bandaging of a jaw fractured in this

[6] Ibid. 32; Engl. transl. Vol. 3, p. 259
[7] Ibid. 33; Engl. transl. Vol. 3 p. 259f.

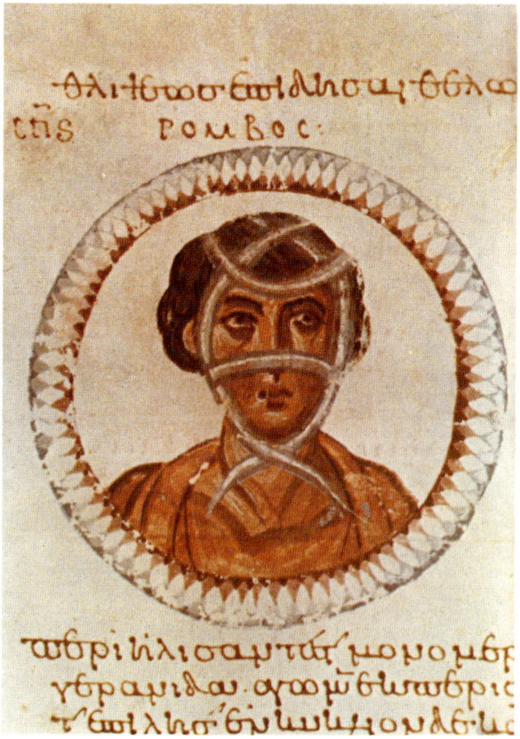

Fig. 1-3 *Soranos*: Facial bandage (Florence, Codex Laurentianus pl. LXXIV, 7 fol. 233ʳ).

way tends to turn the fragments inwards at the lesion rather than bring them to their natural position."[8]

The patient is best placed on his back for reduction of the mandible, with his head supported on a leather-covered pillow or

"someone should hold the patient's head, while the operator grasping the jaw with his fingers inside and out near the chin—the patient keeping it open as wide as he conveniently can—should move the jaw this way and that with his hand, and bid the patient keep it relaxed and assist the movement by yielding to it as far as possible. Then suddenly do a side-slip, having in mind three positions in the manœvre. For the deviation must be reduced to the natural direction, the jaw must be pressed backwards, and following this, the patient must close his jaws and not gape."[9]

Such a procedure is shown, surely based on the picture provided by the Nicetas Codex of *Apollonios* of Citium (approximately 100 B.C. Fig. 1-2). This code is a work dated from before 1000 A.D. Bilateral dislocation is treated similarly. Here the chin is out even further but lateral displacement, as demonstrated by the position of the teeth, is absent.

"If not reduced, there is risk of death from acute fever and deep coma; ...These patients, then, die about the tenth day."[10]

This unusual prognosis has been adopted by the Arabs and transferred to the period of scholastic medicine of Europe of the 16th century. We find it two millennia after its origin in the works of *Ambroise Paré* (1585); it is quoted critically first by the Paris surgeon *Petit* in the 18th century.

Hippocrates' warning against the effects of pressure is even stronger in reference to fractures of the nasal bone than in jaw fractures:

"If the nose is broken, which happens in more than one way, those who delight in fine band-

[8] Ibid. 33; Engl. transl. Vol. 3 p. 263
[9] Ibid. 30; Engl. transl. Vol. 3, pp. 255f.
[10] Ibid. 31; Engl. transl. Vol. 3, p. 257

aging without judgement do more damage than usual. For this is the most varied of bandagings, having the most adze-like turns and diverse rhomboid intervals and vacancies... But such bandaging acts in every way contrary to what is proper; for first, in cases where the nose in rendered concave by the fracture, if more pressure is applied from above, it will obviously be more concave."

He proposes application of a hardening dough made of wheat flour following repositioning with the finger or a probe inserted into the nose and checked by external palpation. He does not demand that the nose be packed as strictly as the Egyptian physician.[11] Traces of this text again may be found in the work of *Soranos* about bandages (Fig. 1-3).

The second grand period of Greek medicine began in the third century B.C. and was called the Alexandrian. It is not known to us directly except through the previously quoted work of *Apollonios* of Citium. Nonetheless, the knowledge of this school was collected in the first half of the first century A.D. in Latin—there never having been an autonomous Roman medicine—by the Roman encyclopedist *Aulus Cornelius Celsus*. In dealing with treatment of fractures of the jaw, however, he and his documents did not advance beyond the followers of *Hippocrates:*

"Next, if the lower jaw has been broken across, in which case generally one tooth stands higher than its neighbour, when it has been put back into position tie together with horsehair the two adjacent teeth, or if these are loose, teeth further away."

Then, at first, only liquids are given, followed by a soft diet

"until the formation of callus has rendered the lower jaw quite firm."

During the reduction of the mandible, the head is held by an aide, as suggested by *Hippocrates*, but a number of positive variations are provided:

"Then the surgeon's thumbs, which have been wrapped around with strips of linen or bandages so that they may not slip, are inserted into the mouth whilst the fingers are applied outside. When the jaw has been grasped firmly, if it has slipped forwards to one side, the chin is to be pressed downwards toward the throat with a jerk. Then simultaneously the head is firmly held, and the chin being raised the jaw is forced back to its place, and the mouth is closed so that all this is done almost (simultaneously)."[12]

For the support of the reduced nasal bone, he introduced

"a roll of folded linen with thin leather sewn on over it.... or some sort of dry pad similarly shaped; or a large quill smeared with gum or joiner's glue, and wrapped round with soft thin leather, which will prevent the cartilage from sinking in again."[13]

The man from antiquity who was most important in the development of medicine in the Europe of the Middle Ages and more important even than *Hippocrates*, was the Greek *Galen* of Pergamon (129-199). He functioned as court physician to the emperor Marcus Aurelius. Although six hundred years separate him from his countryman, *Galen* knew of nothing to add to the instructions of the Hippocratics. Thus, even superfluous trifles such as Carthagian leather are described extensively.[14]

2. The Middle Ages and the Beginnings of Modern Times

Following the final disruption of the West Roman Empire through the onslaught of Germanic tribes in 476, the traditions of Greek medicine were continued in the Byzantine Empire, if in somewhat sterile ways. Surgically most significant among the Byzantine physicians, *Paul* of Aegina worked in the 7th century in Alexandria, and as he expressly admitted, adopted the procedures of the Hippocratic school almost word for word for the treatment of mandibular fractures and dislocations. His only addition was to advocate that probing be used to remove bone chips in complicated fractures, and that wounds shown be sutured. He worked similarly in treating nasal bone fractures,[15] noting the use

[11] Ibid. 35; Engl. transl. Vol. 3, pp. 267f.
[12] *Celsus* VIII 7,2; Engl. transl. Vol. 3, p. 525; VIII 12, 2-4; Engl. transl. Vol. 3, p. 565
[13] Ibid. VIII 5, 1-6; Engl. transl. Vol. 3, pp. 519f.
[14] *Galen* Hipp. Art comment. 2, 25. XVIII 1, p. 455, 1-10 Kühn.
[15] *Paulos* VI 92, 3; VI 112, 2-3; VI 91

Figs. 1-4 A and B *Abu l-Qasim* (Albucasis): Wire splinting of loose teeth.

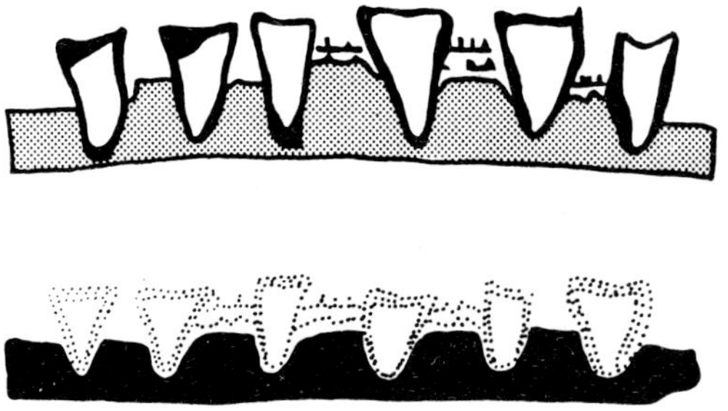

Fig. 1-4 A Redrawn by H. Huntington (from Spink/Lewis).

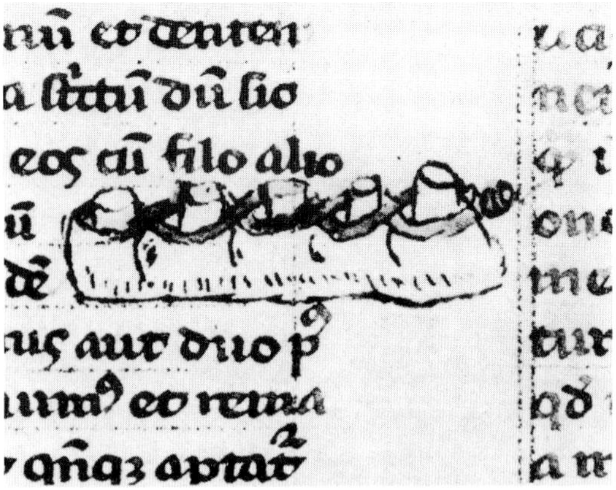

Fig. 1-4 B In the Latin translation of Gerard of Cremona (Stadtbibliothek Bamberg Ms LIII 15).

of quills (in his case from geese), known from the time of *Celsus*.

When Alexandria surrendered to the Arabs without a battle in 643, *Paul* remained, with full honors, but medical life ended there about 700. The true successors to this Alexandrian medicine were the founders of Islamic culture. In the ninth century, Arab scholars translated not only the works of *Paul*, but also the Hippocratic writings as well as those of *Aristotle*, *Galen* and other Greeks into their language. In a marvelous synthesis with their own knowledge, they formed the fundamental base for the flowering of medical science in the occident too.

Among the most important Islamic physicians, from the surgical point of view, of the 10th and 11th centuries was *Abu l-Qasim* who lived in Arab-occupied Spain. He was born in Cordoba, worked there and died after 1009. His method for the care of the reduced fractured mandible was completely in the ancient tradition:

> "If any of the teeth be loosened or broken away, bind those that you hope may be preserved with a gold or silver or silken ligature (Fig. 1-4); then put wax upon the fractured mandible, and upon that a doubled dressing, and upon the dressing a large and strong splint or a piece of shoe-sole leather the length of the jaw; then cover that bandage in such wise as you conveniently can and as will conduce to drawing it together so as not to loosen."

In general, he leaned strongly on *Paul* of Aegina, as is clearly shown especially in the treatment of a complicated fracture:

> "If the fracture be with an open wound, examine it, and if one or more splinters have been detached from the bone, gently remove the pieces of splinter with any convenient instrument. If the opening of the wound be narrow, open it up with a scalpel as much as you need. When you have removed these pieces, letting no trace of them remain, suture the opening of the wound if it is wide; otherwise apply one of the ointments that are suitable for that purpose and will encourage the growth of flesh over the wound, until it heals."

Abu l-Qasim also adopted the Hippocratic prognosis of danger of death in the event of delayed adjustment from *Paul* of Aegina.[16]

The works of the Islamic physicians were translated in Salerno and Toledo into Latin in the 11th and 12th centuries, and were willingly accepted in Europe. This led to the decline of the so-called "monk's medicine" and to the development of a scientific medicine based on an Arab-influenced Greek tradition.

Gerard of Cremona (1114-1187), who was the

[16] *Abu l-Qasim* XXX 3,24, p. 600, 11f.; Albucasis Engl. transl. Spink and Lewis pp. 716f.; p. 790

chief of the Toledan school, translated among others the surgical opus of *Abu l-Qasim (Albucasis)* and the dominating "Canon medicinae" of *Ibn-Sina (Avicenna*, 980-1037). Both of these works had decisive influence on the surgery of the occident—at first especially on that of northern Italy.

Among the northern Italian surgeons who adopted the writings of *Albucasis* and *Avicenna*, the important Bolognese surgeon *Teoderico Borgognoni (Theodericus* of Cervia, approximately 1205-1298) added the advice that an assistant should pull forward on the fragments of a double mandibular fracture while the wire ligature was being placed.[17] *William* of Saliceto (approximately 1210-1280), who was active in Bologna and Verona, provided a particularly plastic description of jaw splinting, for which he used waxed, twisted silk threads:

> "...and bind the teeth with it as if you were weaving a hurdle and continue this interlacing between the teeth of the injured jaw and those of the uninjured jaw, going from one tooth to another in such a way that the part be immobilised."

The Lyon edition of 1492 includes the following addition:

> "This done, tie the teeth of the uninjured jaw to the teeth of the injured jaw in this way."

Here for the first time we find the suggestion that the fractured mandible be splinted to the intact maxilla. But because this phrase is absent from the remaining handwritten manuscripts of the 13th century, and also does not appear in the early prints of *William*—one that was prepared from the such handwritten versions—the extra phrase might well be an isolated addition made in the 15th century.[18] In any case, such a suggestion from that time is significant, because the thought was not brought up again until the end of the 19th century. *William* was the first to mention the rare upward dislocation.

Lanfranchi (d. approximately 1306), a student of *William*, and later a Milanese surgeon, was banned from Milan in 1250 and worked with extraordinary fruitfulness in Paris. He proposed a new method for reduction of the mandible: An assistant sitting behind the patient pulls a sling placed around the patient's chin backwards while the surgeon pushes two wedge-shaped blocks of wood serving as levers as far back between the dental arches as possible.[19]

Most of this Greek-Arabic-Italian knowledge appears again in the writings of *Guy de Chauliac* (d. 1368), who was surgeon in Montpellier and papal court physician in Avignon. His works influenced *Ambroise Paré* (1510-1590) of Paris, who was court surgeon to four French kings, and who may be said to have prepared the way for modern surgery. In other respects an important innovator, he added nothing to the treatment of jaw fractures. In discussing dislocations of the TMJ, he notes the previously described Hippocratic thesis of death on the tenth day after failure of reduction; he also described *William*'s method with a backward pull on a sling and the sling-wedge method of *Lanfranchi*. *Paré* restored the fractured nasal bone with the externally palpating hand and a covered spatula inserted into a nostril. Then he placed pieces of sponge or black oakum into the nostril. He also supported the nasal skeleton with gold, silver or lead tubes which he fastened to a head cap with bands.[20]

William's comparison of the wrapped teeth "with a hurdle" was illustrated graphically by the Strasbourg surgeon *Hieronymus Brunschwig* (approximately 1450-1512/13) in his "Buch der Cirurgia," printed for the first time in 1497 (Fig. 1-5). Following splinting, he shaped a wooden chin for immobilization, sewed a cloth over it, and fastened 3 or 4 further cloths to it with flour glue. This chin cup arrangement was fitted to the chin and held in place by bands running around the top of the head. Dislocations were treated according to *Lanfranchi*'s method with sling and wooden wedges.[21] The wire splint dressing devised by *Walther Ryff* (d. 1562), also from Strasbourg, gives a much more solid impression. It is described in his "Gross Chirurgei" published in 1545, with the notation that the wire should be annealed beforehand[22] (Fig. 1-6).

The usually thoroughly practical surgeon and doctor of medicine of the Hague, *Cornelius Solingen* (1641-1687), repeated *Paré*'s instructions about nasal fractures in his own "Hand-

[17] *Theodoricus* Cerv. (1400) II 28, p. 110b^{V}, 35-50
[18] *William of Saliceto* (1546) III 18; III 2; see *Rowe*
[19] *Lanfranchi* (1400) IV 2,2, p. 211a^{V}, 41-60
[20] *Paré* (1585) XV 7, pp. 536f.; XVI 8-10, pp. 556f.; XV 6, pp. 535f.
[21] *Brunschwig* (1497, 1518) Fol. 59b^{V}-60b^{r}; Fol. 112a^{V}-113a^{r}
[22] *Ryff* (1559) Fol. 38^{r}

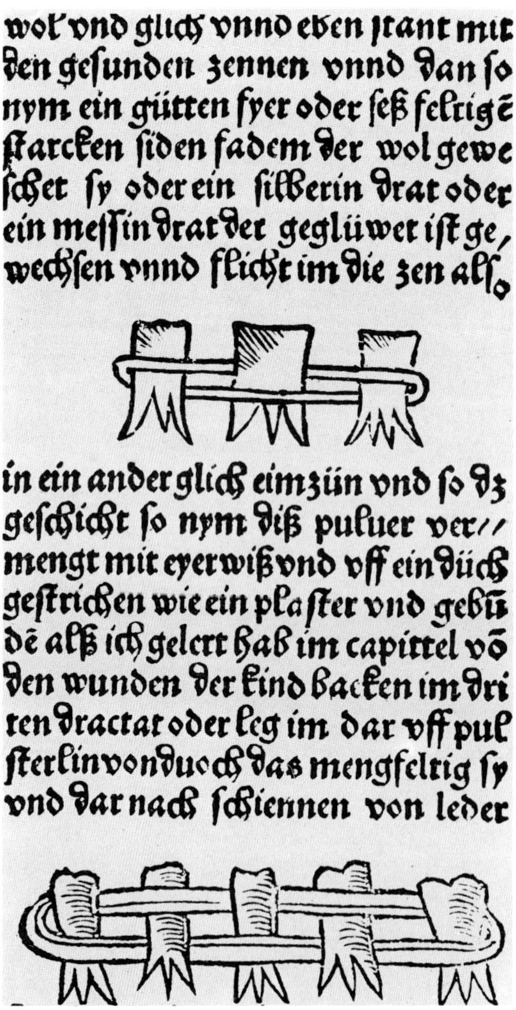

wol vnd glich vnnd eben stant mit
den gesunden zennen vnnd dan so
nym ein gütten syer oder seß seltigē
starcken siden fadem der wol gewe
schet sy oder ein silberin drat oder
ein messin drat der geglüwet ist ge/
wechsen vnnd flicht im die zen also

in ein ander glich eim züin vnd so dz
geschicht so nym diß puluer ver//
mengt mit eyerwiß vnd vff ein düch
gestrichen wie ein pflaster vnd gebū
dē alß ich gelert hab im capittel vō
den wunden der kind backen im dri
ten tractat oder leg im dar vff pul
sterlin von duech das mengseltig sy
vnd dar nach schiennen von leder

Fig. 1-5 *Brunschwig:* Woodcut of a splinted jaw fracture in the "Buch der Cirurgia," 1497; below, the illustration in the 1518 impression.

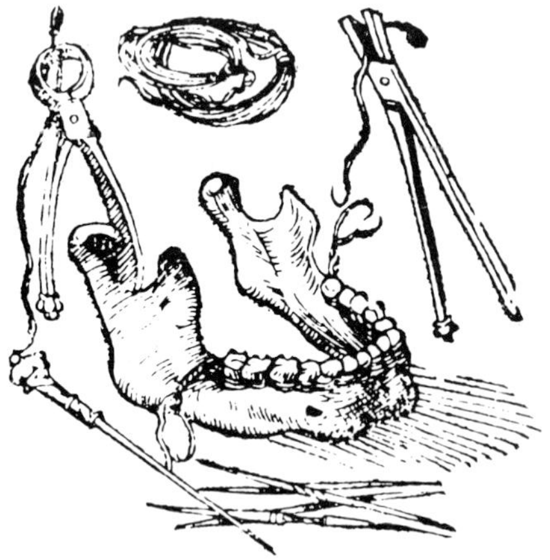

Fig. 1-6 *Ryff:* Wire splinting of a mandibular fracture, 1559.

griffe der Chirurgie" whose first edition was published in 1684. In support of the repositioned framework, however, he limited himself to individually fitted lead tubes affixed with thread to a cap. In diagonal fractures of the mandible, to the contrary, which in his view were invariably accompanied by loss of teeth, he had a new (perhaps) idea. A piece of soft wood (called "palm wood" in another writing) was placed over the fracture site, this wood having been hollowed out on its bottom surface and at its ends so that it adapted to the gingiva and adjacent teeth. The piece of wood was fastened to each of the adjacent distal and mesial teeth—which must thus be present—with cord: an early intraoral splint. The whole device is held in place with a dressing. He deems this "instrument" to be more protective than that proposed by his Amsterdam colleague *Hendrik von Roonhuyze* (1625-1672): a beaten copper plate that appears rather more suitable today, covering the region of the fracture site and the teeth.

"This (the device) is fastened with an annealed copper wire the thickness of a needle being

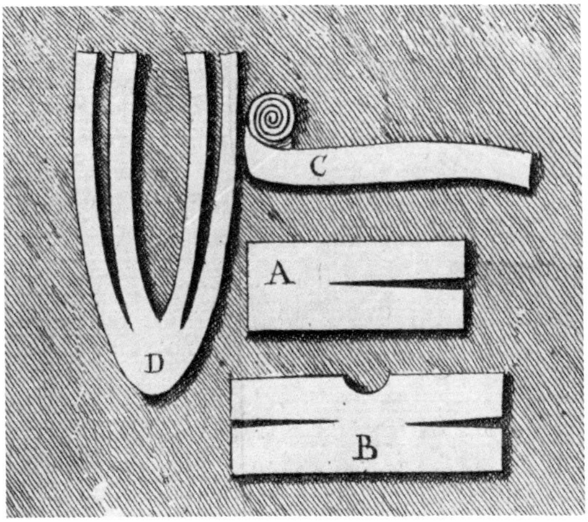

Fig. 1-7 *Petit:* Bandaging material for treatment of jaw fractures, 1723.

drawn around four teeth and pulled through holes prepared for the purpose in the instrument."[23]

The Arnheim surgeon *Johannes Muys* (b. 1654), proposed, in his "Praxis medico-chirurgica rationalis" of 1695, an instrument of ivory whose hollowing took up four teeth (namely two on each side), and with its (a bandage) help made the fractured mandible immobile; in 20 days it was completely healed.[24] —Was this an early version of a kind of cap splint?

3. The 18th Century

The combined intra- and extraoral therapy of mandibular fractures practiced since the time of antiquity (e.g., *Charles Gabriel Le Clerc* in Paris in 1700, *Lorenz Heister* in Helmstedt in 1718) was brought a true step backward by *Jean Louis Petit* (1676-1750), an otherwise important Parisian surgeon. In his two-volume "Traité de maladies des os" (A treatise on the diseases of the bone), contrary to the warnings of the Hippocratics against the displacing effects of bandages, he determined that the fractured mandible would no longer change its position after reduction and that therefore one could restrict treatment to an external bandage (Fig. 1-7). In fractures of the nasal bone too, whose care he undertook exactly as prescribed by *Paré*, he deemed a special bandage as more important than support through packing with lint. He believed that more force is required for the redisplacement of the broken bone than to reduce it. Treatment of mandibular dislocation was described in principle as it is in textbooks of today, but *Petit*'s writings show the first signs of doubt of the truth of the Hippocratic prognosis of death on the tenth day following neglected reduction of the mandible.[25]

As we have read, treatment of trauma of the jaws had been almost exclusively the province of the surgeon in the Middle Ages. This non-academically but almost exclusively mechanically trained, guild-organized craft slowly became established parallel to physicians through the fact that priests, who made up the bulk of physicians, were not allowed to undertake surgical measures. This was the result of an order of the IVth Lateran Council of 1215, forbidding priests anything that might have death as a consequence of their actions. The step, however, led to slow separation of academic medicine from practice, coming to rest in the following centuries in the rigid authoritarian beliefs of Greco-Arabic

[23] *Solingen* (1693) pp. 496-498
[24] *Muys* (1695) pp. 400f.
[25] *Le Clerc* (1700) pp. 82f.; *Heister* (1724) pp. 161f.; *Petit* (1725) 2, pp. 52f.

authors, especially that of the "Canon medicinae" of *Avicenna*. This cleavage of the medical arts into academic physicians and artisan-surgeons continued in most of the nations of Europe until the middle of the 19th century, e.g., in Prussia to 1852. At that time the surgeons joined the medical profession.
The profession of dentistry, slowly rising above the third and lowest level of the healing arts, was filled by charlatans and travelling journeymen, tooth drawers, cataract cutters, bone setters and lithotomists and herniotomists, leaving treatment of fractures in the hands of the surgeons exclusively at first. Thus there is not a single word in the two-volume work "Le Chirurgien Dentiste" by the Parisian dentist *Pierre Fauchard* (1678-1761), although it provided the cornerstone for an autonomous specialty of dentistry in 1728. For example, the book devotes many pages to closure of palatal perforations with obturators, however.
A comprehensive literature was initiated through *Fauchard*'s epochal work; yet, like him, his successors were silent on the subject. *Robert Bunon* (1702-1748), whose scientific interests and truly progressive drive distinguished him from his fellow chirurgiens dentistes, was an exception.[26] In his report of investigations of ricketts in Parisian hospitals, he indicated, in 1746, the care of a bilateral mandibular fracture with waxed silk ligatures. Here, two molars that disturbed the occlusion were extracted with little ceremony. When he saw the patient later, he found no "inégalité." More important is another instance quoted from 1733, in which the teeth adjacent the fracture site were missing. *Bunon* placed a piece of walrus bone (chevalmarin) into the gap, fastening it with silk threads through holes at its ends. With continuous slings about the adjacent teeth, he immobilized the splint and the fracture, a procedure that we have seen together with other material from *Solingen*.[27]
In his comprehensive volume "Tabulae ossium morbosorum" (Tables of bone diseases) of 1788, *Andreas Bonn* (1738-1818), professor of anatomy and surgery in Amsterdam, depicted typical fractures of the facial skeleton, but neither the text nor the illustrations include a suggestion for treatment or an attempt at classification, so that this richly produced atlas was of little practical use.[28]

4. The 19th and 20th Centuries

4.1 Conservative and Surgical Treatment of Mandibular Fractures

In the late 18th century the Industrial Revolution began its move into manufacturing establishments, and treatment of fractures began to be mechanized as well. The Parisian surgeons *Chopard* and *Desault* (1779), the Prussian military physician *Rütenick* (1799) and the Briton *Francis Bush* (1822) constructed complicated, but in principle similar devices which, according to reports of contemporaries (e.g., *Malgaigne*[29]) could be worn for only short periods because of the development of pressure points. Despite many variations and attempts at improvement, none of them proved worthwhile. They enclosed the dental arch with metal splints which were screwed into a wooden plate placed under the chin; clamps were used for this purpose (Fig. 1-8). The method of *Rütenick* was distinguished from the others in that it used a headcap in addition (Fig. 1-9). The Braunschweig dentist *Fr. Hartig* improved the device in 1830 by combining the many single components into a closed, hinge-connected apparatus (Fig. 1-10).[30]
The Parisian surgeon *Alexis Boyer* (1757-1833) led a return to simple methods when he proposed, in 1803, the placement of two equally thick cork lamellae on each side between the dental arches. The teeth were to press into these and to immobilize the fractured components in their positions. Now the mandible was to be immobilized in a head sling.[31] Commenting on this technique in 1836, the Nürtingen physician *Johann Paul Späth* (1770-1857) noted that the material was too soft and that it soon smelled

26 *Hoffmann-Axthelm* (1967, 1973, pp. 200f.; 1981, pp. 207f.)
27 *Bunon* (1746) pp. 272f.
28 *Bonn* (1788) pp. 2f.; Tab. IV-VII
29 *Malgaigne* (1847) p. 395
30 *Chopart/Desault* (1795) pp. 216f.; *Branco* (1825); *Graefe* (1822); *Michaelis* (1823); *Richter* (1828) pp. VIf., Tab. VI 9 *Rütenick* (1799); *Michaelis* (1823); *Richter* (1828) p. VIII, Tab. VI 10 *Bush* (1822); *Hartig*, 1830
31 *Boyer* (1804) p. 77; (1807) p. 93

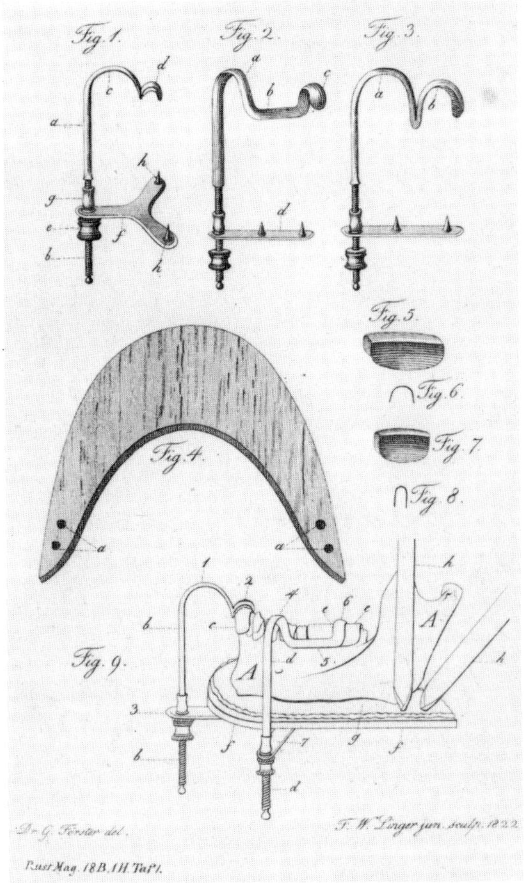

Fig. 1-8 *Rütenick:* Device for splinting a mandibular fracture, 1799.

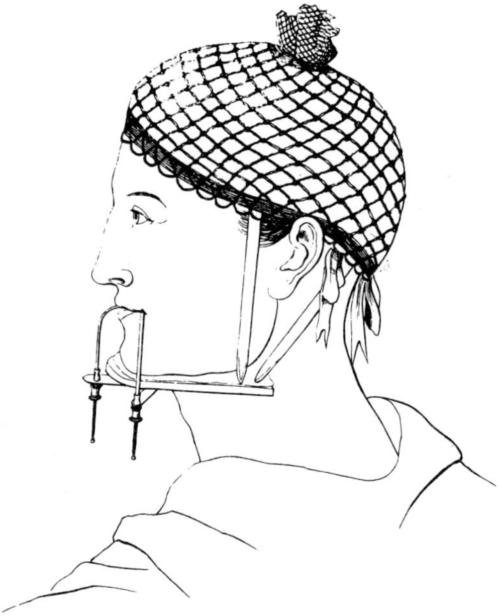

Fig. 1-9 *Rütenick:* Device in place with a head cap, 1799.

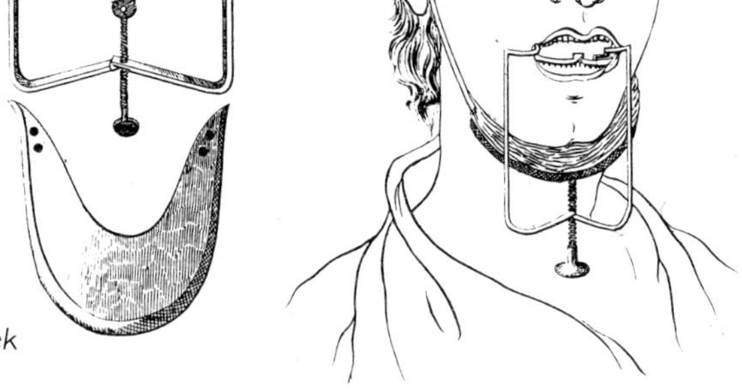

Fig. 1-10 *Hartig:* Development of the *Rütenick* device, 1830.

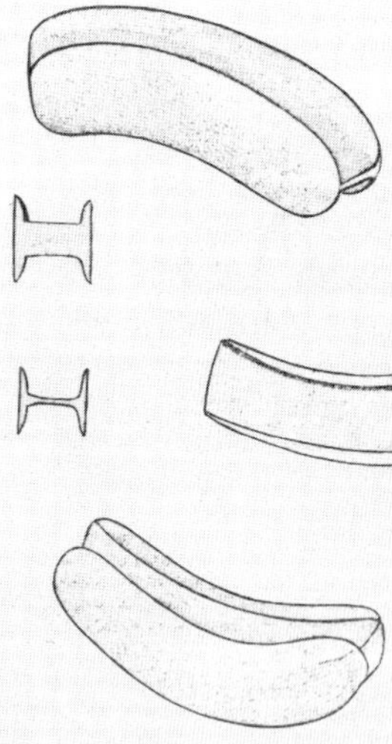

Fig. 1-11 *Späth:* Horn splints for splinting the mandible, 1836.

quite bad. Instead, therefore, he had a turner make two double channels of horn, one each for the diseased and the sound side[32] (Fig. 1-11).

A fundamentally new approach was made in 1840 by *Jean-Baptiste Baudens* (1804-1857) when he demonstrated to the Paris Academy of Medicine an oblique fracture of the body of the mandible treated with a cord carried around the bone with a needle and knotted above the teeth, an early variety of circumferential wiring.[33]
The latter was carried out, in fact, in 1852 in Paris when *Alphonse Robert* (1801-1862) placed silver wire around the dental arch and the body of the mandible over a lingually adapted lead (later zinc) plate and knotted it over a tampon under the chin (Fig. 1-12).[34] An early, perhaps the first, wire ligature placed for immobilizing an edentulous mandible through two holes drilled into the fractured pieces had been described in 1847 by New York Hospital surgeon *Gurdon Buck* (1807-1877).[35]

Important for further development was a method described in 1855 to the Paris Academy by *Victor Morel-Lavallée* (1811-1865). Following reduction and immobilization, he pressed gutta percha previously heated in a water bath against the dental arches, leaving a feeding gap at the center. Then he placed a chin cap. He also made an apparatus consisting of a kind of impression tray (moule) which, filled with gutta percha, was held in place under the chin with a spring and compression plate (poínt d'appui, Fig. 1-13). The Berlin surgeon *Ernst Gurlt* (1825-1899) recommended this procedure as the first one in his thorough "Lehre von den Knochenbrüchen" (Textbook of bone fractures) in 1864.[36]
Later medical inspector in the American Civil War, *Frank Hastings Hamilton* (1813-1886), described a similar technique in 1855. He softened two pieces of gutta percha and surrounded therewith the posterior teeth on each side of the mouth; taking care, of course, that on the fractured side the splint extended sufficiently far forward to traverse thoroughly the line of fracture. Then he placed a 4-tailed chin splint bandage. Later, in 1857, he had a dentist make a kind of impression tray, a silver cap, that he filled with gutta percha.[37]
The dental textbooks of the first half of the

[32] *Späth* (1836)
[33] *Baudens* (1844)
[34] *Robert* (1852)
[35] *Hamilton* (1860) pp. 127f.; *Schwartz* (1944)
[36] *Morel-Lavallée* (1855, 1860, 1862); *Gurlt* (1864) II pp. 426f.
[37] *Hamilton* (1860) pp. 130f.

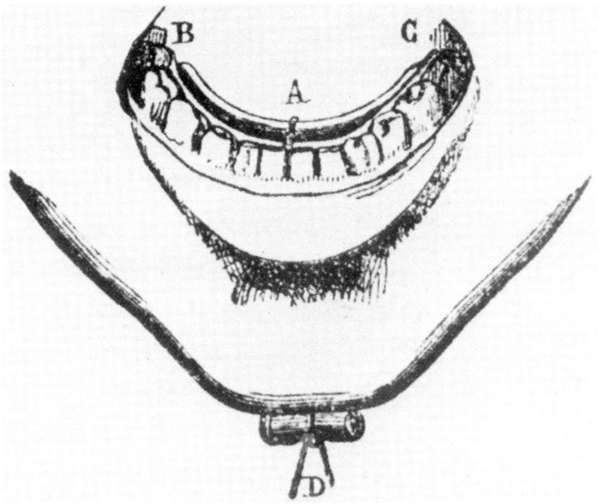

Fig. 1-12 *Robert:* Circumferential wiring of the mandible and a lingually positioned metal plate (according to the author, the wire in front of the dental arch is missing in the illustration), 1852.

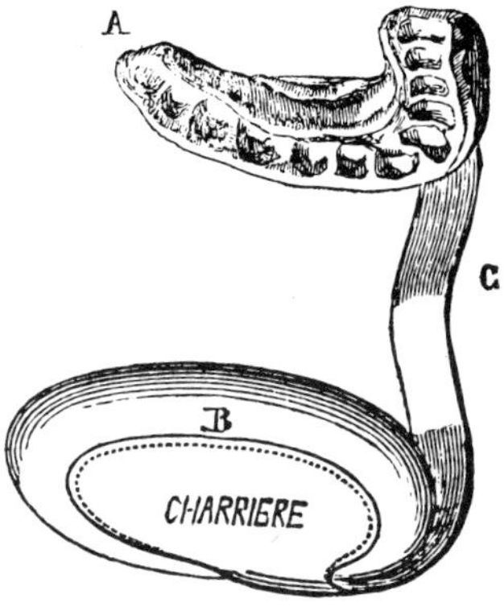

Fig. 1-13 *Morel-Lavallée:* Apparatus for fixation of a gutta percha-filled metal splint, 1855.

19th century treated jaw fractures only peripherally as complications of tooth extractions. Thus, if an author such as the Chirurgien Dentiste du Roi *Malagou Antoine Désirabode* (1781-1851) devoted some pages of his textbook (1843) to therapy, his recommendations were simply quotations of surgeons, among which the procedure of *Baudens* was rejected because of the pain with which it was associated.[38]

The treatment of mandibular fractures passed to the hands of dentists only in the second half of the century through the use of hard rubber as a splinting material with which the dentist had become skilled. Its introduction was probably the work of two Americans separated at the time by the front of the Civil War. One of them was *Thomas Brian Gunning* (1813-1889), born in London and practicing in New York; the other was the Southerner *James Baxter Bean* (1834-1870). The former reduced the mandible as the first step, held it in place with well-stretched silk and then made an impression from which an enveloping rubber splint was vulcanized. *Gunning* anchored it with screws placed in pre-drilled molars.

> "It so happened that Mr. G. was (1862) the first to receive the benefit of his ingenuity, fracturing his lower jaw by being thrown from his horse."

Gunning himself notes:

> "A Vulcanite splint was applied thirteen hours after injury (Fig. 1-14 A). It inclosed all the lower teeth, and was fastened by gold screws to the first molars. It held the fragments so well that I was able to attend to patients in the afternoon..."

Later he constructed a splint of the second class, or those in which the jaw is held still, because now the maxilla is included as well (Fig. 1-14 B). *Gunning* was probably the first to recognize that changes in shape of the mandibular body were less caused by trauma than by muscular forces.[39]

The former medical inspector of the (defeated) Confederate Army, *E. M. Covey*, reported in 1866 about *Bean*, noting that the latter had treated mandibular fractures with an interdental splint made of hard rubber during the last months of the war. *Bean* made wax impressions of the fragments and placed the plaster casts in occlusion with the maxilla. Insertion of the splint encompassing the maxillary and mandibular arches made from this model led to reduction

38 *Désirabode* (1843) pp. 530f.
39 *Sands* (1864, quotation); *Gilmer* (1881/82); *Kingsley* (1880) pp. 348f.; *Fraser-Moodie* (1869); *Schwartz* (1944, quotation)

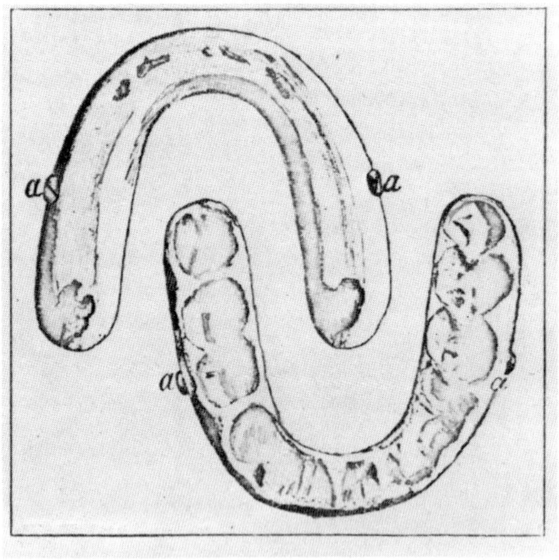

Fig. 1-14 A *Gunning:* Rubber splint with which the author's own jaw fracture was treated (a : gold screws), 1862.

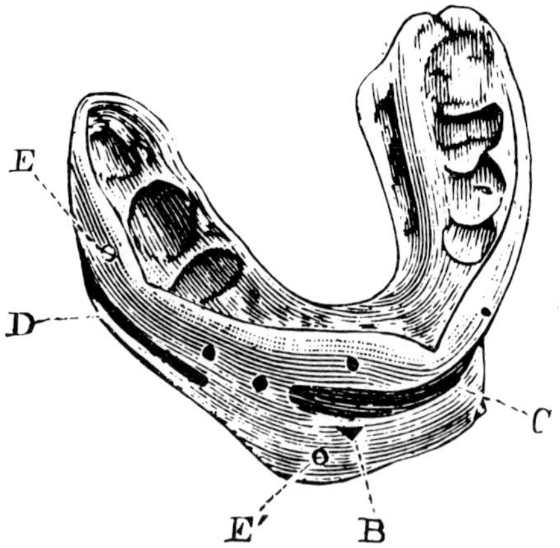

Fig. 1-14 B *Gunning:* Rubber splint encompassing the mandible and the maxilla.

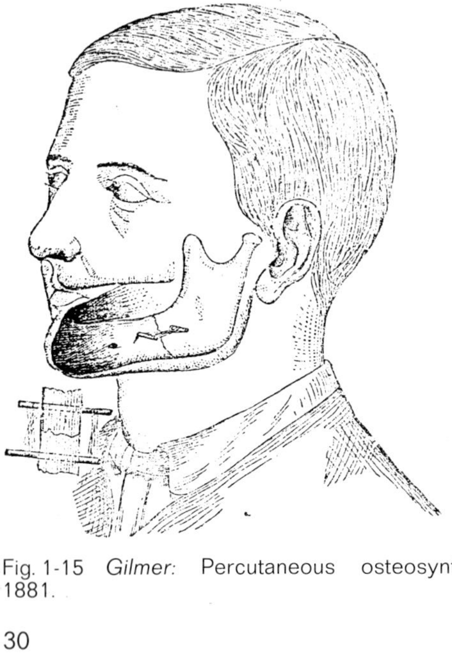

Fig. 1-15 *Gilmer:* Percutaneous osteosynthesis, 1881.

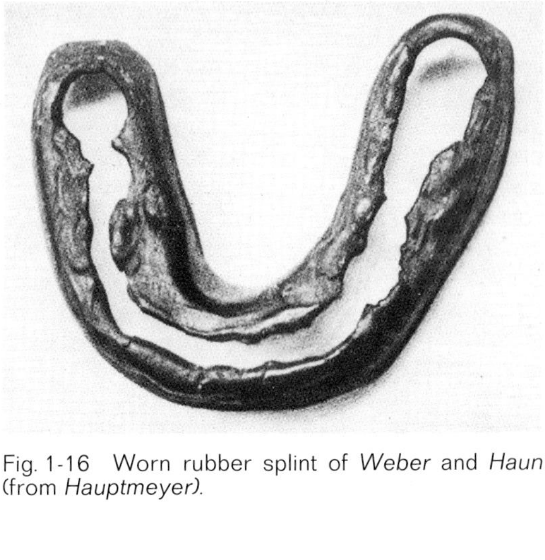

Fig. 1-16 Worn rubber splint of *Weber* and *Haun* (from *Hauptmeyer*).

of the mandibular fracture. Immobilization followed with a mental compress and an occipitofrontal bandage. In principle, *Bean*'s splint corresponded to that of *Gunning*'s second class.[40]
The physician and dentist of Quincy, Illinois, and later co-founder of the Dental School of Northwestern University (Chicago) *Thomas Lewis Gilmer* (1849-1931) in 1881 described the attachment of a lower rubber splint via wiring around the mandible, as had been proposed by *Robert* in 1852 for a metal splint. Furthermore, we have *Gilmer* to thank for what is probably the first description of a percutaneous osteosynthesis of the jaws: Two posts were introduced into prepared holes adjacent to the fracture line; their lingual, skin-piercing ends were laced together with wire (Fig. 1-15).[41]
More important, however, is *Gilmer*'s (1887) proposal that the fractured mandible be immobilized to the maxilla. A bilateral fracture was treated first on one side by interosseous wiring, whereafter he tied all the remaining teeth of the maxilla and the mandible with iron wire.

> "The ends of each wire were brought together and twisted, fastening it securely to the teeth. This being done, the teeth of the lower jaw were exactly articulated with those of the upper and the wires of the lower teeth secured to those of the upper by bringing them together and twisting, thus firmly lashing the lower to the upper jaw."

There reappears here for the first time, at least to author's knowledge, a procedure first intimated in an early publication from 1492.[42]
The first European hard rubber splint was demonstrated in 1865 at a dental meeting in Leipzig by the Parisian dentist *J. A. C. Weber*. He made an impression while trying to hold the fractured parts in the best possible position. His splint included only the mandibular arch, whose incisal edges and occlusal surfaces remained exposed so that, as he said, the patient was soon able to chew—in contrast to the interdental splints. After three weeks, there appeared to be complete healing.[43] This principle was perfected in 1867 by the Erfurt dentist *Carl Haun* (1832-1899), who lined the rubber splint with softened gutta percha (Fig. 1-16).[43] Entirely independently, *Bean*'s divided impression was redeveloped again for use in the wounded of the Franco-Prussian war (1870/71) by *Friedrich Süersen* (1827-1919), the personal dentist of the first German Kaiser. New, however, was his idea of placing ever longer hickory posts between two rubber splints holding each fracture separately, thus separating the fractured pieces which tended to heal in poor position over each other (Fig. 1-17).[45] At approximately the same time, the British dentist *Alexander Nasmyth* (1789-1848) adapted *Gunning*'s splint more conservatively by fastening it in the interdental spaces with screws.[46]
Extraoral splinting of mandibular fractures was developed further in London by *Henry Hayward* in 1858. He shaped a metal plate to surround the fracture from an impression, and provided it with external bars (Fig. 1-18). This technique was perfected around 1880 by the use of rubber plates whose occlusal surfaces were shaped as masticatory surfaces, by *Norman William Kingsley* of New York (1829-1913), so important in the growth of orthodontics. The external bars were immobilized with a chin strap (Figs. 1-19 and 1-20).[47]
Claude Martin (1843-1911), Medicin-Dentiste and teacher at the Ecole du Service de Santé militaire in Lyon, took particular interest in the development of the shell splint. His method, described in a book devoted to the subject, rested on the principle proposed by *Morel-Lavallée* (see Fig. 1-13), except that he used hard rubber in place of gutta percha and that instead of a simple button he fitted a plate adapted to the margin of the mandible; a steel spring was mounted in the plate (Figs. 1-21 and 1-22). The plate bore a hook for rubber bands; these were attached to a headcap so that the splint and the maxillary arch were forced against each other.[48]
Martin perceived the advantage of this rather complicated device in that the patient could open his mouth to eat, an advantage soon lost by the development of intermaxillary fixation provided by elastic bands or tie wires. Many similar devices were developed in the Old World as well as in the New.

40 *Covey* (1866); *Schwartz* (1944)
41 *Gilmer* (1881/82)
42 *Gilmer* (1887)
43 *Weber* (1865)
44 *Haun* (1867)
45 *Süersen* (1871)
46 *Kingsley* (1880) pp. 388f.
47 *Kingsley* (1880) pp. 398f.
48 *Martin* (1887)

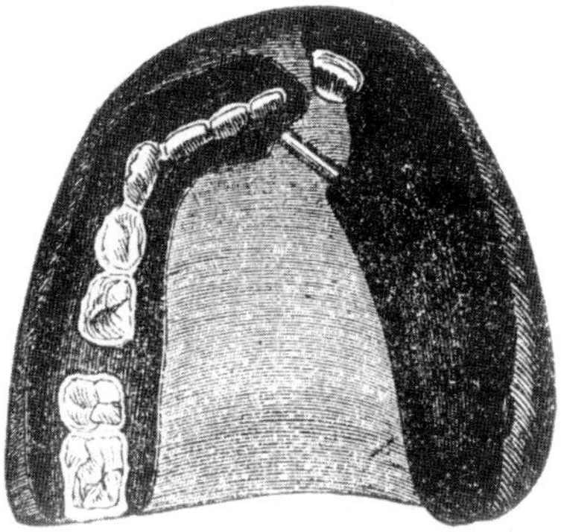

Fig. 1-17 *Süersen:* Separation of displaced healing fragments with hickory posts, 1871.

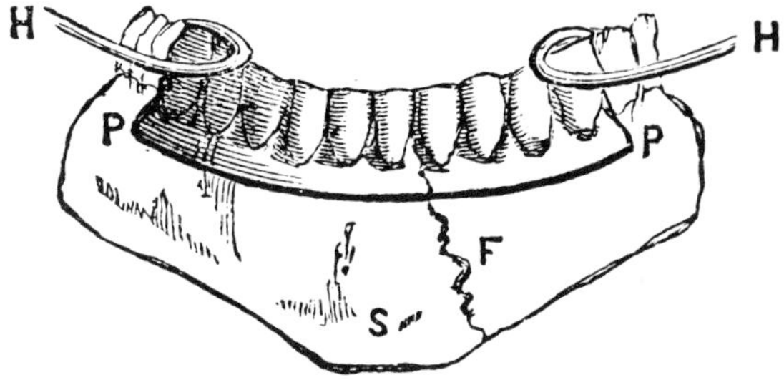

Fig. 1-18 *Hayward:* Extraorally retained metal splint, 1858 (from Kingsley).

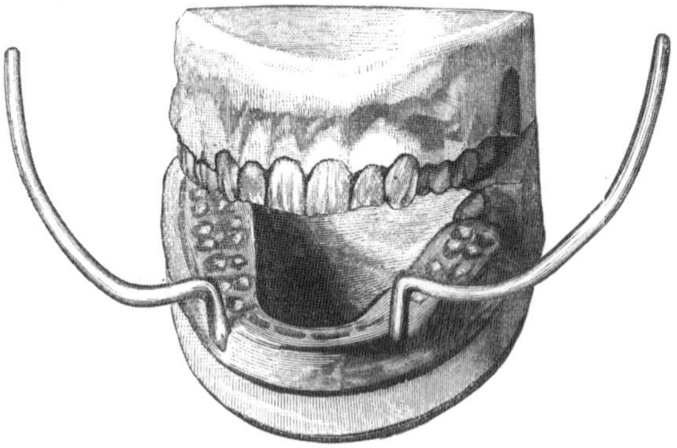

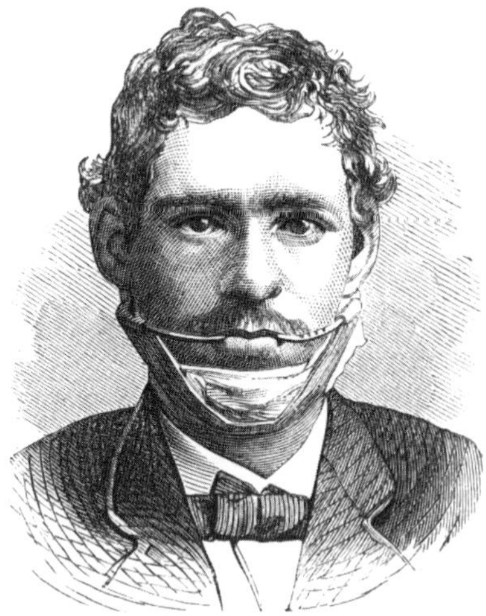

Figs. 1-19 and 1-20 *Kingsley:* Extraorally retained rubber splint, 1880.

The first arch bar in the sense that term is used today may have been devised by *Gurnell E. Hammond*, a London dentist, when he placed a steel wire around the dental arch of the wounded in occupied Paris in 1871, and fixed this in place with twisted dental wires (Fig. 1-23);[49] he used a model to bend the arch bar. The technique was significantly improved and standardized to a usable method by *Carl Sauer* (1835-1892), a dentist and first prosthodontist—from 1884—at the Berlin University Dental Institute. In 1880, he split his—preferably gold—circumferential arch bar, connected it to a lingual tube, and left final reduction to the effects of spring forces, a technique especially suitable for fractures showing initial callus formation (Fig. 1-24).[50] In fractures characterized by loss of bone, *Sauer* proposed in 1887 that an inclined plane be soldered to the

[49] *Hammond* (1872/73)
[50] *Sauer* (1881)

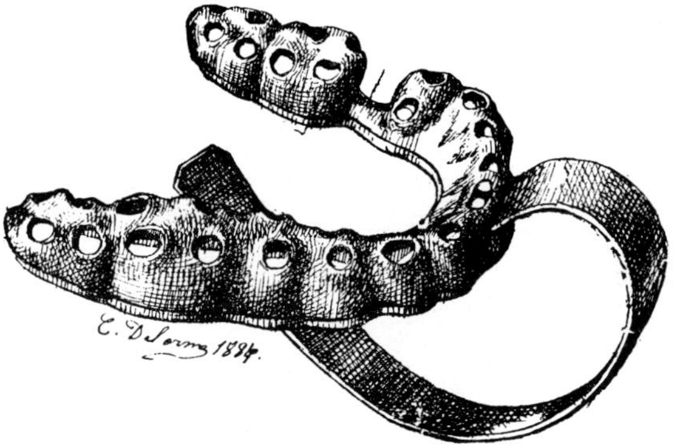

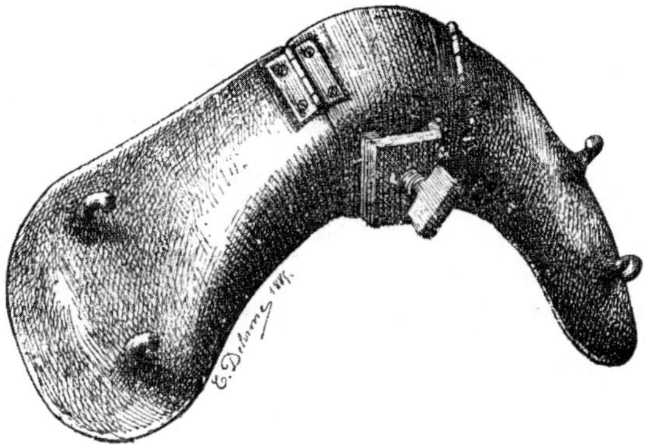

Figs. 1-21 and 1-22 *Martin:* Comprehensive rubber splint with spring and support plate on the mandible, 1887.

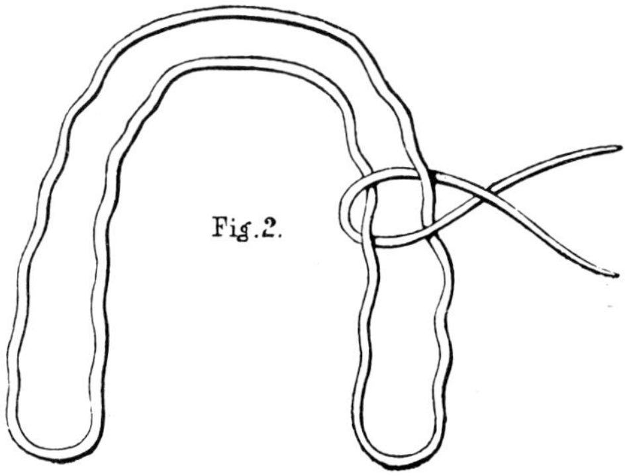

Fig. 1-23 *Hammond:* Circumferential arch bar, 1871.

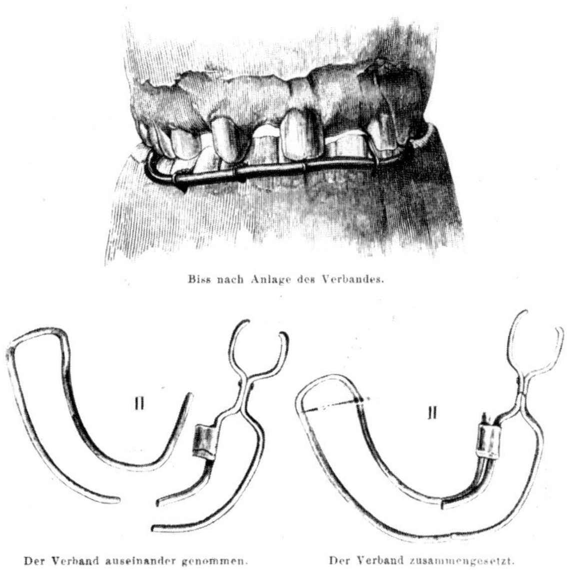

Fig. 1-24 *Sauer:* Spring-fitted circumferential arch bar, 1881.

splint,[51] and in 1889 he suggested that a labial arch bar be tied as an emergency measure, having been shaped free-hand into the desired ideal form. Reduction was effected through systematic tightening of the ligatures[52] (Fig. 1-25).

In the United States, the famous orthodontist *Edward Hartley Angle* (1850-1930) attempted to make his orthodontic system of bands and arch wires serviceable in the treatment of fractures, but his proposal did not prove out because it required that the reduced mandible be wired rigidly to the maxilla (Fig. 1-26),[53] as *Gilmer* had done before. Perhaps stimulated by these efforts, *Heinrich Löhers,* a Heidelberg dentist, in 1893 devised a ring-nut dressing, a screwable

51 *Schnoor* (1887)
52 *Sauer* (1889)
53 *Angle* (1900) pp. 285f.

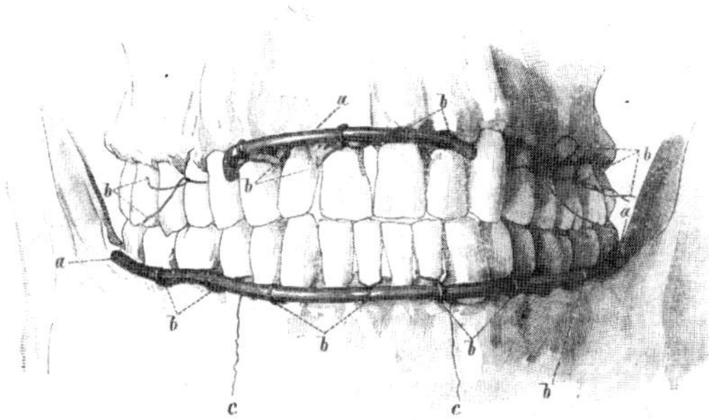

Fig. 1-25 *Sauer:* The iron wire emergency arch bar, 1889.

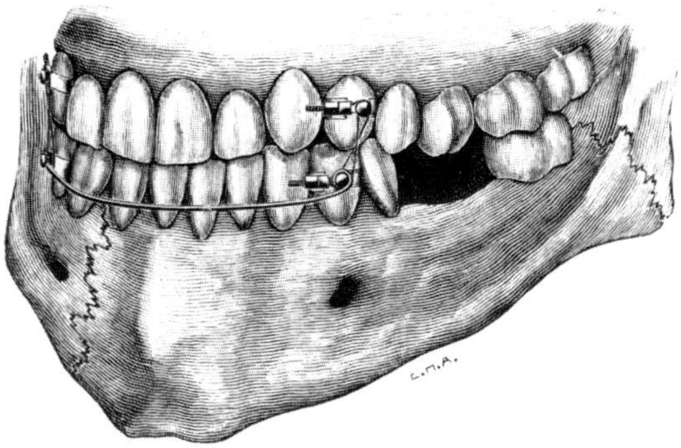

Fig. 1-26 *Angle:* Retention via orthodontic bands, around 1890.

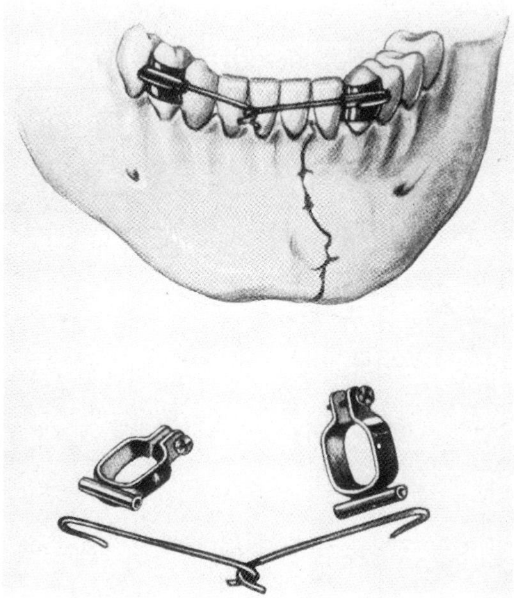

Fig. 1-27 *Löhers:* Ring-nut arch bar, 1893.

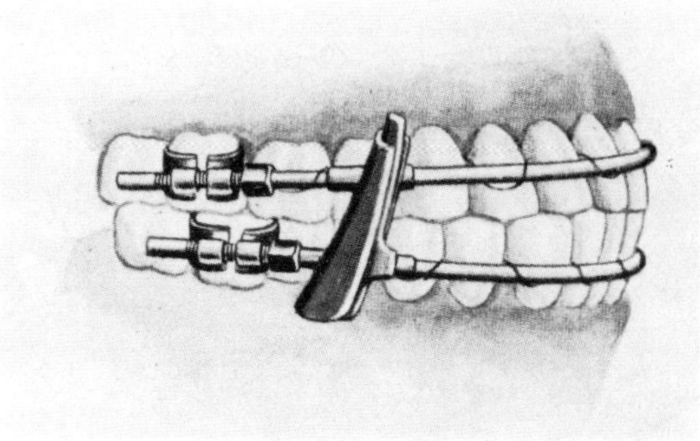

Fig. 1-28 *Schröder:* Modified ring-nut arch bar and sliding splint, 1910.

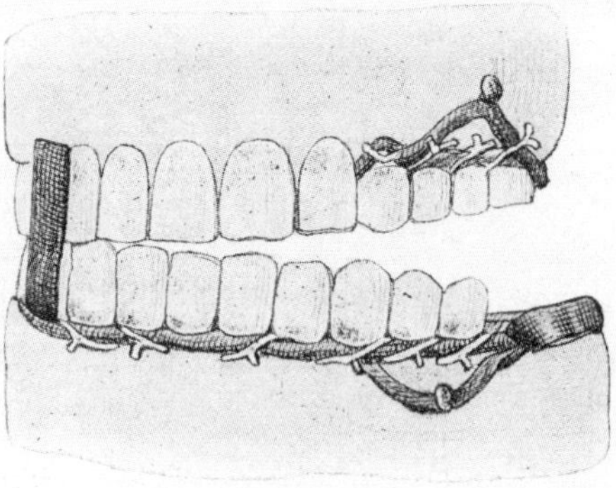

Fig. 1-29 *Heitmüller:* Maxillary auxiliary splint to support rubber bands, 1897.

band to fasten an arch bar (Fig. 1-27).[54] This technique was adopted in 1911 by *Hermann Schröder* (1876-1942), a Berlin prosthodontist, who improved it through the addition of a "sliding splint" that was to guide the uninjured portion of the jaw rigidly in a correct course of motion, especially in fractures involving missing bone (Fig. 1-28).[55] The device, developed jointly with *Franz Ernst* (1887-1947), an oral surgeon, was produced commercially; in the course of the years, many other devices were proposed.

A great advance in the use of arch bars for treatment was made with the introduction of rubber bands, used in orthodontics by the New York dentist *Elisha Gustavus Tucker* (1808-1895) in 1852. Adaptation of these bands to treatment of jaw fractures might be the work of *Karl Heitmüller* (1864-1951) of Göttingen, who suggested in 1897 that a supplemental splint be placed in the maxilla, with the aid of which the sunken fragment be drawn into occlusion through rubber bands (Fig. 1-29).[56] Independently, *William L. Darnall* (1889-1941), a U.S. Navy dentist, in 1923 suggested the use of intermaxillary rubber bands, for the first time in the U.S.[57] Thus, the problem of functionally appropriate treatment of simple mandibular fractures was solved in principle.

The Berlin maxillofacial surgeon *Martin Wassmund* (1892-1956) combined orthodontic tubes with his intraorally shaped arch bar made of semicircular annealed bronze wire. This splint was tied to each individual tooth with ligatures. Thus he developed a treatment system independent of the dental laboratory in the 1920s.[58] During the second world war, molar bands came to be seen as superfluous in practice.

Arch bars, tooth-holding plates and cap splints developed in a rich variety simultaneously. Arch bars were found especially useful in emergency cases and in war surgery. If the arch bar is covered with cold-curing acrylic today after being fitted by means of dental wire ligatures, this development may be seen as a movement of the two techniques toward each other with the advantages of both being largely combined.[59]

4.2 Fractures of the Midface

Guidelines for the treatment of maxillary fractures appear rather late in the surgical literature. *Richard Wiseman* (1622-1676), personal physician to British kings, was probably the first to deal with them, in 1676. In his book "Severall Chirurgicall Treatises" he recalls being summoned to attend a boy who was a victim of a horse's kick, his face being beaten in, and the lower jaw jutting out. With his finger moving from behind the uvula, he pulled the maxilla forward. Upon being released, however, it sank back at once. He formed an instrument bent up at one end, that he called "my extender", but the fractured segment relapsed again. Thereupon he devised an improved, but not otherwise described, instrument with which the child, his mother and the servants alternately pulled forward the maxilla until callus formation was initiated.[60]

Treatment of a partial fracture of the maxilla was described for the first time by the important Parisian surgeon *Henry-François Le Dran* (1685-1770) in 1731. Having been run over, the maxillary four last molars and the alveolus (premolars often were not distinguished at the time) were tipped palatally and the mandible was fractured multiply in the region of the chin. To immobilize the wobbly fragment of the maxilla, *Le Dran* had the Dentiste du Roi *Jean-François Caperon* (d. 1763) wrap the four teeth still firmly rooted in the alveolus with cords and bind them to a fifth. Following placement of a chin cap, the six mandibular anteriors were ligated similarly. The cords dropped away after as little as 10-12 days, but the fragments had become firm in the interval.—An early example of dental-surgical cooperation.[61]

Compared to these rather primitive experiments, it was a significant advance when, in 1822, the Berlin surgeon *Carl Ferdinand (von) Graefe* (1787-1840) had a doctoral student describe an apparatus in which the fixation on the

54 *Röse* (1893) pp. 48f.; *Löhers* did not describe this device himself, but left its publication to *Carl Röse*, a physician and dentist then teaching dentistry in the University of Freiburg.
55 *Schröder* (1911) pp. 78f.; (b)
56 *Heitmüller* (1897)
57 *Thoma* (1943)
58 *Wassmund* (1927)
59 *Schuchardt* (1956)
60 *Wiseman* (1676 p. 472f.
61 *Le Dran* (1731) pp. 9-17

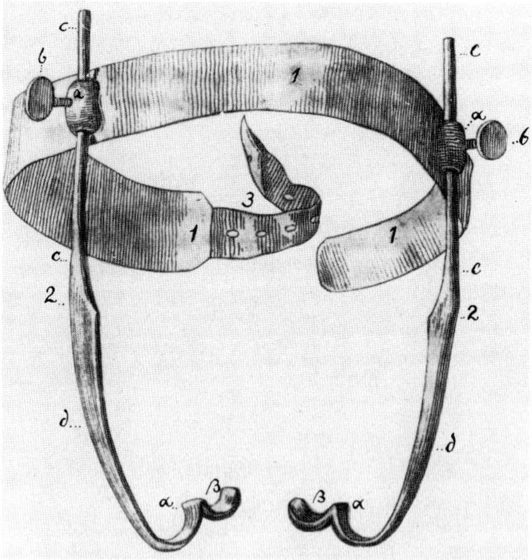

Fig. 1-30 *C. F. Graefe:* Retention device for fractures of the maxilla, 1822.

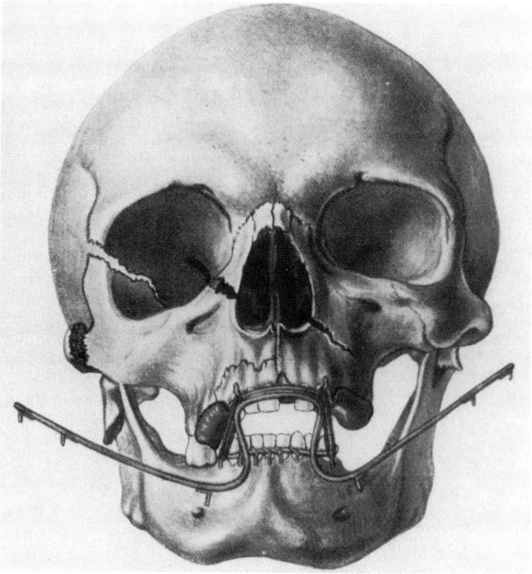

Fig. 1-31 Maxillary splint with side bars (Hirschgeweih, antlers) which are directed outward through the angle of the mouth and attached to a head cap (from *Wassmund*).

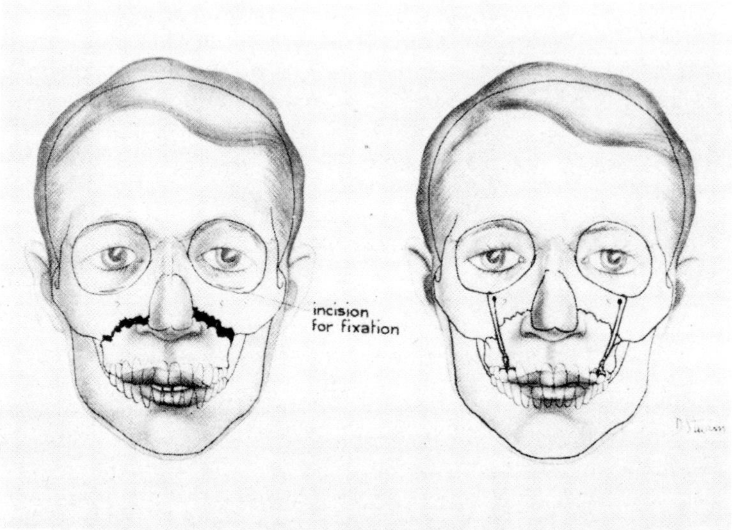

Fig. 1-32 *Adams:* Wire suspension of the fractured maxilla, 1942.

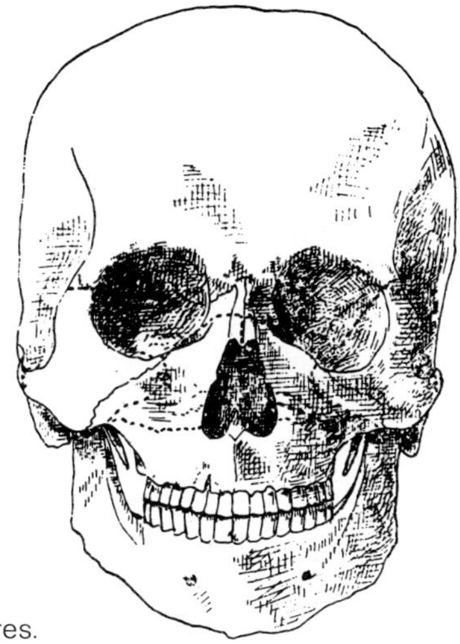

Fig. 1-33 *Le Fort:* Typical weak lines of maxillary fractures.

head proposed by *Rütenick* was taken up again, this time, however, for immobilization of the fractured maxilla. A lined chin band of steel bore two adjustable bars which held the fragment in its proper position (Fig. 1-30).[62]

In accordance with *Kingsley*'s procedure on the mandible (see Figs. 1-19 and 1-20), one could encompass the maxillary arch with a rubber splint and fasten it with external bars to a head cap. This initially rigid design was replaced toward the turn of the century by rubber bands, as had been proposed in 1898 by the Frankfurt dentist *Ernst Moeser*, who placed a strip of rubber dam across the top of the patient's head; a technique still used, in principle, today (Fig. 1-31).[63] This procedure predominated until 1942, when the American oral surgeon *William Milton Adams* (1905-1957) proposed that the maxillary fragment be suspended on wires running subcutaneously along the lower margin of the orbit (Fig. 1-32). This surgical procedure has undergone several modifications and has become well established, together with the conservative methods.[64]

Classification of midface fractures is the work of two French surgeons. In Paris in 1886, *Alphonse Guérin* (1817-1895) described the fracture of the tooth-bearing portion of the maxilla without displacement, a condition still bearing his name.[65] In 1901, Lille's surgeon, *René Le Fort* (1869-1951) noted that the fracture without displacement is the rule. This finding, which probably explains the low level of clinical interest in such fractures theretofore, had been made on the facial skeletons of 35 cadaver skulls that he had subjected to a variety of traumata and then dissected. Above all else, however, he found the typical three classes of weak lines of midface fractures, landmarks still bearing his name today (Fig. 1-33).[66]

The helplessness characterizing every approach to fractures of the zygoma until the first half of the 19th century is remarkable. *Joseph François Malgaigne* (1816-1865), the great theoretician of modern surgery, failed for anatomical reasons, as he notes in his 1842 special work devoted to bone fractures, to reduce such fractures with his finger from within the oral cavity; he avoided the technique already used by others—surgical exposure and reduction.[67] In 1844, the surgeon *Louis Stromeyer* (1804-1876), then working in Freiburg, in his "Handbuch der Chirurgie" (Handbook of surgery), recommended that the zygoma be repositioned

62 *Reiche* (1822); *Graefe* (1822)
63 *Moeser* (1898)
64 *Adams* (1942); see *Thoma* (1944), for example; *Mac Intosh/Obwegeser* (1967)
65 Guérin (1866)
66 *Le Fort* (1901)
67 *Malgaigne* (1847) I pp. 352f.

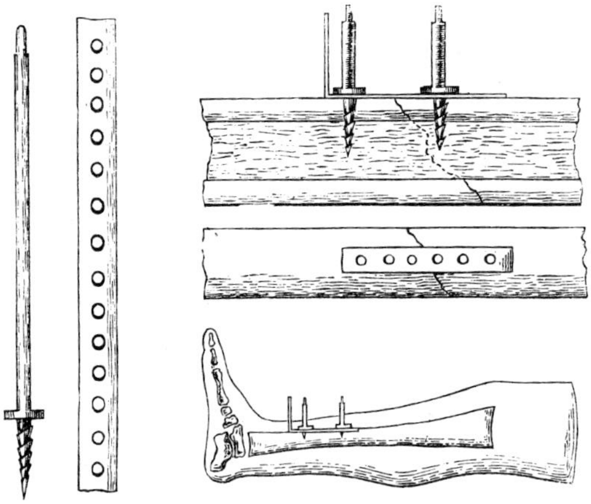

Fig. 1-34 *Hansmann:* Plate osteosynthesis, 1886.

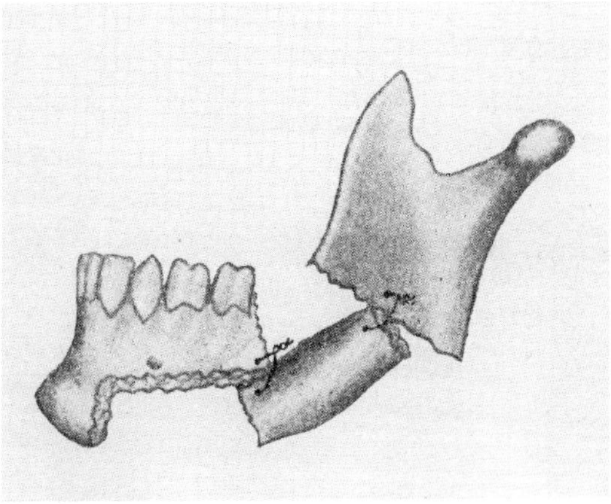

Fig. 1-35 *Wildt:* Osteoplasty via transposition of a pedicled flap, containing bone, 1896.

through the external skin with the aid of a sharp hook, a technique still used today but criticized severely by *Gurlt* in 1864. However, the antiseptic era had not yet begun, and *Stromeyer* had not been able to test his proposal in practice because of the absence of opportunity.[68]

In discussing fractures of the nasal bone—about which the *Smith* papyrus, the Corpus Hippocraticum, and *Celsus* from ancient times, and *Paré* and *Petit* in the modern era already had reported[69] —*Malgaigne* referred particularly to the ancients, especially to *Hippocrates*, because the more recent sources in fact only followed him. *Malgaigne* criticized *Petit*'s belief that intranasal support following realignment was superfluous. *Gurlt*, to the contrary, placed great value on stable splinting with lead foil and gutta percha.[70]

4.3 Surgical Methods in the Antiseptic Era

Surgical treatment begun around the middle of the last century for fractures of the edentulous mandible was no longer used, or limited exclusively to emergency cases. One attempted to solve the problems prosthodontically, initially with existing dentures and compression with a chin cup, or, in subjects who did not have dentures, by the fabrication of appropriate rubber—later plastic—splints. Only after the introduction of antibiotic drugs did surgical techniques, now denominated osteosynthesis, find wider application. Because this (still incomplete) development properly does not belong in an historical analysis, it is only noted here. Attempts at marrow pinning, made in 1939 by the Kiel surgeon *Gerhard Küntscher*, failed because of the anatomical conditions prevailing in the mandible. Interosseous wiring introduced in 1847 by *Buck* for the edentulous mandible, was taken up again in the twenties under aseptic conditions, as was the circumferential wiring proposed by *Baudens* (1844) and *Robert* (1852), the latter with an intraoral prosthetic splint when appropriate. Percutaneous osteosynthesis (pin fixation), described in principle for use in the mandible by *Gilmer* in 1881 (see Fig. 1-15), was proposed for surgery of the extremities with screw connections of the single pins by several surgeons: *C. Parkhill* (1897), *Albin Lambotte* (Antwerp, 1907), and *Roger Anderson* (Seattle, 1936). It was practiced in mandibular fractures by *Jean G. Ginestet* (Paris, 1934) and *John Marquis Converse* (New York, 1942). *Erwin Becker*, a Berlin

68 *Stromeyer* (1844) I pp. 703f; Gurlt II pp. 484f.
69 See pp. 17, 20f., 23, 25
70 *Malgaigne* (1897) I pp. 360f.; *Gurlt* (1864) II p. 517

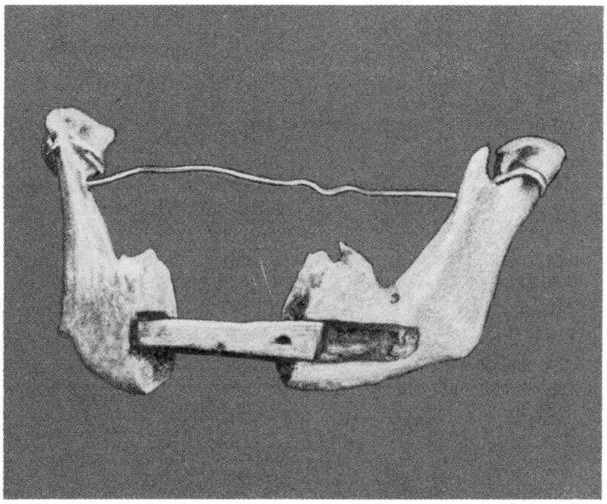

Fig. 1-36 *Sykoff*: Free bone grafting, 1900.

veterinarian, replaced extraoral pin fixation by a cold-curing resin bar in 1958.[71]

An even more favorable stabilization was sought by bridging the fracture site with a corrosion-free metal plate screwed into the bone, a technique already used for splinting the lower extremities in 1886 by the Hamburg surgeon *Hansmann* (Fig. 1-34) and in 1895 by the British surgeon Sir *William Arbuthnot Lane* (1856-1943).[72] Further improvements in this technique are being tested and are the subject of lively discussion.

The relatively recently instituted surgical measures for treatment of midface fractures are detailed in volume 2.[73]

The problem of replacing defects in fractures of the mandible with endogenous material may be said to have been solved in principle during the First World War, with the introduction of antibiotics significantly improving the success rate since that time. The surgical mentor of *Claude Martin*, the Lyon surgeon *Louis Ollier* (1830-1900), was one of the first to deal with the problem of autologous bone transfer, in 1867. He recognized the importance of transplanting the periosteum at that time, but practical application became possible only after the introduction of aseptic surgical techniques. At first one did not attempt free plasty, but bridged the mandibular defect with a pedicled dermis-periosteum flap from the forehead, as indicated by the Cologne surgeon *Bernhard Bardenheuer* (1839-1913) in 1892. He treated two additional patients with mucoperiosteal flaps containing bone from the external surface of the mandible.[74] In 1896, *Bardenheuer*'s successor, *August Wildt* described a similar procedure (Fig. 1-35).[75] As early as 1892, *Ludwig Ritter von Rydygier* (1850-1920), then surgeon in Cracow, transferred material from the clavicle to the region of the chin with a pedicled flap.[76] The first truly free bone transplantation in the mandible was probably carried out in 1900 by the Moscow surgeon *W. Sykoff*. The bone graft, 4 cm long, was taken from the anterior margin of the ascending ramus of the mandible and placed into the damaged region of the chin[77] (Fig. 1-36). Later, rib and especially tibial grafts were used, and in 1908, *Erich Lexer* (1867-1938), then working in Freiburg, reported on covering mandibular defects with homologous bone taken from a fresh, warm cadaver or a newly amputated leg.[78]

71 *Anderson* (1936), *Kazanjian/Converse* (1974), *Converse* and *Waknitz* (1942), *Becker* (1958)
72 *Hansmann* (1886); *Lane* (1895)
73 See chapters 10 and 11
74 *Bardenheuer* (1892)
75 *Wildt* (1896)
76 *Rydygier* (1908)
77 *Sykoff* (1900)
78 *Lexer* (1908, 1920)

In the same year, 1908, *Georg Axhausen* (1877-1960), a surgeon and later maxillofacial specialist at the University of Berlin, demonstrated the genetic capacity of bone marrow experimentally.[79] During the first world war, *Rudolf Klapp* (1873-1949) of Berlin and *August Lindemann* (1880-1970) of Düsseldorf introduced the use of iliac grafts as autologous material,[80] a procedure that soon won worldwide use despite the war-closed borders, and one that continues to be of primary importance today. Only at viable sites,[81] e.g., small defects having surface contact with vital, freshened bone stumps, is insertion of banked homologous bone permitted today, a procedure occasionally used in recent times.

Thus we have come to the point—in surgical therapy of fractures and in conservative treatment as well—at which are met the contemporary problems that make up the further content of this book.

79 *Axhausen* (1908)
80 *Klapp* (1916); *Lindemann* (1916)
81 *Lexer* (1924)

References

Abu l-Qasim (Albucasis)
De Chirurgia, arabice et latine. Cura Joh. Channing. Oxonii 1778. On surgery and instruments. Ed., transl. M. S. Spink/G. L. Lewis, London 1973

Adams, William Milton (1942)
Internal wiring fixation of facial fractures. Surgery 12: 523-540

Anderson, Roger (1936)
An ambulatory method of treating fractures of the shaft of the femur. Surg. Gynec. Obstet. 62: 865-873

Angle, Edward Hartley (1900)
Treatment of malocclusion of the teeth and fractures of the maxillae. Philadelphia

Apollonios of Citium
Kommentar zu Hippokrates über das Einrenken der Gelenke (Corpus medicorum graecorum XI 1,1). Ed. Jutta Kollesch/Friedolf Kudlien. Berlin 1965

Axhausen, Georg (1908)
Histologische Untersuchungen über Knochentransplantationen am Menschen. Dtsch. Z. Chir. 91: 388-428

Bardenheuer, Bernhard (1892)
Über Unter- und Oberkieferresektion. Verh. dtsch. Ges. Chir. 21: 123-130

Baudens, Jean Baptiste Lucien (1844)
Communications verbales. Bull. Acad. Méd., Paris 230 f., 341 f.

Bean, James Baxter
Quoted by Covey, E. M. (1866) and Schwartz, L. L. (1944)

Becker, Erwin (1958)
Ein Instrumentarium zur extracutanen Osteosynthese.... Chirurg 29: 63-67

Bonn, Andreas (1788)
Tabulae ossium morbosorum. Amstelaedami

Boyer, Alexis
a) Vorlesungen über die Krankheiten der Knochen. Transl. Georg August Spangenberg. Vol. 1 Leipzig 1804. b) The lectures of Boyer upon diseases of the bones. Vol. 1. Arr. A. Richerand, transl. M. Farell. London 1807

Branco (1825)
Über die Fractur des Unterkiefers nebst Beschreibung und Abbildung der Rütenickschen Maschine. (Rust's) Magazin ges. Heilk. 18: 3-59

Breasted, James Henry (1930)
The Edwin Smith surgical papyrus. Vol. 1, Chicago

Brunschwig, Hieronymus (1497 and 1518)
a) Dis ist das Buch der Cirurgia. Handwirckung der Wundartzny. Straßburg 1497. b) idem Rostock 1518

Buck, Gurdon
Quoted by Hamilton, F. H. (1860)

Bunon, Robert (1746)
Expériences et démonstrations faites á l'Hôpital de la Salpêtrière... Paris

Bush, Francis
Quoted by Malgaigne, J. F. (1847)

Caperon, Jean-François
Quoted by Le Dran, H.-F. (1731)

Celsus, Aulus, Cornelius
Corpus medicorum lat. Vol. 1. A. Cornelii Celsi quae supersunt rec. Fridericus Marx. Lipsiae et Berolini 1915. – De medicina. Engl. transl. W. G. Spencer. Vol. 3 London/Cambridge (Mass.) 1961

Chopart, François and Pierre Joseph Desault (1795)
Traité des maladies chirurgicales,... Vol. 1. Paris

Converse, J. M. and F. W. Waknitz (1942)
External skeletal fixation in fractures of the mandibular angle. J. Bone Jt. Surg. 24: 154

Covey, E. M. (1866)
The interdental splint. Brit J. dent. Sci. 19: 145-153

Darnall, W. L.
Quoted by Thoma, K. H. (1943)

Désirabode, Malagou Antoine (1843)
Nouveaux éléments complets de la science et de l'art du dentiste. 2 Vols. Paris

Ernst, Franz (1927)
Die zahnärztliche Behandlung der Unterkieferbrüche. In Kirschner, M. and O. Nordmann: Die Chirurgie. Berlin – Wien, Urban & Schwarzenberg

Fauchard, Pierre (1728)
Le chirurgien dentiste. Paris

Fraser-Moodie, W. (1869)
Mr. Gunning and his splint. Brit. J. Oral Surg. 7: 112-115

Galen
Claudii Galeni opera omnia. Ed. C. G. Kühn. Hipp. Art. comment. Tomus XVIII 1. Leipzig 1829

Gerard of Cremona (1507)
Liber canonis Avicenne. Venetiis

Gilmer, Thomas Lewis (1881/82)
Fractures of the inferior maxilla. Ohio St. J. dent. Sci. 1: 309-320; 2: 14-25, 57-104, 112-122

Gilmer, Thomas Lewis (1887)
A case of fracture of the lower jaw with remarks on the treatment. Arch. Dent. 4: 388-390

Ginestet, J. G. (1934)
Quoted by Kazanjian, V. H. and J. M. Converse (1974)

Graefe, Carl Ferdinand von (1822)
Jahresbericht. J. Chir. Augenhk., Berlin 4: 692-693

Guérin, Alphonse (1866)
Des fractures du maxillaire supérieur. Arch. gén. Méd. 6. série 8: 5-13

Gunning, Thomas Brian
Quoted by Sands A. L. (1864), Gilmer, T. L. (1881/82), Kingsley, N. W. (1880), Fraser-Moodie, W. (1889), Schwartz, L. L. (1944)

Gurlt, Ernst. (1864)
Handbuch von der Lehre von den Knochenbrüchen. Vol. 2, Hamm

Guy de Chauliac (1400)
Chirurgia magna. In: Guido de Cauliaco, Cyrurgia, p. 1^r-74^r. Venetiis

Hamilton, Frank Hastings (1860)
A practical treatise on fractures and dislocations. Philadelphia

Hammond, Gurnell E. (1872/73)
New treatment of fractured maxillae. Mth. Rev. dental Surg. 1: 547-550

Hansmann (1886)
Eine neue Methode zur Fixierung der Fragmente bei complicirten Fracturen. Verh. dtsch. Ges. Chir. 15: 134-136

Hartig, Fr. (1830)
Beschreibung eines neuen Apparates zur Retention des Unterkiefers. J. Chir. Augenhk., Berlin 14: 496-506

Haun, Carl (1867)
Mittheilung über einen Verband, die Körperbrüche des Unterkiefers zu heilen. Dtsch. Vjschr. Zahnhk. 7: 213-222

Heister, Laurentius (1724)
Chirurgie,... 2nd Ed., Nürnberg

Heitmüller, Karl (1897)
Die Verwendung des elastischen Gummibandes bei Kieferbrüchen,... Dtsch. Mschr. Zahnhk. 15 (1897) 523-529

Hippocrates
Oeuvres complètes. Trad. et ed. par É(mile) Littré, Tome 4. Paris 1844. – Übers. Richard Kapferer/Georg Sticker, Band 4. Stuttgart 1933-1940. – Engl. Transl. E. T. Withnington, Vol. 3, Cambridge (Mass.)/London 1928

Hoffmann-Axthelm, Walter (1967)
Robert Bunon (1702-1748), der erste Krankenhauszahnarzt. Zahnärztl. Mitt. 57: 1110-1112

Hoffmann-Axthelm, Walter (1973, 1981)
Die Geschichte der Zahnheilkunde. Berlin; Amer. Ed.: History of dentistry. Chicago-Berlin, Quintessence Publishing Co.

Kazanjian, V. H., and J. M. Converse (1974)
Surgical treatment of facial injuries. Baltimore, Williams & Wilkins

Kingsley, Norman William (1880)
A treatise on oral deformities... New York

Klapp, Rudolf (1916)
Über chirurgische Behandlung der Kieferschußbrüche. Zahnärztl. Fortbild. 13: 325-332

Köcher, F. (1979)
Oral communication

Lane, William, Arbuthnot (1895)
Some remarks on the treatment of fractures. Brit. med. J. 6: 861-863

Lanfranchi (1400)
Chirurgia magna. In: Guido de Cauliaco, Cyrurgia. Venetiis pp. 176^r-216^v

Le Clerc, Charles Gabriel (1700)
L'appareil commode en faveur des jeunes chirurgiens. Paris

Le Dran, Henry-François (1731)
Observations de Chirurgie. Vol. 1, Paris

Le Fort, René (1901)
Étude expérimentale sur les fractures de la mâchoire supérieure. Rev. Chir., Paris 23: 208-227; 360-379; 479-507

Lexer, Erich (1908)
Die Verwendung der freien Knochenplastik... Chir. Kongreß Verh. II 188-203

Lexer, Erich (1920)
Wiederherstellungschirurgie. Leipzig

Lexer, Erich (1924)
Die Verpflanzung von Knochen und Mark. In Lexer, E.: Die freien Transplantationen. Vol. 2 pp. 1-285. Stuttgart

Lindemann, August (1916)
In Bruhn, C.: Die gegenwärtigen Behandlungswege der Kieferschußverletzungen. Part. 4-6. Wiesbaden

Löhers, Heinrich
Quoted by Röse, C. (1893)

MacIntosh, Robert B. and Hugo L. Obwegeser (1967)
Internal wiring fixation. Oral Surg. 23: 703-708

Malgaigne, Joseph François (1847)
Traité des fractures et des luxations. Vol. 1, Paris

Martin, Claude (1887)
Du traitement des fractures du maxillaire inférieur par un nouvel appareil. Paris

Michaelis, Heinrich (1823)
Beschreibung der neuerdings angegebenen Maschinen zur Heilung der Kinnladenbrüche. J. Chir. Augenhk. Berlin 5: 346-355

Moeser, Ernst (1898)
Apparat zur Behandlung eines schweren Oberkieferbruches. Dtsch. Mschr. Zahnhk. 16: 62-64

Morel-Lavallée, Victor Auguste François (1855)
Nouvel appareil pour les fractures des mâchoires. Gaz. Hôp., Paris 28: 404

Morel-Lavallée, Victor Auguste François (1860)
Gaz. Hôp., Paris 33: 576

Morel-Lavallée, Victor Auguste François (1862)
Appareil en gutta-percha pour les fractures des mâchoires... Bull. gén. Thérap., Paris 63: 246-248; 352-358; 398-399

Muys, Johannes (1695)
Praxis medico-chirurgica rationalis,... Amstelaedami

Nasmyth, Alexander
Quoted by Kingsley, N. W. (1880)

Ollier, Louis (1867)
Traité expérimentel et clinique de la régénération des os et de la production artificielle du tissu osseux, Paris, G. Masson

Paré, Ambroise (1585)
Les oeuvres... en vingt huit livres. Paris

Paulos of Aigina
Ed. J. L. Heiberg (= Corpus medicorum graecorum IX 1-2). Leipzig/Berlin 1921-1924. - Des besten Arztes sieben Bücher. Transl. I. Berendes. Leiden 1914. – The seven books of Paulus Aegineta. Transl. Francis Adams. London 1844

Petit, Jean Louis (1725)
Abhandlung von denen Krankheiten derer Knochen... Berlin

Petit, Jean Louis (1726)
A treatise on the diseases of the bones. London

Petit, Jean Louis (1767)
Traité des maladies des os. Paris

Reiche, Carolus Fridericus Cuilelmus (1822)
De maxillae superioris fractura. Med. Diss. Berlin

Richter, Adolph Leopold (1828)
40 lithographierte Tafeln nebst Erklärung und Erläuterung derselben... Berlin

Robert, Alphonse (1852)
Nouveau procédé de traitement des fractures de la portion alvéolaire de la machoire inférieure. Bull. gén. Thérap., Paris 42: 22-25

Roonhuyze, Hendrik von
Quoted by Solingen C. (1693)

Röse, Carl (1893)
Über Kieferbrüche und Kieferverbände. Jena

Rowe, Norman Lester (1971)
The history of treatment of maxillofacial trauma. Ann. Roy. Coll. Surg. England 49: 329-349

Rütenick
Quoted by Branco (1825)

Rydygier, Ludwig Ritter von (1908)
Zum osteoplastischen Ersatz nach Unterkieferresektion. Zbl. Chir. 35: 1320-13222

Ryff (Rivius), Walther Hermann (1559)
Die groß Chirurgei, oder vollkommene Wundartzeney... Franckfurt

Sands, Austin L. (1864)
Fracture of lower jaw, treated by intra-dental splints. Dent. Cosmos 5: 124-127

Sauer, Carl (1881)
Herstellung eines neuen Verbandes bei Unterkieferbrüchen. Dtsch. Vjschr. Zahnhk. 21: 362-375

Sauer, Carl (1889)
Nothverband bei Kieferbrüchen aus Eisendraht. Dtsch. Mschr. Zahnhk. 7: 381-392

Schnoor, Gustav (1887)
Professor Sauer's Anwendung der schiefen Ebene... Dtsch. Mschr. Zahnhk. 5: 217-219

Schröder, Hermann (1911)
Frakturen und Luxationen der Kiefer. Berlin

Schuchardt, Karl (1956)
Ein Vorschlag zur Verbesserung der Drahtschienenverbände. Dtsch. Zahn Mund-Kieferhk. 24: 39-44

Schwartz, Laszlo L. (1944)
The development of the treatment of jaw fractures. J. Oral Surg. 2: 193-221

Smith papyrus
Transl. by Westendorf (1966) and Breasted (1930)

Solingen, Cornelis (1693)
Handgriffe der Wund-Artzney. Franckfurt/Oder

Soranos of Ephesos
De fasciis. Ed. Johannes Ilberg, Corp. med. graec. IV, Leipzig and Berlin 1924

Späth, Johann Paul (1836)
Komplicirte Fraktur des Unterkiefers. Med. Corresp. bl. württemb. ärztl. Verein 6 276-277

Strohmeyer, Louis (1844)
Handbuch der Chirurgie, Vol. 1, Freiburg im Breisgau

Süersen, Wilhelm (1871)
Über Verletzungen resp. Fracturen des Ober- und Unterkiefers Dtsch. Vjschr. Zahnhk. 11 261-273

Sykoff, W. (1900)
Zur Frage der Knochenplastik am Unterkiefer. Zbl. Chir. 35 881-883

Theodoricus Cerviensis (1400)
Chirurgia. In: Guido de Cauliaco, Cyrurgia. Venetiis pp 97^{r}-134^{v}

Thoma, Kurt H. (1943)
A new method of intermaxillary fixation for jaw fractures... Amer. J. Orthodont. oral Surg. 29: 433-441

Thoma, Kurt H. (1944)
A historical review of methods advocated for the treatment of jaw fractures,... Oral Surg. 30 399-504

Tucker, Elisha Gustavus
Quoted by Heitmüller, L. (1897)

Wassmund, Martin (1927)
Frakturen und Luxationen, Berlin

Weber, J. A. C. (1865)
Adhäsionsgebisse und über Unterkieferbrüche. Dtsch. Vjschr. Zahnhk. 5: 285:292

Westendorf, Wolfhart (1966)
Papyrus Edwin Smith. Bern/Stuttgart

Wildt, A. (1896)
Über partielle Unterkieferresektion mit Bildung einer natürlichen Prothese durch Knochentransplantation. Zbl. Chir. 23: 1177-1182

William of Saliceto (1546)
Chirurgia. In: Ars chirurgica Guidonis Chauliaci. Venetiis pp. 303-361

Wiseman, Richard (1676)
Severall chirurgicall treatises. London

Chapter 2

Maxillofacial Injuries—Statistics and Causes of Accidents

Jürgen Lentrodt

In the era of increasing motorization, industrialization, and technology, the treatment of maxillofacial injuries, the most frequent form of therapy in our specialty, has attained a prominent position. Traffic accidents, which are becoming more and more frequent, particularly have brought about an increase in maxillary and facial injuries, as the head, the exposed part of the body, is involved in the highest percentage of injuries of all body regions. Numerous statistical data confirm that head trauma, at more than 70%, definitely predominates among injuries caused by traffic accidents, whereas in other accidents, the skull is involved in one-third of the cases (*Sheldon*, 1955; *Braunstein*, 1957; *Gögler*, 1962; *Dingman* and *Natvig*, 1964; *Cornell*, 1969). Among 100 traffic fatalities, 70.3 (among motorcyclists, 93.7) are due to the sequelae of skull and brain trauma.

1. Frequency of Maxillofacial Injuries

Over a 30-year interval (1946-1975), a total of 6173 fractures of the facial skeleton were treated at the Nordwestdeutsche Kieferklinik in Hamburg. Analysis of this extensive series of traumatized patients permits insights into this development and makes possible detection of trends which are of great clinical interest.

Grouping of our fractures of the facial skeleton according to years reveals a distinct trend toward increasing frequency. In the years immediately following the war, on the average 130 such injuries were treated annually while now there are 302; i.e., the number of cases has increased 2.3-fold.

In addition to the increased incidence of fractures of the facial skeleton, statistical studies show primarily that there is a rapid increase in fractures in the middle third of the face and in composite injuries. A total of 2782 fractures in the midface (45% of all fractures) were observed, of which 17% occurred in combination with a mandibular fracture. During the late 1940s, the yearly average of treated fractures in the middle third of the face was 32.6, whereas now this figure is 180.6, i.e., the increase is 554%. A comparable increase in frequency of fractures of the floor of the orbit has occurred (*Blümel* and *Pfeifer* 1977). The increased severity of the injuries is evident from the fact that combined fractures of the midface and of the mandible formerly occurred in 4% and now are seen in 10% of traumatized patients. Although the percentage of mandibular fractures has decreased from 75% to the present figure of 40%, the absolute numbers show a small increase.

The relationship between fractures of the midface and those of the mandible varies widely in a large number of publications. *Bolle* (1962), *Hermann* et al. (1960), *Müller* (1969), as well as *Paschke* and *Berz* (1961) report a ratio of 1:3, *Gischler* and *Lücke* (1962) 1:2, *Rowe* and *Killey* (1968) 1:1.6, and *McCoy* et al. (1962) as well as *van Hoof* et al. (1977), 1:1. As can be seen in Table 2-I, for our patients in the first twelve years after the war, the ratio was 1:3; during 1958-66, 1:1.5; and during the last nine years, 1:0.67; the overall relationship is 1.22 mandibular fractures for one fracture in the midface.

It would be wrong, when comparisons are made

Table 2-I **Frequency increase of facial skull fractures in a 30-year period at the University of Hamburg's Nordwestdeutsche Kieferklinik**

Three Patient Groups	I 1946-1957	II 1958-1966	III 1967-1975	Total
Midface	1 (324 = 21 %)	2.6 (627 = 33 %)	5.6 (1351 = 50 %)	2.302 = 37 %
Midface + Mandible	1 (69 = 4 %)	2.7 (137 = 7 %)	5.4 (275 = 10 %)	480 = 8 %
Midface total	1 (392 = 25 %)	2.6 (764 = 40 %)	5.5 (1626 = 60 %)	2.782 = 45 %
Mandible	1 (1174 = 75 %)	1.3 (1127 = 60 %)	1.2 (1090 = 40 %)	3.391 = 55 %)
All types of fractures	1 (1566)	1.6 (1891)	2.3 (2716)	6.173

with the statistics of other hospitals or other countries, to draw conclusions retrospectively regarding motorization or industrialization from this global compilation, without giving more detailed data. The figures are greatly influenced, for example, by the area served by a department of maxillofacial surgery, and by the number of oral and maxillofacial surgeons for this region who treat mandibular fractures on an outpatient or inpatient basis. However, if one surveys individual publications, one finds that statistical data with relatively low proportions of fractures in the middle third of the face usually go back to earlier dates, whereas more recent papers consistently cite high percentages of fractures in the midface. This increase is evident not only in our own cases (Table 2-I), but, for example, also in those of *Rowe* and *Killey* (1968), who report that while the number of fractures has doubled over the years, the ratio of fractures in the middle third of the face to mandibular fractures has shifted from 1:2.33 to 1:1.33.

The ratio of male to female patients affected fluctuates considerably in the individual studies. Whereas in our patients, fractures occurred 7.3 times more frequently in males than in female patients, other authors do not report such a large difference. The greater the proportion of fractures resulting from fistfights, the higher the number of male patients.

Reports agree that the peak age of patients with fractures of the facial skeleton occurs in the third decade (*Lindström*, 1960; *Blomquist* and *Kassel*, 1964; *Schuchardt* et al., 1966; *Rowe* and *Killey*, 1968; *Müller*, 1969). Only *van Hoof* et al. (1977) report the highest frequency to lie between 11 and 20 years of age.

2. Causes of Maxillofacial Injuries

In 1966, a paper from our department discussed in detail the causes of facial skeleton fractures (*Schuchardt* et al., 1966). According to this report, for our patients traffic accidents, at 35.6 %, contributed the greatest etiologic share; almost as frequent were fistfights at 31.8 %; work-related accidents contributed 11.6 %, whereas sports accidents, at 3.3 %, played a subordinate role.

By analyzing the individual groups, we were able to show that fractures caused by automobile accidents have increased over the years, whereas fractures caused by motorcycle accidents have decreased. In contrast, in Holland, mandibular fractures due to moped accidents constitute the highest percentage (*van Hoof* et al., 1977).

Compared with other statistics, the number of

fractures of the facial skeleton caused by fistfights is very high in our patients. Only in the German Democratic Republic (*Müller*, 1969) and in the Scandinavian literature (*Lindström*, 1960; *Blomquist* and *Kassel*, 1964) is the percentage slightly higher; otherwise, it is consistently reported to be substantially lower (*Rowe* and *Killey*, 1968; *van Hoof* et al., 1977). We ascribe our high figures in this area to the particular circumstances of Hamburg as a port city (Reeperbahn red light district). It is significant in this connection that fractures produced by the impact of blows also have increased in percentage.

The increase in fractures of the middle third of the face caused by automobile accidents, and also by fistfights, is particularly notable. Since the amount of traffic in the German Federal Republic continues its increasing trend, it must be anticipated that injuries of the facial skeleton, and especially the fractures in the middle third of the face thus created, caused by traffic accidents will experience a further increase. As it has been proved experimentally that automobile accidents involve primarily an impact of the upper half of the face on the dashboard, it remains to be seen whether the increased use of safety belts, which has now become obligatory by law, will lead to a reduction in these injuries.

3. Fracture Sites

In mandibular fractures, the condylar process is involved most frequently. Among our patients, 25 % (*Schuchardt* et al., 1966) and 29 % (*Lentrodt* and *Luhr*, 1969) of those with mandibular fractures had fractures of the condylar process. Fractures of the angle of the mandible occupy the second place, with 19 % and 26 %. The remaining fractures are distributed, in decreasing frequency, among the following mandibular segments: canine region, premolar region, molar region, and symphysis region (*Müller*, 1969). The alveolar crest in our patients accounted for barely 5 % and the ascending ramus, for a good 4 % of mandibular fractures. The least frequent fractures observed are those of the coronoid process.

These figures are basically in agreement with data from other countries. Only in Holland is the proportion of condylar fractures extremely high at 47 %; as foot- or motor-propelled bicycles are the most frequent means of transportation there, according to *van Hoof* et al. (1977), this high percentage can be explained in terms of the lack of protection of the driver who impinges, for example, with his chin from a considerable height onto the street surface.

Among fractures in the middle third of the face, Le Fort II fractures predominate at 23 % and zygomatic bone fractures at 22 %. Next are fractures of the Le Fort I and Le Fort III type, fractures of the alveolar process, fractures of the nasal bone, as well as sagittal fractures of the maxilla. It should be emphasized, particularly in fractures in the middle third of the face, that one often encounters a combination of the different types of fractures as well as atypical forms.

Our data are essentially in agreement with the figures of other investigators. An exception is the surprisingly high proportion of zygomatic bone fractures of 51 % reported by *Rowe* and *Killey* (1968), which is not explained in detail by these authors.

4. Combined Bone and Soft-Tissue Injuries

Although injuries of the soft tissues of the face are more frequent in Great Britain, at 40 % of facial skeleton fractures (*Rowe* and *Killey*, 1968) and in the Netherlands, at 33 % (*van Hoof* et al., 1977), among our patients as well as those in the German Democratic Republic (*Müller*, 1969) about every fifth fracture of this type is associated with more or less extensive injury to the soft tissues covering the bones. The percentage of cuts, tears, contusions and defect wounds is, of course, greatest in combined fractures of the midface and the mandible and least in isolated mandibular fractures. Of course, these soft-tissue wounds also occur without fractures of the facial skeleton. We have made the interesting observation in our traumatized patients that in automobile accidents, isolated injuries of the facial soft tissues occur almost exclusively, and combined soft tissue-bone trauma predominantly in patients who were not wearing safety belts at the time of the accident. Today it can be considered certain that injuries to facial soft tissues, which are not exactly infrequent and are often quite extensive, can be avoided to a large extent by the use of safety belts in the car.

5. Injuries Associated with Maxillofacial Trauma

The most frequent injury that accompanies maxillofacial injuries is traumatic brain damage in the form of brain concussion. This occurred in more than 22 % of our injured patients. *Paschke* and *Berz* (1961), *Müller* (1969) and *Deutschländer-Wolff* et al. (1976) report similar percentages. Only in the report by *van Hoof* et al. (1977) does traumatic brain damage occur in almost every second patient with fractures of the facial skeleton. The frequency of brain concussion is highest with fractures in the middle third of the face and with combined fractures, but is naturally lower with isolated mandibular fractures.

Müller (1969) as well as *van Hoof* et al. (1977) observed aditional fractures in other parts of the body in 6.9 % and 16.9 % of cases, respectively. According to *Müller* (1969), 11 % of displaced mandibular fractures result in traumatic damage to the mandibular nerve. In contrast, in terms of percentages, fractures of the base of the skull, frontal bone and sinuses, and ethmoid bone as well as direct injuries of the eyeball play a subordinate role, even though such types of trauma are very important in individual cases, since optimal treatment ordinarily calls for team approach by various specialists. During the last few years we have observed a distinct increase in such secondary injuries, chiefly because of the increase in severe traffic accidents; these injuries include trauma to the thorax, abdomen, and extremities; and require close interdisciplinary cooperation among all specialists involved with traumatology.

References

Blomquist, K., and T. Kassel (1964)
300 Käkfrakturer analyserade med hänsyn till frevken, uppkomstsätt, diagnos och terapi. (The analysis of 300 jaw fractures, with emphasis on the frequency of causes, diagnosis, and therapy.) Svensk tandläk. T. 57:713

Blümel, J., and G. Pfeifer (1977)
Der Bruchlinienverlauf bei Orbitafrakturen. (The course of the fracture lines in orbital fractures.) Fortschr. Kiefer- u. Gesichtschir. 22:20

Bolle, R. (1962)
Kieferbruchbehandlung an der zahnärztlichen Klinik und Poliklinik der Universität Göttingen. (Treatment of jaw fractures in the Dental College of the University of Göttingen.) Stoma 15:116, 133

Braunstein, P. W. (1957)
Medical aspects of automotive crash injury research. J. Amer. med. Ass. 163:249

Cornell (1969)
cited by Müller, W. (1969)

Deutschländer-Wolff, J., W. Veigel, and V. Castillejos (1976)
Begleitverletzungen bei Gesichtsschädelfrakturen. (Injuries accompanying facial skull fractures.) Fortschr. Kiefer- u. Gesichtschir. 21:294

Dingman, R. O., and P. Natvig (1964)
Surgery of facial fractures. Philadelphia, Saunders

Gischler, E., and R. Lücke (1962)
Beitrag zur Häufigkeit der Frakturen im Bereich der Kiefer- und Gesichtsschädelknochen. (Contribution to the study of frequency of fractures of the bones of the jaw and facial skeleton.) Dtsch. zahnärztl. Z. 17:649

Gögler, E. (1962)
Unfallopfer im Straßenverkehr. (Accident victims in traffic accidents.) Documenta Geigy, Series Chirurgia, Basel, Geigy

Hermann, M., H.-H. Grasser, and I. Bleisiegel (1960)
Die Kieferbrüche an der Zahn-, Mund- und Kieferklinik in Mainz von 1949-1959. (Jaw fractures at the Mainz Dental College in the period 1949-1959.) Dtsch. zahnärztl. Z. 15:657

van Hoof, R. F., C. A. Merkx, and E. C. Stekelenburg (1977)
The different patterns of fractures of the facial skeleton in four European countries. Int. J. oral Surg. 6:3

Lentrodt, J., and H. G. Luhr (1969)
Indications for conservative and surgical treatment of facial bone fractures. Panminerva med. 11:88

Lindström, D. (1960)
Jämförande översikt av käkfrakturerna under aven 1948-58. (Comparative investigations of jaw fractures in 1948-1959.) Suom. Hammastääk. Toim. 56:16

McCoy, F. J., R. A. Chandler, C. G. Magman, J. R. Moore, and G. Siemsen (1962)
An analysis of facial fractures and their complications. Plast. reconstr. Surg. 29:381

Müller, W. (1969)
Häufigkeit, Sitz und Ursachen der Gesichtsschädelfrakturen. (Frequency, site and causes of facial skeleton fractures.) In Reichenbach, E. (ed.): Traumatologie im Kiefer-Gesichts-Bereich. (Maxillofacial traumatology.) Munich, Barth

Paschke, H., and A. Berz (1961)
Die Frakturen der Kiefer-Gesichtsknochen und die statistische Auswertung derselben am Krankengut der Universitätsklinik für Zahn-, Mund- und Kieferkranke in Erlangen von 1950-1960. (Fractures of the facial skeleton and their statistical evaluation in patients of the University of Erlangen's Dental College.) Dtsch. Zahnärztebl. 15:681

Rowe, N. L., and H. C. Killey (1968)
Fractures of the facial skeleton. 2nd ed., Edinburgh-London, Livingstone

Schuchardt, K., N. Schwenzer, B. Rottke, and J. Lentrodt (1966)
Ursachen, Häufigkeit und Lokalisation der Frakturen des Gesichtsschädels. (Causes, frequency and localization of fractures of the facial skeleton.) Fortschr. Kiefer- u. Gesichtschir. 11:1

Sheldon, C. H. (1955)
Prevention, the only cure for head injuries resulting from automobile accidents. J. Amer. med. Ass. 159:981

Chapter 3

Radiographic Diagnosis of Fractures of the Facial Skeleton

Bernhard Rottke

1. Introduction

Optimal care of patients with injuries of the facial skull can be planned, managed and supervised only where facilities exist for accurate radiographic diagnosis.

This chapter proposes radiographic methods which take into account the equipment available and the state of the patient, under both emergency and optimum conditions. Moreover, attention is given to variations likely to facilitate the procedures followed. Radiographs are discussed to demonstrate their indications, information content and faults.

2. Radiographic Methods and Indications for their Use

The following equipment is recommended for visualising the regions affected in traumatic lesions of the facial skeleton:

1. mobile tank unit (variable kV)
2. panoramic unit
3. skull unit
4. rotating-anode tube, mobile, with generator
5. tomograph
6. accessories (grids, collimators, cassettes, etc.)

In a well-equipped department it should be possible to perform the following examinations (*Clementschitsch*, 1948, 1955, 1963; *Beutel* and *Tänzer*, 1963; *Grashey* and *Birkner*, 1964; *Zimmer* and *Brossy*, 1974):

- 2.1 Intraoral radiographs
  - 2.1.1 dental films
  - 2.1.2 occlusal radiographs
    - 2.1.2.1 maxillary occlusal view, median and lateral
    - 2.1.2.2 mandibular occlusal view, mandible axial, and survey of floor of the mouth
- 2.2 Extraoral projections of the mandible
  - 2.2.1 chin region
  - 2.2.2 horizontal ramus
  - 2.2.3 ascending ramus
  - 2.2.4 TMJ by *Parma* technique
- 2.3 Panoramic survey radiographs
  - 2.3.1 panoramic tomograms
  - 2.3.2 panoramic enlargement radiographs
- 2.4 Skull radiographs
  - 2.4.1 sagittal projections
    - 2.4.1.1 skull, posterior-anterior (PA)
    - 2.4.1.2 skull, AP and PA eccentric
    - 2.4.1.3 paranasal sinuses
    - 2.4.1.4 orbital survey
    - 2.4.1.5 TMJ, transorbital
  - 2.4.2 axial (inferosuperior) projections
    - 2.4.2.1 skull, axial
    - 2.4.2.2 comparative views of both zygomatic arches
    - 2.4.2.3 isolated zygomatic arch
  - 2.4.3 lateral projection
    - 2.4.3.1 skull, lateral
    - 2.4.3.2 skull, teleradiograph, cephalometric lateral view, with simultaneous visualization of soft tissue
    - 2.4.3.3 nose, lateral
    - 2.4.3.4 TMJ by *Schüller* technique
- 2.5 Tomography

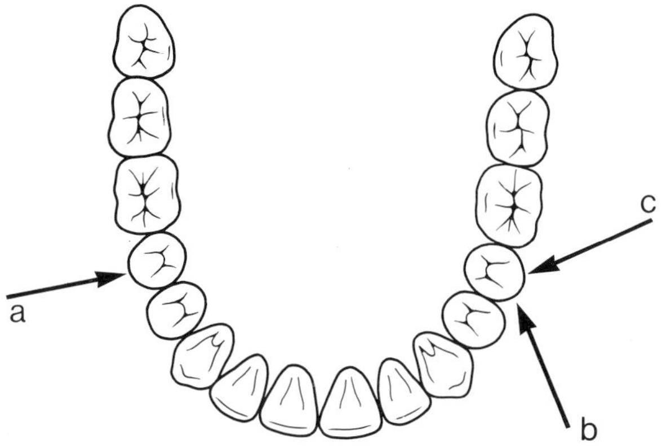

Fig. 3-1 Adjustment of the central beam for dental radiographs:
a. orthoradial (*Pordes*, 1919)
b. mesial-eccentric
c. distal-eccentric

2.1 Intraoral Radiographs

2.1.1 Dental Films

Equipment:	Dental unit (**Oralix, Heliodent**) films 2 × 3 cm, 3 × 4 cm, 4 × 5 cm no screen
Technique:	Positioning: orthoradial (Fig. 3-1) as well as half-angle (Fig. 3-2) or right-angle technique (Fig. 3-3)
Information:	Provides sharpest image of dental region
Indications:	Tooth fractures, fractures of the alveolar process

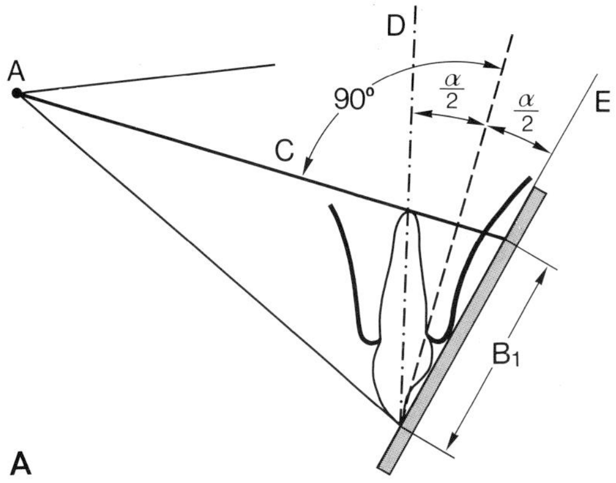

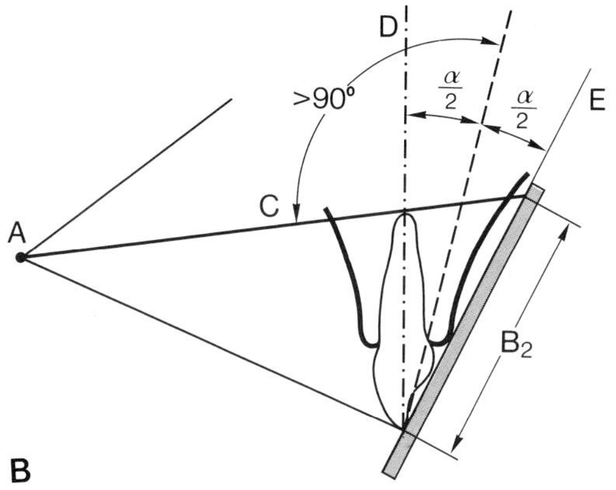

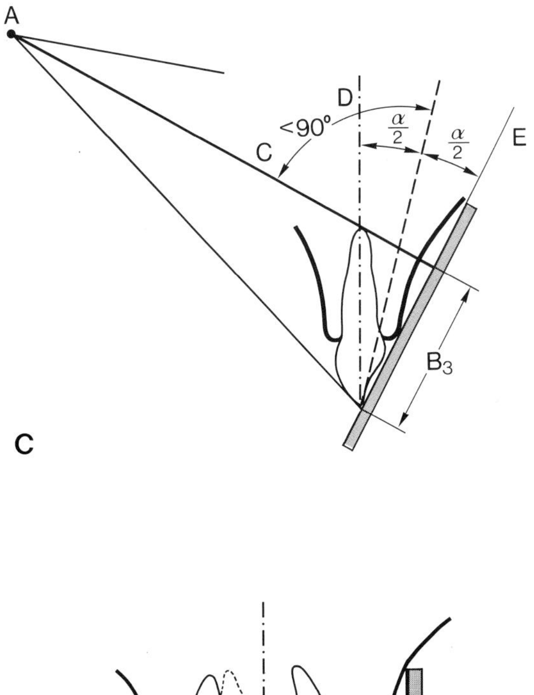

Figs. 3-2 A to C Half-angle technique for dental radiographs.

Fig. 3-2 A Proper adjustment.

Fig. 3-2 B Adjustment too flat.

Fig. 3-2 C
Adjustment too steep.

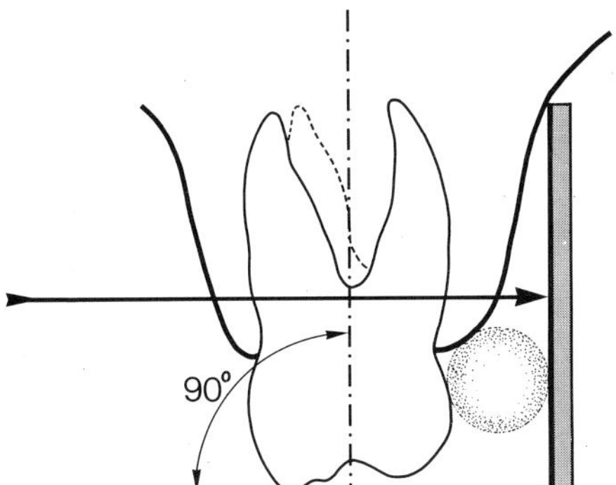

Fig. 3-3 Right angle technique for dental radiographs. (*Fitzgerald*, 1947; *Hielscher*, 1954; *van Aken*, 1969).

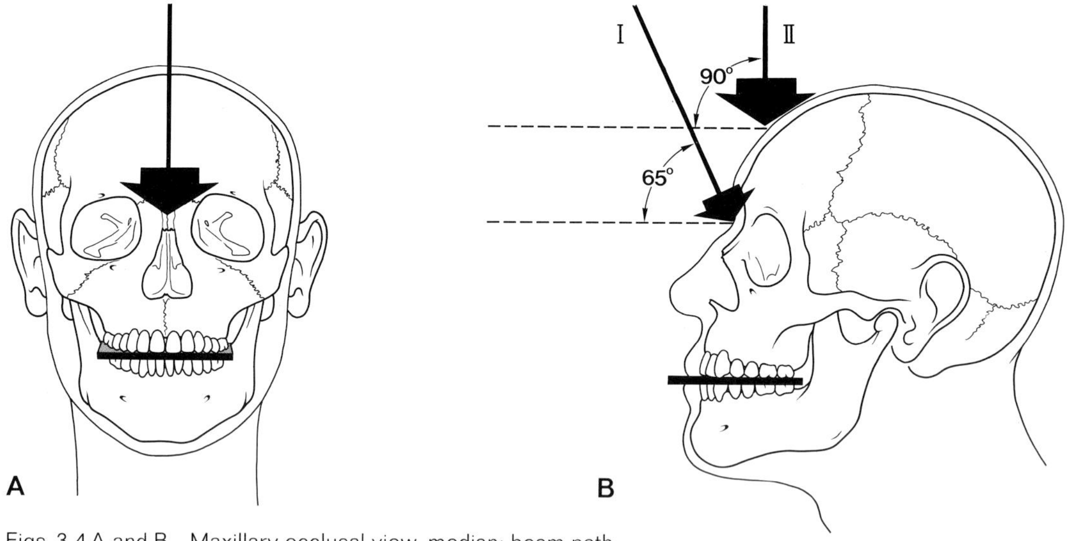

Figs. 3-4 A and B Maxillary occlusal view, median; beam path.
I. Flat adjustment.
II. Steep adjustment.

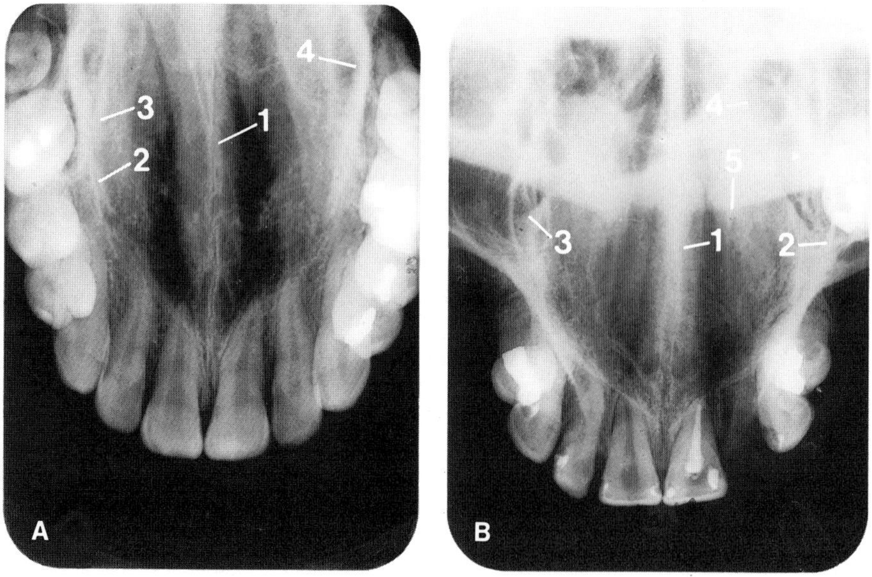

Figs. 3-5 A and B Maxillary occlusal view, median.

Fig. 3-5 A Flat adjustment.
Fig. 3-5 B Steep adjustment.

1. nasal septum
2. lateral wall of the nasal cavity
3. medial wall of the alveolar recess
4. naso-lacrimal duct
5. frontal bone

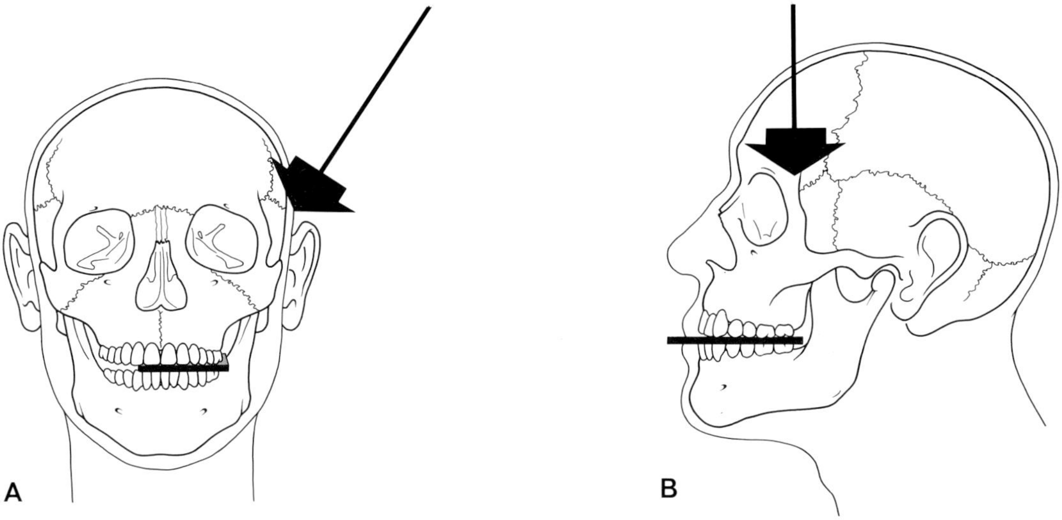

Figs. 3-6 A and B Maxillary occlusal view, lateral; beam path.

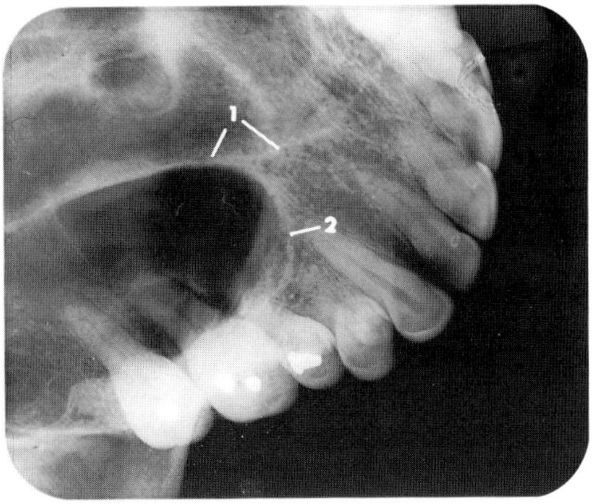

Fig. 3-7 Maxillary occlusal view, lateral.
1. wall of the nasal cavity
2. anterior limit of the alveolar recess of the maxillary sinus

2.1.2 Occlusal Radiographs (*Balters*, 1925; *Schindler*, 1927)

2.1.2.1 Maxillary Occlusal View

Equipment:	Dental unit, occlusal film (**Kodak**), non-screen (7.5 × 5.5 cm)
A. Median	
Technique:	Film in occlusal plane, median Central ray passes through root of nose at flat (65°) or steep (90°) angle (Fig. 3-4)
Information:	Good visualization of the anterior part of the alveolar process and hard palate (Fig. 3-5)
Indication:	Fractures in this region
Errors:	Excessively steep projection causes superimpositioning of frontal bone
B. Lateral	
Technique:	Film in occlusal plane, moved toward side to be visualised, central ray passes obliquely through the malar bone (Fig. 1-6)
Information:	Relevant half of the maxilla from anterior teeth to molar region including alveolar process as well as part of the nasal cavity wall and the alveolar recess of the maxillary sinus (Fig. 3-7)

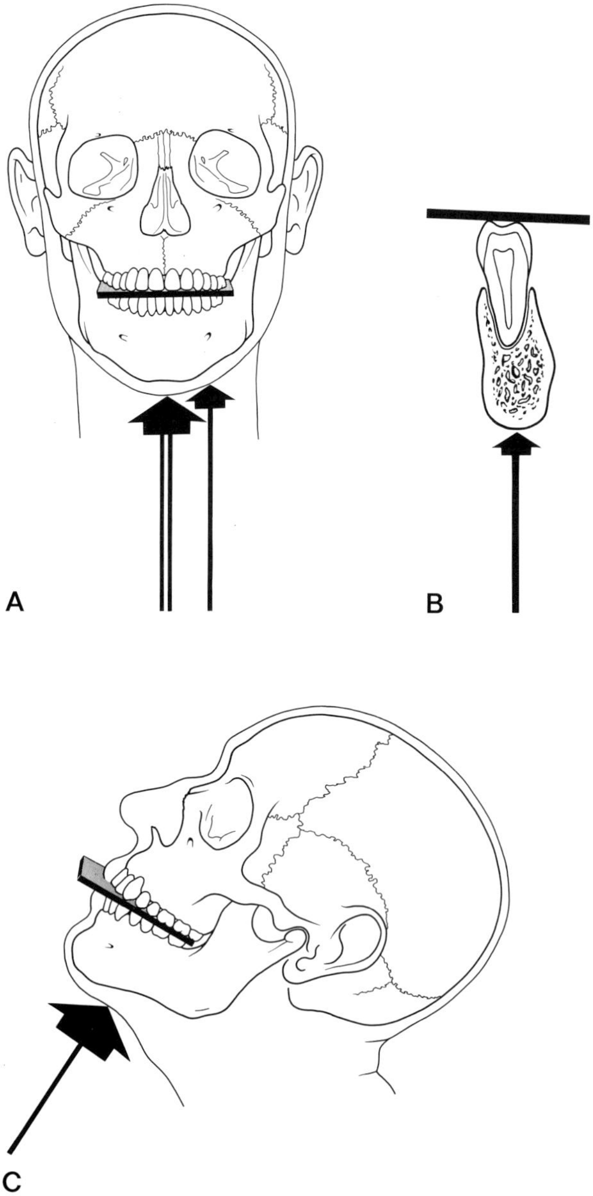

Figs. 3-8 A to C Mandibular occlusal view, axial, and survey of floor of the mouth (double arrow); beam path.

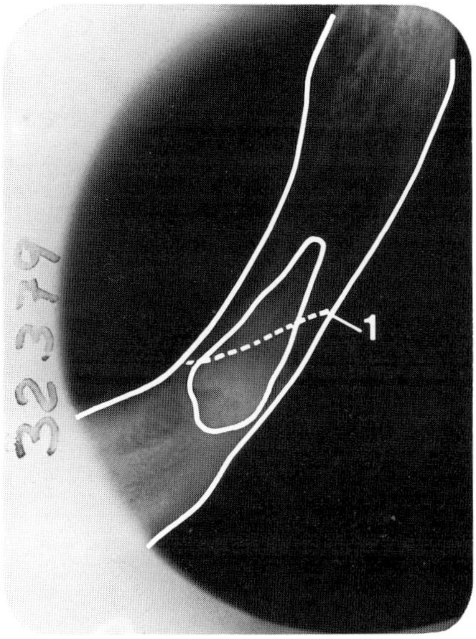

Fig. 3-9 Mandibular occlusal view, axial. Translucent line (1) in the region of the impacted 35 as an expression of a non-displaced fracture of the mandible.

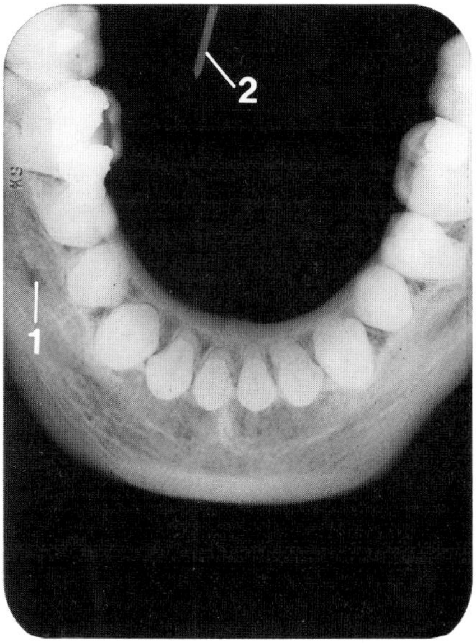

Fig. 3-10 View of the floor of the mouth.
1. mental foramen
2. shadow of metal injection needle in the floor of the mouth

2.1.2.2 Mandibular Occlusal View

A. Mandible, axial

Equipment:	Dental unit
Technique:	Film lies against region of occlusal plane to be visualized, central ray passes axially through mandible (Fig. 3-8)
Information:	Lingual and buccal mandibular bone with displacement in this direction
Indication:	Oblique fractures located latero-medially (Fig. 3-9)
Errors:	Inaccurate axial positioning, so teeth do not appear round

B. Survey of floor of the mouth

Equipment:	Dental unit
Technique:	Film in occlusal plane, head tilted dorsally, central ray passes through middle of floor of mouth (Fig. 3-8 A)
Information:	Visualization of soft parts of floor of mouth and tongue (Fig. 3-10)
Indication:	Localization of foreign bodies
Errors:	Film has not been pushed far enough into the oral cavity

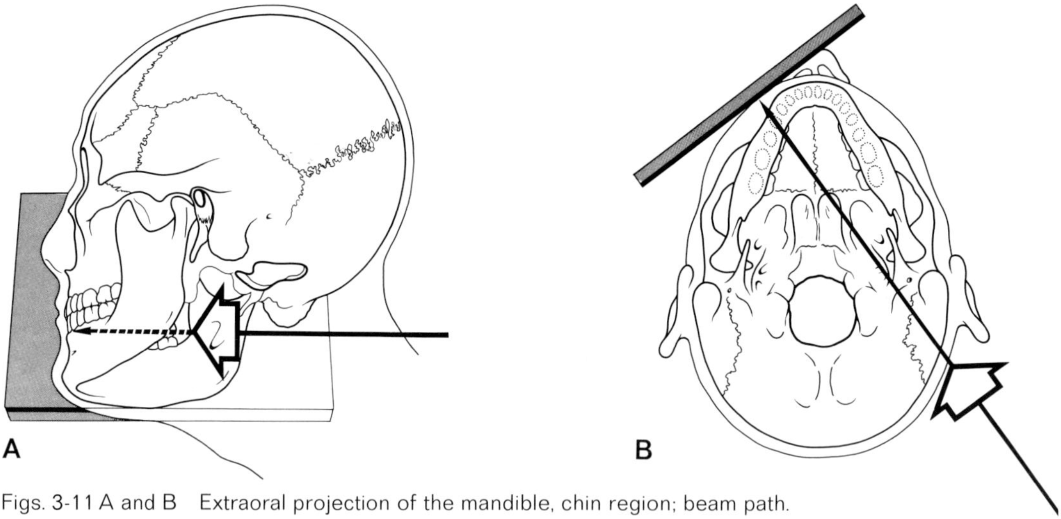

Figs. 3-11 A and B Extraoral projection of the mandible, chin region; beam path.

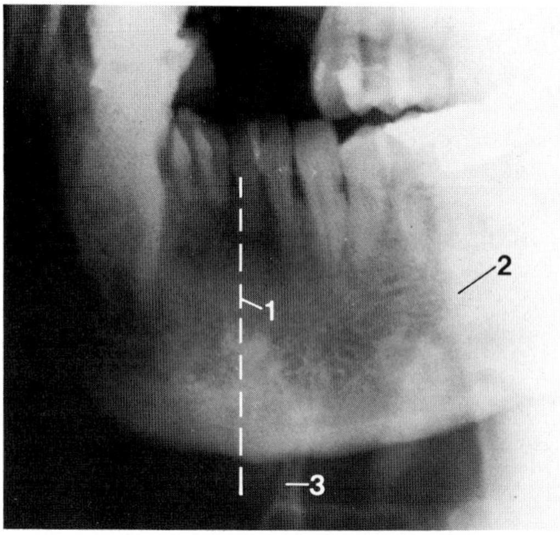

Fig. 3-12 Extraoral projection of the mandible, region of the chin.
1. mid-line
2. lateral limit of the spinal column
3. hyoid bone

Fig. 3-14 (see page 57) Extraoral projection of the mandible, horizontal ramus.
1. mandibular canal
2. angle of the mandible
3. hyoid bone
4. fracture line
5. maxillary tuberosity
6. alveolar recess of the maxillary sinus
7. inferior border of the opposite side of the mandible

2.2 Extraoral Projections of the Mandible (*Cieszynski*, 1911, 1926; *Balters*, 1925)

Equipment: Dental unit (**Oralix, Oralix 65, Heliodent, Explorer 500**), cone, corresponding kV value, cassettes 9 × 12 or 13 × 18 cm, screen ultra or fine, depending on rating of X-ray tube

2.2.1 Chin Region

Technique: Cassette fixed in front of chin, central ray projected from opposite side past spinal

Information: Visualization of left or right half of chin (Fig. 3-12)
Indication: Chin fractures, in the absence of a PEU (panoramic enlargement unit)
Errors: With patient recumbent, spinal column often is superimposed

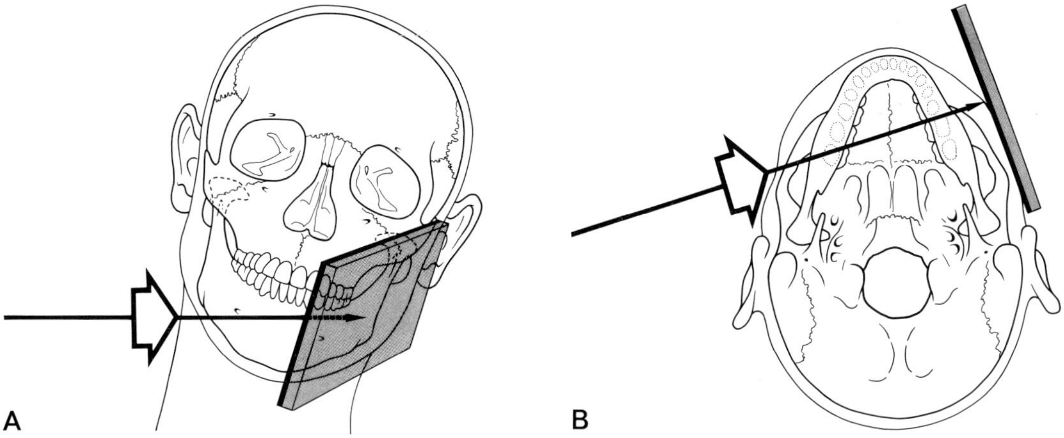

Figs. 3-13 A and B   Extraoral projection of the mandible, horizontal ramus; beam path.

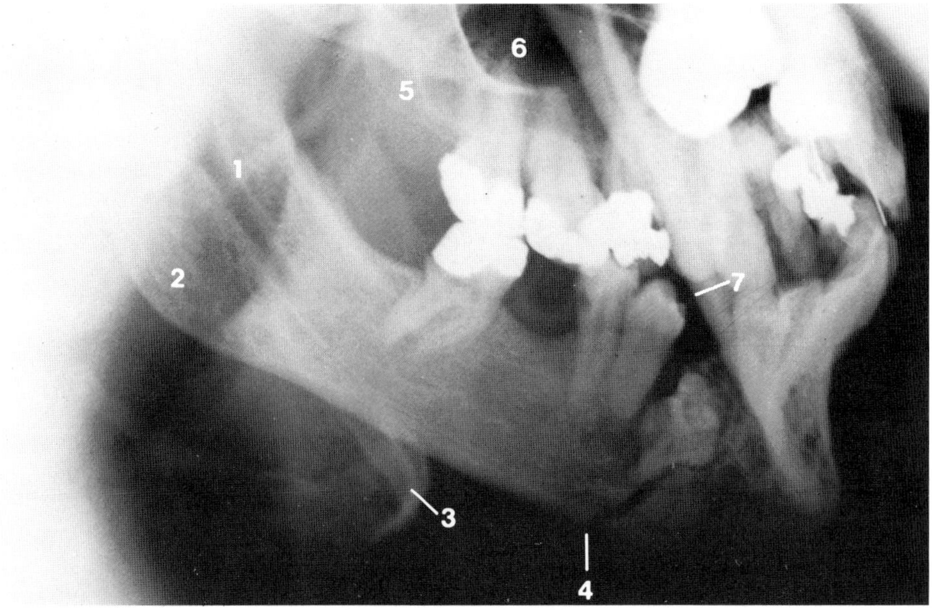

Fig. 3-14
Legend on page 56

2.2.2 Horizontal Ramus

Technique: Cassette is placed laterally against mandible, head is tilted slightly laterally, central ray passes below border of mandible (Fig. 3-13)

Information: Visualization of the mandible between canine and angle (Fig. 3-14)

Indication: Fractures of mandible in the absence of a panoramic tomograph; recumbent patient

Errors: Insufficient tilting results in superimpositioning of opposite side; excessive tilting has the effect of foreshortening and inclusion of hyoid bone in field

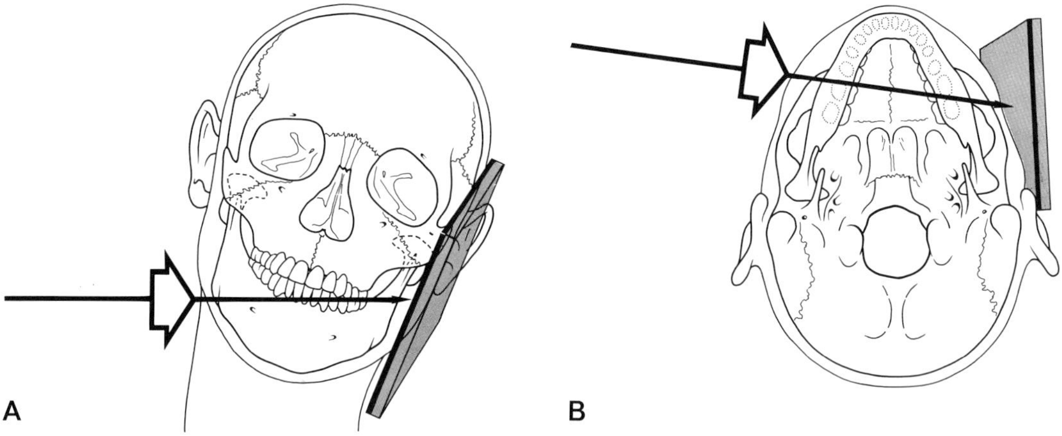

Figs. 3-15 A and B Extraoral projection of the mandible, ascending ramus, beam path.

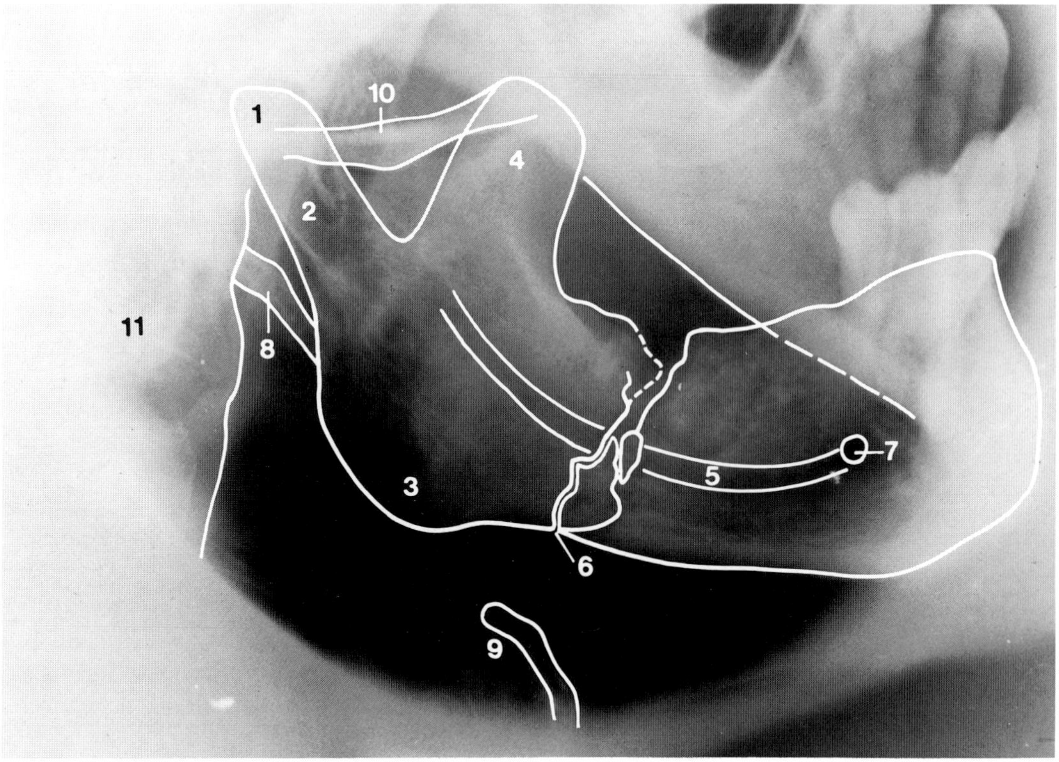

Fig. 3-16 Extraoral projection of the mandible, ascending ramus.

1. condyle
2. neck of the condyle
3. angle of the mandible
4. coronoid process
5. mandibular nerve
6. fracture line with 2 bone splinters
7. mental foramen
8. styloid process
9. hyoid bone
10. zygomatic arch
11. cervical vertebrae

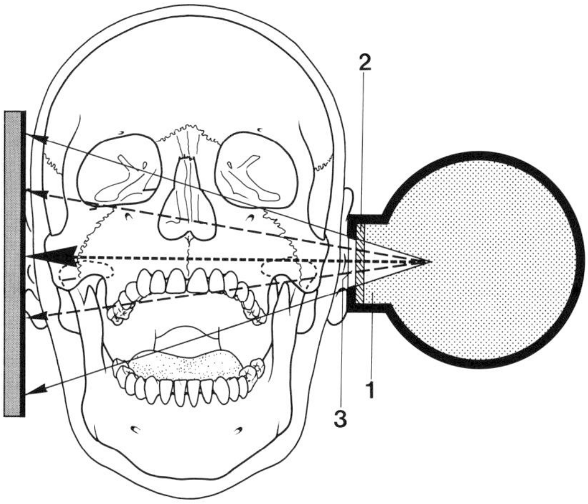

Fig. 3-17 Lateral temporomandibular joint (TMJ) projection (*Parma*), beam path.
1. short tube (*Reckow*)
2. supplemental (3 mm thick) aluminum filter
3. diaphragm

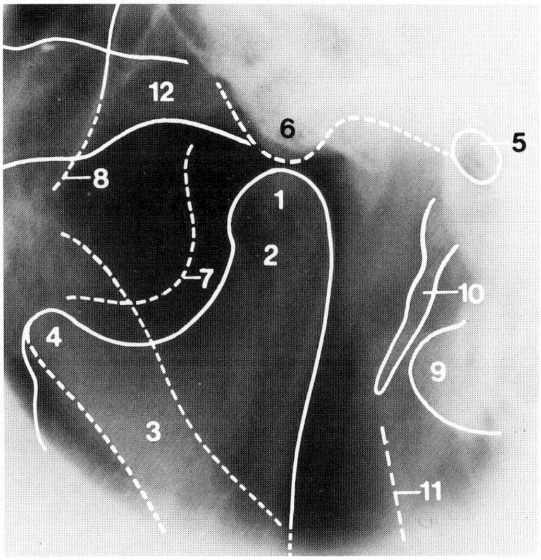

Fig. 3-18 Lateral TMJ projection (*Parma*).
1. condyle
2. neck of the condyle
3. soft palate
4. coronoid process
5. acoustic meatus
6. articular eminence
7. pterygoid process
8. wall of the maxillary sinus
9. atlas
10. styloid process
11. posterior wall of the pharynx
12. zygomatic arch

2.2.3 Ascending Ramus

Technique: Cassette upright against ascending ramus, central ray projected onto it from mesio-caudal direction (Fig. 3-15)

Information: Angle of the mandible and ascending ramus up to region of TMJ (Fig. 3-16)

2.2.4 Temporomandibular Joint (TMJ) by Parma Technique (1932, 1942)

Equipment: Dental unit, short cone with extra Al filtration (3 mm), annular collimator (2.5 cm), cassette 9 × 12 cm

Technique: Cassette is laid against joint to be visualized, tube is in contact with opposite site, mouth fully opened (Fig. 3-17)

Information: Good lateral view of the condylar process together with adjacent regions (Fig. 3-18)

Indication: Fractures of the condylar and coronoid process

Errors: Moderate diagnostic value if mouth not fully open, frequent over-exposure (pharynx), superimpositioning of uvula and base of tongue

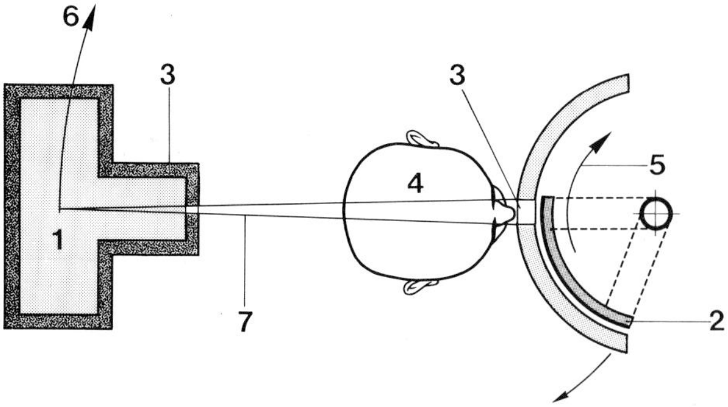

Fig. 3-19 Principle of laminagraphy for the production of panoramic tomograms with the orthopantomograph (from *Rottke* et al., 1974).

1. X-ray unit
2. film holder
3. wedge-shaped shutter
4. patient
5. direction of movement of the film holder
6. direction of movement of the tube
7. beam

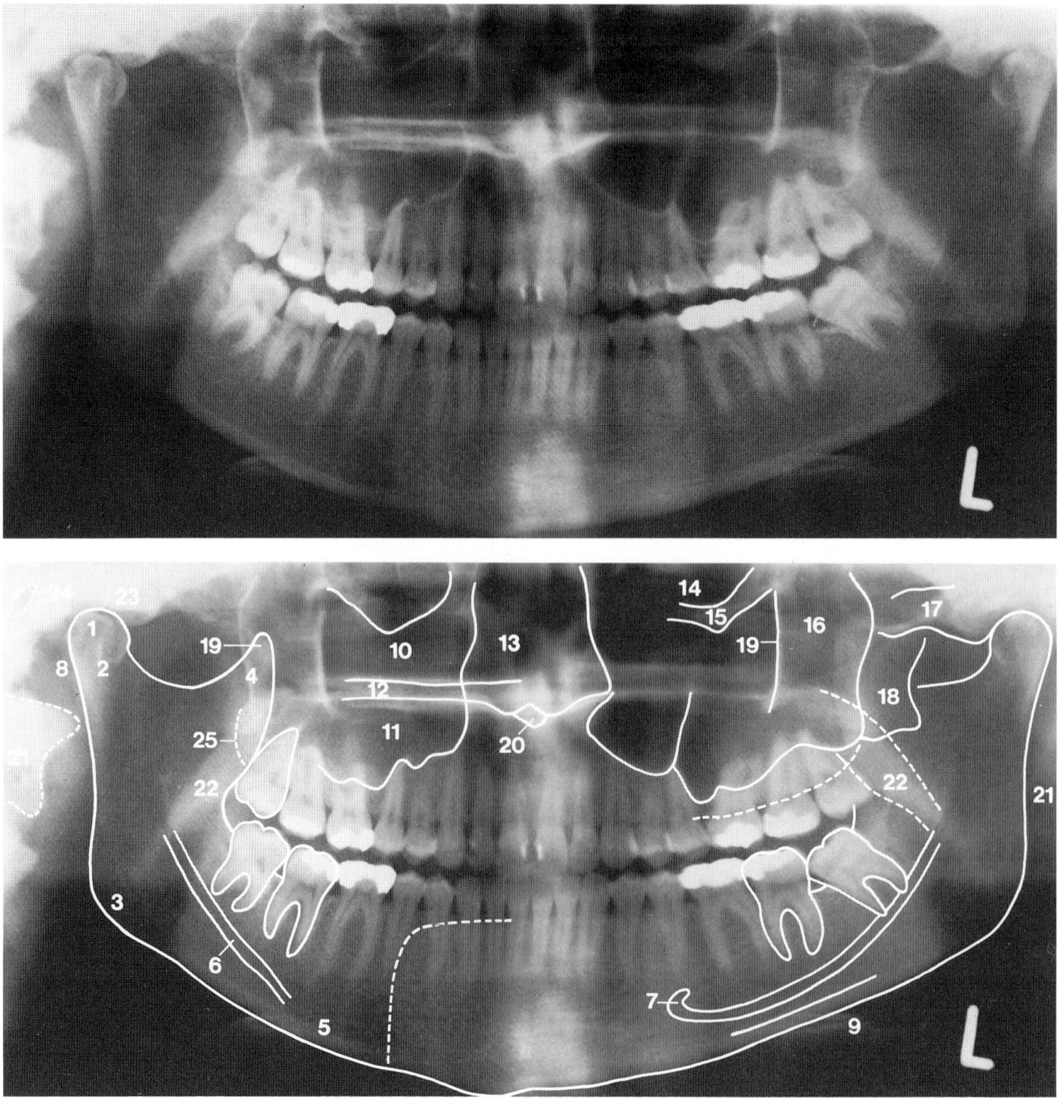

Fig. 3-20 Legend on page 61.

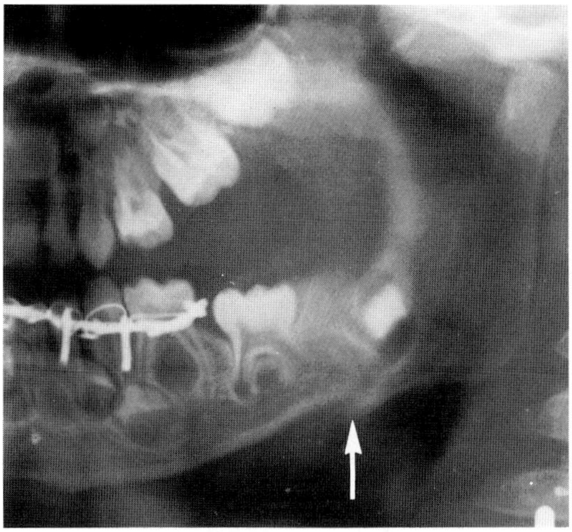

Fig. 3-21 A Orthopantomogram. Potential source of error: Shoulder on the left side of the mandible simulating a fracture, caused by motion during exposure of film.

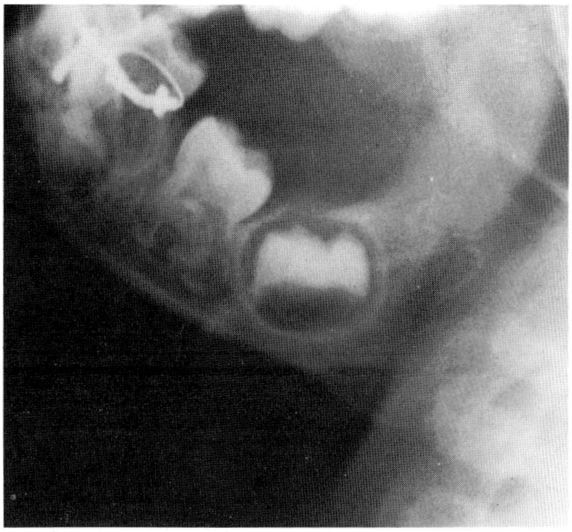

Fig. 3-21 B Check film of the left side of the mandible: no shoulder visible.

Fig. 3-20 (see page 60) Orthopantomogram.

1. condyle
2. neck of the condyle
3. angle of the mandible
4. coronoid process of the mandible
5. horizontal ramus of the mandible
6. mandibular canal
7. mental foramen
8. styloid process
9. hyoid bone
10. maxillary sinus
11. alveolar recess
12. hard palate
13. nasal septum
14. orbit
15. floor of the orbit
16. zygoma
17. zygomatic arch
18. pterygoid process
19. wall of the maxillary sinus
20. anterior nasal spine
21. cervical spine
22. soft palate
23. articular eminence
24. acoustic meatus

2.3 Panoramic Survey Radiographs

2.3.1 Panoramic Tomograms (PT; *Numata,* 1933; *Heckmann,* 1939)

A. Equipment:	Unit with three axes of rotation (**Orthopantomograph, Orth-Oralix**; *Paatero,* 1949)
Technique:	The patient is positioned standing in the unit; points of importance: edge-to-edge bite position; bite rim is used if necessary, naso-auricular plane horizontal, tongue against palate, slight bending of cervical spine (Fig. 3-19)
Information:	In addition to the central regions, the dentigerous parts of the maxilla and mandible are visualized clearly (Fig. 3-20; *Jung,* 1972)
Indication:	Fractures of the mandible and maxilla
Errors:	Malpositioning results in marked blur in the region of the anterior teeth and tilts the palate line mesially or distally; brief movement may simulate fracture (Fig. 3-21; *Ando,* 1971; *Buchmann,* 1974)

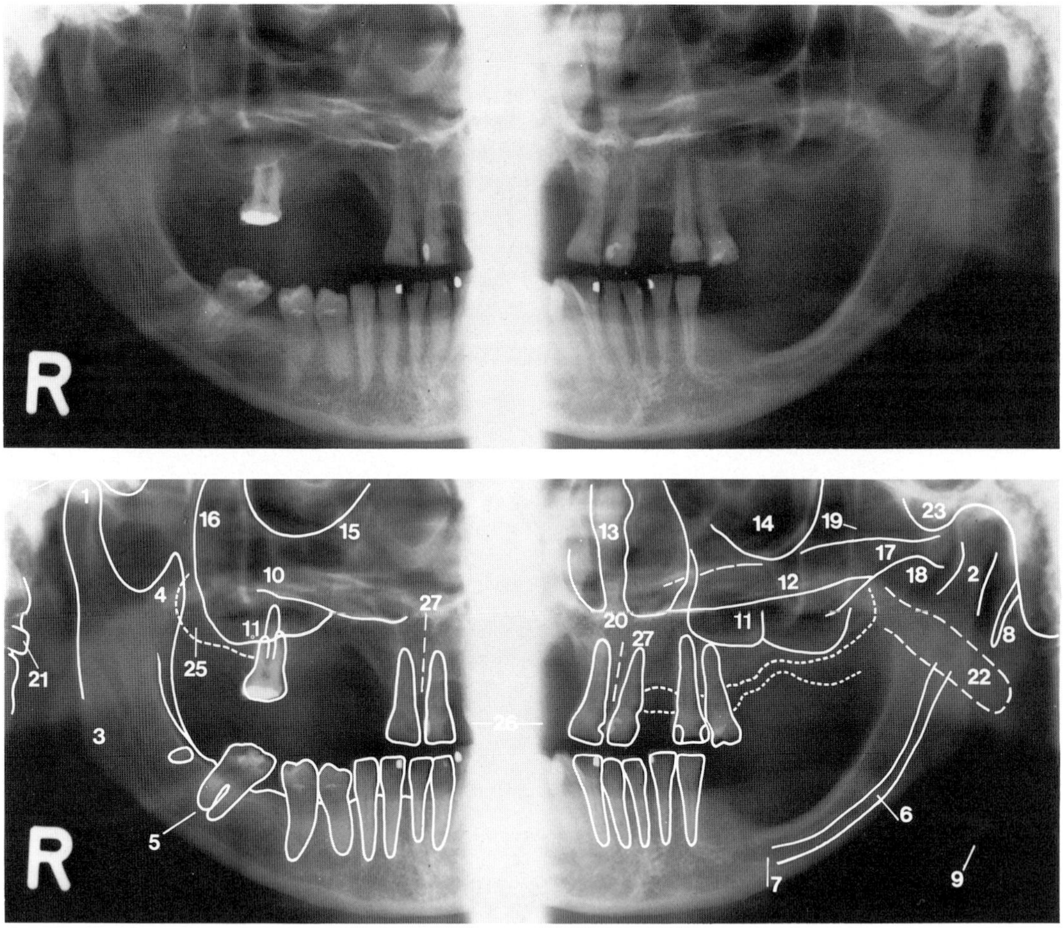

Fig. 3-22 Panorex film.

1. condyle
2. neck of the condyle
3. angle of the mandible
4. coronoid process of the mandible
5. horizontal ramus of the mandible
6. mandibular canal
7. mental foramen
8. styloid process
9. hyoid bone
10. maxillary sinus
11. alveolar recess
12. hard palate
13. nasal septum
14. orbit
15. floor of the orbit
16. zygoma
17. zygomatic arch
18. pterygoid process
19. wall of the maxillary sinus
20. anterior nasal spine
21. cervical spine
22. soft palate
23. articular eminence
24. acoustic meatus
25. maxillary tuberosity
26. non-irradiated zone, caused by cutting current off
27. midline, doubly depicted

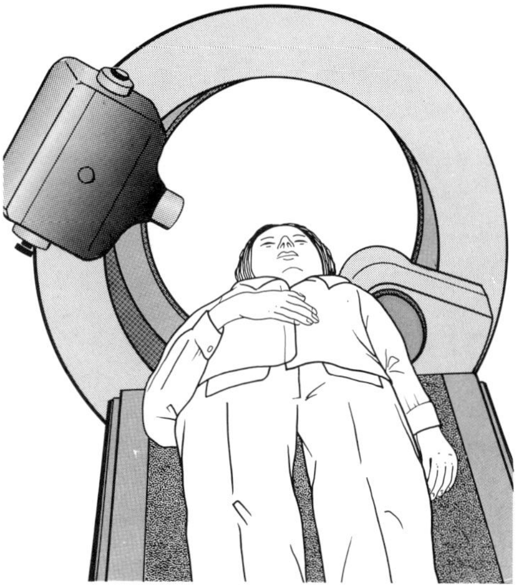

Fig. 3-23 Tomorex, panoramic tomogram taken with the patient reclining.

B. Equipment: Unit with two axes of rotation (**Panorex**; *Hudson* et al., 1957)

Technique: The patient is positioned seated in the unit, chair is moved while X-radiation is cut off briefly

Information: Double visualization of the frontal region excludes drawbacks of other panoramic tomographs. Sharp definition and slight, uniform enlargement of jaw region (Fig. 3-22)

Errors: Tube may jam with short-necked patients. Malpositioning of center line

C. The development of the **Tomorex** represents an important step forward. It permits panoramic tomograms to be made of recumbent patients (Fig. 3-23)

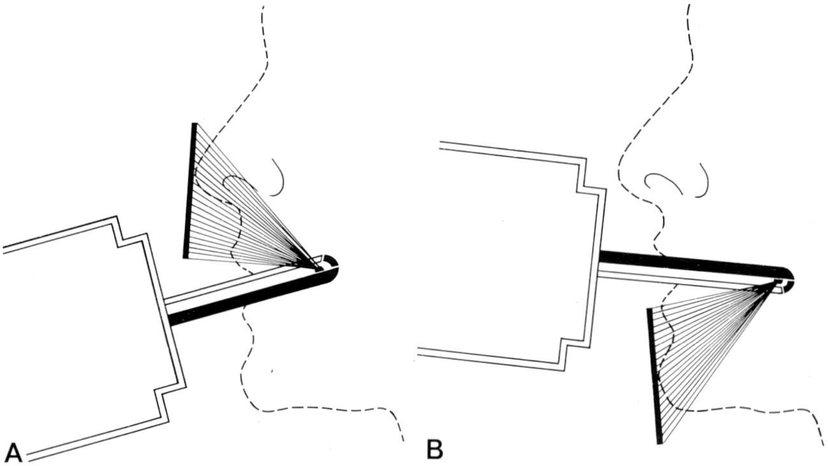

Figs. 3-24 A and B
Central beam in panagraphy.

Fig. 3-24 A Maxilla.

Fig. 3-24 B Mandible.

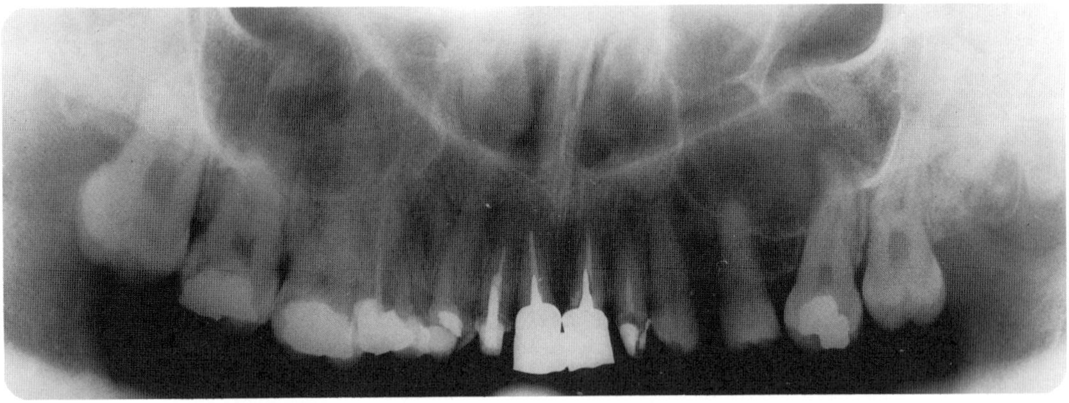

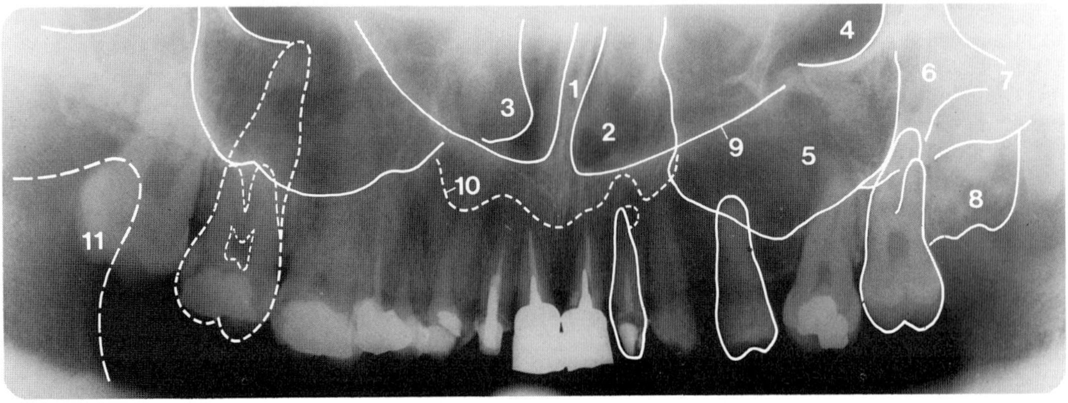

1. nasal septum
2. nasal sinus
3. nasal concha
4. orbit
5. alveolar recess of the maxillary sinus
6. zygoma
7. zygomatic arch
8. maxillary tuberosity
9. border of the maxillary sinus
10. shadow of nasal soft tissue
11. coronoid process of the mandible

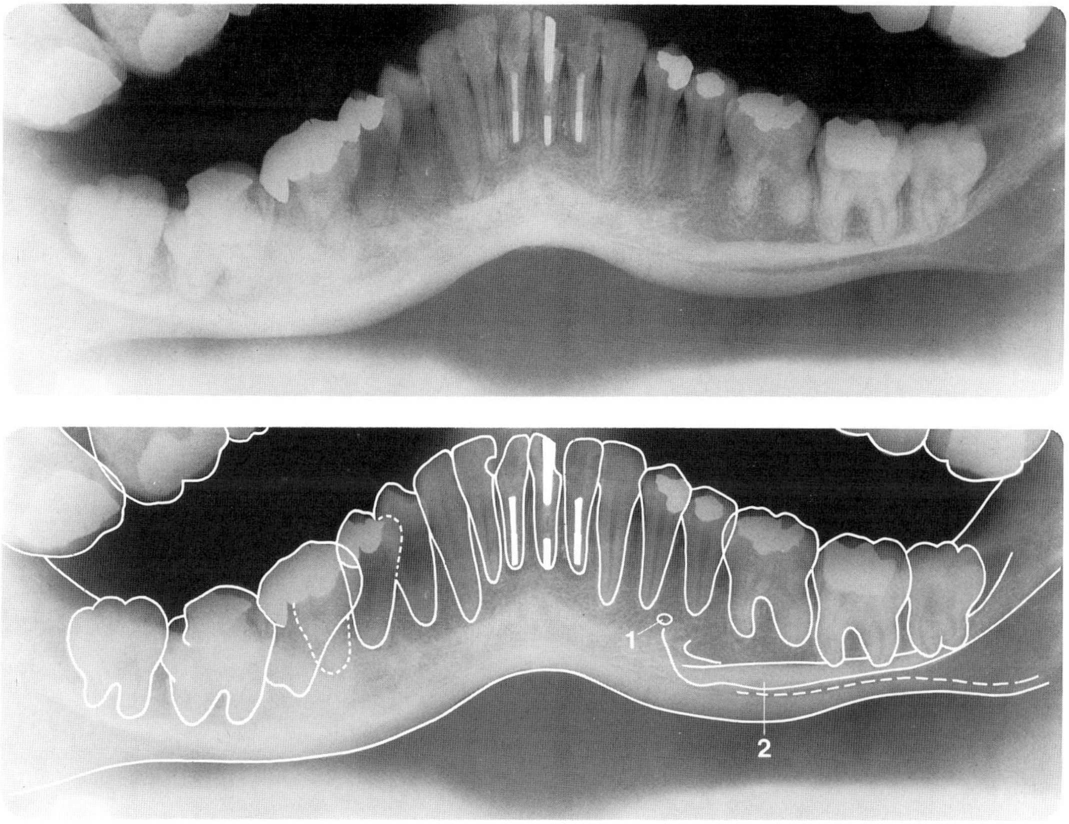

Fig. 3-26 Panoramic radiograph, mandible.
1. mental foramen 2. mylohyoid line (projected over the mandibular canal)

2.3.2 Panoramic Enlargement Radiographs (PER; *Berger*, 1943; *Ott*, 1960)

Equipment: Unit with intraoral focal spot (**Status-X, Stat-Oralix, Panoramix**)

Technique: Patient is seated, the jaw to be visualized is positioned horizontally, and then the window of the X-ray tube is turned in the appropriate direction. Tube is inserted into the oral cavity (up to the mark provided), tilted 5° cranially in the maxilla, 5° caudally in the mandible. Film is brought into position and held by patient (Fig. 3-24)

Information: Excellent visualization of middle sections of the maxilla or mandible (Fig. 3-25 and 3-26)

Indication: Fractures in the anterior part of the maxilla and mandible.

Errors: Enlargement and considerable blur of the region of the posterior teeth, poor visualization of oblique fractures, slight lateral deviation causes nonuniform enlargement and simulates unilateral shadowing of the alveolar recess.
As compared with other procedures, the high X-ray exposure of the mucous membrane is a disadvantage. (*Aken* and *Linden*, 1966; *Regulla* et al., 1972; *Sonnabend*, 1972; *Rottke* et al., 1974)

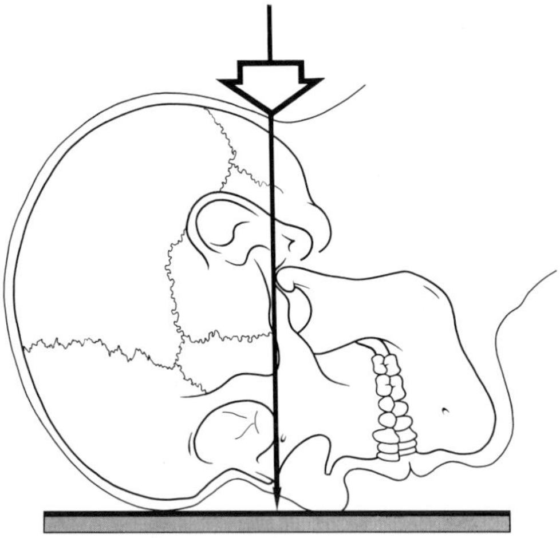

Fig. 3-27 P-A skull projection; beam path.

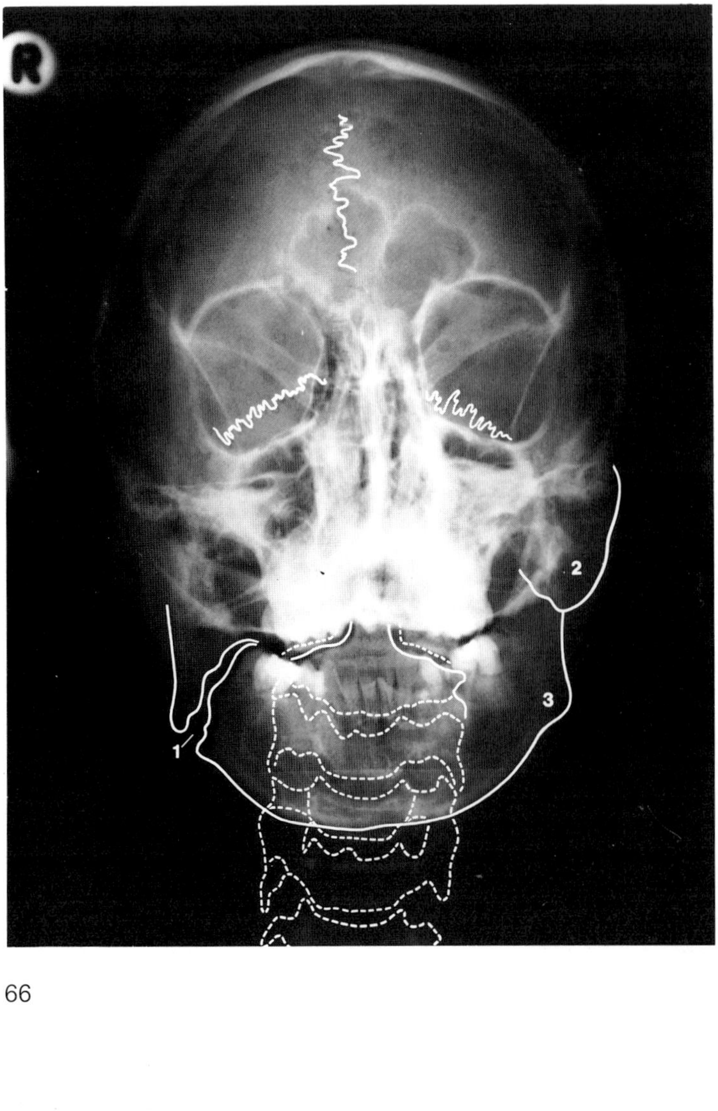

Fig. 3-28 P-A skull projection.
1. fracture line
2. mastoid process
3. angle of the mandible

2.4 Skull Radiographs

2.4.1 Sagittal Projection

2.4.1.1 Skull, Posterior-Anterior (PA; Stenhuis; Carlsten, 1971)

Equipment: Skull unit (**Lysholm, Orbix, Cranio-Diagnost**), cassette 24 × 30 cm set upright, fine intensifying screen

Technique: Cassette rests against forehead and tip of nose. The orbito-meatal line is vertical, the central ray passing through it and the median sagittal plane from dorsal to root of nose (Fig. 3-27)

Information: Petrous bone is projected in orbita, mastoid process covers temporomandibular joint and coronoid process. Good visualization of vault of cranium, frontal sinuses, ethmoid cells and nasal cavity. Equally good perception of the upper edge of the orbit (Fig. 3-28)

Indication: Fractures of vault of cranium

Errors: Malpositioning in the sagittal projection, recognizable from pyramid position. Lateral tilting noticeable from position of lamina papyracea.

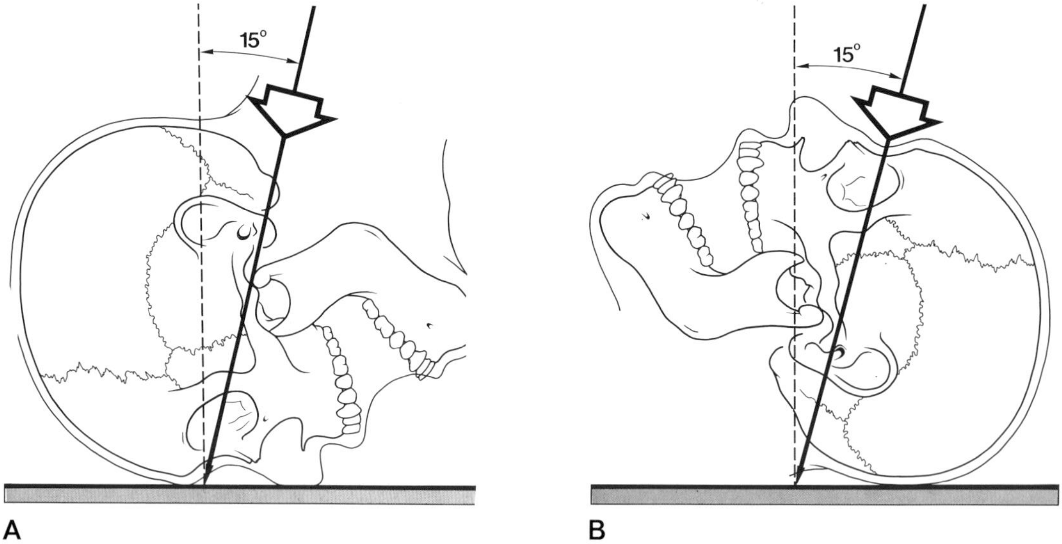

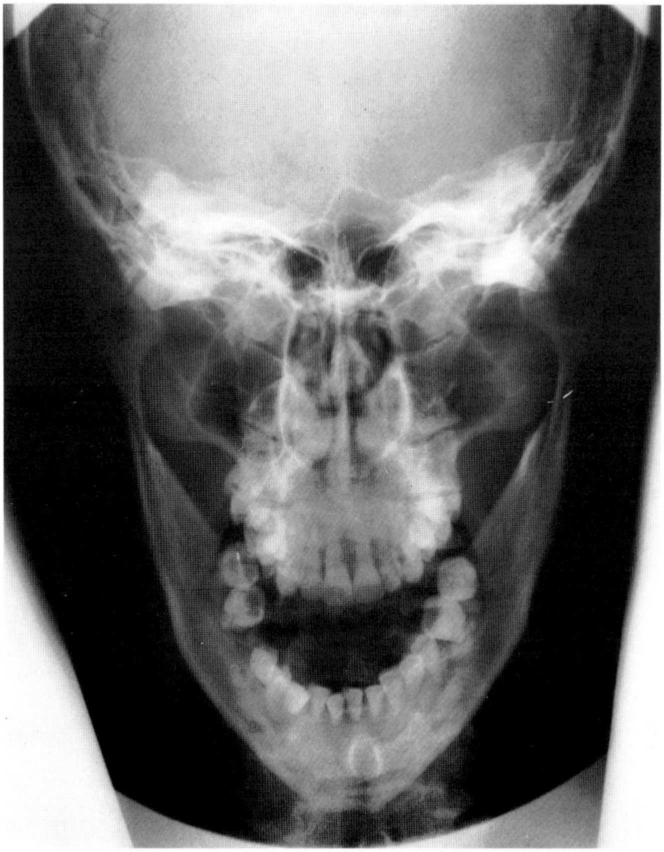

Fig. 3-29 A P-A skull projection, 15° eccentric; beam path.

Fig. 3-29 B A-P skull projection, 15° eccentric; beam path.

Figure 3-30

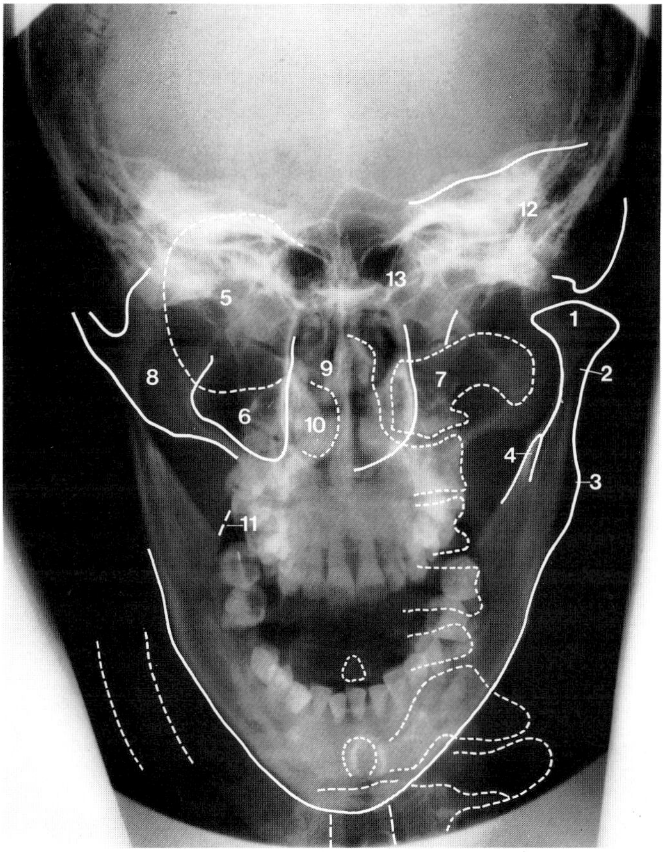

Fig. 3-30 A-P skull projection, 15° eccentric; good depiction of the region of the temporomandibular joint.
1. condyle
2. neck of the condyle
3. angle of the mandible
4. coronoid process
5. orbit
6. maxillary sinus
7. spine
8. zygoma
9. nasal sinus
10. nasal concha
11. border of the oral cavity
12. petrous bone
13. ethmoid cells

2.4.1.2 Skull, PA and AP Eccentric (*Carlsten*, 1917; *Haas*, 1932; *Clementschitsch*, 1941)

Equipment: Same as described in 2.4.1.1

Technique PA: Cassette resting against forehead and nose (Fig. 3-29 A). The orbito-meatal line is vertical, mouth is open, tube tilted 15° down, so that X-ray beam exits at root of nose

AP: Radiograph is taken similarly in anterior-posterior direction (Fig. 3-29 B)

Information: Free projection of the condyle and condylar process as well as the ascending ramus. Oblique projection of the horizontal ramus (Fig. 3-30)

Indication: Fractures of the mandible, particularly in condylar process and ascending ramus

Errors: Insufficient tilting, mouth not properly opened, overexposure, lateral rotation

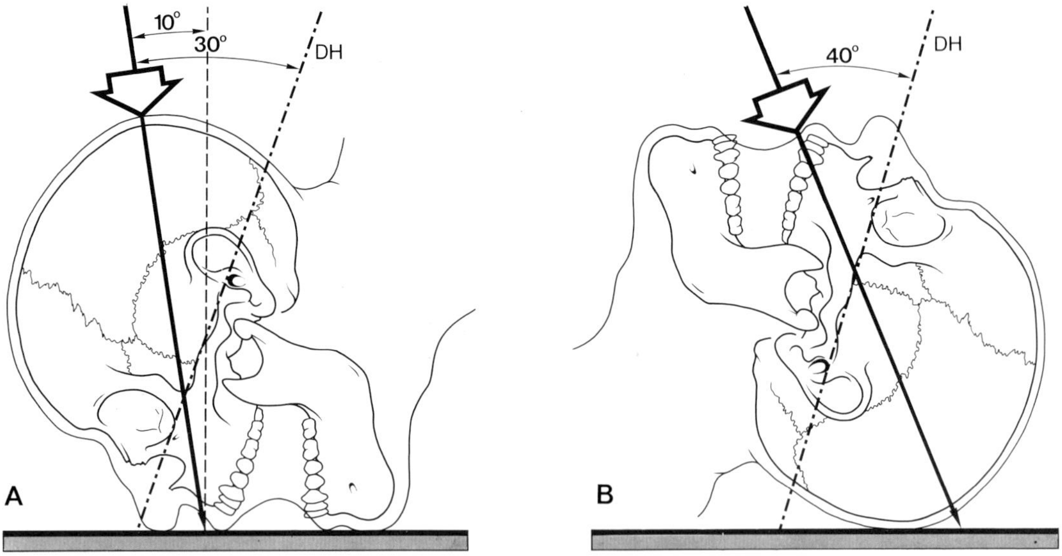

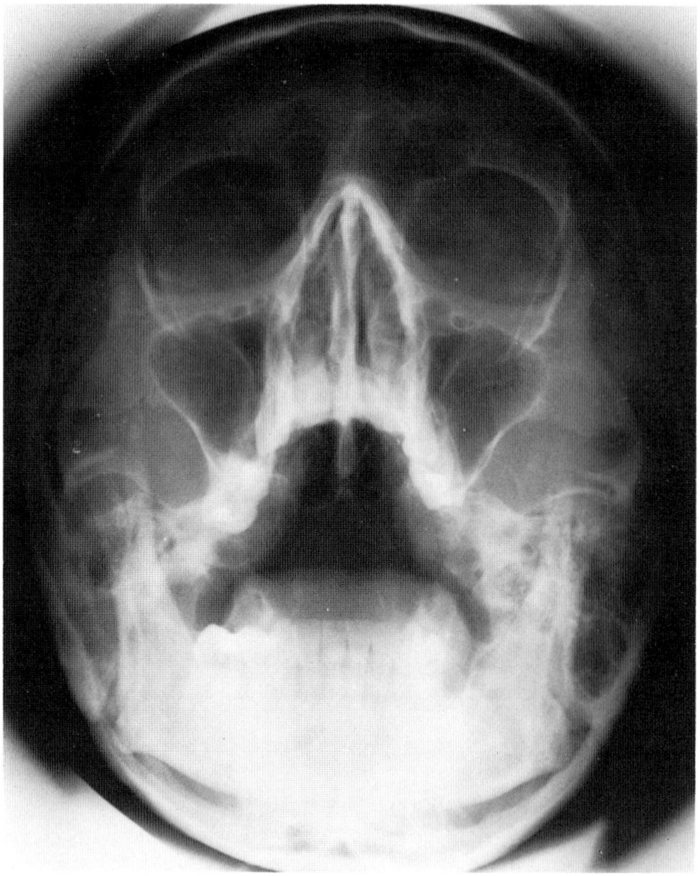

Fig. 3-31 A P-A projection of paranasal sinuses; beam path. The central beam forms a 30° angle cranially with the Frankfort horizontal plane, corresponding approximately to a cranial tilting of 10° for the tube.

Fig. 3-31 B A-P projection of paranasal sinuses, patient supine; beam path. The central beam passes through the oral cavity and forms an angle of approximately 40° caudally with the Frankfort horizontal plane.

Figure 3-32

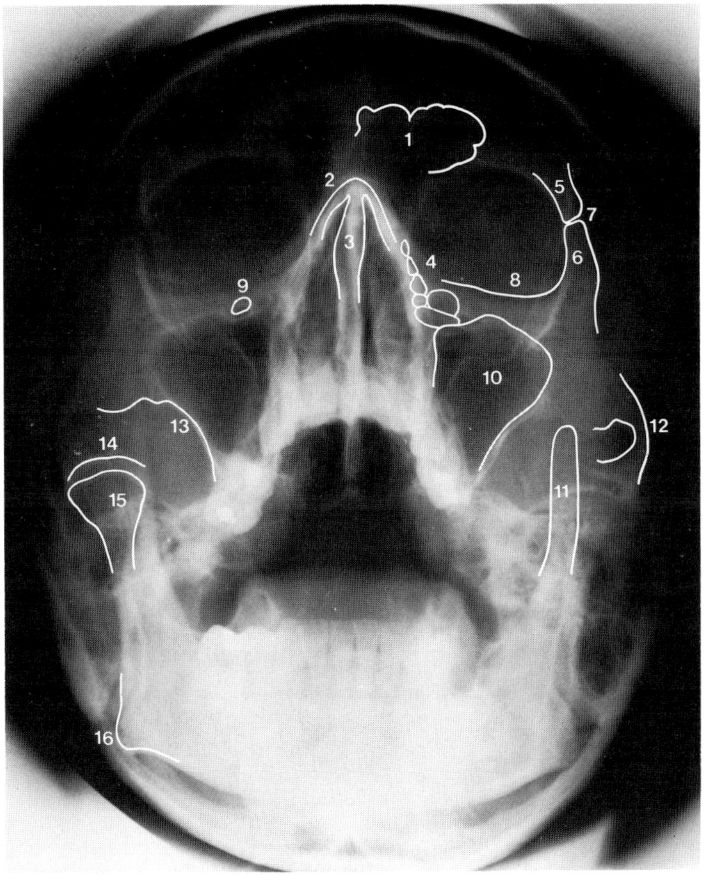

Fig. 3-32 P-A projection of paranasal sinuses.
1. frontal sinus
2. nasal bone
3. nasal septum
4. ethmoid cells
5. zygomatic process of the frontal bone
6. frontal process of the zygoma
7. frontozygomatic suture
8. floor of the orbit
9. infraorbital foramen
10. maxillary sinus
11. coronoid process of the mandible.
12. zygomatic arch
13. zygomatico-alveolar crest (lateral wall of the maxillary sinus)
14. glenoid fossa
15. condyle
16. angle of the mandible

2.4.1.3 Paranasal Sinuses (Waters and *Waldron,* 1915; *Tschebull,* 1921)

Equipment: Skull unit, cassette 18 × 24 cm, screens

Technique: Head in dorsal flexion, tip of nose and point of chin against cassette, mouth open. Centering is on glabellar region. Tube is tilted 10° towards head (Fig. 3-31 A)
The film can be prepared with the patient recumbent if he is seriously injured. The central beam is at a 40° angle from the orbito-meatal line (Fig. 3-31 B)

Information: Good assessment of both maxillary sinuses and their walls, of the malar bone and its processes, as well as the frontal edge of the orbits. Foreshortened presentation of the zygomatic arch. Sometimes the articular space is visualized sagittally (Fig. 3-32); petrous bones are shown caudally to the maxillary sinuses

Indication: Fractures of the maxilla, malar bone and zygomatic arch, orbits and the nasal bone

Errors: The most serious error occurs with inadequate dorsal flexion, which causes superimpositioning of the petrous bones on the lower sections of the maxillary sinuses so that basal shadowing and any fractures in this region cannot be diagnosed

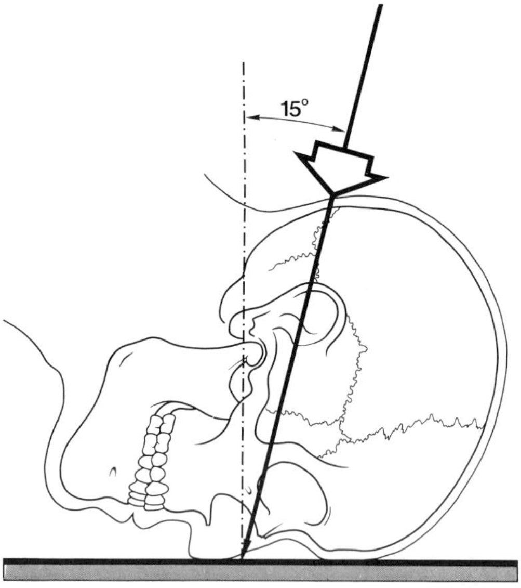

Fig. 3-33 P-A orbital projection (orbital survey); beam path.

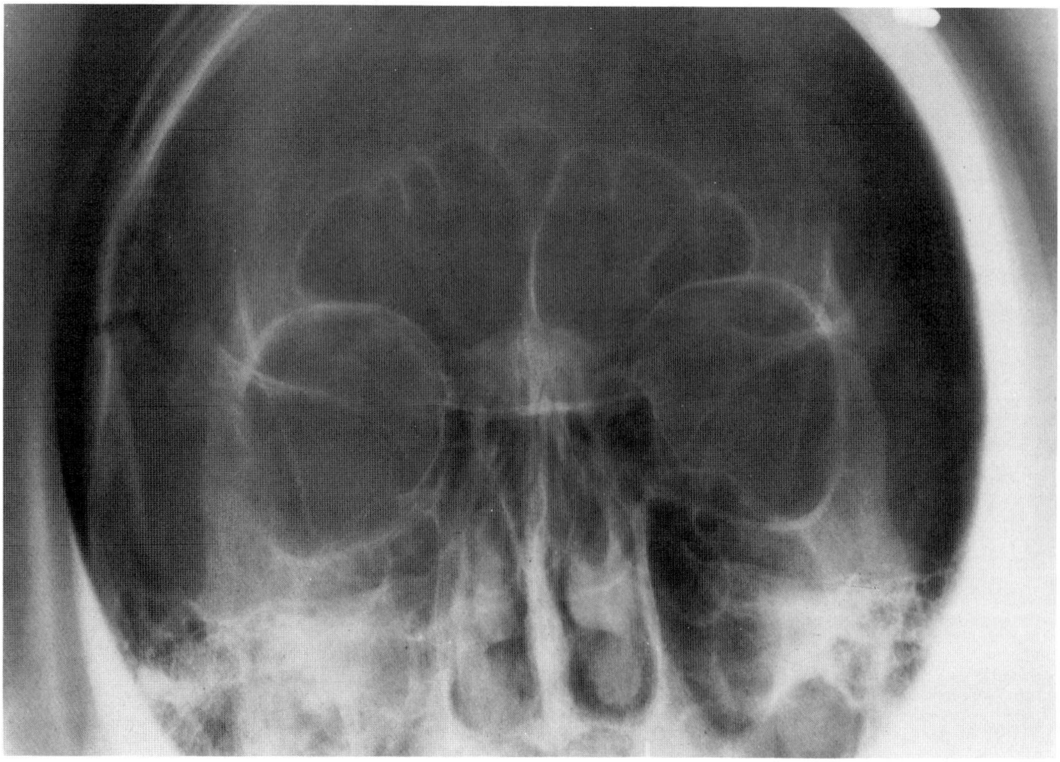

Figure 3-34

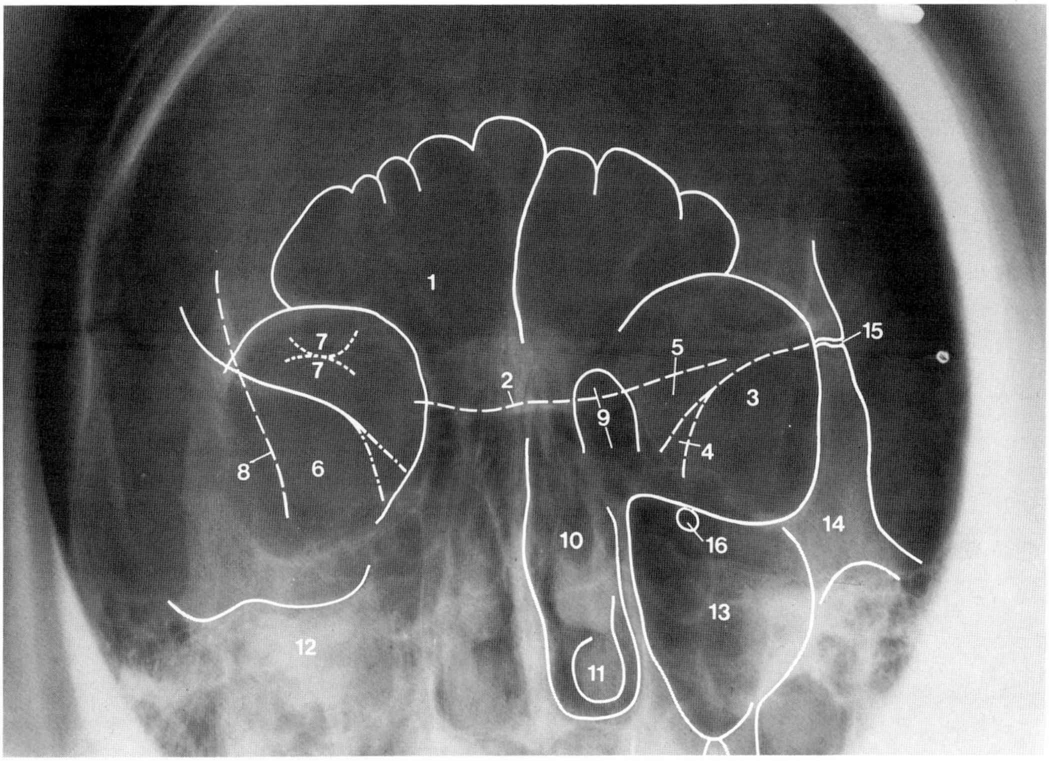

Fig. 3-34 P-A orbital survey.
1. frontal sinus
2. sphenoid plane
3. orbit
4. superior orbital fissure
5. small wing of the sphenoid bone
6. large wing of the sphenoid bone
7. cerebral ridges of the cranium
8. innominate line
9. ethmoid cells
10. nasal sinus
11. nasal concha
12. petrous bone
13. maxillary sinus
14. zygoma
15. frontozygomatic suture

2.4.1.4 Orbital Survey

Equipment: Skull unit

Technique: Forehead and nose against cassette. Orbito-meatal line vertical. Tube is tilted 15° towards the head, central ray projected on root of nose (Fig. 3-33)

Information: Upper pyramidal edges are projected closely below the orbital edge. The contour of the orbit is shown as a vertical oval, and as a circle when the central ray is projected vertically onto the film (Fig. 3-34)
Flat visualization of vault and lateral edge of orbit, floor and median wall of orbit are shown in orthogonal projection

Indication: Fractures of the orbital region

Errors: As a rule, the lambdoid suture is projected in the orbit; in normal projection of the paranasal sinuses, it is visualized in the region of the maxillary sinuses. Nonetheless, the anterior lower edge of the orbit and the infraorbital foramen are well visualized

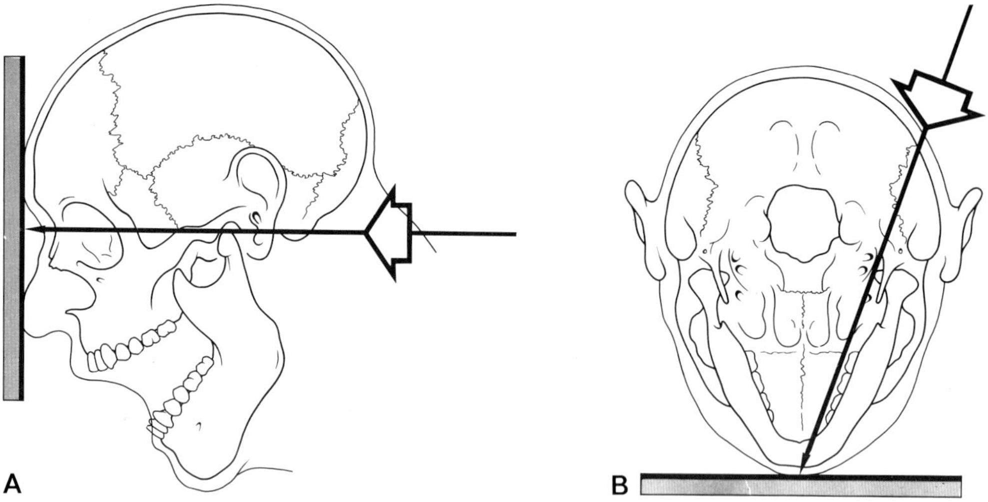

Figs. 3-35 A and B Transorbital TMJ projection (*Hofrath*); beam path.

Fig. 35 A Lateral view.

Fig. 35 B Caudal view.

2.4.1.5 Temporomandibular Joint (TMJ), Transorbital (*Hofrath*, 1931)

Equipment: Skull unit, cassette 13 × 18 cm, screens

Technique: Head rests with forehead and bridge of nose against cassette. Central ray passes from mastoid process on the side to be radiographed to the middle of the orbit on that same side. Mouth open (Fig. 3-35)

Information: Mandibular condyle and condylar process can be seen in cranial and both lateral sections; but glenoid fossa is not visible (Fig. 3-36)

Indication: Fractures of condyle and condylar process

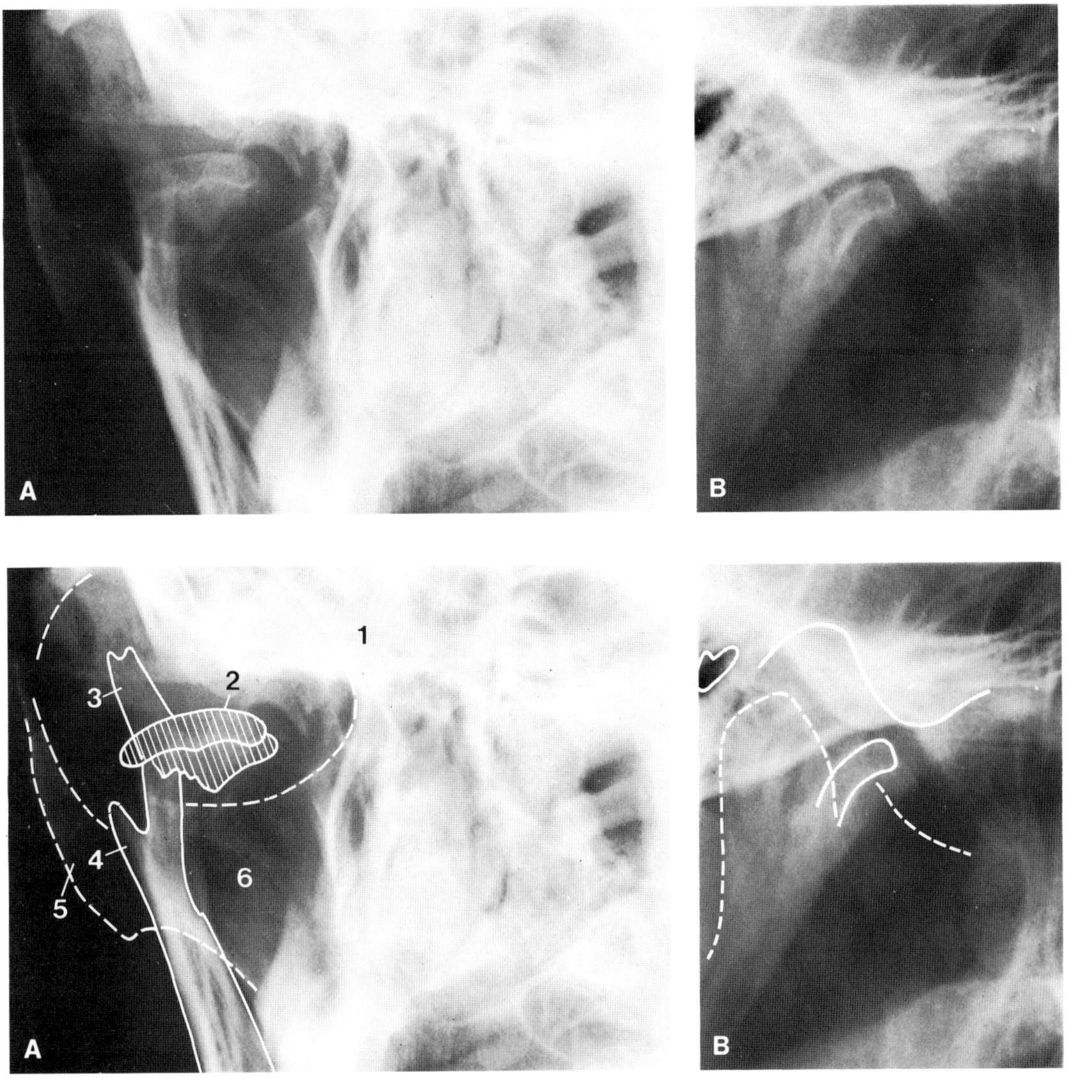

Fig. 3-36 A Transorbital view of the TMJ (*Hofrath*) in condylar fracture.
1. limit of the orbit
2. condyle, dislocated medio-caudally
3. neck of the condyle
4. coronoid process
5. zygomatic arch
6. maxillary sinus

Fig. 3-36 B *Parma* TMJ projection for comparison.

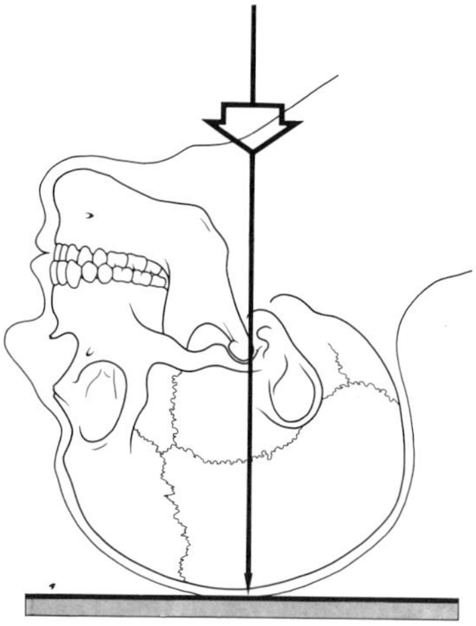

Fig. 3-37 A Inferosuperior (axial) skull projection, "hanging head"; beam path.

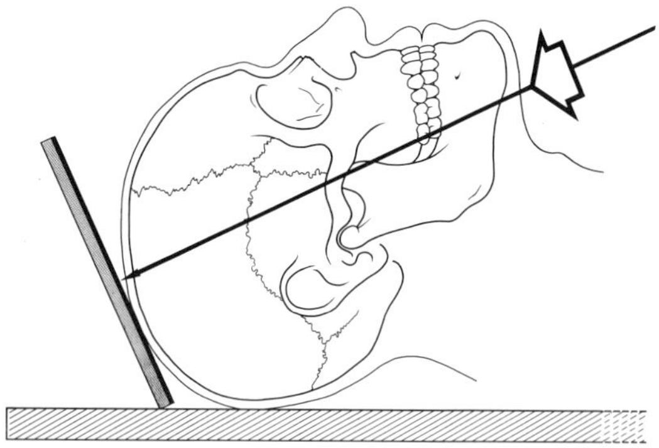

Fig. 3-37 B Inferosuperior (axial) skull projection in poor dorsal reflection; beam path.

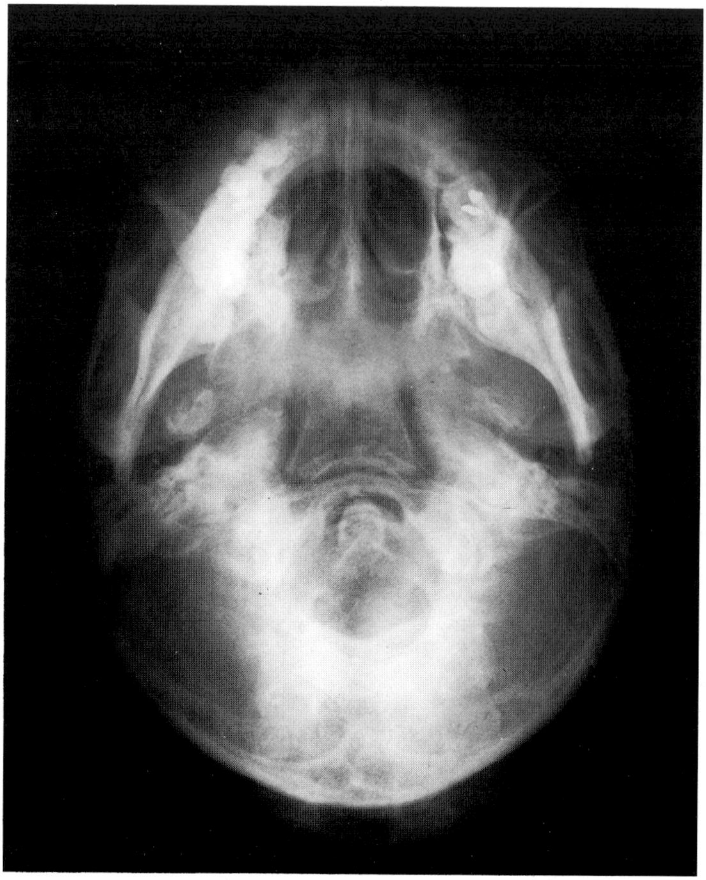

Figure 3-38

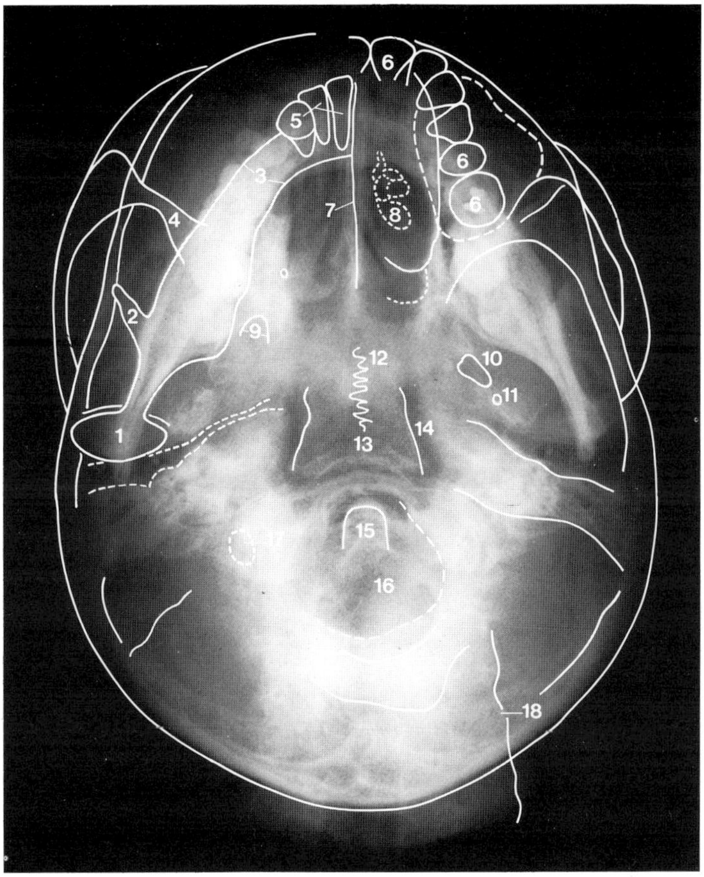

Fig. 3-38 Inferosuperior (axial) skull projection.
1. condyle
2. coronoid process
3. corpus mandibulae
4. zygomatico-alveolar crest (lateral wall of the maxillary sinus)
5. mandibular teeth
6. maxillary teeth
7. bony septum of the nose
8. ethmoid cells
9. pterygoid process
10. oval foramen
11. spinous foramen
12. sagittal suture
13. clivus
14. foramen lacerum
15. odontoid process of the axis
16. greater occipital foramen
17. transverse foramen of the atlas
18. cervical spine

2.4.2 Axial Inferosuperior Projections

2.4.2.1 Skull Axial (Inferosuperior)

Equipment:	Skull unit, cassette 24 × 30 cm, fine screen
Technique:	Patient supine (Fig. 3-37 A) with head in maximum dorsal flexion, cassette as closely parallel as possible to vault of cranium and perpendicular to central ray. Advantageous use can be made of vertically adjustable film carrier In the event of restricted dorsal flexion, the X-ray tube must be tilted footwards (Fig. 3-37 B)
Information:	Visualization of the base of the skull, part of the rear wall and the lateral edges of the maxillary sinus and nasal cavity, and the trochleae of the mandible. Part of the front edge of the maxillary sinus also can be distinguished (Fig. 3-38)
Errors:	Mostly caused by inadequate tilting

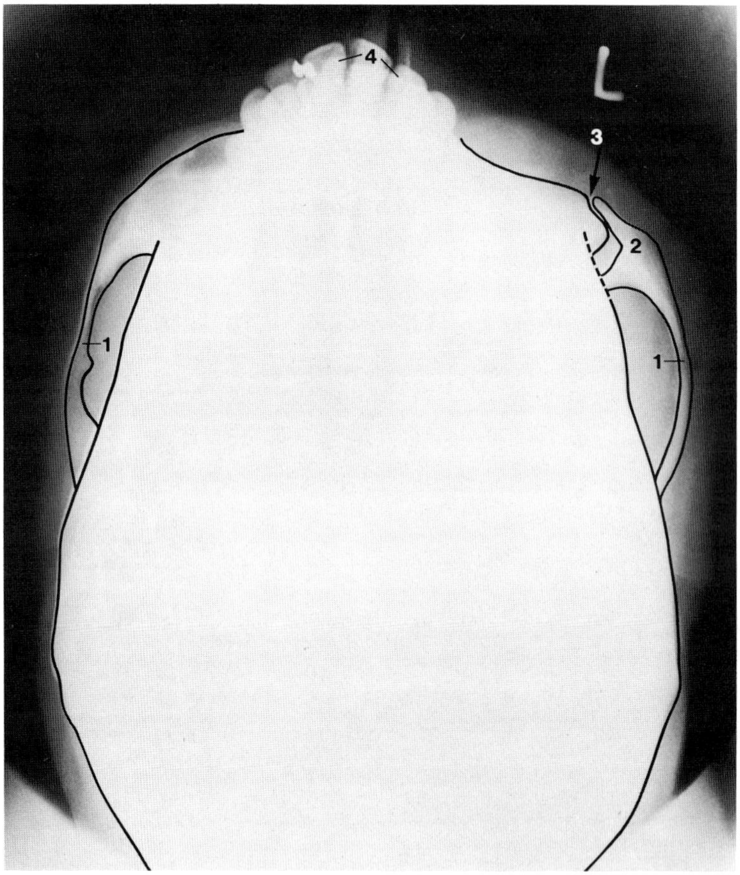

Fig. 3-39 Comparative view of both zygomatic arches.
1. zygomatic arches
2. zygoma
3. fracture line
4. incisors

2.4.2.2 Comparative View of Both Zygomatic Arches

This radiograph differs from the preceding one solely by requiring a lower radiation dose.

Information: Because of the low radiation dose used, this view precludes evaluation of all solid parts of the skull; only the zygomatic arches—provided they protrude beyond the skull—can be visualized well, particulary in the event of medial or lateral displacement (Fig. 3-39)

Indication: Zygomatic arch fractures

Errors: Positioning not exactly central

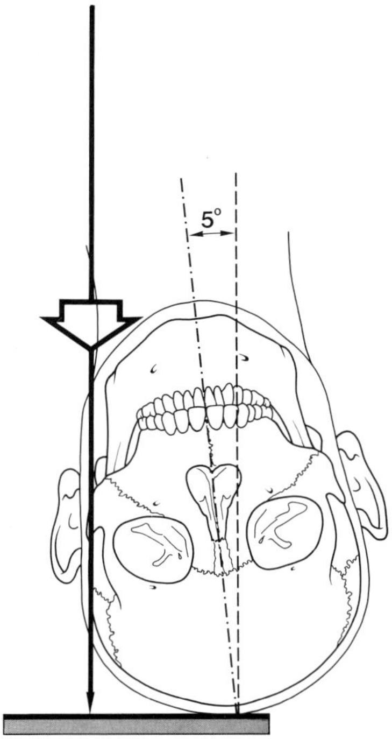

Fig. 3-40 Isolated zygomatic arch; beam path.

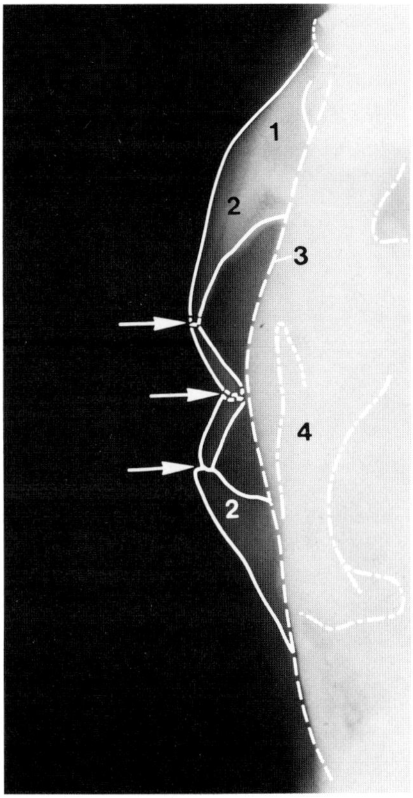

Fig. 3-41 Isolated projection of the zygomatic arch.
1. zygoma
2. fractured zygomatic arch
3. lateral limit of the skull
4. mandible

2.4.2.3 Isolated Zygomatic Arch (Bronner and *Koch,* 1930; *Zimmer,* 1937)

Equipment: Skull or dental unit, cassette 13 × 18 cm, fine screen

Technique: Skull is placed so that the central beam is tangential to the zygomatic arch to be visualized (Fig. 3-40)

Information: Both lateral and medial displacement of a zygomatic arch can be diagnosed (Fig. 3-41)

Errors: Because of insufficient rotation, other parts of the skull may be superimposed on the zygomatic arch

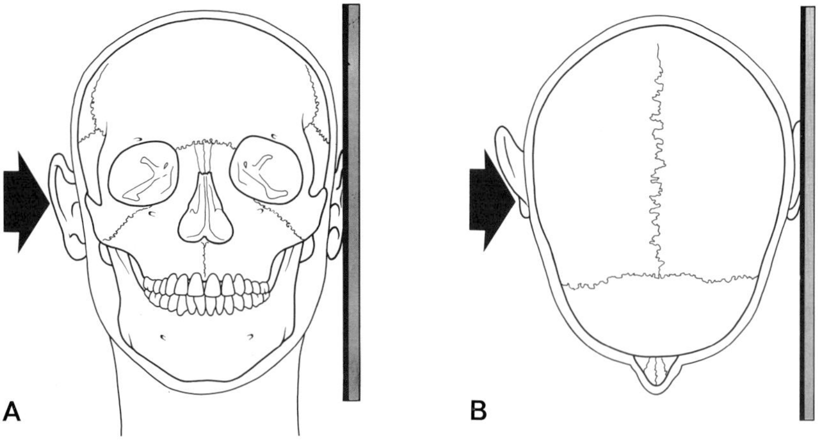

Figs. 3-42 A and B Lateral skull projection; beam path.

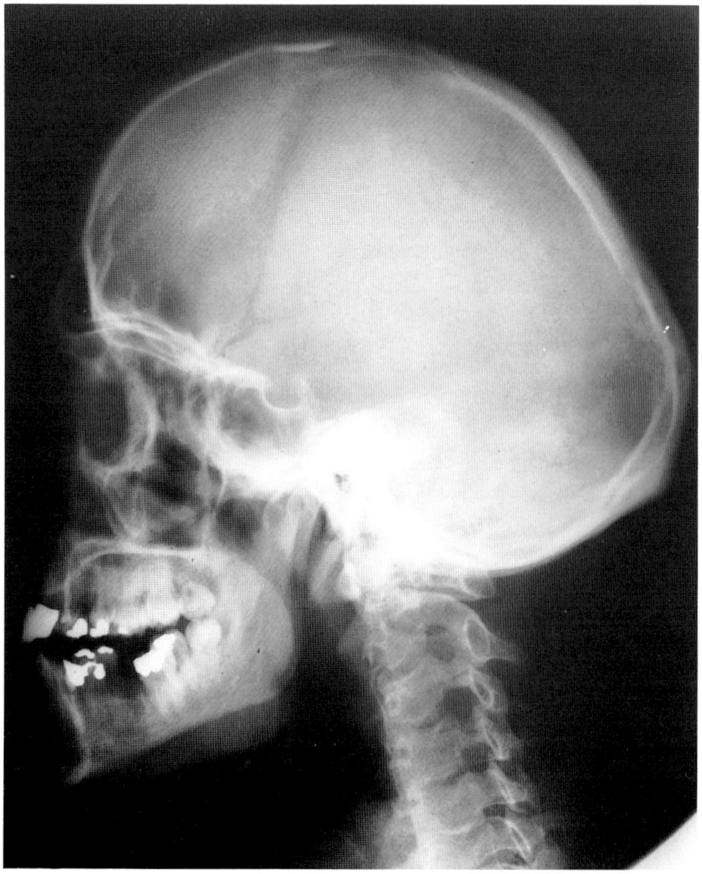

Figure 3-43

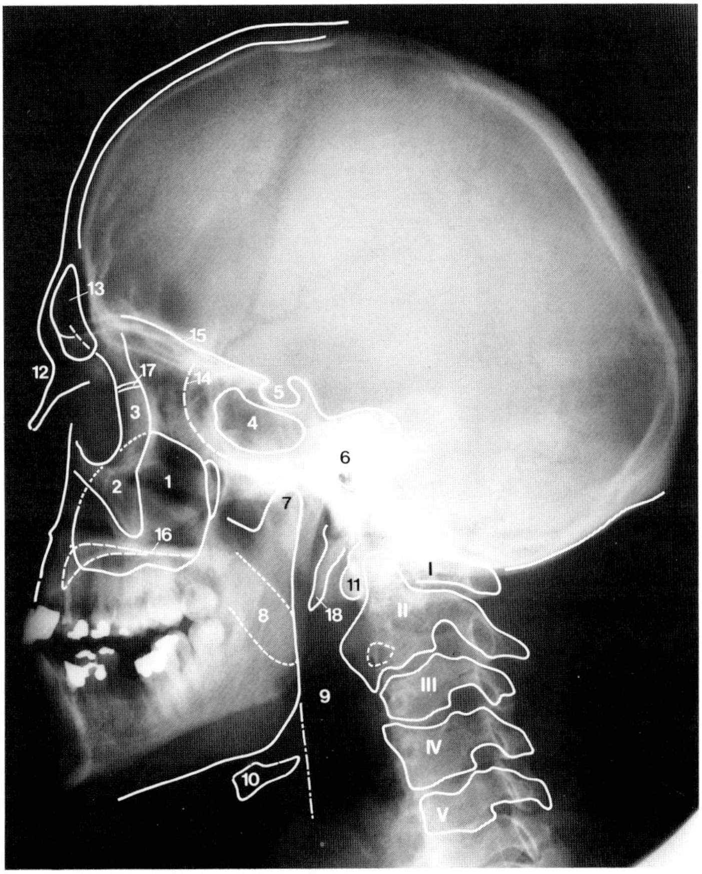

Fig. 3-43 Lateral skull projection.
1. maxillary sinus, nasal cavity with turbinates
2. zygoma
3. frontal process of the zygoma
4. sphenoid sinus
5. sella turica
6. pars petrosa with external acoustic meatus
7. condyle
8. soft palate
9. pharynx
10. hyoid bone
11. anterior arch of the atlas
12. nasal bone
13. frontal sinus
14. floor of the middle cranial fossa
15. floor of the anterior cranial fossa
16. hard palate
17. frontozygomatic suture
18. styloid process

2.4.3. Lateral Projection

2.4.3.1 Skull Lateral

Equipment: Skull unit, cassette 24 × 30 cm (upright), fine screen

Technique: Median plane parallel to cassette (Fig. 3-42). Central beam perpendicular thereto, entry portal at skull varies depending on whether visualization is required of

a) **Vault of cranium:** Central beam just above sella. Cassette horizontal

Information: Good visualisation of vault edges as well as sella turcica and sphenoid sinus. Owing to the relatively low radiation absorption and higher radiographic density of the facial skeleton, evaluation of the latter is hardly possible

b) **Facial skull:** Central beam passes through bony auditory meatus. Reduced exposure required

Information: Due to the superimposed projection of both sides, the diagnostic value in the region of the maxilla and the maxillary sinuses is limited (Fig. 3-43)

Indication: Fractures with rearward displacement of the midfacial region or the mandible (bilateral fractures of the condylar process)

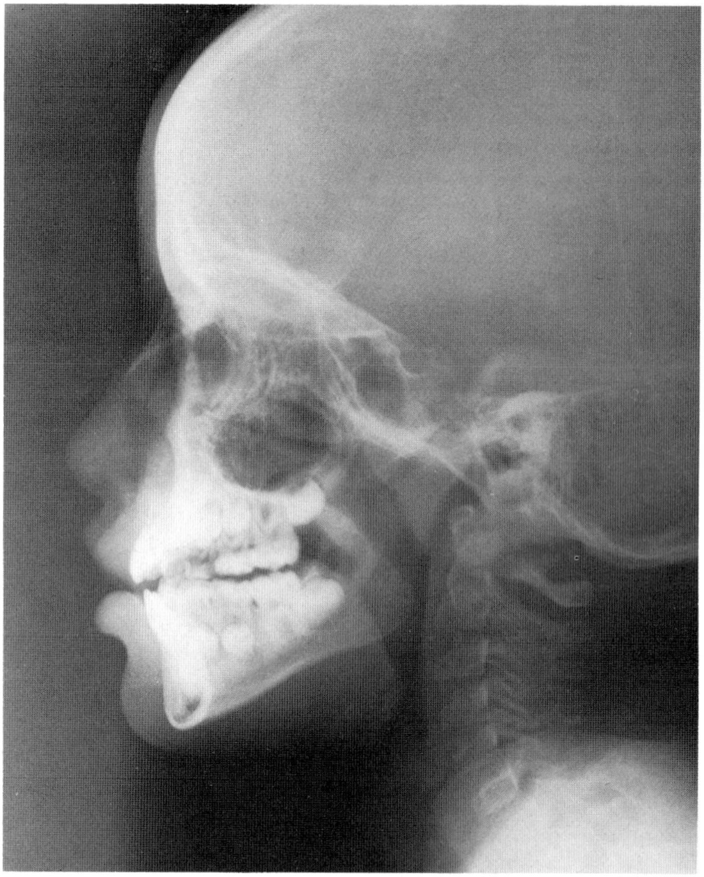

Figure 3-44

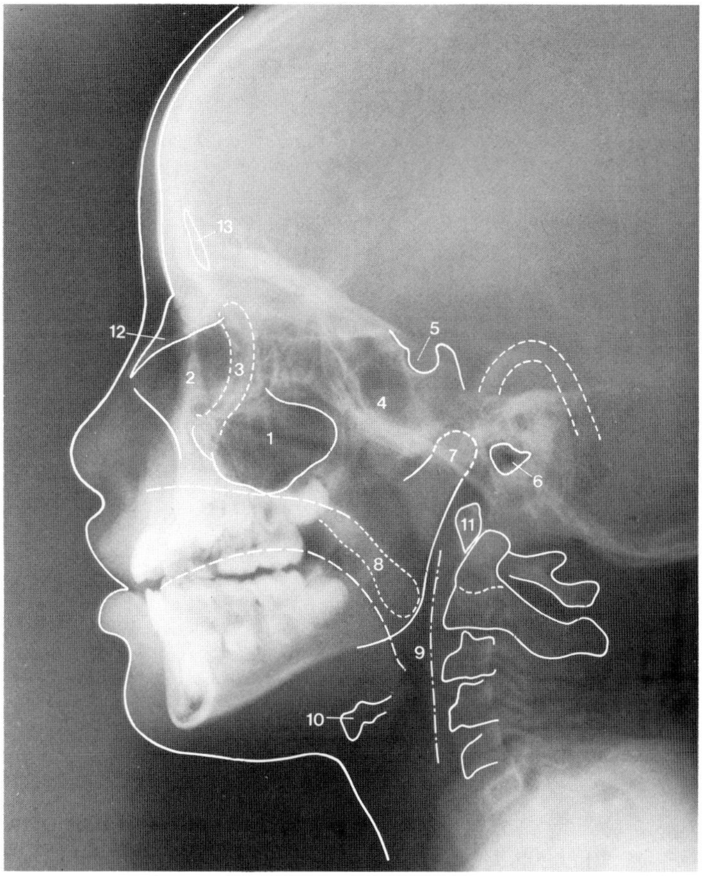

Fig. 3-44 Teleradiograph, lateral cephalometric view.
1. maxillary sinus
2. lacrimal bone
3. lateral border of the orbit
4. sphenoid sinus
5. sella turica
6. acoustic meatus
7. condyle
8. soft palate
9. pharynx
10. hyoid bone
11. atlas
12. nasal bone

2.4.3.2 Skull, Teleradiograph, cephalometric lateral view, with simultaneous visualization of soft tissue (*Hofrath*, 1931)

Thanks to the radiograph being taken from a distance and the parallel beam incidence, uniform visualization of both parts of the skull is achieved. Proper collimation and the use of a plus/minus cassette, i.e. attenuation of the front of the face, ensure good visualization of soft tissue parts. The exposure is made with the cassette upright (Fig. 3-44)

Errors: Excess radiation of the facial skeleton, malpositioning resulting in uneven exposure of the sides

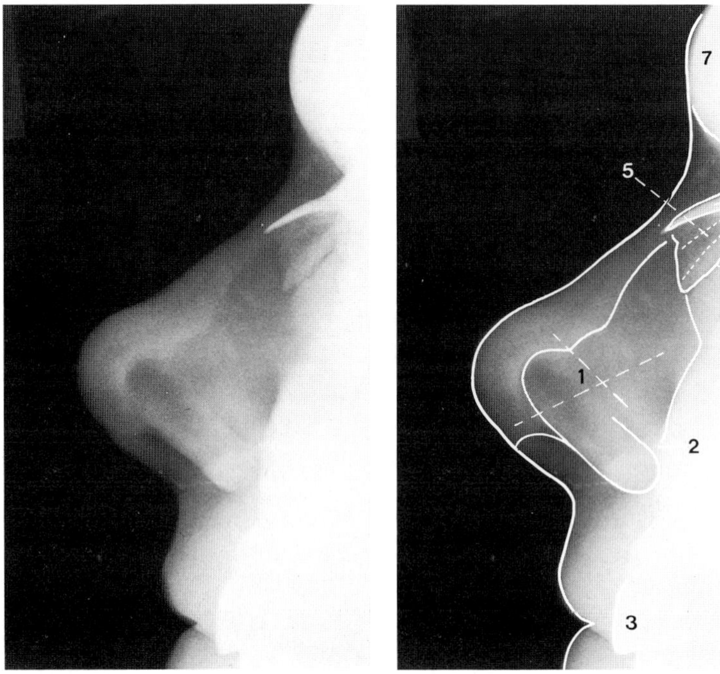

Fig. 3-45 Nose, lateral view.
1. soft tissue of the nose
2. anterior nasal spine
3. maxillary incisors
4. nasal bone
5. ethmoid sulcus
6. nasomaxillary suture
7. frontal bone

2.4.3.3 Nose, Lateral

Technique: With the aid of an occlusal film or cassette-screen film, it is possible to make a lateral study; for this purpose the film is laid against the side of the nose, and the nasal bone is visualized with the aid of a dental unit with a cone

Information: Visualization of frame of nose (Fig. 3-45)

Indication: Fractures of nasal bone

Errors: The normal structure of the nasal bone is furrowed (sulcus ethmoidalis); consequently an erroneous diagnosis of fracture easily can be made

2.4.3.4 Temporomandibular Joint (TMJ) by *Schüller* Technique (1905)

Equipment: Skull unit, cassette 13 × 18 cm, long side horizontal (in order to expose both sides on one film), small collimation (approx. 6 cm diameter), fine screen

Technique: Patient is positioned lying on his side; median plane parallel to film plane, entry portal of beam is first centered on articular space, then tube is tilted 25° towards the head (Fig. 3-46)

Information: Visualization of a cross section through the articular space in the latero-cranial region. Diagnostic value very limited, many sources of error (Fig. 3-47)

Indication: Suspected articular effusion, dislocation of the temporomandibular joint

Errors: Imprecise angulation, chin not sufficiently drawn in, unbalanced positioning of sides

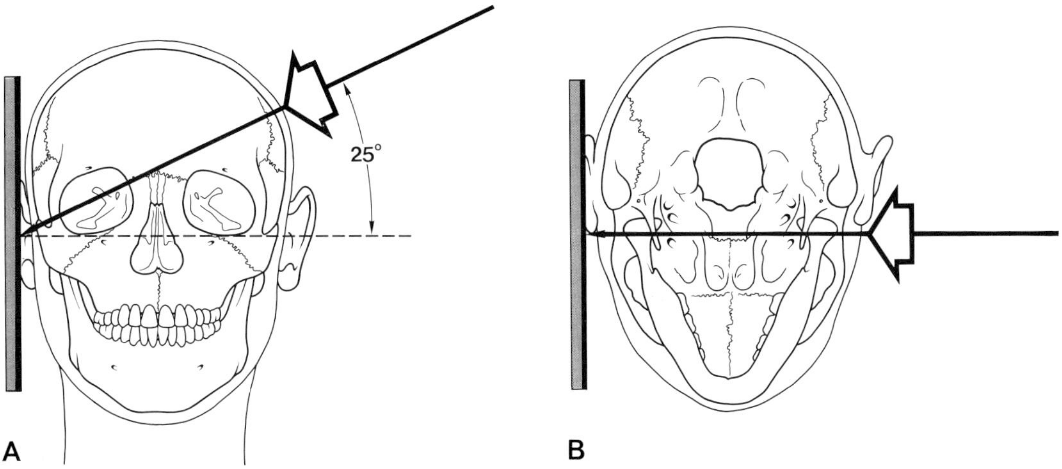

Figs. 3-46 A and B Lateral TMJ projection (*Schüller*); beam path.

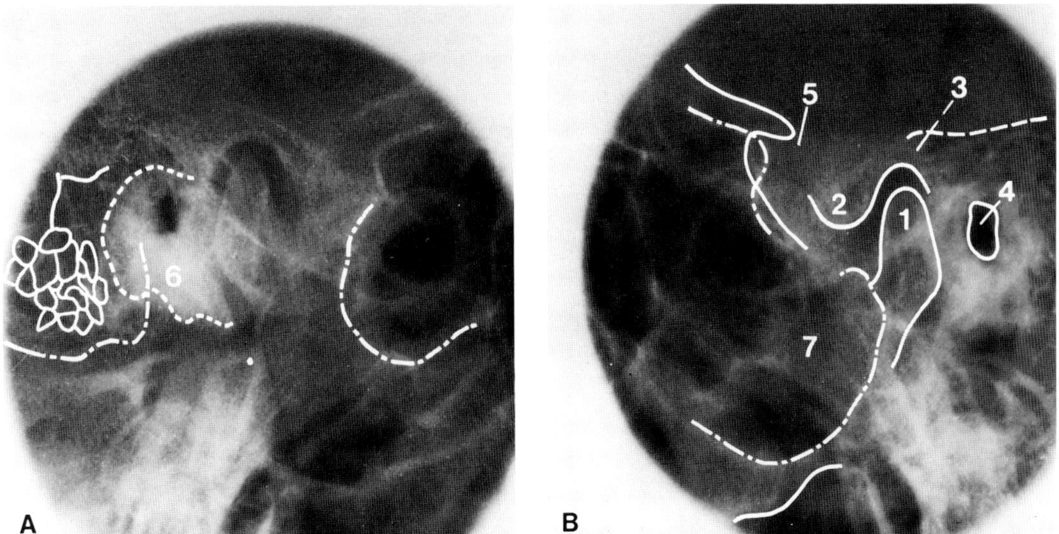

Figs. 3-47 A and B Lateral TMJ projection (*Schüller*).
1. condyle
2. articular eminence
3. interarticular space
4. external acoustic meatus
5. sella turica
6. pars petrosa of the temporal bone
7. sphenoid sinus

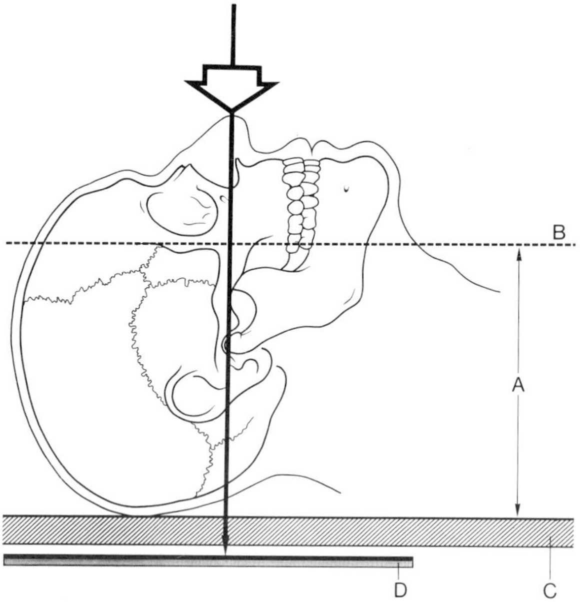

Fig. 3-48 Position in sagittal tomography.
A: layer depth (distance BC in cm)
B: plane of the layer
C: table
D: film

Fig. 3-49 (below and on page 87) A-P tomogram of the midface (16.5 cm distance between plane of the layer and plane of the table).

1. bony nasal septum
2. nasal concha
3. hard palate
4. tongue
5. mandibular molar
6. maxillary molar
7. alveolar process
8. maxillary sinus
9. zygoma
10. frontozygomatic suture
11. orbit
12. Blow-out fracture of the orbital floor with caudal displacement of orbital contents
13. ethmoid cells
14. crista galli
15. ascending ramus of the mandible

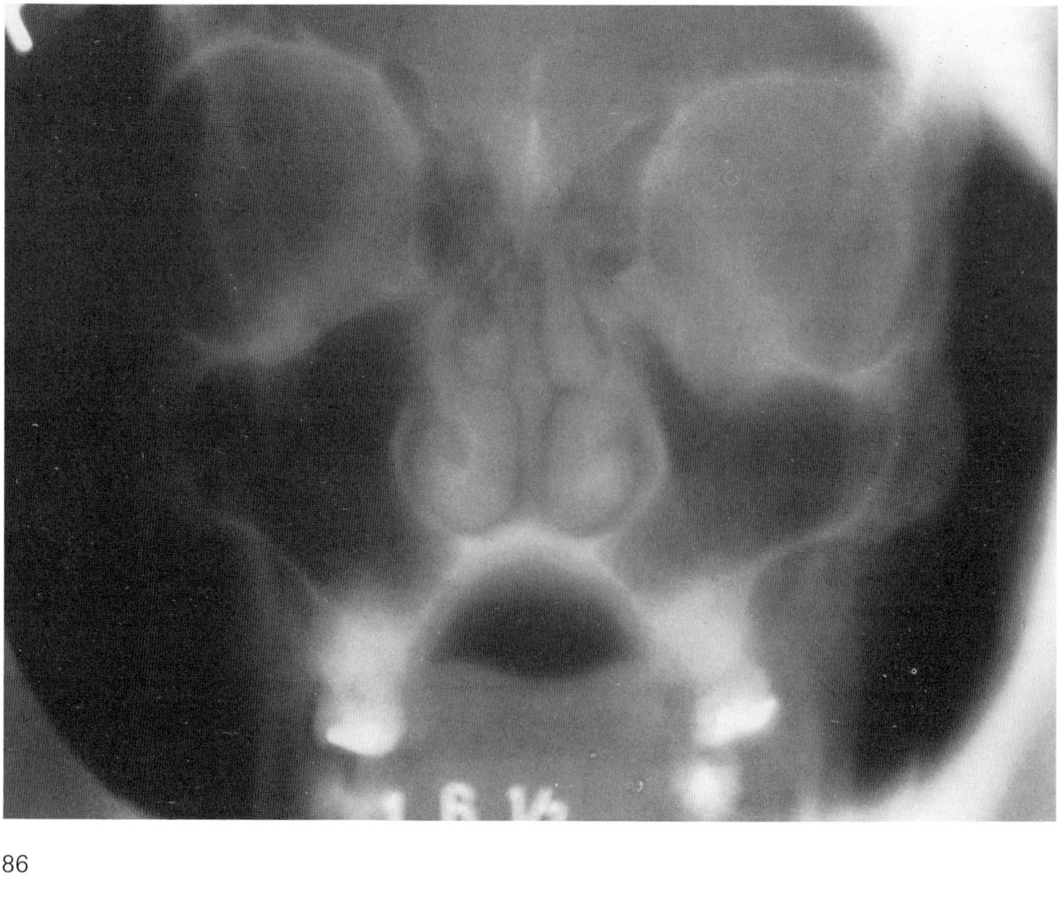

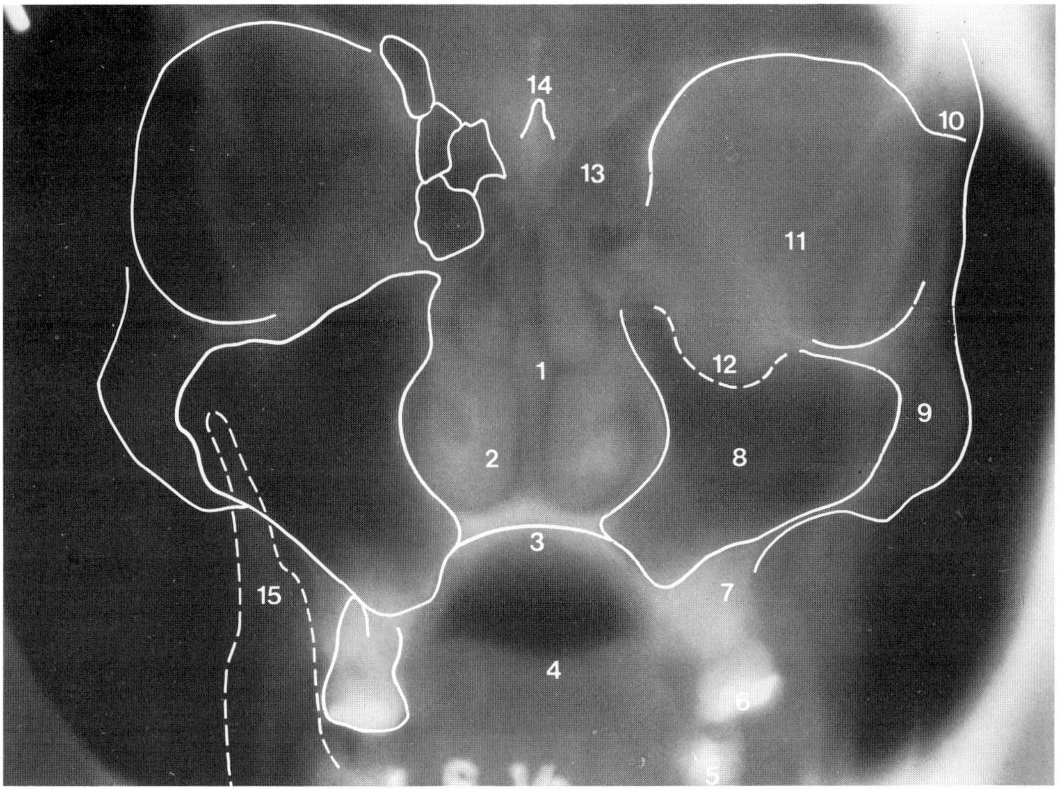

Fig. 3-49 Legend on page 86

2.5 Tomography (*Bocage*, 1921)

Equipment: Special tomograph, preferably with pluridirectional (hypocycloidal) blurring movement (**Polytome**; *Buchmann*, 1963; *Nickol*, 1964; *Ritter*, 1970)

Technique: The design of the apparatus is such (Fig. 3-48) that no more than a thin layer (approx. 1 mm) of the object is visualized sharply. This is achieved by coordinated movement of tube and film with a sharp image being produced only in the point of rotation of the X-ray beam. Furthermore, those parts of the object located outside the tomographic layer are eliminated by blurring. As this layer is fixed for each unit, the patient's position must be changed to vary the level of the tomographic layer. This, however, requires no more than a vertically adjustable table. The procedure is sparing of the patient and is therefore especially recommended for the examination of the seriously injured.

The most suitable types of tomograph are those which, in addition to hypocycloidal blurring, incorporate facilities for conventional radiodiagnostic examination (e.g., **Horizontal Polytome**) and with which good radiographs can be made by inserting a bucky into the field without the patient's position having to be shifted (*Rottke*, 1971).

As a rule, with anterior-posterior projection, it is adequate to "dissect" the facial skull into several layers at intervals of 0.5 to 1 cm. The specific layer thickness interval and the number of tomograms to be made depend on the findings. For midfacial fractures, the average is seven separate tomograms (Fig. 3-49).

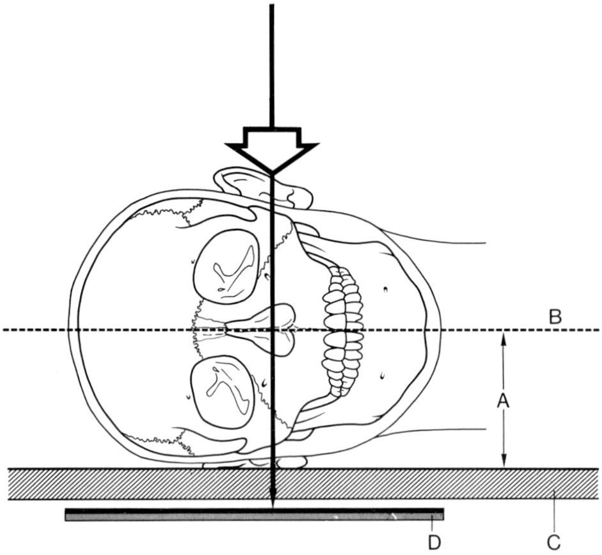

Fig. 3-50 Positions in lateral tomography.
A: layer depth (distance BC in cm)
B: layer plane
C: table
D: film

Figs. 3-51 A and B (see page 89) Tomogram of the midface, lateral beam path.

Fig. 3-51 A: 9 cm distance between exposed plane and table.

Fig. 3-51 B: 9.5 cm distance between exposed plane and table.

1. frontal sinus
2. orbit
3. anterior cranial fossa
4. ethmoid cells
5. shadows of soft tissue (in blow-out fracture)
6. maxillary sinus
7. sphenoid sinus
8. pterygopalatine fossa
9. hamulus
10. pterygoid process (medial plate)
11. maxillary molar
12. mandibular molar
13. anterior wall of the maxillary sinus

In some instances lateral layering may be necessary, e.g., fractures of the orbital floor. Here best results are obtained with the patient lying prone with the head turned fully sideways (Fig. 3-50). It is advisable to use a smaller field (9 × 12 cm) than with AP tomography (13 × 18 cm)

Information: The major benefit of tomography is the possibility it offers of producing images of any part of the skull without superimpositioning (Fig. 3-51), while hardly any stress is imposed on the patient from whom practically no cooperation is required

Indication: Midfacial fractures with suspected orbital involvement

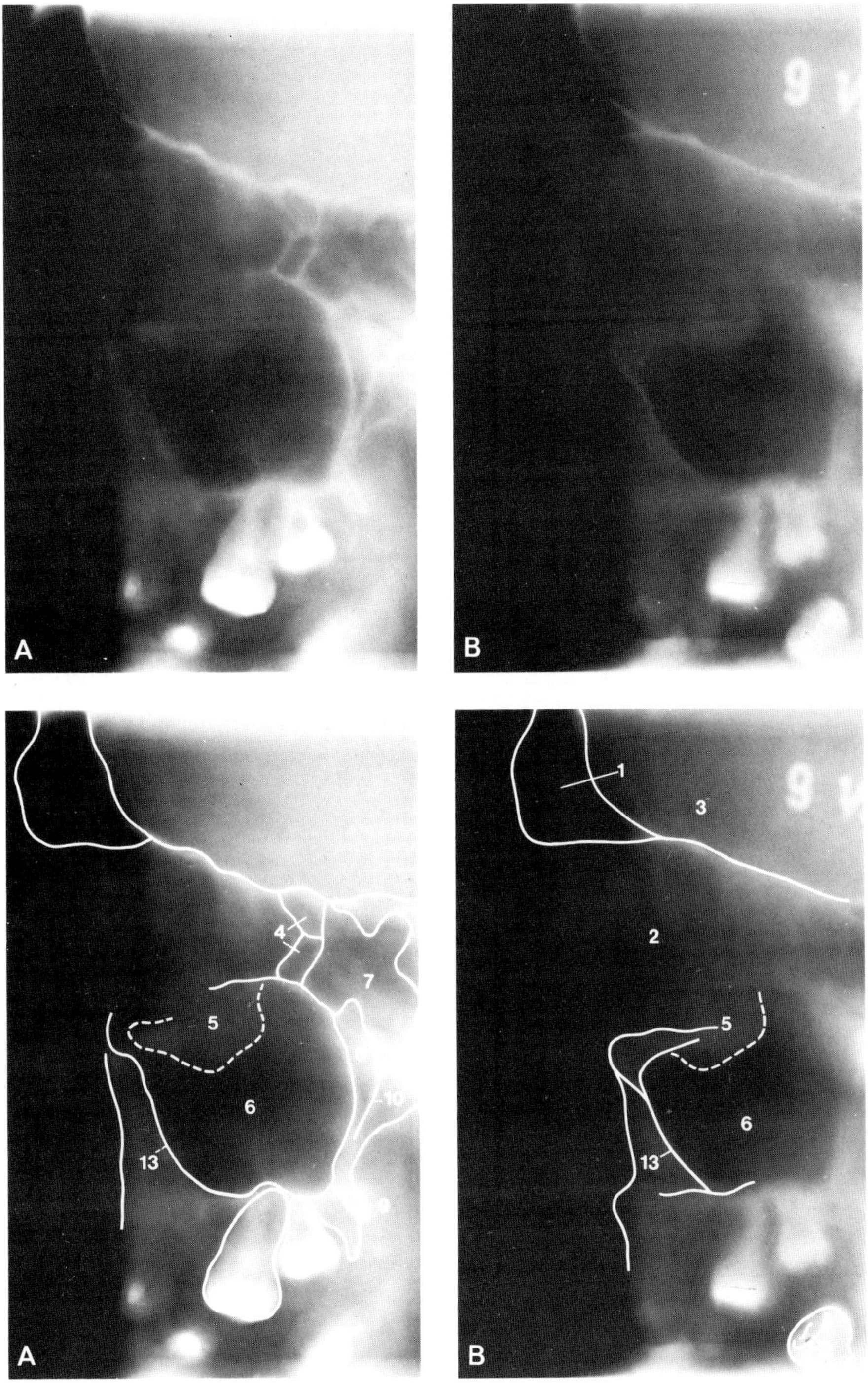

Figs. 3-51 A and B   Legend on page 88

3. Procedure for Visualization of the Facial Skull

3.1 Fundamentals

The various radiographic procedures require different degrees of cooperation from patients and subject them to distress of varying extent. The doctor requesting the radiograph must have a sound grasp of the technique so that he can judge whether it is not too demanding: a patient suffering from cerebral trauma can be radiographed only while recumbent, for example. Another important point is whether the patient is unconscious or can respond to questioning. Due consideration also has to be given to the time that has elapsed since the injury occurred. Once post-traumatic swelling has begun, the resulting increased absorption of radiation necessitates a considerably higher X-ray dose, while the higher amount of scattered radiation leads to poorer image quality. It should be left to the surgeon to decide, therefore, whether a detailed diagnosis is required then and there or whether it can be postponed until later, when the swelling has subsided.

3.2 Fractures of the Mandible

The procedure depends on the general condition of the patient who, as a rule, can stand briefly, or at least sit. Under these circumstances a panoramic tomogram (**Orthopantomogram, Orth-Oralix, Panorex**) should always be the first step. It provides the best visualization of the entire mandible.
Only the region of the chin may be blurred, as this is where the layer thickness inherent in the unit is small and the individual patient variations from the assumed standard jaw are great. Thanks to the feature of double reproduction of the chin region, the **Panorex** procedure provides more information. Other panoramic tomography procedures may call at times for additional studies (panoramic enlargement, extraoral projection of mandible).
Often it is not possible to assess fractures in the region of the temporomandibular joint on the basis of panoramic tomograms. In such instances an additional *Parma* radiograph has to be made, and if uncertainty persists, we resort to a tomographic series. The *Schüller* technique for visualization of the articular space only provides clear information when there is a contusion of the joint with enlargement of the articular space, or in the presence of a dislocation when the empty space is visualized.
If the patient has to radiographed while recumbent, only the panoramic enlargement procedure (**Status-X, Stat-Oralix, Panoramix**) can be used to provide a survey of the anterior region. For the rest we have to rely on extraoral projections of the mandible which require little sophistication as regards equipment, but which are more demanding as regards method.
As a recent development, mention should be made of the **Tomorex**, a panoramic tomograph suitable for examination of even the recumbent patient.
A second plane (skull, PA 15°) has to be visualized in any case. The condition of the patient is of relatively minor importance here, since both supine and prone positioning are feasible. The latter, however, is preferred because of the more advantageous object-film distance.
In this way, when there is a mandibular fracture, zones of reduced density and dislocations of fragments can be visualized in the mediolateral region of the horizontal and ascending rami. For reproduction of the condyle it is essential that the mouth can be opened so that the condyle emerges from the glenoid fossa. If this is not feasible, then in the case of condylar fractures it may be useful to visualize it transorbitally (*Hofrath*, 1931). On very rare occasions a tomographic series may be worthwhile.
In fractures of the mandible, the third plane is visualised by means of the axial radiograph. It is recommended for oblique fractures in the horizontal ramus and chin region, which might otherwise escape detection.
For assessing the coronoid process, the panoramic tomogram or *Parma* study again is the first method of choice, while in the second plane it appears in the radiograph of the paranasal sinuses and the PA skull study.

3.3 Fractures of the Maxilla

The radiograph of the paranasal sinuses is of paramount importance for visualizing a maxil-

lary fracture. It should therefore be the first to be made, irrespective of the patient's condition. Seriously injured subjects can be radiographed in the recumbent position without suffering distress, nor is any cooperation required from them. In addition to providing information about the degree of ventilation in the paranasal sinuses, it shows zones of reduced density and fragment displacement in the sinus walls, except for the facial and dorsal parts.
The malar bone and its processes with their many weak spots prone to fracture can be assessed well.

3.4 Fractures of the Orbit

With orbital fractures the primary procedure is radiography of the paranasal sinuses. We have to watch particularly for caudal displacements which may consist of bone or discrete swellings of the mucous membrane, and may occasionally even be simulated by a retention cyst of the mucous membrane of the maxillary sinus. Displacement also can occur in the direction of the ethmoid cells. Sometimes it is difficult to recognize these changes. It is advisable, therefore, to supplement the examination with an orbital survey radiograph. This should be adopted as routine practice when fractures are suspected in this region. With its aid we obtain good orthogonal visualization of the orbital floor and the medial orbital wall.
In contrast, the orbital roof and the lateral orbital wall are visualized in planar presentation.
In almost all instances, however, tomography of the orbital region is useful. It clears up doubtful findings in the lateral orbital region due to superprojection of the frontal zygomatic suture. If doubt persists, surgical exploration is indicated.
The second plane in the form of a lateral skull radiograph is of limited diagnostic value only, because the sides are superimposed. In the caudal sections the panoramic tomogram is more informative, e.g., regarding the alveolar recess, the wall of the maxillary sinus and the zygomatic arch.
For the third plane in axial projection, preference is mostly given to a comparative study of both zygomatic arches or of one zygomatic arch. This is a good method for the detection of incomplete bending fractures of the vault of the cranium.
The more highly exposed axial skull radiograph is but seldom required for diagnosing maxillary fractures.
In all cases of doubt, a tomographic series of the midfacial region is the most informative technique.

References

Aken, J. van (1969)
Optimum conditions for intraoral roentgenograms. Oral Surg. 27: 475

Aken, J. van, and L. W. J. van der Linden (1966)
The integral absorbed dose in conventional and panoramix complete mouth examination. Oral Surg. 22: 603

Ando, S. (1971)
Orthopantomography. Tokyo

Balters, W. (1925)
Leitfaden der zahnärztlichen Röntgenkunde. (Guidelines for dental radiography.) Berlin, H. Meusser

Berger, H. (1943)
Einrichtung zur Herstellung von Körperhöhlen-Röntgenaufnahmen, insbesondere zahnärztliche Röntgenaufnahmen. (Equipment for radiography of body cavities, with special reference to dental radiographs.) German Patent Nr. 765871, dated 12.5.1943, RGBL II, p. 150

Beutel, A., and A. Tänzer (1963)
Röntgendiagnostik der Orbitae, der Augen und der Tränenwege. (Radiographic diagnosis of the orbits, the eyes and the tear ducts.) In: Olsson, O., F. Strnad, H. Vieten, and A. Zuppinger: Handbuch der Medizinischen Radiologie. (Handbook of medical radiology.) Vol. VII/2, p. 673, Berlin – Göttingen – Heidelberg, Springer

Bocage, A. E. M. (1921)
Procédé et dispositifs de radiographie sur plaque on mouvement. (Procedure and apparatus for plate radiography in motion.) French Patent Nr. 536464

Bronner, H., and C. E. Koch (1930)
Die Röntgendarstellung der Jochbögen. (Radiographic depiction of the zygomatic arch.) Röntgenpraxis 2: 754

Buchmann, F. (1963)
Detailwiedergabe und Schichtdicke bei der Tomographie. (Detail reproduction and layer thickness in tomography.) Röntgen-Bl. 18: 361

Buchmann, F. (1974)
Die Prinzipien des Dental-Tomograph. (The principles of the dental tomograph.) Röntgenstrahlen 31: 24

Carlsten, B. (1917)
Röntgenologie der Nasennebenhöhlen. (Radiology of the paranasal sinuses.) Stockholm, Marcus

Cieszyński, A. (1907)
Über die Einstellung der Röntgenröhre bei Zahnaufnahmen. (Adjustment of X-ray tubes for dental radiographs.) Korresp.bl. Zahnärzte 36: 158, 289

Cieszyńsky, A. (1911)
Über extraorale Kieferaufnahmen. (Extraoral skull radiographs.) Fortschr. Röntgenstr. 18: 1

Cieszyński, A. (1926)
Zahnärztliche Röntgenologie. (Dental radiology.) 2nd ed. Leipzig. J. A. Barth

Clementschitsch, F. (1941)
Mitteilung einer symmetrischen Aufnahme beider Kiefergelenke in posteriorer-anteriorer Richtung. (Report of a symmetrical depiction of both temporomandibular joints in posterior-anterior direction.) Z. Stomat. 23: 877

Clementschitsch, F. (1948)
Die Röntgendarstellung des Gesichtsschädels. (Radiographic depiction of the facial skull.) Wien, Urban & Schwarzenberg

Clementschitsch, F. (1955)
Über die Röntgendarstellung bei Erkrankungen und Verletzungen der Kiefer. (Radiography in diseases and injuries of the jaws.) Dtsch. zahnärztli. Z. 10: 380

Clementschitsch, F. (1963)
Die Röntgendarstellung der Kiefergelenke. (The radiographic depiction of the temporomandibular joints.) In Olsson, O., F. Strnad, H. Vieten, and A. Zuppinger: Handbuch der Medizinischen Radiologie. (Handbook of medical radiology.) Vol. VII/2, p. 819, Berlin – Göttingen – Heidelberg, Springer

Fitzgerald, G. M. (1947)
Dental Roentgenography II: Vertical angulation, film placement and increased object-film distance. J. Amer. dent. Ass. 34: 160

Grashey, R., and R. Birkner (1964)
Atlas typischer Röntgenbilder vom normalen Menschen. (Atlas of typical radiographs of normal humans.) Munich, Urban & Schwarzenberg

Haas, L. (1932)
Über die nucho-frontale Aufnahme. (The nucho-frontal view.) Fortschr. Röntgenstr. 45: 532

Heckmann, K. (1939)
Die Röntgenperspektive und ihre Umwandlung durch eine neue Aufnahmetechnik. (Radiographic perspective and its change via a new exposure technique.) Fortschr. Röntgenstr. 60: 144

Hielscher, W. (1954)
Winkelhalbierungs- oder Rechtwinkeltechnik. (Half-angle or right angle technique.) Zahnärztl. Welt 9: 693

Hofrath, H. (1931)
Die Bedeutung der Röntgenfern- und Abstandaufnahme für die Diagnostik der Kieferanomalien. (The significance of teleradiographic views in the diagnosis of anomalies of the jaw.) Fortschr. Orthodont. 1: 232

Hudson, D. C., J. W. Kumpula, and G. Dickson (1957)
A panoramic dental X-ray machine. U. S. armed Forces med. J. 8: 46

Jung, T. (1972)
Die Wiedergabe der Frontzahnregion auf Panorama-Schicht-Aufnahmen. (The reproducibility of the region of the anterior teeth on panoramic tomograms.) Dtsch. zahnärztl. Z. 27: 972

Nickol, H.-J. (1964)
Über die diagnostischen Möglichkeiten mit Hilfe des Schichtverfahrens mit hypocycloidaler Verwischung unter besonderer Berücksichtigung des Kiefergelenkes. (The diagnostic possibilities afforded by tomography with hypocycloid blurring, with special reference to the temporomandibular joint.) Dtsch. zahnärztl. Z. 19: 257

Numata, H. (1933)
A consideration on parabolic radiography in dental examination. J. Shimazu Studies 10: 13

Ott, W. (1960)
Panorama-Röntgen. (Panoramic radiography.) Schweiz. Mschr. Zahnheilk. 70: 822

Paatero, Y. V. (1949) A new tomographical method for radiographing curved outer surfaces. Acta Radiol. 32: 177

Parma, C. (1932)
Die Röntgendiagnostik der Kiefergelenke. (Radiographic diagnosis of the temporomandibular joint.) Röntgenpraxis 4: 633

Parma, C. (1942)
Die Tomo- und Nahaufnahmen der Kiefergelenke. (Tomographic and contact exposures of the temporomandibular joints.) Z. Stomat. 40: 391

Pordes, F. (1919)
Die radiographische Darstellung der einzelnen Zähne und der Kiefer. (Radiographic depiction of individual teeth and the jaw.) Berlin, Urban & Schwarzenberg

Regulla, D. F., A. Ricci, and E. Sonnabend (1972)
Dosismessungen bei Panorama-Röntgenaufnahmen des Gebisses mit Thermolumineszenzdosimetern. (Dose measurement in panoramic radiography of the teeth with thermoluminescence dosimeters.) Dtsch. zahnärztl. Z. 27: 14

Ritter, W. (1970)
Das Schichtverfahren mit hypozycloidaler Verwischung als diagnostische Hilfe in der Kieferchirurgie. (The tomographic technique with hypocycloid blurring as a diagnostic aid in oral surgery.) Dtsch. zahnärztl. Z. 25: 170

Rottke, B. (1971)
Die Bedeutung der Röntgenschichtuntersuchung für die Zahn-, Mund- und Kieferheilkunde. (The significance of X-ray tomography for dentistry.) Deutscher Zahnärztekalender. p. 101, München, C. Hanser

Rottke, B., F. Buchmann, and B. Gossau (1974)
Strahlenschutzverhältnisse an einem Panorama-Schichtgeräte. (Radiation protection conditions in a panoramic X-ray unit.) Quintessenz 25: 10/127, Ref. 5112

Schindler, J. (1927)
Leitfaden der zahnärztlichen Röntgentechnik. (Guidelines for dental radiographic techniques.) Leipzig, G. Thieme

Schüller, A. (1905)
Die Schädelbasis im Röntgenbild. (The base of the skull in the radiograph.) Hamburg, Lucas, Gräge, and Sillem

Sonnabend, E. (1972)
Zur Dosis bei Panorama-Röntgen-Aufnahmen. (The dose in panoramic radiography.) Dtsch. zahnärztl. Z. 27: 984

Stenhuis: Quoted by Grashey, R. and R. Birkner (1964)

Tschebull, H. (1921)
Eine neue Darstellung der Nebenhöhlen. (A new visualisation of the paranasal sinuses.) Fortschr. Röntgenstr. 28: 222

Waters, J. W., and C. W. Waldron (1915)
Roentgenology of accessory nasal sinuses describing modifications of occipito-frontal positions. Amer. J. Roentgenol. 2: 633

Zimmer, E. A. (1937)
Der normale und der gebrochene Jochbogen in neuen Aufnahmerichtungen. (The normal and the fractured zygomatic arch in new radiographic views.) Fortschr. Röntgenstr. 55: 67

Zimmer, E. A., and M. Brossy (1974)
Lehrbuch der röntgen-diagnostischen Technik. (Textbook of radiographic diagnostic techniques.) Berlin, Springer

Chapter 4

General Principles of Treatment in Maxillofacial Injuries

Eberhard Krüger and Wilfried Schilli

Injuries of the face and jaw are frequently associated with other injuries. In planning treatment, therefore, one should be aware that care of fractures and injuries of the maxillofacial region is a part of the total treatment plan. Such care must fit into the broader plan for comprehensive treatment. Cooperation with surgeons, neurosurgeons, otorhinolaryngologists and ophthalmologists is often necessary. Severely injured patients should be taken to intensive care facilities immediately, where constant observation of respiration and circulation is possible and where treatment in all specialties can be arranged.

Emergency treatment centers, in which all specialties including oral and maxillofacial surgery are represented, offer the best assurance for optimal patient care. Because such centers are found only in larger metropolitan regions, however, numerous patients with injuries of the face and jaw are taken initially to local hospitals. Thus arises the question of transfer of the patient to a specialized center: yes or no?

Fractures of the alveolar process and simple fractures of the mandible can be cared for, fundamentally, in local hospitals by consulting oral surgeons or dentists who have completed a course of training in oral and maxillofacial surgery not shorter than three years in duration. Such dentists must not only be able to provide optimal care of such fractures, but must also have sufficient experience in maxillofacial trauma diagnosis to be able to recognize those injured patients whose conditions require referral to a more specialized center (*Schüle*, 1976).

Treatment of maxillofacial injuries should be definitive whenever possible; it may be undertaken immediately on the day of the injury or delayed for a few days. Emergency care measures should be limited to those absolutely necessary; in the first instance they are necessary for preservation of vital functions (respiration and circulation) and to prepare the patient for transportation. Occasionally, emergency measures for fracture treatment may be indicated when the total condition of the patient is such (brain complications, thoracic contusions, abdominal trauma, fat embolism, etc.) that definitive care is not possible.

1. Emergency Care

1.1 Measures at the Accident Site and During Transport

First aid is administered by lay personnel as well as by trained aides (ambulance drivers) and emergency physicians (surgeons or anesthesiologists). The most important measures are maintainance of patent airway, temporary cessation of hemorrhage, and provision of blood fluid replacement to support circulation.

Maintenance of patent airway requires first of all that the oral cavity be cleared of blood coagula and vomitus. At the same time, dentures and severely loosened teeth should be removed. Then the patient must be placed in a position such that blood seepage and fresh vomitus can flow out; this is achieved through the stable lateral position. As the danger of aspiration of stomach contents is less in the left sided than in the right sided position

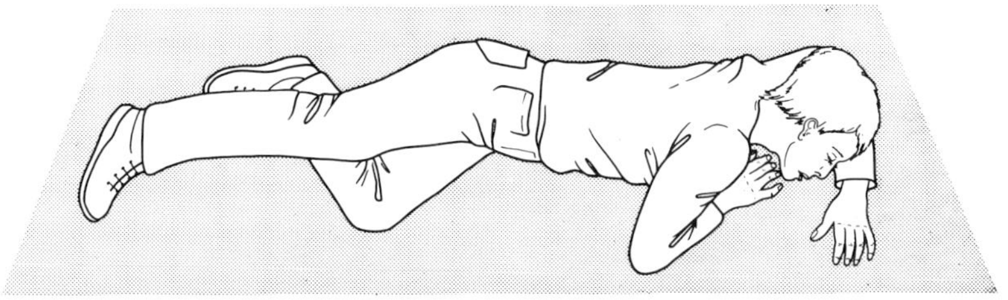

Fig. 4-1 Stable left-sided lateral position.

(*W. Vogler* and *M. Vogler*, 1966), the patient always should be placed in a **stable, left-sided lateral position** (Fig. 4-1). This position, otherwise used only for the unconscious subject, should be used for the maxillofacially injured patient who remains conscious if blood seepage from the oral cavity and from the oropharyngeal space is likely during transport. The supine position is contraindicated in the transport of patients with maxillofacial injuries (*Grimm*, 1969).

A patent airway can be maintained in bilateral mid-mandibular fractures and in the presence of hematomas and severe lingual swelling through the placement of an oropharyngeal *(Guedel)* or nasopharyngeal *(Wendel)* tube. These devices lie along the back of the pharyngeal wall and therefore stimulate retching and vomiting. Stomach contents therefore must first be aspirated; if that is not possible, placement of the tube is better avoided. In that case, patency of the airway is maintained by extending the head (*Ruben*, 1961). It may be necessary, in crushing fractures of the mandible, to extend the tongue; if so, this can be done with the help of a large safety pin which is drawn through the tongue musculature and which then serves to hold an extension loop. It is better in such cases to intubate the patient; an emergency tracheotomy is also possible at accident sites (see below).

Transport in the sitting position with the head bent forward is indicated for less serious injuries without brain involvement.

Temporary hemostasis includes simple measures and is usually undertaken by the placement of immobilizing external bandages. When there is extensive soft tissue injury; the wound edges are approximated as well as possible and maintained in position with the external bandage placed over them. Temporary immobilization is afforded well by the classical Funda maxillae (chin sling, Fig. 4-2 A) or the barrel bandage (Fig. 4-2 B). These bandages can be placed quickly and with simple materials; they prevent further displacement and enhance hemostasis and analgesia through the immobilization of the fragments. Maxillary fractures can be somewhat immobilized with this bandage as well, as it holds the mandible against the maxilla. Fixation of the maxilla against the base of the skull may be achieved with a spatula dressing (Fig. 4-2 C). A wooden spatula or tongue depressor is placed over the occlusal plane of the maxillary teeth at the level of the premolars. This is pulled against the base of the skull through an elastic bandage or with knotted rubber bands running over the top of the head. Hemorrhages in the region of the oral cavity frequently cease after placement of gauze pads and immobilization of the mandible with a *Funda maxillae* (chin sling dressing).

Pressure bandages generally are insufficient to control hemorrhage from larger arteries. Only digital pressure on the carotid artery serves this purpose. The pulsating artery is located between the thyroid cartilage and the anterior margin of the sternocleidomastoid muscle (Fig. 4-3). The artery is pressed against the deep transverse process of the sixth cervical vertebra. The blood flow of the internal carotid artery also is interrupted by this measure, an event that may lead to cerebral damage. The pressure therefore should be exerted intermittently on the carotid artery, if possible. If bleeding in the pressure-free inter-

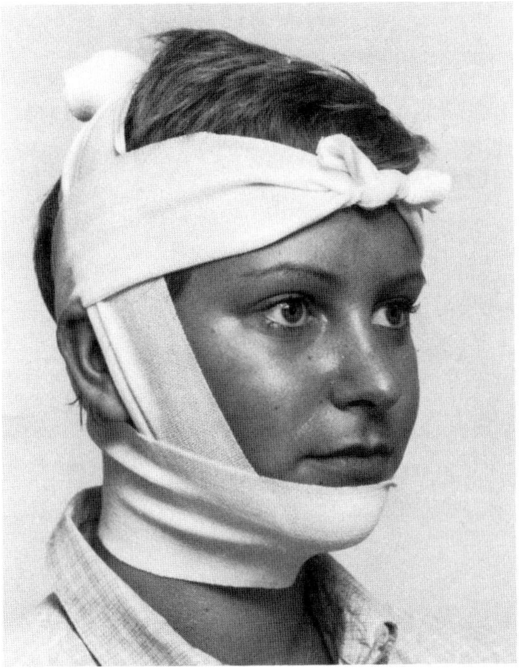

Fig. 4-2 A Funda maxillae.

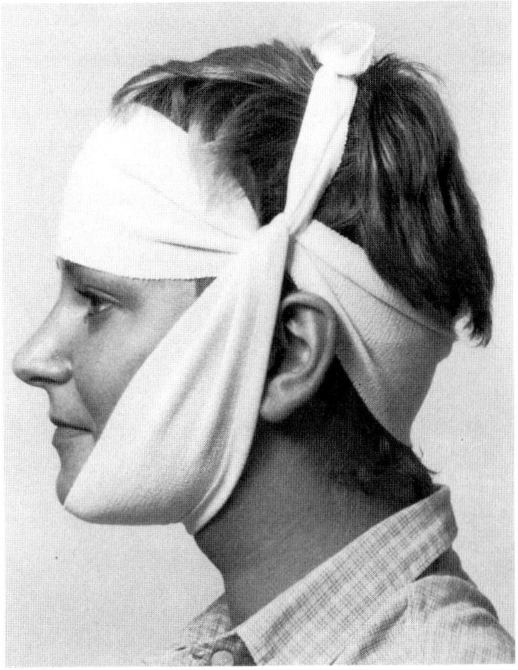

Fig. 4-2 B Barrel bandage.

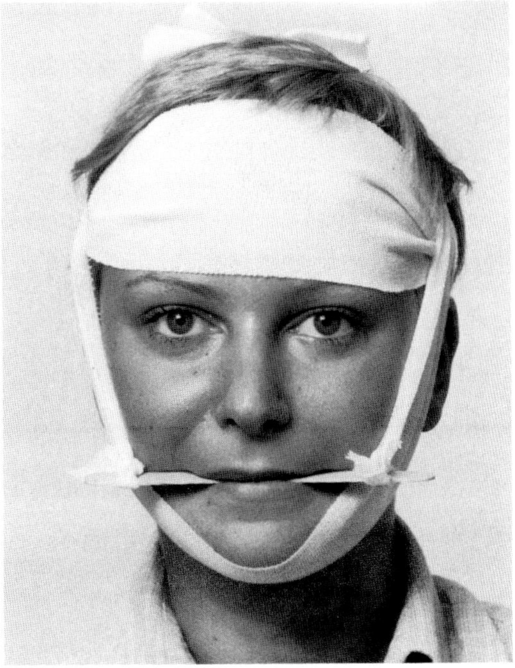

Fig. 4-2 C Spatula dressing for emergency splinting of a fracture of the maxilla.

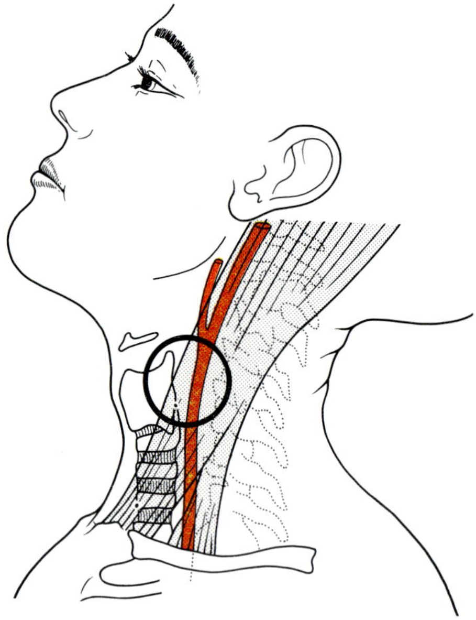

Fig. 4-3 Carotid artery digital compression point.

vals is too great, a pressure bandage should be placed supplementally over the site of the injury. Digital pressure must be provided in such cases during transport of the patient too, until definitive hemostasis can be provided in the surgical suite.

Blood replacement by the provision of fluid is necessary when shock symptoms are present or threatened. The measures necessary for this purpose are generally known and need not be discussed in the framework of this book.

1.2 Hospital Treatment

Immediate emergency surgery following arrival in the hospital is required chiefly by those patients in whom temporary measures at control of bleeding have not been completely successful. Furthermore, a tracheotomy may be indicated to assure an patent airway. Only infrequently, however, are emergency splinting procedures required. Soft tissue injuries also should be attended on the day of the accident, not as emergency measures but rather in the course of definitive immediate treatment to the extent possible.

Surgical hemostatic procedures are best undertaken under general anesthesia with endotracheal intubation. A tracheotomy may be performed under local anesthesia in case of urgency; general anesthesia is better for this purpose. Emergency splinting and nasal tamponade do not require anesthesia in many instances.

Preoperatively, the oral cavity should be cleaned as well as possible. If general anesthesia is required, aspiration of stomach contents through a wide tube is necessary. Ingested food may remain in the stomach up to 24 to 48 hours after an accident because the trauma of the event may cause pyloric spasm. Intubation should be by the nasal route if at all possible so that intermaxillary fixation is not hindered. If a tracheotomy has been performed, intubation may proceed through the tracheostoma.

1.2.1 Definitive Control of Hemorrhage

Immediate measures to control bleeding are necessary if there is hemorrhaging from larger vessels. Massive bleeding from the mouth and nose occur after tearing of the maxillary artery

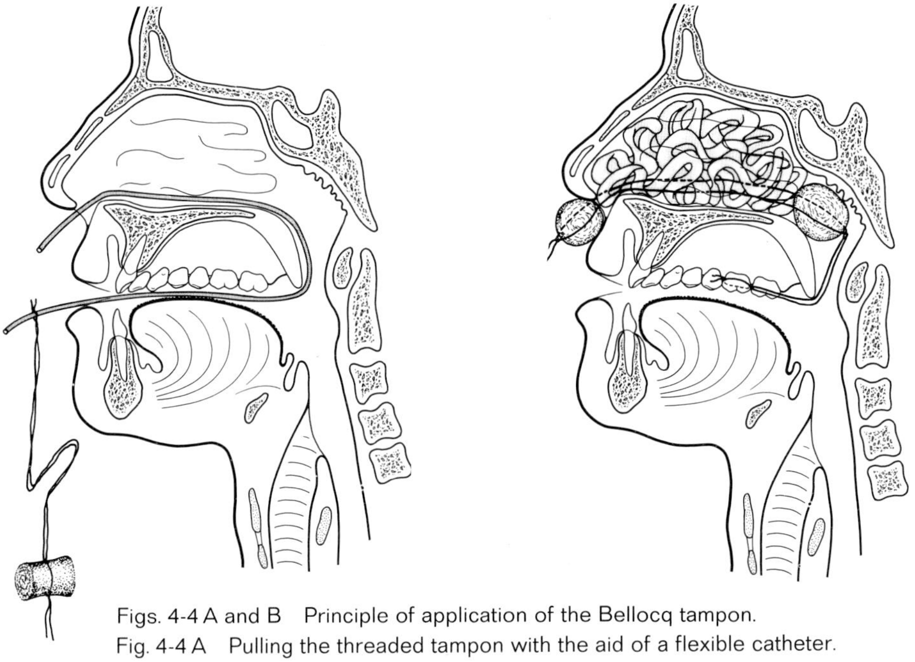

Figs. 4-4 A and B Principle of application of the Bellocq tampon.

Fig. 4-4 A Pulling the threaded tampon with the aid of a flexible catheter.

Fig. 4-4 B Tampon in place. The retention thread has passed the lower nasal meatus and has been tied to a gauze pad at the naris. A second thread passes into the oral cavity via the posterior border of the soft palate and is tied to the penultimate tooth in the arch. This thread is used later to withdraw the tampon. The nasal meatus is tamponaded with a gauze strip.

in midface fractures. Bleeding can arise from branches of the lingual artery and vein after injuries to the floor of the mouth and the tongue, and from branches of the facial artery and vein in soft tissue injuries of the face.

Hemorrhages from soft tissue are controlled by placement of ligatures or purse-string sutures in the course of care of the soft tissue damage. Bleeding from the nasopharyngeal space, except for massive bleeding from the maxillary artery, can be controlled by **nasal tamponade.**

Anterior nasal tamponade is undertaken from the nares. The nasal cavities are plugged bilaterally with gauze strips coated with a mild ointment, e. g. Nebacetin. Packing begins in the upper posterior region and proceeds through the center and anterior nasal passage sections until the anterior portion of the nose is packed as well. To prevent slippage of the gauze into the nasopharyngeal space, *Feldmann* (1973) recommended that a foam rubber pad be inserted into the lower nasal meatus. Gauze strips may be packed against this cushion. The foam rubber cushion should be provided with a looped thread extending out of the nose for safety's sake; the loose end is tied to a gauze pad or a second piece of foam rubber placed at the naris.

Bellocq's **(posterior) tamponade** provides a more rigid tamponade in the rearmost portions of the nose through its application from behind in the nasopharyngeal space. *Bellocq* tampons are made easily by tying gauze pads or pieces of foam rubber together like a package with simple thread; commercially prepared, various sized ones are available as well.* The tampon is placed more sparingly with rubber catheters or stomach probes than with the Bellocq cannula. A catheter is moved from each side

* Manufacturer: Fresenius, D-6300 Bad Homburg, Germany

of the nose through the lower portion into the mesopharynx and the ends are brought out of the oral cavity with a forceps over the posterior border of the soft palate. Now the tampon threads are tied to the catheters and these are drawn back through the posterior nasal apertures and out of the nose; the tampon threads are used to pull the tampons into place. A second thread should remain in the mouth, attached to teeth or a splint so that the tampon can be removed later through the oral cavity. While pulling lightly on the nasal thread, the nose is packed with a gauze strip and the thread ends are tied to a piece of gauze or rubber at the outer edge of the nose (Fig. 4-4).

Nasal tamponades should not remain in place longer than three days if possible. If the *Bellocq* tamponade is applied with too much pressure, necrosis of the nasal mucosa may occur. The danger of middle ear or paranasal sinus infection is no longer as great as it was because of antibiotic protection. In fractures of the central midface, tears in the region of the ethmoid bone mucosa must be assumed to provide a direct connection to the anterior cranial fossa. The danger of ascending infection and the development of nasal meningitis therefore is great. This is especially so if a rigid tamponade leads to accumulation of secretions in the region of the paranasal sinus mucosa, a region normally richly contaminated with microorganisms. For this reason, antibiotic cover is extremly important.

The indication for nasal tamponade is present only infrequently in fractures of the midface. Hemorrhages that do not stop spontaneously usually stop after reduction and fixation of the fractured parts of the jaw. For this reason the treatment of fractures should be undertaken immediately if there is continuous bleeding from the nose. Only occasionally will it then be found necessary to use nasal tamponade. If immediate care of the fracture is not possible in such instances, tamponade may be the only primary treatment undertaken.

Massive bleeding from the maxillary artery usually is not controllable by nasal tamponade. Ligation of the supplying artery is required.

Ligation of the maxillary artery via the antrum through a Caldwell-Luc approach with resection of the posterior wall of the maxillary sinus should be avoided in fractures of the midface because of the additional bone defects that result, and the disturbance of fracture healing associated therewith.

Ligation of the external carotid artery at the angle of the mandible affects the temporal artery and the posterior auricular artery as well as the maxillary artery, a hardly disadvantageous circumstance. The advantage of this approach over the Caldwell-Luc approach lies in the fact that the former is outside the region of the fracture and does not require additional weakening of the midface. The external incision is two fingerbreadths below the angle of the mandible in a natural skin-fold (Fig. 4-5 A). After division of the platysma, one proceeds deep between the angle of the mandible and the lower pole of the parotid gland to expose the upper margin of the stylohyoid muscle and the posterior belly of the digastric muscle. The carotid artery is immediately below (Fig. 4-5 B).

The indication for ligation of the carotid artery is given by massive bleeding from the nasopharyngeal space and from the maxillary portion of the oral cavity uncontrollable by nasal tamponade.

Bleeding from the tongue generally can be stopped when the wounds are treated. Only exceptionally is specific ligation of the lingual artery required.

Ligation of the lingual artery is undertaken via a submandibular incision of the skin lying over the hyoid bone, approximately two fingerbreadths below the lower margin of the mandible in a natural skin-fold. After the lower pole of the submandibular gland and the digastric tendon has been found at the hyoid bone, the gland is turned upward to expose the posterior margin of the mylohyoid muscle. The hypoglossus nerve and the sublingual vein are found lying over the deeply located hyoglossus muscle; the nerve and vein are freed and turned dorsally upwards. Then the hyoglossus muscle is divided immediately over the digastric tendon between the posterior margin of the mylohyoid muscle and the hypoglossus nerve; this exposes the lingual artery (Fig. 4-6) at a point after the branching for the base of the tongue. Should these branches be ligated as well, the hyoglossus incision is extended to the dorsal edge of the muscle.

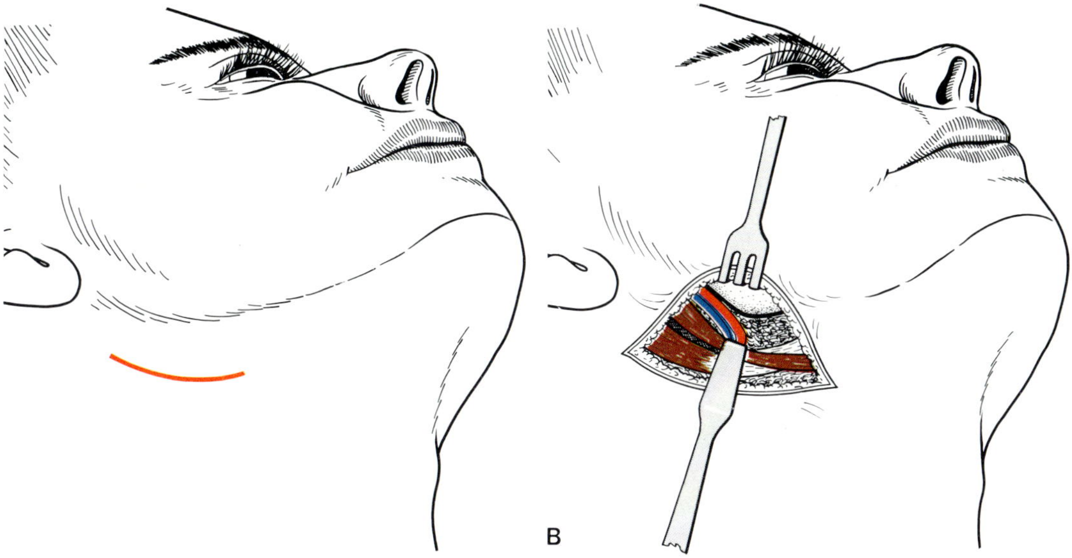

Figs. 4-5 A and B Site for ligating the external carotid artery at the mandibular angle.

Figs. 4-5 A Course of the incision.

Fig. 4-5 B External carotid artery and retromandibular vein have been exposed; they lie beneath the stylohoid muscle and the posterior belly of the digastric muscle.

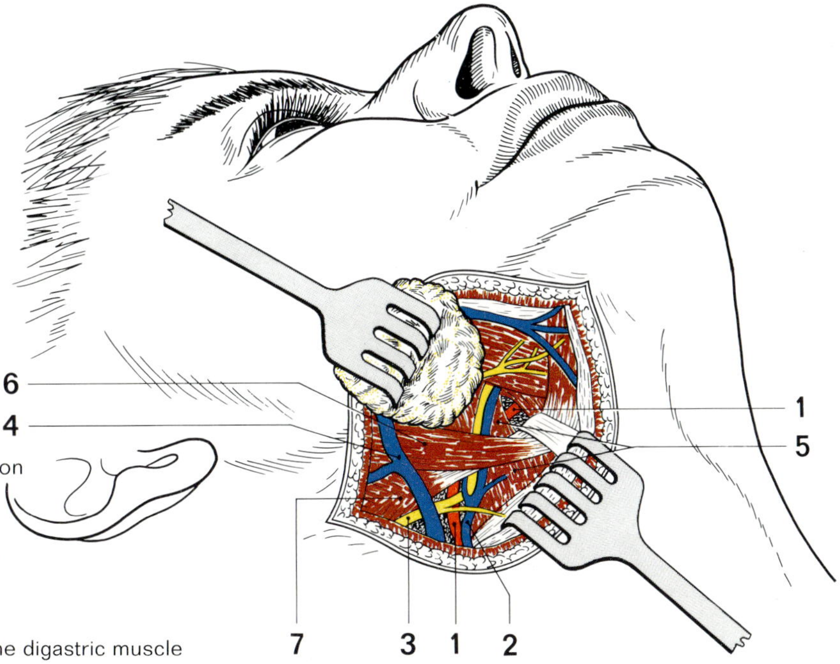

Fig. 4-6 Site for ligation of the lingual artery.
1. lingual artery
2. lingual vein
3. hypoglossus nerve
4. facial vein
5. hyoglossus muscle
6. stylohyoid muscle
7. posterior belly of the digastric muscle

Ligation of the lingual artery is rarely required in tonque injuries. It may be indicated, however, if bleeding persists from the tongue and floor of the mouth **after** repair of the soft tissue damage.

1.2.2 Maintenance of Airway Patency; Tracheotomy

Blood and wound secretions must be aspirated continuously from the oral cavity, the nasopharyngeal space and the pharynx. In the unconscious patient suctioning should include the trachea and the larynx as well. Patients who are not disoriented may be permitted to sit up from time to time so that they may expectorate accumulated blood and secretions into a container from a slightly bent forward position. In unconscious patients and those who cannot sit up because of cerebral trauma, the following possibilities exist for removal of these liquids:

1. stable lateral position
2. naso-pharyngeo-tracheal and oral suction
3. nasotracheal or orotracheal intubation
4. tracheotomy

Patients placed into the stable lateral position should have supplemental suctioning regularly. Supine patients require frequent suction of the nose, oral cavity and pharynx, and of the larynx and trachea if warranted. If this is insufficient for the maintenance of a patent airway, e.g., when there is retrusion of the tongue in a crush fracture in the chin, either tracheotomy or intubation is necessary. In both cases, suction is appreciably simplified; however, the irritation provided by the tube or the cannula causes increased formation of secretions so that more must be suctioned away. In every case, nutrition must be provided parenterally or by means of a stomach tube.

Intubation is best undertaken nasotracheally. The trachea may be anesthetized beforehand with tetracaine in the awake patient. For this purpose, not more than 1 ml of a 2% solution or 2 ml of a 1% solution are injected intratracheally through the cricothyroid ligament (*Grimm*, 1969). *Kwapis* (1954), *Holinger* et al. (1955), as well as *Dingmann* and *Natvig* (1964) also suggest a 5 to 10% solution of cocaine.

The tube should not be left in place longer than 48 hours because otherwise permanent damage may arise from pressure lesions on the vocal cords and the wall of the trachea. Lesions of the mucosa develop within 12 hours and after 36 hours ulcerations may be demonstrated almost routinely. These reach the cartilage after approximately 48 hours (*Rügheimer*, 1977). Some tracheal stenosis must be anticipated after prolonged endotracheal intubation in about 20% of the cases; more serious stenosis is rare, however (*Deane* and *Mills*, 1970). Development of tracheitis and bronchitis is common.

If a prolonged indwelling period is anticipated, tracheotomy is more useful than intubation.

Tracheotomy

By definition, tracheotomy is the surgical formation of an opening in the trachea between the larynx and the jugulum, through which the patient can breathe or be given respiration after introduction of a cannula. The classification of superior, medial, or inferior tracheotomy depends on whether the opening into the trachea is above, in the center of, or below the isthmus of the thyroid gland.

The advantages of tracheotomy over intubation are primarily that mucosal lesions caused by the action of cannulas against the tracheal wall are limited. Resulting stenoses can be dealt with more easily than in the larynx (*Denecke*, 1968, 1971). Therefore, long term treatment is more readily possible than with nasotracheal intubation. On the other hand, the reduction of the dead space hardly comes into consideration; blood gas analyses show only an insignificant reduction of pCO_2 after tracheotomy (*Tyler*, 1961; *Froeb* and *Kimm*, 1964; *Reichel*, 1967; *Rügheimer*, 1977). Reduction of respiratory resistance related to normal respiration arises only if the internal diameter of the cannula is at least 10 mm (*Grazon* et al., 1963).

Indications for tracheotomy arise on the basis of the local situation and for reasons of intensive care. Experience shows tracheotomy to be undertaken too frequently. Almost always, the same effect may be attained by intubation, at least in the first 24 hours.

During the course of the definitive treatment of fractures, tracheotomy can be avoided frequently. Intermaxillary fixation alone is not an indication for tracheotomy. Even when injuries of the tongue and floor of the mouth are present and edema of the laryngeal opening is anticipated, tracheotomy often can be avoided. As a first step, one should intubate rather than perform a tracheotomy. Crushing fractures of the chin in many instances can be so reduced and fixated that even here tracheotomy is required only infrequently. For technical reasons, however, tracheotomy may be necessary if neither nasotracheal nor orotracheal intubation is possible without impeding the surgical procedure. This is the case when there is a combination of soft tissue injury in the region of the nares — requiring orotracheal intubation — and those fractures of the jaws that can be reduced to occlusion only with nasotracheal intubation.

The following situations are indications for tracheotomy:

1. Fractures with retrusion of the tongue, especially comminuted fractures in the chin region, if immediate care is not possible.
2. Injuries in the laryngeal region.
3. Need for suctioning over a longer period in patients with pre-existing diseases of the lungs, contusion of the thorax, or brain trauma.
4. Need for artificial long-term respiration.
5. To provide an anesthetic pathway in jaw fractures combined with soft tissue injury of the nose, if nasal as well as oral intubation would hinder proper care.
6. Long term intubation, if extubation is not possible after 48 hours.

The **surgical technique** varies according to the course of the incision, in the level of the incision (superior, medial, or inferior tracheotomy), and in the shape of the tracheal wall incision. Before the variations possible are considered, the following will describe our preferred technique:

The patient is placed in the dorsal flexion position, with his head extended (Fig. 4-7 A). A median vertical incision is made from the cricoid cartilage to the jugulum (base of the throat).
Blunt dissection of the subcutaneous fatty tissue follows, with ligation of the branches of the ventral superficial jugular vein present here. Separation of the superficial and medial fascia of the neck is followed by displacement of the sternohyoid muscles laterally and exposure of the isthmus of the thyroid gland. The trachea is palpated with the finger before blunt dissection of the prevertebral fatty tissue is accomplished below the isthmus with ligation or lateral displacement of the *venae thyreoideae imae*. The anterior wall of the trachea is exposed immediately below the isthmus (Fig. 4-7 B). The isthmus is separated from the trachea from below and the third and fourth tracheal rings are exposed. A strongly developed isthmus is not easily pulled up over the third tracheal ring, and in that case it must be clamped, ligated, and divided. Before the trachea is opened, bleeding in the entire surgical field should be controlled. When the surgery is done under local anesthesia, the annular ligament is pierced between the third and fourth tracheal ring with a fine injection needle. Then 1 ml of 1 % lidocaine solution is injected into the trachea to reduce the coughing reflex. Two tracheal hooks are inserted laterally between the third and fourth tracheal rings and the trachea is pulled forward. A vertical incision is made through the third and fourth tracheal rings, and an oval window (Fig. 4-7 C) is cut out. In operations under general anesthesia, the intratracheal tube is pulled back until its end is above the tracheal window. A flexible tracheotomy tube with inflatable cuff is introduced (Trachoflex, Figs. 4-7 D and 4-8). In general anesthesia, the anesthesia machine now is attached to the tracheotomy tube and the cuff is inflated to seal the trachea. The muscular layer is sutured loosely, as is the subcutaneous fatty tissue and the skin, so that escaping air can pass between the tube and the tracheal window without being forced into the tissue. The tube shield is underlaid with gauze and supported by a bandage wound about the neck.

Variations are possible in the line of the **incision.** Although the vertical incision described above is preferred by the majority of authors (*Lanz* and *Wachsmuth*, 1955; *Nelson* and *Bowers*, 1957; *Rowe* and *Killey*, 1968; *Messerklinger*, 1972; *Rügheimer*, 1977; among others), some authors (e.g., *Dingman* and *Natvig*, 1964; *Kazanjian* and *Converse*, 1974) prefer a transverse incision. This has the advantage that it follows the skin folds. To its disadvantage is that it leads to

Figs. 4-7 A to D Tracheotomy.

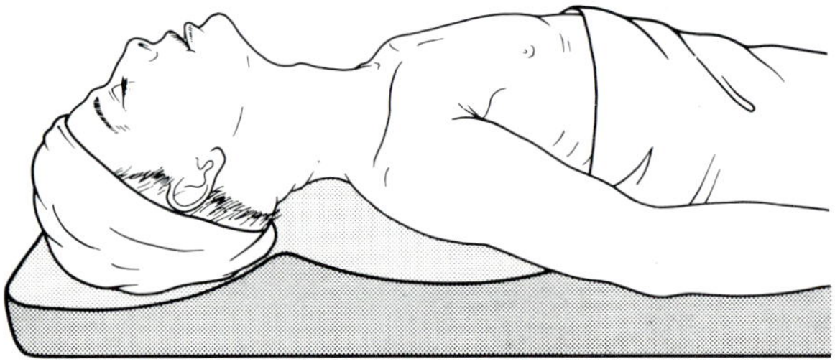

Fig. 4-7 A Dorsal flexion position.

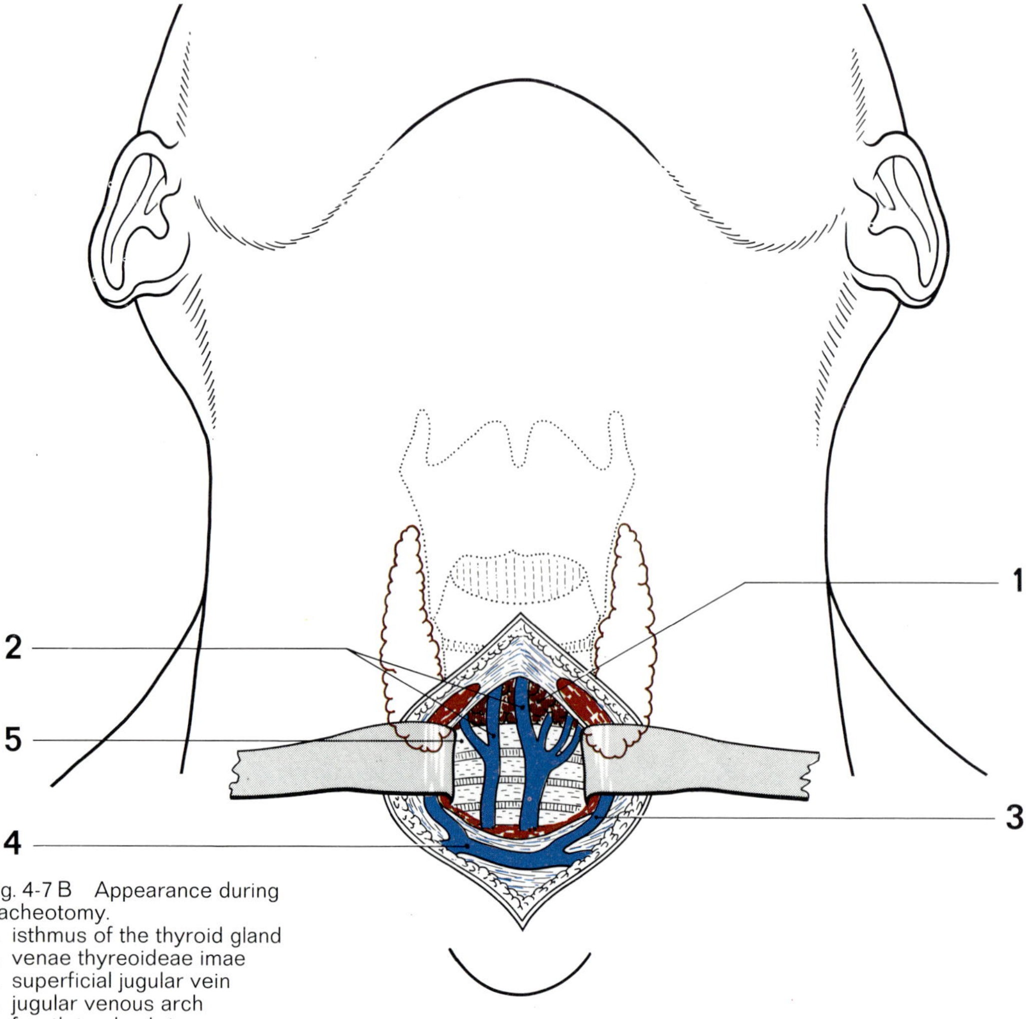

Fig. 4-7 B Appearance during tracheotomy.
1. isthmus of the thyroid gland
2. venae thyreoideae imae
3. superficial jugular vein
4. jugular venous arch
5. fourth tracheal ring

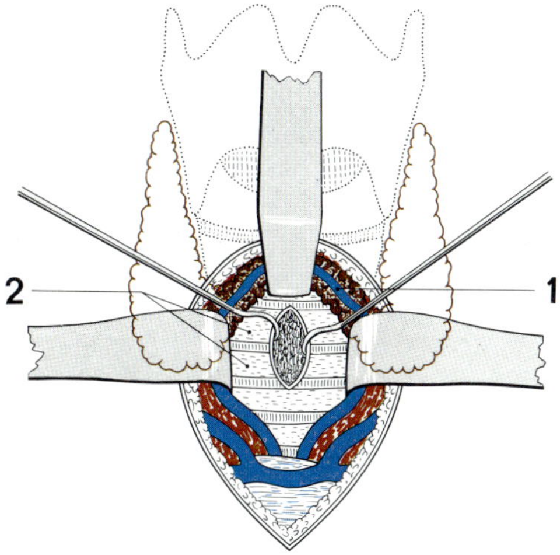

Fig. 4-7 C Appearance following opening of the trachea.
1. venae thyreoideae imae, pulled aside with a hook
2. third and fourth tracheal rings

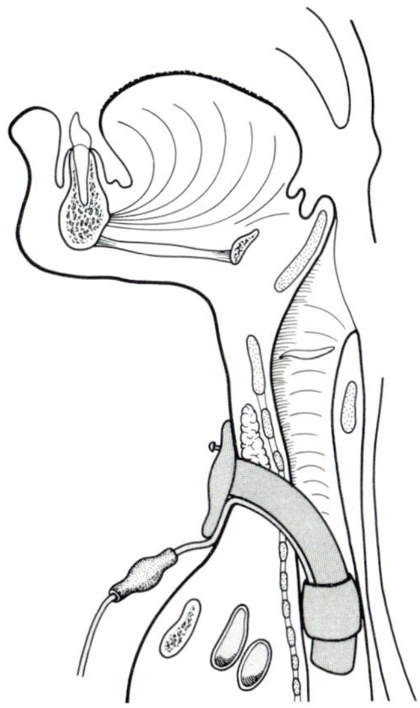

Fig. 4-7 D Position of the tracheal cannula with inflated cuff.

displacement of the tracheal cannula if the plane of the incision is not precisely over the tracheal window. Furthermore, secretions collect easily under the lower skin margin.

Another variation exists in the **height of the tracheal opening.** The technique that we prefer opens the trachea at the level of the third and fourth tracheal ring. The medial tracheotomy, which involves a division of the isthmus, is usually undertaken at the level of the second and third tracheal ring (*Rowe* and *Killey*, 1968; *Messerklinger*, 1972); the inferior tracheotomy, on the other hand, is done in the region of the fifth and sixth rings. The incision described by *Rügheimer* (1977) as a medial tracheotomy with opening of the airway at the third and fourth tracheal rings is really more a high inferior tracheotomy because the division of the isthmus frequently can be avoided. It should be considered, however, that a voluminous isthmus pulled upward during the operation may slide in front of the tracheal window during subsequent changes of the tube, and thus may make introduction of a new tracheotomy tube difficult. If that is to be feared, it is better to divide the isthmus or at least to incise it.

The superior tracheotomy is undertaken at the level of the first and second tracheal ring. Here the danger of injuring the cricoid cartilage or causing damage through pressure exists, with subsequent stenosis and more difficult decannulation (*Rügheimer*, 1977). The inferior tracheotomy has the disadvantage of the longer path: the distance between the skin and trachea here is 4 to 6 cm. This particularly reduces the stability of rigid metal cannulas. Pressure necroses at the tracheal bifurcation and at the anterior trachea, with perforation of the brachiocephalic trunk and fatal erosion hemorrhage, are possible.

The tracheal wall incision should not be made solely through a vertical incision because the cartilage edges can be forced into an abnormal position, to be fixated there for longer periods. This can lead to formation of an additional vertical torus on the posterior wall of the trachea. These disadvantages are avoided by extending

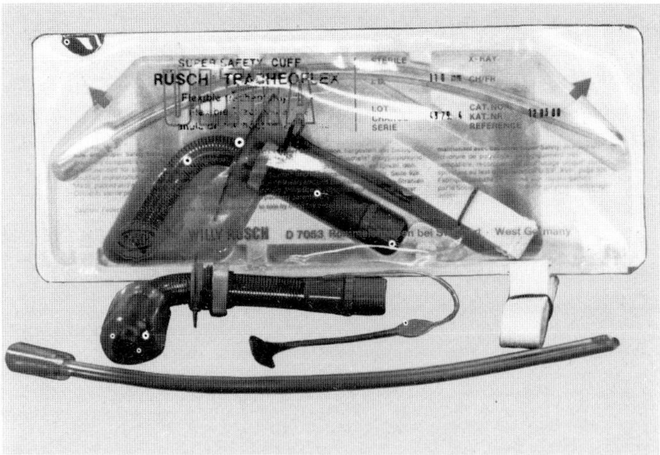

Fig. 4-8 A Tracheoflex cannula and accessories in sterile pack and unpacked.

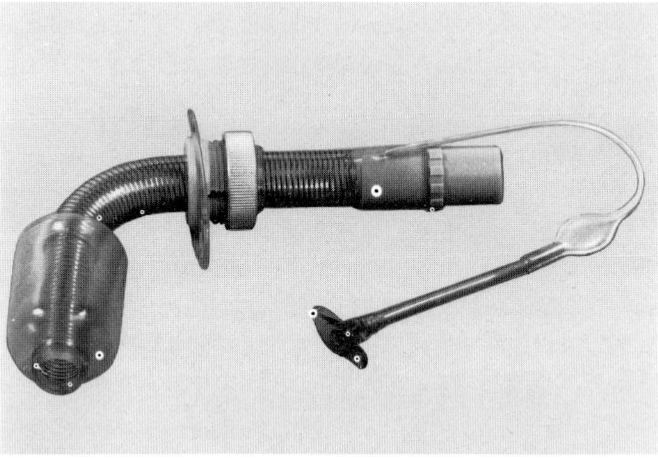

Fig. 4-8 B Tracheoflex cannula with super safety cuff.

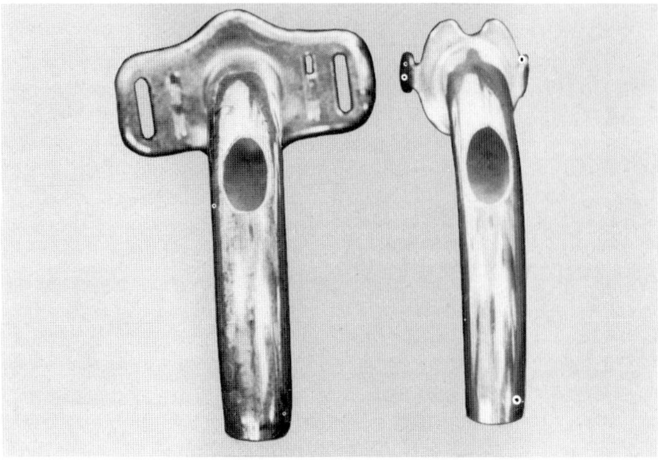

Fig. 4-9 Speech cannula. Left: the external cannula; right: the internal cannula. The additional opening affords air entry to the larynx. As a rule, the external opening must be closed with a fingertip or a cork during speech.

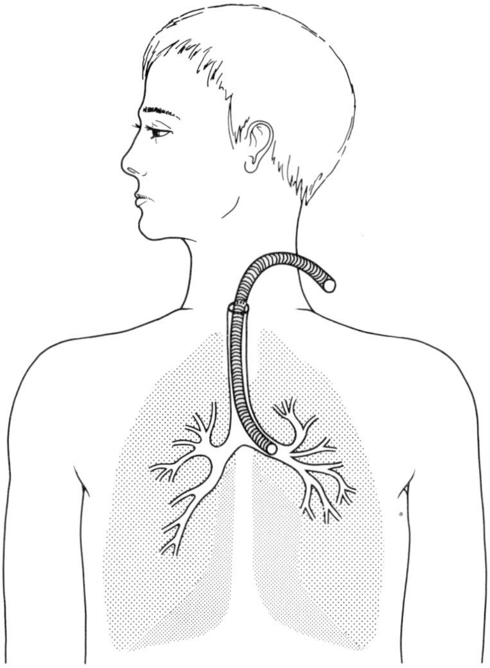

A

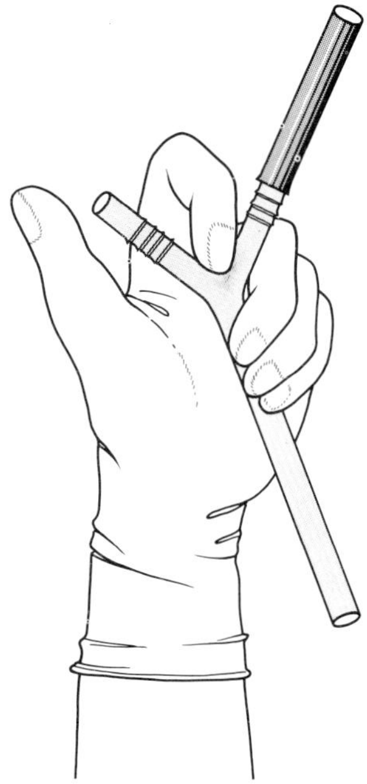

B

Figs. 4-10 A and B Bronchial toilet.

Fig. 4-10 A Evacuation of bronchial secretion on the left side. The head is turned to the right. The aspirating tube then slides into the left primary bronchus. To aspirate the right side, the head is turned to the left.

Fig. 4-10 B A Y-tube simplifies aspiration. The open end can be opened and closed alternately with the thumb. While the aspirating catheter is introduced into the trachea, the opening is not covered.

the vertical incision to an oval window. In addition, placement of a circular window having precisely the size of the tube is suggested (*Messerklinger*, 1972; *Rügheimer*, 1977). *Dingman* and *Natvig* (1964) and *Kazanjian* and *Converse* (1974) prefer a cruciate incision. Here too, the danger exists that the four triangular flaps developed can be pushed into the trachea. A transverse incision should be rejected in any case because the upper margin of the incision is pushed into the trachea by the cannula while the lower margin slides outward; this leads to formation of a transverse torus in the membranous posterior wall of the trachea.

The type of **tracheotomy tube** has special significance. In the event artificial respiration is necessary, the tube must have an inflatable cuff. Furthermore, it is necessary that the cannula be flexible and adapt well to the wound, the tracheal stoma and the tracheal wall. These requirements are fulfilled best by the Tracheoflex tube with cylindrical cuff, which has a standard 15 mm connector to adapt to every respiration and anesthesia unit (Fig. 4-8). It is available in all the common sizes.* Before decannulation, the Tracheoflex should be replaced with a "speech cannula." This is a metal cannula with a hole on its convex side (Fig. 4-9) that permits passage of air over the nasopharyngeal space.

Postoperative care following tracheotomy or intubation requires an attentive nursing staff. Because the patient is unable to speak, he must have access to a calling system and to writing

* Manufacturer: Willy Rüsch, P.O.Box 1620, D-7050 Waiblingen, Germany

instruments so that he can call for help and describe his needs. The absence of the nasopharyngeal space as a dust filter and heating and humidifying system, and of the glottis as a vent for excess pressure in coughing and as an obstruction to bacteria leads to increased production of secretions and increased risk of infection.

The following measures, therefore, are necessary:
1. bronchial toilet
2. air conditioning and humidification of the inspired air
3. antibiotic therapy.

Bronchial toilet refers to the aspiration of secretions from the trachea and large bronchi at regular intervals. Each aspiration requires sterile disposable gloves, sterile disposable aspirating catheters with a separation between the oral and tracheal catheter, and sterile Ringer's solution to moisten the catheter. Aspiration is done as required, i.e., when secretions have collected (stridor, coughing, rales). For aspiration in the left side of the bronchial tree, the patient's head is turned to the right, and the reverse for aspiration of the right side (Fig. 4-10 A). The use of a Y-tube between the aspirating catheter and the vacuum source has proven worthwhile (*Glas* et al., 1962). The open end of the "Y" is alternately covered and opened with the thumb (Fig. 4-10 B). The aspirating catheter is rotated slowly as it is pulled out with the period of aspiration being less than 15 seconds. An inflated cuff must be collapsed briefly at intervals of two hours to avoid injury to the tracheal wall.

The tracheotomy tube should be changed daily from the third postoperative day on to avoid formation of crusts from secretions.

To **condition and humidify the inspired air**, it is best to use an ultrasonic atomizer that produces steam-saturated air at body temperature or discharges a secretolytic aerosol into the region of the tracheotomy tube.

Antibiotic therapy is provided to prevent infection of the respiratory system, primarily by gram negative organisms. Identification of microorganisms present requires bacteriological screening with sensitivity tests of the sputum. Until the results of these tests are known, broad-spectrum antibiotics (carbenicillin, gentamycin, azlocillin) should be given. A physical pneumonia prophylaxis is indicated in addition.

Decannulation should be done as soon as possible. Sufficient oxygenation of the blood (blood gas analysis) during spontaneous respiration is prerequisite to this step. It is sensible to replace the Tracheoflex tube before decannulation with a "speech cannula" and to close its external opening with a cork. If the patient is then able to breathe without any difficulty, the speech cannula, too, can be withdrawn. The tracheotomy opening heals as a rule without any further surgery.

Complications following tracheotomy are elicited by slippage of the cannula, emphysema, infections consequent to foreign body irritation with hypersecretion, and by mechanical lesions of the tracheal wall caused by long-term placement of the cannula.

Dislodgement of the tracheotomy tube is possible if the tube is held too loosely by the neck sling. It may be dislodged through strong coughing. If this occurs after the third day, as a rule it causes no problems to reintroduce the tube. If the event occurs shortly after the operation, however, the situation is less favorable. Then the wound still gives way and tissue may fall over the tracheal window, preventing reintubation. In that event the wound must be opened to provide a better view. After exposure of the tracheal window, the tube may be inserted again.

If the tracheal window is too large and the skin incision was sutured too tightly, air may be pressed into the tissue. If such a **skin emphysema** forms, the skin incision must be opened.

Development of **bronchial pneumonia** is promoted by poor bronchial toilet and insufficient antibiotic cover. **Mechanical lesions** lead to necroses of the tracheal wall. If the tube is in place only for a short period, the damage does not lead to diminished function. If it is in place longer, severe complications are possible. If the ulceration rate is greater than the repair rate, a **tracheo-esophageal fistula** may form from pressure on the back wall of the trachea; pressure on the lateral wall leads to a **tracheo-pleural** fistula; and pressure on the anterior wall to **erosion of the brachiocephalic trunk** with lethal bleeding. If the rate of repair is greater than the rate of ulceration, **granulation tissue** may form and later **scar stenoses.** The loss of large sections of cartilage leads to **malacia.** In such cases decannulation is no longer possible. The resulting stenoses frequently can be treated surgically.

Tracheotomy in children involves a special risk of complications. *Oliver* et al. (1962) found a mortality of 20.1 % in childhood following tracheotomy; 3.4 % of the deaths were ascribed to the surgery. The complication rate in surgical, postsurgical and decannulation problems was 31 % overall. Eighty to 100 % of all complications were seen in children under age 5 years. *Kornmesser* (1972) suggests that the diameter of the tracheotomy tube should not exceed two-thirds of that of the trachea. Only in this manner is it possible to keep the wall defect small and to reduce the number of scar necroses.

Emergency tracheotomy

Emergency tracheotomy in acute dyspnea has been replaced largely by emergency intubation today. Only in laryngeal injury and displacement of the vocal chords by a foreign body or acute glottal edema may an emergency tracheotomy be indicated.
The simplest procedure is **puncture of the conic ligament.** Several sharp cannulas having internal diameters of 1.5 to 2 mm are used to puncture the trachea between the thyroid and cricoid cartilages. Oxygen administration eases breathing for the patient. The method is not dangerous and may be used by a person with little experience in emergency medicine without much risk. The duration of effectiveness is limited because of the increased difficulty of expiration. In many instances, however, it may be used during the period of transport to the hospital and until the time of definitive tracheotomy (*Nicholas* and *Rumer*, 1960).
If the desired result does not occur within three minutes, **coniotomy** must be undertaken. This procedure, already described in 1805 by the Frenchman *Vicq d'Azyr* and later by *Tandler* (1923), is the classical life-saving incision into the trachea in acute obstruction of the inlet of the larynx: the head is overextended in dorsal flexion as for tracheotomy and the cricothyroid notch corresponding to the conic ligament is palpated in midline; the left index finger is used and the fingertip is placed on the right margin of the cartilage. A transverse incision is made in the skin from the fingertip to the left margin of the cartilage. The skin margins are separated with sharp hooks. When bleeding has been stopped, the conic ligament is divided over the cricoid cartilage (Fig. 4-11) and a tracheotomy tube or other non-collapsible hollow tube is introduced. In place of the transverse skin incision (*Dingmann* and *Natvig*, 1964; *Rowe* and *Kelley*, 1968), a vertical incision may be made (*Lanz* and *Wachsmuth*, 1955; *Messerklinger*, 1972). The conic ligament is incised transversally in any event.
When there is acute danger of suffocation, a transverse incision can be made simultaneously through the skin and mucosa (*Tandler*, 1923). If no tube is available, the wound margins should be held apart with adhesive tape to assure an air passage.
The emergency tracheotomy can be undertaken with a trocar, over which the tracheotomy cannula is pushed. The trocar, serving as introducer, is pushed through the conic ligament carrying the cannula (Fig. 4-12).
An emergency airway set is available for emergency tracheotomy (Fig. 4-13). It consists of a puncture dilator with sharply pointed forceps, a two-bladed external cannula whose spring arms can be forced together, and an internal cannula. Manipulation is as simple as possible: the puncture dilator is pushed through the skin and conic ligament into the trachea with the forceps closed. The instrument is spread until air can enter and leave. The closed external cannula is introduced while the puncture site is held open with the spread dilator. The dilator is removed and the internal cannula is introduced. Both cannulas are held in place with a neck sling.
Significant bleeding may arise during blind coniotomy and in the trocar or dilator puncture of the ligament. The fine branches of the arteries lying over the thyroid cartilage are not injured as a rule by an incision over the upper margin of the cricoid cartilage. Hemorrhage from these vessels usually stops spontaneously. More severe hemorrhage can arise from injury of the cricothyroid vein (Fig. 4-11). Bleeding also is possible if a pyramid process of the thyroid happens to overlie the conic ligament.

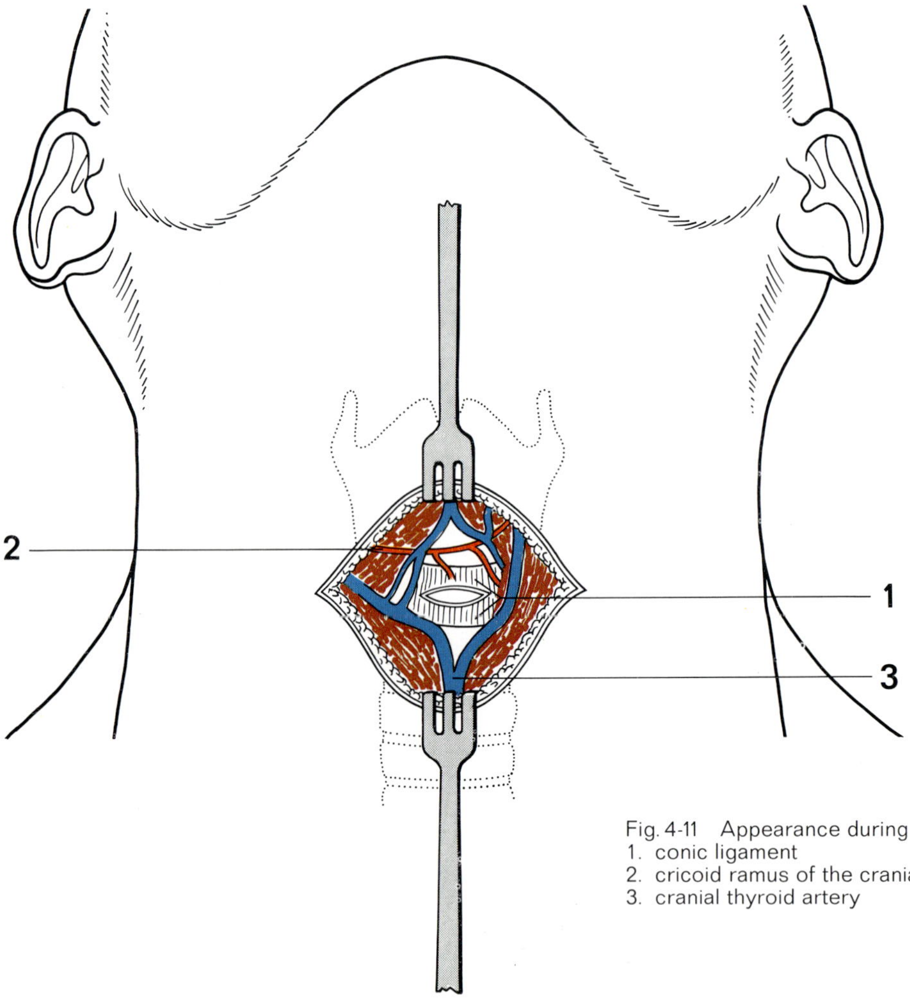

Fig. 4-11 Appearance during coniotomy.
1. conic ligament
2. cricoid ramus of the cranial thyroid artery
3. cranial thyroid artery

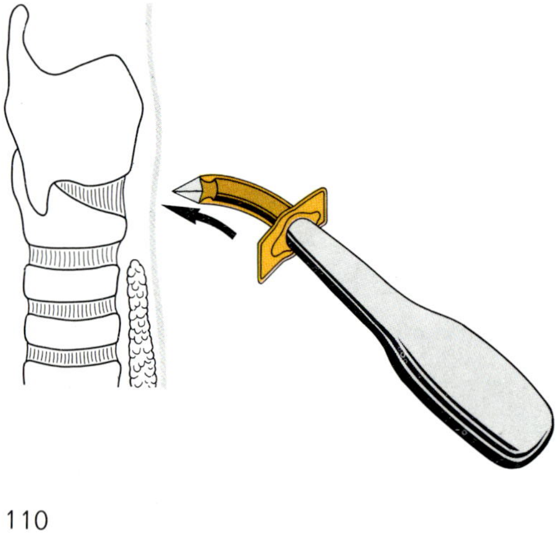

Fig. 4-12 Emergency tracheotomy with a trocar, above which a tracheotomy cannula has been inserted. Following puncture of the soft tissue covering and the conic ligament, the trocar and the cannula are guided into the trachea. Then the trocar is removed while the cannula remains in place.

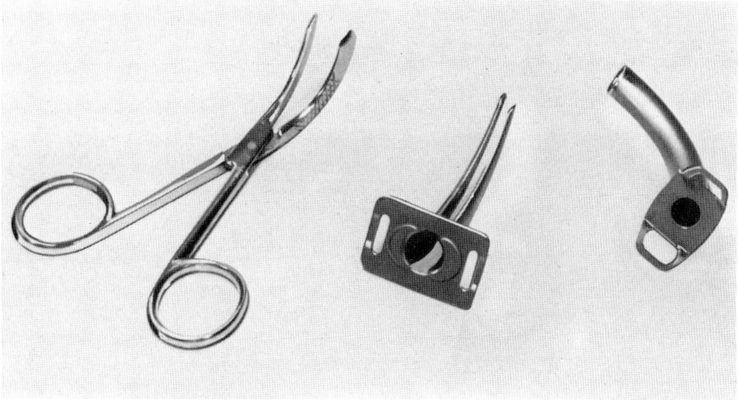

Fig. 4-13 Emergency airway set for coniotomy, with puncture dilator (left), two-bladed external cannula (center) and internal cannula (right).

In view of the possibilities for damaging these vessels, blind coniotomy and puncture of the ligaments with a trocar or puncture dilator should be used only in extreme emergency, and never through any thyroid gland tissue overlying the ligament. Any hemorrhage that arises must be brought under control by digital compression.

Coniotomy and puncture of the conic ligament are not definitive measures. Air flow through piercing injection needles is insufficient over the long term. A coniotomy tube leads to pressure necrosis if left in place for a longer period, with circular diminution of the subglottal space that is correctable only with difficulty. For these reasons, a tracheotomy should be undertaken within 12 to 24 hours.

1.2.3 Emergency Splinting Measures

In jaw injuries, one strives, as a rule, for definitive treatment through splinting or surgical measures, or both, forthwith. Emergency fixation appliances therefore are indicated only in certain exceptional situations.

The **indication** for emergency splinting exists especially when the general condition of the patient does not permit any tedious fracture manipulation in the facial skull because of other injuries or general complications. Occasionally it may be desirable to immobilize the fractured jaw components for transport from a general hospital to a specialized center. This may be particularly useful if the individual fragments are greatly displaced and mobile, with consequent severe fracture pain and increased danger of hemorrhage and infection.

External bandages, like the previously mentioned chin sling (see Fig. 4-2 A) and the barrel bandage (see Fig. 4-2 B) are appropriate for temporary immobilization of jaw fragments only to a limited degree. Thus, they are considered only as first aid at the accident site, especially if there are simultaneous soft tissue injuries. Broken fragments only can be supported tolerably under especially favorable conditions. The **plaster head-chin cap** (Fig. 4-14) and the **rubber chin sling** (*Ernst,* 1927, 1932), consisting of a rubber binding about the chin and top of the head, can be evaluated somewhat more favorably; these bandages are most likely to be appropriate for support of the fractured maxilla in that they force the mandible against it. With the spatula dressing (see Fig. 4-2 C), the displaced maxilla also can be forced against the base of the skull and thus immobilized. In comminuted fractures, one must expect significant additional displacement in the process. All of these emergency bandages, however, cannot replace the emergency wire fixation tied to the teeth in mandibular fractures.

Interdental wire ligatures with intermaxillary fixation are used as emergency appliances for immobilization of the mandible.

The *Gilmer* **method** (1887) is a direct wiring between the maxillary and mandibular teeth.

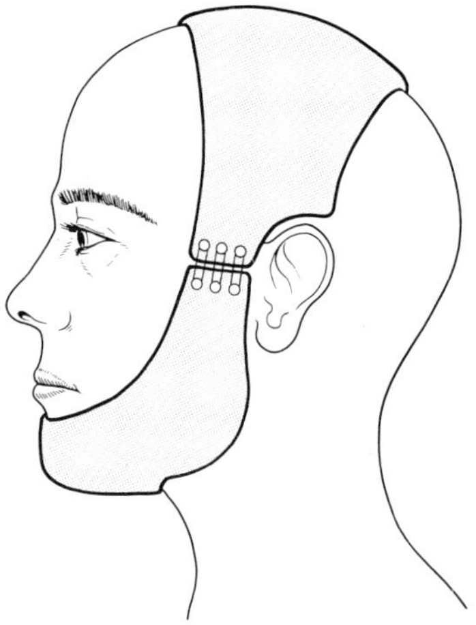

Fig. 4-14 Plaster head-chin cap.

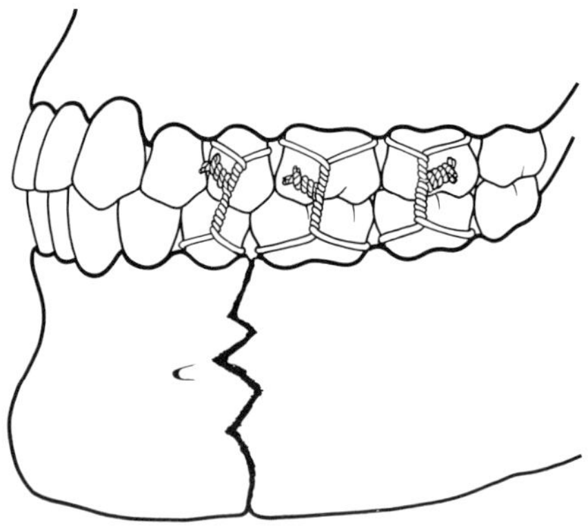

Fig. 4-15 Interdental wire ligatures with Gilmer's intermaxillary fixation.

Individual ligatures are placed on several teeth of the mandible and the maxilla. Intermaxillary fixation is established by twisting the upper wires to the lower ones (Fig. 4-15).

The *Kazanjian* **button** (1933) is made from two individual ligatures from adjacent teeth. The two twisted wires are retwisted. The end, shortened to 2.5 cm, is then shaped with forceps into a small button that serves to hold intermaxillary ligatures or rubber bands (Fig. 4-16).

The **eyelet method** (*Eby*, 1920; *Ivy*, 1922) also may be used for intermaxillary fixation in emergency situations. A wire is twisted about an instrument, e.g., a bur, to establish a loop. Both ends of the wire are drawn through the interproximal space of two adjacent teeth so that the loop lies vestibularly. One end of the wire is then drawn around the anterior tooth, the other around the posterior tooth. The posterior wire end is passed through the loop or between the interdental wires and twisted together with the anterior wire. Tie wires are drawn through the loops of the opposing upper and lower eyelet wires for intermaxillary fixation (Fig. 4-17).

The *Ernst* **ligature** (1927, 1932) is the one most frequently used for emergency wire fixation in Germany. Two adjacent teeth are looped in a figure of 8 with a wire. One wire end is drawn from the vestibule through the anterior interproximal space, the other through the posterior interproximal space; together they are returned to the vestibule through the central interproximal space. The ends, twisted together over the vestibular wire loop, are cut to approximately 5 mm and adapted to the gingival margin so that a hook is formed to take up intermaxillary tie wires of rubber bands (Fig. 4-18). The hook may be coated with cold-curing acrylic for better stabilization (*Grimm*, 1969). Not infrequently, the wire ends from opposing maxillary and mandibular ligatures are twisted together as in the *Gilmer* method.

Ligatures to bridge fracture lines in the mandible are usually insufficiently stable without intermaxillary fixation. The attempt, noted from time to time, to immobilize fragments by bridging the fracture site with ligatures from adjacent teeth (Fig. 4-19) should be rejected. This sort of "fixation" is entirely insufficient; in addition, the forces acting on the fragments lead to rapid loosening of the teeth involved.

When an emergency appliance becomes necessary for combined maxillary and mandibular fractures, it is best to combine intermaxillary

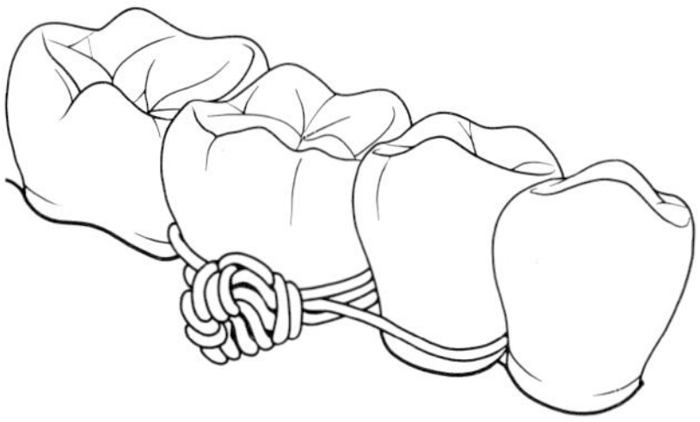

Fig. 4-16 Kazanjian button.

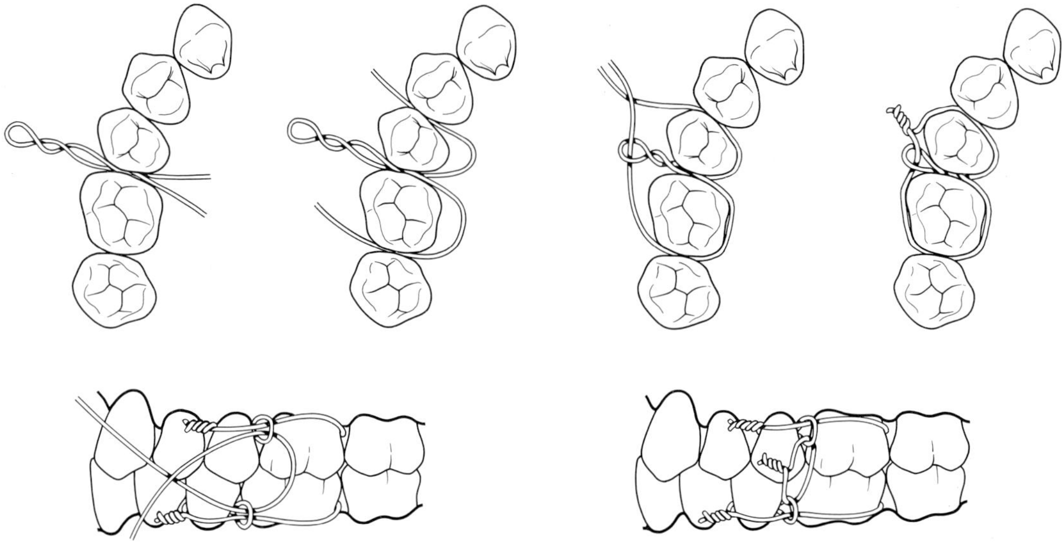

Fig. 4-17 Eyelet wires.

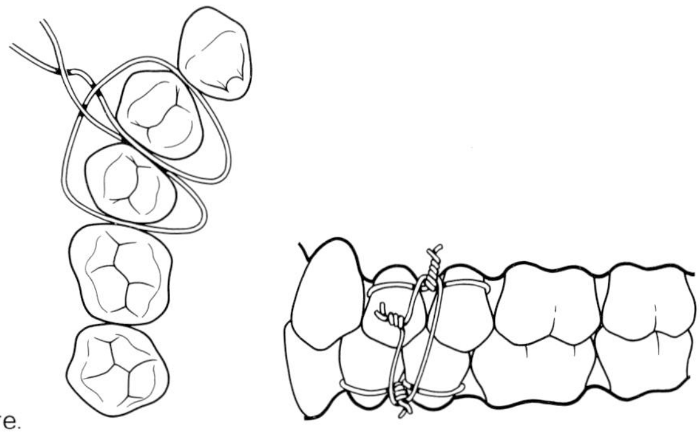

Fig. 4-18 Ernst ligature.

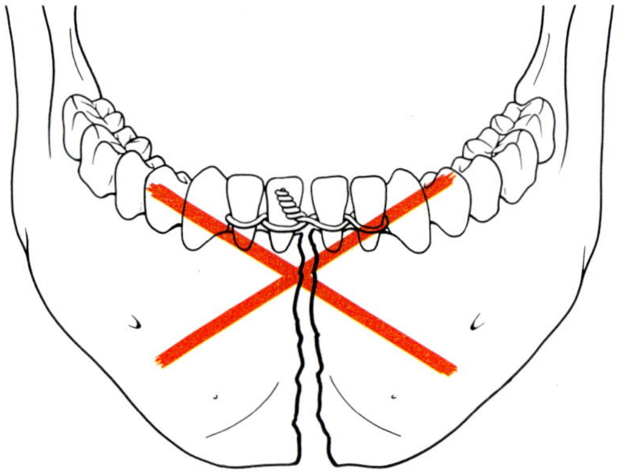

Fig. 4-19 Improper technique of emergency splinting! Ligatures which bridge the fracture gap are insufficiently stable without intermaxillary fixation. The fragments largely retain their mobility and the affected teeth become mobile in a short time.

fixation via ligatures with a head-chin cap. Given an intact zygomatic arch, circumzygomatic wiring may be used because this procedure can be carried out in a few minutes under ultra-short intravenous anesthesia.

1.2.4 Emergency Care of Soft Tissue Injuries

Soft tissue injuries should be treated definitively immediately, to the extent possible. Note should be taken in the maxillofacial region, however, that bone injuries must be reduced and immobilized simultaneously. An anatomically exact restoration of the facial skeleton is an unalterable prerequisite for optimal reconstruction of the soft tissues of the face, functionally and esthetically. The principle of proceeding from within to the outside was enunciated by *Ganzer* (1943) on the basis of his experiences in military surgery in the first and second world wars; similarly, *Schuchardt* (1966) as well as *Reichenbach* and *Grimm* (1969) promote it insistently. Unfortunately, in local hospitals—and even in specialized centers—the principle is often violated in that facial injuries are treated during the course of first aid; the surgeon providing the treatment believing that his care is definitive. Only then is the patient referred to a department of maxillofacial surgery, placing the maxillofacial surgeon in the position of having to decide whether to divide the soft tissue—now thoroughly edematous—in order to care properly for the jaw fracture, or to delay treatment of the fracture until the soft tissue is healed to the extent that the maxillofacial region is approachable without having to tear up the soft tissue.

For this reason, definitive care of soft tissue injuries in the region of the facial skeleton should be undertaken, when at all possible, where the potential exists for treatment of the jaw fractures by a department of maxillofacial surgery. Local hospitals not staffed in this way should be the site only of emergency care of soft tissue injuries, with the goal of bridging the period to the definitive care.

The **emergency treatment of soft tissue injuries** includes the following measures:

1. Hemostasis; gentle cleansing of the wound edges by rinsing with physiological saline solution or careful sponging with fine, moist pads. Necrotic and badly torn pieces of tissue, as well as foreign bodies (e.g., glass splinters) are removed. Dislocated teeth, the bony alveoli of which are destroyed and thus have become unsuitable for replantation, are extracted. Bone splinters, however, which remain connected to vital tissue, are retained. The otherwise customary wound excision is omitted.

2. The wound edges are adapted with sutures. Only atraumatic needles and sutures, to size 3-0, should be used in the region of the face. Injuries that cannot be treated definitively immediately may be adapted with wound dressings (e.g., Leukostrip, Steristrip) so that temporary adaptational sutures do not cause additional damage. Spaces should be covered with iodoform gauze or salve strips, loosely.
3. Antibiotic prophylaxis. This is especially required in open mandibular fractures and in all those instances in which there is suspicion of central midface fractures with the danger of opening of the intracranial space. In such cases, antibiotic therapy with a broad spectrum antibiotic is indicted.
4. Tetanus prophylaxis. If previous vaccination against tetanus can be established with certainty, a 0.5 ml tetanus toxoid injection serves as a booster dose. In the absence of such certainty, and in seriously injured persons even when certainty exists, 250 i.u. hyperimmunoglobulin (and for most seriously injured patients, 500 i.u.) and 0.5 ml tetanus toxoid are injected on contralateral body points.

The patient then should be transferred to a hospital with a department of maxillofacial surgery as soon as possible.
If immediate simultaneous definitive care of the soft tissue and bone injuries is not possible because of the poor general condition of the patient (brain trauma, severe thoracic or abdominal injuries, fat embolism), contrary to the rule, definitive soft tissue repair may be undertaken separately; treatment of the fracture then must be delayed until the soft tissue trauma has healed. The decision for such a procedure should be made in the specialized center in consultation with the maxillofacial surgeon. Local hospitals should be the site of definitive soft tissue repair without simultaneous fracture treatment only if the patient is absolutely unable to withstand transfer. Note here, however, that today even the most critically ill, multiply traumatized patient may be transported under the care of a specialist physician, with artificial respiration if necessary. The timely transfer of even polytraumatized subjects to a hospital with a department of oral and maxillofacial surgery therefore is almost always possible.

2. Definitive Treatment

2.1 General Diagnostic Procedures; Determination of Priorities in Multiple Injury Patients

The first treatment of maxillofacial injuries should be the definitive care whenever possible. As outlined above, emergency measures going beyond that required by the ability of the patient to withstand transfer are indicated only in special cases. As a rule, then, treatment planning does not revolve about the question of what must be done immediately and what may be delayed. Rather, the question should be posed as: Is **immediate treatment** necessary and possible, or may—or must—one wait **(delayed treatment)?**

This decision must be based on the general condition of the patient. Maintenance of respiration and circulation is usually the responsibility of the anesthesiologist. In cases of severe blood loss or anticipated lengthy surgery, the availability of adequate amounts of blood must be considered. Following the stabilization of vital functions, developing central complications must be excluded. This can lead to great difficulties in the unconscious patient if the eyes and their pupillary reflexes cannot be relied upon as diagnostic aids because of massive facial injuries. Often the condition of the patient does not permit thorough radiographic examination. But even simple survey films of the skull made in two planes generally are enough to demonstrate depressed fractures of the cranium. Such fractures are absolute indications for neurosurgical intervention. The availability of these films therefore is an absolute prerequisite for the decision to begin surgical maxillofacial treatment. If there is any indication at all of central nervous system involvement, a neurosurgical consultation should be requested. This is true especially whenever is any rhinorrhea, often recognizable from the formation of a watery pool in blood flowing out of the nose.

Because these preoperative examinations do not always permit establishment of the complete extent of the injuries, definitive surgical care should be undertaken only after all possible diagnostic measures have been completed and the quick availability of other potentially required specialists is assured. This is especially true of injuries in the region of the eyes; these must be treated without delay by a surgically experienced ophthalmologist.

If additional specialists must be consulted for diagnosis and treatment, a treatment plan with precise timing is prepared. Following maintenance of the vital functions of the central nervous system, treatment of eye injuries follows in priority. The care of facial and jaw injuries may be undertaken simultaneously with surgical treatment of extremities under some conditions. It is astounding again and again, how quickly recovery proceeds after definitive treatment of all injuries, even when the procedures have required many hours of time. In the establishment of priorities and the related planning of surgery and time, one should always remember that the face is important for identification of the human individual. Facial disfigurement can disturb a person more than crippling of an extremity. Errors and missed opportunities for reconstruction in the facial region cannot be covered with clothes. For later integration into society, a person with a facial disfigurement is incomparably more damaged than one with a crippled limb. Careful reconstruction of the esthetics of external facial expression must be seen in this sense as restoration and maintenance of a function of vital importance to the patient. The esthetics of the face here serves an important function. This should never be forgotten in the establishment of priorities.

2.2 Immediate Treatment

Immediate treatment is given on the day of the accident or no later than the following day. As a rule, it takes place outside the regular operating program. Indications for immediate treatment are provided largely by the type and extent of soft tissue injuries present. Jaw fractures without coexisting soft tissue injuries only under unusual conditions, as in continuing hemorrhage from the nose in maxillary fractures, require immediate reduction and immobilization.

An indication for immediate rigid internal fixation of mandibular fractures is provided by the collapse of the floor of the mouth and the tongue, with obstruction of the airway. In such cases definitive, stable fixation may be life-saving. It makes tracheotomy with all of the possible damage arising from it superfluous.

A further indication for immediate care may be based on accompanying injuries. Even when the injuries in the facial region, e.g., closed fractures, do not require immediate care, it may be desirable to make use of long-duration anesthesia administered, for example, for treatment of injuries to the extremities.

The treatment of combined bone-soft tissue injuries is undertaken in accordance with the principles of *Ganzer* (1943) from the inside to the outside (*Schuchardt*, 1966; *Reichenbach* and *Grimm*, 1969). It begins with care of tongue, floor of the mouth, and palatal injuries. Reduction and immobilization of bone fragments follows. The decision about conservative or surgical fracture treatment being necessary depends on the conditions. In every case, exact and stable reconstruction of the bony skeleton should be sought, leading to restoration of function as quickly as possible.

Soft tissue injuries of the mandible and in the periorbital region not infrequently permit access to the underlying bone. Such "natural" approaches should be used to the extent possible in surgical treatment of the fractures.

The reconstruction of the facial skeleton is the indispensable prerequisite for the subsequent care of injuries of the soft components of the face. The extraordinarily good blood supply of the facial region affords good conditions for the healing of torn tissue fragments. For this reason, maintenance of every piece of tissue still reasonably supplied with circulation is necessary. Wound excision to eliminate microorganisms is not necessary; careful cleansing by washing with hydrogen peroxide solution suffices. Glass splinters lying deep in a wound sometimes are not recognizable even after careful washing and sponging. If suspicion of deep glass splinters exists, the wound should be palpated carefully with the fingertips. Completely crushed soft tissue is excised. Portions of the face that have been torn away may be preserved by microsurgical measures, by anastomosing the supplying and draining vessels. Tissue defects resulting in spite of such measures should be closed with local flaps whenever possible. An esthetically satisfactory restoration of the surface of the skin requires close closure with the finest atraumatic needles; the strain on the closure should be relieved by the placement of adhesive strips. Discharge of secretions must be assured through placement of suction drains (Redon, Minivac) in extensive soft tissue injuries.

Soft tissue damage not involving the lips and the nares may be restored without previous restoration of the facial skeleton in an emergency. Nevertheless, in such cases too, bone and soft tissue injuries should be treated in a single procedure if possible, to spare the patient multiple surgeries.

2.3 Delayed Treatment

The treatment of injuries of the maxillofacial region should, in principle, be undertaken as early as possible. This is particularly true of soft tissue injuries, although here too it is possible—accepting certain disadvantages—to wait a few days after temporary measures if the circumstances demand it (*Schuchardt*, 1966). *Reichenbach* and *Grimm* (1966) reported successfully treating facial wounds 48 or more hours after injury. In many cases, it is possible, then, to wait until the bone fractures can be treated as well. Premature treatment of soft tissue injuries without simultaneous restoration of the continuity of the facial skeleton therefore is indicated only if the general condition of the patient is so poor that fracture reduction cannot be undertaken within the first week.
Bone fractures without soft tissue injury need not be treated immediately. Such therapy can follow within the framework of the normal surgical program. But here too, the principle holds: As early as possible. Waiting too long increases the danger of fracture line infection, quite apart from the delay of healing. Jaw fractures within the dental arch are open fractures as a rule. The relatively thin gingiva of the alveolar process tears in most instances, or the fracture surfaces have a connection to the oral cavity through the discontinuity in the periosteum of a tooth in the fracture line or the pericoronal space of an impacted third molar. In this way, detritus or bacteria can find their way into the fracture gap. Even with barely noticeable displacement, the fragments move against each other with each swallow or speaking motion, thus pumping saliva contaminated with bacteria into the fracture line. Only rarely is the open mandibular fracture free of infection two or three weeks after the injury in untreated patients. Fracture line infections in the mandible frequently lead to chronic osteomyelitis and in the healing stage to a pseudoarthrosis.
The danger of infection is not as great in fractures of the midface. Nonetheless, the danger exists of the development of meningitis here, if there is a fracture of the base of the skull simultaneously. If the orbital floor is disrupted in midfacial fractures, displacement of the eyeball may occur, with resulting double vision. The treatment of such fractures becomes increasingly difficult if one waits too long. It is therefore of special significance that such orbital injuries be recognized quickly, and treated. The surgical reduction and immobilization of a sunken orbital floor and the surgical revision of the orbit, with freeing and repositioning of the jammed and possibly herniated (into the sinus) orbital tissue are procedures that should be undertaken early during the course of the entire treatment, if possible.

Delayed care must not be postponed too long. If possible, it should be undertaken within the first week and not later than 10 days after the injury (*Krüger*, 1972, 1974). During this time the general condition of a severely injured patient either has improved so much that definitive treatment becomes possible or it is so bad that complete restoration cannot be carried out within a foreseeable period. An important prerequisite for delayed treatment of mandibular and midface fractures is prevention of infection through the administration of high doses of antibiotics immediately after the accident. This holds for all fractures opening into the mouth and frontobasal skull fractures. This therapy must be continued for at least a week after definitive treatment of the fractures.

2.4 Principles of Treatment of Mandibular, Condylar and Midface Fractures

Mandibular fractures are treated either indirectly with immobilizing splints or directly by osteosynthesis of the fracture fragments.

Indirect fixation by means of monomaxillary fixation is sufficient, only if both—or all—fragments can be grasped securely by the splint elements. In a large fraction of the cases, however, this is not possible; then intermaxillary fixation must be undertaken with the maxilla in centric occlusion. This is done either rigidly with wires or elastically with rubber bands. In another option, many very small bands are used to provide rigid immobilization; the force of contraction then attained is so great that movement of the mandible is prevented. Usually, rigid fixation is used for three weeks and elastic immobilization for three weeks thereafter.

Direct fixation is undertaken either with interosseous wiring or rigid internal fixation with the aid of bone plates and screws. Intermaxillary fixation is not required with functionally stable osteosynthesis, while interosseous wiring needs supplemental intermaxillary fixation as a rule.

In **fractures of the condylar process,** one differentiates between functional therapy with activator-guided mouth opening exercises (*Reichenbach*, 1957, 1958) and intermaxillary fixation. The latter is indicated in condylar fractures with minor displacement, in which healing in the anatomically correct position may be anticipated. The treatment is not different from that of conservative therapy of mandibular fractures. Functional therapy is used in all displaced and dislocated condylar fractures which cannot be reduced, the majority of cases. The emphasis here is on the maintenance of a tolerable degree of function with anatomical restoration being waived. If there is some occlusal disturbance simultaneously, short-term intermaxillary fixation is indicated before functional therapy. The occlusion is adjusted with tight intermaxillary rubber bands; these are used for approximately 8 days and then replaced by elastic bands. Two or three weeks later, activator therapy is initiated.

Direct fixation with wire sutures or bone plating is indicated only in deep, displaced condylar process base fractures. Bilateral condylar process fractures tend to induce dorsal displacement of the mandible. As a rule, extension therapy is necessary, in which the mandible is drawn forward. Later, activator therapy must be provided.

Midface (*Le Fort*) **fractures** require approximately six weeks of fixation to the skull. This may be attained with an external fixation appliance on a head cap or with internal or interosseous wiring. As a rule, intermaxillary wire fixation in centric occlusion also is necessary for approximately three weeks. A maxilla consolidated in a displaced position may be mobilized with intermaxillary rubber bands even three to four weeks following an accident and thus be repositioned. Following such mobilization in older fractures, placement of bone grafts at the fracture sites is frequently necessary in addition to skull fixation and intermaxillary wire fixation.

In selected instances, the Haloframe may be used for immobilization of the maxilla. This is a metal ring attached to the cranial vault with transcutaneous screws, through which the maxilla is suspended on transbuccal wires (see Fig. 6-30).

Rigid internal fixation by means of bone plates and screws is also possible in midface fractures; in this case intermaxillary fixation is not required.

These fundamentals of therapy, to be expanded in the following chapters, must be modified when **combined fractures** exist. The usual treatment does not change much when there are simultaneous fractures of the maxilla and mandible. The replacement of intermaxillary wires with elastic rubber bands, customary in fractures of the mandible, should be avoided because the maxilla would be mobilized through movements of the mandible. Intermaxillary guidance is no longer possible, therefore, after removal of the intermaxillary wires. When there is a bilateral fracture of the mandible in the molar region or outside the dental arches, the intermaxillary wires are left in place somewhat longer. Following their removal, the mandibular fixation appliance may be removed as well. If there is a fracture within the dental arch, the mandibular splint remains in place without intermaxillary fixation until the maxillary appliance is removed.

Dorsal displacement of the midface is prevented by intermaxillary wires if the mandible is supported securely against the skull by the condylar processes. In bilateral condylar process fractures and displaced fractures in the ascending rami, this support is missing, so that the maxilla and the mandible can slip dorsally together. If it is not possible to assure adequate support through osteosynthesis, the dorsal displacement must be prevented through the use of an extension bar as suggested by *Stenzel* (1902). In treatment with intra- and extraoral appliances this extension bar is attached additionally to the head cap. A special head cap for mounting the extension bar must be prepared after internal wire fixation. The maxillary splint or arch bar is attached by means of a lightly tensed wire to the extension bar mounted sagittally in the midline in front of the face (see Fig. 6-28).

Functional treatment of condylar process fractures cannot be carried out immediately if there is a simultaneous maxillary fracture requiring intermaxillary fixation. A compromise must be struck in this situation: functional therapy is delayed until the intermaxillary wires are removed. An activator may be inserted even when the splint or the arch bar of the maxilla must remain with internal wire fixation.

Mandibular as well as maxillary fractures can be treated with rigid internal fixation by means of bone plates and screws when they are combined with fractures of the head or neck of the condyle which require functional therapy. This type of stabilization is advantageous because intermaxillary fixation is not necessary and functional treatment of the condylar fracture can begin at once.

After completion of definitive treatment, radiographic films should be prepared as quickly as possible in two planes. These are required for documentation and determination of the need for any further treatment. If the films provide any indication of inadequate reduction of the fragments, further measures—including an open reduction—may be necessary, particularly after conservative treatment.

2.5 Nutrition and Aftercare

Feeding of patients after treatment of jaw fractures demands that the special condition of the oral cavity be considered. Splints, intermaxillary fixation, mucosal injuries, and postoperative edema hinder food uptake significantly. Only **clear liquids** can be taken orally, including tea, bouillon and fruit juices. Because this diet is inadequate in calories, supplemental intravenous infusions containing amino acids, fructose, fat emulsions, electrolytes and vitamins must be given. A gastric feeding tube is the best means to provide adequate caloric intake in these patients; it is introduced through the nose and may remain for longer periods. The tube feedings can be compounded from ordinary foods such as milk, eggs, sugar, flour and oil in the kitchen. Commercially produced diets are available as well, often as dried powders. The stomach tube often irritates the esophageal and gastric mucosa, leading to gastritis and reflux esophagitis. The patient may complain of heartburn. When gastric tubes are left in situ for longer periods, therefore, antacids should be given routinely.

A stomach tube should not be placed in an unconscious patient for purposes of feeding because that would increase the risk of vomiting. For this reason, nutrition is provided to unconscious patients only by parenteral infusion.

Following completion of healing of intraoral wounds, the patient can take calorie-rich fluids orally. The **liquid jaw fracture diet** is prepared in kitchen mixers and strained. Each day, 150 to 200 g protein, 300 to 350 g carbohydrate and 80 to 100 g fat should be given (*Smith*, 1965; *Perko*, 1966). Supplementing this diet, one should give regular doses of vitamin C and the B vitamin group, as well as the fat-soluble vitamins A, D and K. The liquid diet, containing at least 2000 ml of water each day, should be given to the patient with a feeding cup (Fig. 4-20). *Rheinwald* (1965) suggests a plastic bottle, the contents of which are squeezed into the oral cavity through a tube. Even when the mandible is absolutely immobilized with intermaxillary wire ligatures, it

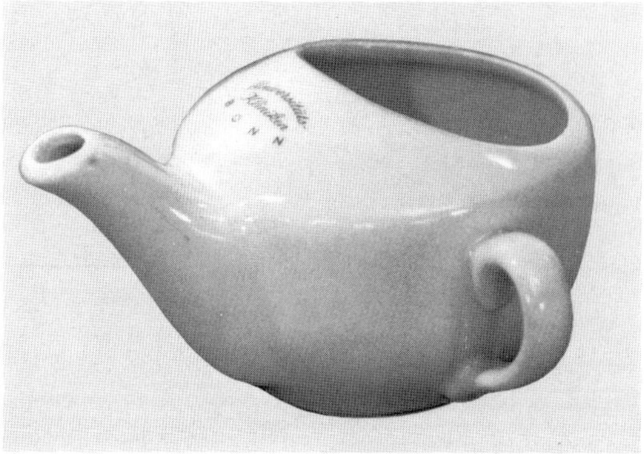

Fig. 4-20 Feeding cup for liquid feedings during intermaxillary fixation.

is possible for the patient to swallow liquids through gaps in the dentition or distal to the teeth when the nutrient has been placed into the vestibule. It is important that the liquid be appetizing and varied and that flavor be adjusted so that the patient is not dependent on a monotonous diet for several weeks.

This kind of nutrition from a liquid diet demands a significant adjustment on the part of the patient, one that may lead to psychological damage. Young patients. especially, complain of constant hunger pangs that arise from physical inactivity and that are only increased by inability to work (*Schönberger*, 1969). Appetite-reducing drugs are proposed for such patients by *Rheinwald* (1965) and *Scheunemann* (1957); *Schönberger* (1969) believes the provision of filling materials to be superior. As most of the patients lose weight initially, *Geddes* (1963) proposes regular weighing.

Special problems arise in the feeding of diabetics. The required changes in diet can complicate the adjustment of blood sugar immensely and thus lead to increased sensitivity to infections, with all the negative consequences that may have on healing of bone and soft tissue.

Following the replacement of intermaxillary ligatures with rubber bands, patients can take **semi-solid diets**. The patient removes the rubber bands while eating, and then replaces them. After increasing the chewing stress slowly, the patient is returned to a **normal diet** following the final removal of the splints.

Careful **oral hygiene** is required during the entire period of fracture treatment with intraoral devices. The oral cavity, the teeth, and the splints themselves must be kept meticulously clean. At first this is done by the nursing staff. After each meal, the teeth and devices are cleaned carefully with a spray. In addition, rinses with oral disinfectants are required.

As soon as conditions permit, the patient should become personally responsible for his oral hygiene. From the oral vestibule, the splints can be scrubbed with a toothbrush until all food debris is removed, even with intermaxillary fixation. The patient must convince himself with a mirror that everything is clean; then he rinses with an oral rinse. Only when the patient has learned the technique of keeping the intraoral devices clean is he discharged from the hospital.

If oral hygiene is neglected during the time that the devices are worn, **gingivitis** or **stomatitis** may arise. When the fracture gap extends into the mouth, the danger of its infection is especially great.

Soiling of the devices furthermore favors the development of dental caries; such lesions cannot always be avoided entirely, even with careful oral hygiene. The narrow spaces between the arch bar and the enamel surface of the teeth is not accessible to mechanical cleaning with toothbrush and oral sprays. Thus, bacteria and food debris may become lodged here, to elicit demineralization processes. Following removal

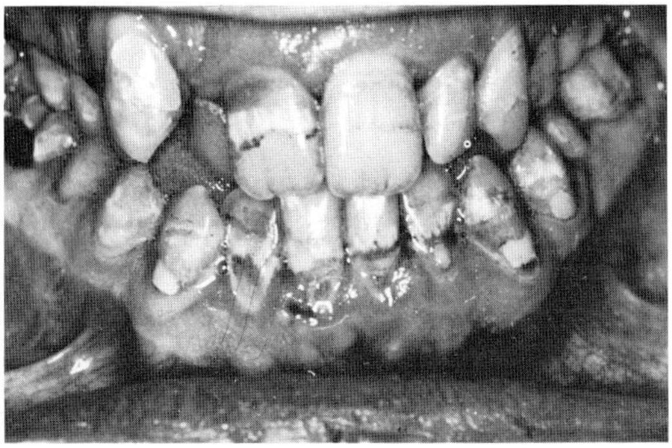

Fig. 4-21 A Demineralization processes and dental caries after treatment with arch bars for six weeks.

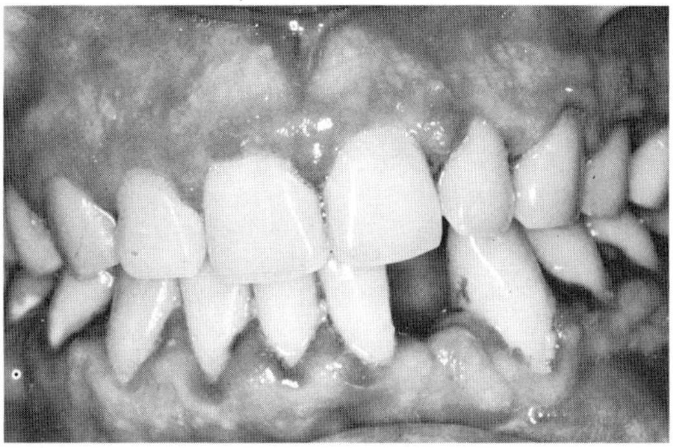

Fig. 4-21 B Undamaged enamel after pretreatment of the tooth crowns with a fluoride solution before placing the arch bars which had remained in place for six weeks.

of the arch bars, these regions appear as white spots or, after long periods of wear of the arch bars, as frank caries on the vestibular coronal surfaces at those sites where the device touched the dental arch (*Krüger* and *Chrissafis*, 1971; Fig. 4-21 A). When placing the arch bars, therefore, one should try to keep these areas as small as possible and also to assure that soiling of the inaccesible spaces be reduced to a minimum by regular, careful cleaning of the accessible areas after each meal.

In addition, intensive pretreatment of the tooth crowns with a fluoride solution can reduce the acid solubility of dental enamel to the extent that the caries-promoting devices can remain in place for six weeks or more without damage to the enamel, provided that careful oral hygiene is practiced and that a dentifrice containing fluoride is used (*Krüger* and *Chrissafis*, 1971, Fig. 4-21 B). The topical application of fluoride, furthermore, should be repeated at weekly intervals until the arch bars or splints are removed.

The cleaning problem in the oral cavity is significantly reduced after rigid internal fixation. In the presence of oral mucosal injuries, a clear liquid diet or a special diet is indicated for the period of wound healing, i.e., for the first 8 to 10 days. When the soft tissue has healed, no special care is required any longer, although maximal chewing force should not be exerted. A diet containing excessively hard substances should be avoided for the first three weeks.

All fracture patients should be seen regularly once or twice each week following their discharge from the hospital. At that time, occlusal relationships, seat of the splints, condition of the oral mucosa and teeth, and progress in reduction of soft tissue swelling should be checked. Teeth, gingiva and devices should be cleaned thoroughly with a spray and the teeth treated with a fluoride preparation as described above. After rigid internal fixation, these measures are required only if a tension band arch bar was placed.

Occlusion should be checked again following removal of the devices in all patients. Sometimes functionally generated path (FGP) is required. If occlusal disturbances are found, grinding is required. Sometimes prosthodontic measures must be used to supplement grinding. Dentures must be replaced in many instances.

Before the patient is discharged from treatment, another radiographic study should be made. As a rule, the fracture line is still easily recognizable six weeks after the accident, even when the fracture is clinically solid. Sometimes after conservative treatment of mandibular fractures, some spring remains in the fragments after removal of the splints.

Functional activator treatment of temporomandibular joint fractures can extend for a period

of three months or more. Functional disturbances such as lateral deviation when the mouth is opened, clicking, and joint pain, if present, should be noted in the discharge diagnosis.
The removal of dynamic compression plates (DCP) should be undertaken no earlier than after three months. Lag screws, miniplates and wire ligatures as a rule need not be removed.

All patients should be checked again six months after the accident. A further radiographic follow-up examination should be done. Occlusion and function should be checked again. If indicated, further grinding or prosthetic balancing may be necessary. In addition, it must be decided whether scars or soft tissue injuries require further revision.

References

Deane, R. S., and E. L. Mills (1970)
Prolonged nasotracheal intubation in adults: a successor and adjunct to tracheotomy. Anesth. Analg. Curr Res. 49: 89

Denecke, H. J. (1968)
Die Tracheotomie in der Unfallchirurgie des Gesichtes und des Halses. (Tracheotomy in accident surgery of the face and the neck.) Arch. Ohr.-, Nas.- u. Kehlk.-Heilk. 191: 352

Denecke, H. J. (1971)
Fehler und Gefahren bei der Tracheotomie. (Errors and dangers in tracheotomy.) Arch. Ohr.-, Nas.- u. Kehlk.-Heilk. 199: 393

Dingman, R. O., and P. Natvig (1964)
Surgery of facial fractures. Philadelphia, W. B. Saunders Co.

Eby, J. D. (1920)
Principles of orthodontia in the treatment of maxillafacial injuries. Intern. J. Orthodont. 6: 273

Ernst, F. (1927)
Die zahnärztliche Behandlung der Unterkieferbrüche. (Dental treatment of mandibular fractures.) In Kirschner M. and O. Nordmann: Die Chirurgie. (Surgery.) Urban & Schwarzenberg, Berlin, vol. 4,1, p. 842

Ernst, F. (1932)
Die Schienenverbände bei Unter- und Oberkieferbrüchen. (Splints in fractures of the mandible and the maxilla.) In Bruhn, C., A. Kantorowicz, and C. Partsch: Handbuch der Zahnheilkunde. (Handbook of dentistry.) 4th. ed. Munich, J. F. Bergmann, vol. 1, p. 115

Feldmann, H. (1973)
Nasenbluten als Notfallsituation. (Nosebleed as an emergency.) Z. Laryng. Rhinol. 52: 314

Froeb, H. F., and B. M. Kim (1964)
Tracheotomy and respiratory dead space in emphysema. J. appl. Physiol. 19: 92

Ganzer, H. (1943)
Die Kriegsverletzungen des Gesichts und des Gesichtsschädels. (War injuries of the face and the facial skull.) Leipzig, J. A. Barth

Garzon, A. A., B. Seltzer and K. E. Karlson (1963)
Influence of tracheotomy cannula size on work of breathing. Surg. Forum 14: 219

Geddes, D. A. M. (1963)
Diets for patients with maxillo-facial injuries. Brit. dent. J. 115: 235

Gilmer, T. L. (1887)
A case of fracture of the lower jaw with remarks on treatment. Arch. Dent. 4: 388

Glas, W. W., D. J. King and A. Loi (1962)
Complications of tracheotomy. Arch. Surg. 85: 56

Grimm, G. (1969)
Allgemeine Grundsätze der Versorgung Kiefer-Gesichts-Verletzter. (General principles in the care of the maxillofacially injured.) In Reichenbach, E.: Traumatologie im Kiefer-Gesichts-Bereich. (Traumatology of the maxillofacial region.) Munich, J. A. Barth, p. 113

Holinger, P., K. Johnston and G. Anison (1955)
Tracheotomy. Surg. Clin. N. Amer. 35: 21

Ivy, R. H. (1922)
Observations of fractures of the mandible. J. Amer. med. Ass. 79: 295

Kazanjian, V. H. (1933)
Treatment of automobile injuries of the face and jaws. J. Amer. dent. Ass: 20: 757

Kazanjian, V. H., and J. M. Converse (1974)
Surgical treatment of facial injuries. 3rd ed. Baltimore, Williams & Wilkins Co.

Kornmesser, H. J. (1972)
Über die Tracheotomie im Kindesalter und konsekutive Stenosen. (Tracheotomy in childhood and consecutive stenoses.) HNO (Berl.) 20: 136

Krüger, E. (1972)
Grundsätzliche Bemerkungen zur Versorgung von Kiefer- und Gesichtsverletzungen. (Fundamentals in the care of maxillofacial injuries.) In Gütgemann, A. and P. Eckert: Besondere Probleme bei Erstversorgung von schwerverletzten Patienten. (Special problems in immediate care of seriously injured patients.) Bad Homburg v.d.H., Wissenschaftliche Informationen Fresenius, p. 23

Krüger, E. (1974)
Lehrbuch der chirurgischen Zahn-, Mund- und Kieferheilkunde. (Textbook of oral and maxillofacial diseases.) 1st ed. 1974, 3rd. ed. 1979 Berlin, Buch- und Zeitschriften-Verlag „Die Quintessenz", vol. 2

Krüger, E., and S. Chrissafis (1971)
Kariesprophylaxe durch lokale Anwendung von Aminfluoriden bei der Versorgung von Kieferbruchpatienten mit der Drahtkunststoffschiene nach Schuchardt. (Caries prevention through topical application of amine fluoride in jaw fracture patients treated with Schuchardt's wire acrylic arch bar.) Dtsch. zahnärztl. Z. 26: 1227

Kwapis, W. (1954)
Early management of maxillofacial war injuries. J. oral Surg. 12: 293

Lanz, T., and W. Wachsmuth (1955)
Praktische Anatomie. (Practical anatomy.) Berlin – Göttingen – Heidelberg, Springer

Messerklinger, W. (1972)
Chirurgie der Luftröhre. Tracheotomie. (Surgery of the trachea. Tracheotomy.) In Naumann, H. H.: Kopf- und Hals-Chirurgie. (Head and neck surgery.) Stuttgart, G. Thieme, vol. 1, p. 337

Nelson, T. G., and W. F. Bowers (1957)
Tracheotomy–Indications, advantages, techniques, complications and results. Analysis of three hundred ten recent operations. J. Amer. med. Ass. 164, 1530

Nicholas, T. H., and G. F. Rumer (1960)
Emergency airway–a plan of action. J. Amer. med. Ass. 174: 1930

Oliver, P., J. R. Richardson, W. R. Clubb and C. A. Flake (1962)
Tracheotomy in children. New Engl. J. Med. 267: 631

Perko, M. (1966)
Das Ernährungsproblem nach kieferchirurgischen Operationen oder Verletzungen im Kieferbereich. (Feeding problem following oral surgery or injuries in the region of the jaw.) Schweiz. Mschr. Zahnheilk. 76: 396

Reichel, G. (1967)
Krankheitszustände mit respiratorischer Insuffizienz. (Disease states with respiratory insufficiency.) Z. prakt. Anästh. Wiederbeleb. 2: 77

Reichenbach, E. (1957)
Verletzungen der Kiefer- und Gesichtsknochen und der benachbarten Weichteile. (Injuries of the maxillofacial bones and the adjacent soft tissues.) In Häupl, K., W. Meyer, and K. Schuchardt: Die Zahn-, Mund- und Kieferheilkunde. (Dentistry.) Munich – Berlin, Urban & Schwarzenberg, vol. III/1, p. 639

Reichenbach, E. (1958)
Probleme der Frakturenbehandlung beim wachsenden Schädel. (Problems of fracture therapy in the growing skull.) Fortschr. Kiefer- u. Gesichtschir. 4: 213

Reichenbach, E., and G. Grimm (1969)
Grundzüge der Versorgung von mit Frakturen einhergehenden Weichteilverletzungen des Gesichts. (Guidelines for the care of soft tissue injuries concurrent with fractures in the face.) In Reichenbach, E.: Traumatologie im Kiefer-Gesichts-Bereich. (Traumatology of the maxillofacial region.) Munich, J. A. Barth, p. 169

Rheinwald, U. (1965)
Die Ernährung des durch Trauma an der Nahrungsaufnahme behinderten Patienten. (The diet of the patient hindered in eating because of trauma.) Dtsch. zahnärztl. Z. 20: 610

Rowe, N. L., and H. C. Killey (1968)
Fractures of the facial skeleton. 2nd ed. Edinburg, Livingstone

Ruben, H. (1961)
Investigation of upper airway problems in resuscitation. Anesthesiology 22: 271

Rügheimer, E. (1977)
Die Tracheotomie. (Tracheotomy.) In Benzer, H., R. Frey, W. Hügin, and O. Mayrhofer: Lehrbuch der Anaesthesiologie, Reanimation und Intensivtherapie. (Textbook of anesthesiology, reanimation and intensive care.) 4th ed. Berlin, Springer, p. 671

Scheunemann, H. (1957)
Klinische Untersuchungen über therapeutische Möglichkeiten mit Preludin in der Kieferchirurgie. (Clinical studies of the therapeutic possibilities of Preludin in maxillofacial surgery.) Dtsch. zahnärztl. Z. 12: 1240

Schönberger, A (1969)
Pflege und Ernährung Kiefer-Gesichts-Verletzter. (Care and feeding of the maxillofacially injured.) In Reichenbach, E.: Traumatologie im Kiefer-Gesichts-Bereich. (Traumatology in the maxillofacial region.) Munich, J. A. Barth, p. 407

Schuchardt, K. (1966)
Grundsätzliches zur Versorgung von kombinierten Weichteil-Knochenverletzungen im Gesichts-Kieferbereich. (Fundamentals of care of combined soft tissue-bone injuries in the maxillofacial region.) Fortschr. Kiefer- u. Gesichtschir. 11: 25

Schüle, H. (1976)
Fortschritte und Schwerpunkte der Behandlung von Mund-Kiefer-Gesichts-Verletzungen. (Advances and emphasis of treatment of oral and maxillofacial injuries.) Fortschr. Kiefer- u. Gesichtschir. 21: 272

Smith, J. F. (1965)
Nutritional maintenance of the oral fracture patient. Oral Surg. 19: 705

Stenzel (1902)
Demonstrationen eines Extensionsverbandes für gewisse Brüche des Unterkiefers. (Demonstrations of an extension bandage for certain fractures of the mandible.) Verh. Dtsch. Ges. Chir. 31: 83

Tandler, J. (1923)
Topographische Anatomie dringlicher Operationen. (Topographic anatomy of urgent operations.) Berlin, Springer

Tyler, J. M. (1961)
Failure to improve effective ventilation on shifting from mouth to tracheotomy breathing in clinically stable emphysema. New Engl. J. Med. 265: 414

Vicq d'Azyr, F. (1805)
Quoted by Dingman, R. O. and P. Natvig (1964)

Vogler, W., and M. Vogler (1966)
Der Einfluß der Notfallslagerung auf die Regurgitation von Mageninhalt. (The effect of the emergency position on regurgitation of stomach contents.) Presented at the first Anesthesia Congress of the Anesthesiology section of the Deutsche Gesellschaft für klinische Medizin, Borkum; quoted by Grimm, G., (1969)

Chapter 5

Fundamentals of Healing of Fractures of the Facial Skull

1. Biomechanics

Herbert Niederdellmann

The concept of biomechanics includes, among other things, the biological reaction of bone to certain mechanical stress such as is caused, for example, by muscular forces. In the treatment of fractures, special attention should be given to biomechanics because static and dynamic events may affect the course of fracture healing in a variety of ways (see section 5.2).
The purpose of all therapy of fractures is the restoration of the original form and function. An important requirement to this end is immobilization, which may be achieved through internal or external means. External means include tooth-borne splints and arch bars and extraoral appliances. Internal means include wire ligatures as well as screws and plates for internal fixation; these, in contrast to external appliances, act directly on the bone.
In conservative treatment of fractures, external appliances are used as a rule. Intermaxillary immobilization, oriented exclusively to occlusion, is established with splints attached directly to the teeth. Immobilization of the jaws in their entirety reduces forces acting externally on the fracture gap to insignificance and leads to static relationships for the duration of the treatment, and thus to healing of the fracture with the aid of external appliances.
This treatment alone is insufficient for displaced fractures. In such cases it is necessary to restore as much as possible the anatomic relationships in the region of the bone and then to immobilize the restoration. Such immobilization can be achieved here by a combination of internal and external devices or by internal appliances alone. The latter can be used effectively, however, only when due consideration is given to the biomechanical conditions which exist. For fracture treatment free of problems and for healing free of complications, understanding of muscle function is necessary because muscular functions elicit the characteristic deformations of bone; these explain the force relationships.
All bones are stressed toward bending by contractions of the musculature; in some regions of bone the forces are predominantly compressive and in others tensile forces predominate. Accordingly, the internal appliances must be located at those sites where tensile forces are to be absorbed, thus to reduce the compressive forces appearing simultaneously on the opposite side and thereby distributing the forces equally over the entire fracture surface (Fig. 5.1-1). This placement of the force-transferring device corresponds to the tension band principle known in mechanics (*Pauwels*, 1940). The principle is usually attainable in long bones, but in the region of the facial skull it is not achievable, as a rule, because of topographic circumstances.

1.1 Mandible

Its elasticity of shape in its various functions is a decisive parameter for the biomechanical constellation of the mandible.
The deformation of the mandible during mouth opening may be described as follows: At maximal mouth opening, the forces of the mylohyoid muscle, the geniohyoid muscle, and the mandibular branch of the digastric muscle lead to an upward bending and fanning out of the teeth in the region of the alveolar process of the hori-

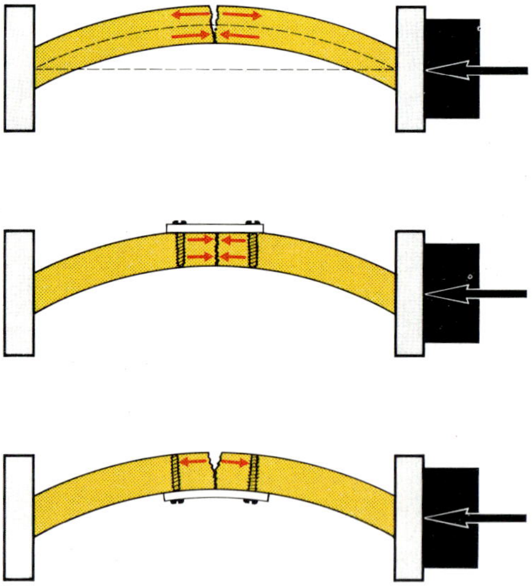

Fig. 5.1-1 Tension band principle, explained with a transverse beam that is stressed on its upper surface by tension and on its lower surface by pressure forces. Placement of an osteosynthesis plate at its upper edge only eliminates tension strains.

zontal rami while the masseter-pterygoid muscles and the temporal muscles are elongated maximally (Fig. 5. 1-2)

In addition, the condyles move medially through the action of the pterygoid muscles which pull at an angle of about 35° medially (*Schumacher*, 1961). This leads to lingual narrowing of the dental arch and related inward tilting of the coronal tooth segments. Anteriorly, the result is closer approximation of the single teeth to each other. The significance of all of this is that in maximal opening, compressive strains are exerted in the anterior section of the mandible in the alveolar process region to the level of the canines, while tractive forces are exerted distal thereto.

Quite similar conditions are found in edge-to-edge bite and in centric relation. In edge-to-edge bite, the mandible, supported by the temporomandibular joints and by the incisal edges of the anterior teeth, is deflected cranially by the masseter-pterygoid sling and the temporalis muscle. In forceful closure of the dental arches to closed bite, the support of the mandible by the posterior teeth and the strong mesiocranial pull of the masseter muscles lead to deflection of the horizontal mandibular rami. Simultaneously there is torsion of the body of the mandible with a lateral movement of the angle of the mandible and the basal portions of the horizontal ramus. This implies that compression occurs in the anterior region of the alveolar process to the region of the canines and tension occurs distally when these functions are carried out.

In swallowing and in maximal mandibular protrusion, as well as in all lateral excursions, there is a fanning out of the entire dental arch (Fig. 5. 1-3). Under such functional loads, therefore, tractive forces are exerted on the entire mandibular arch.

Although there are differences of opinion about the situation of the muscles in these functions, there is unanimity about the resulting forces (*Weber-Thedy*, 1964; *Marx*, 1966; *Jung*, 1952; *Köck* and *Sander*, 1978; *Siebert*, 1978; *Niederdellmann* et al., 1979).

In molar occlusion, the teeth of the maxilla and the mandible close to each other on the working side. This approximation of individual teeth decreases continuously across the midline so that a condition characterized by the existence of an interocclusal gap results. For the region of the alveolar process on the working side, this leads to development of compressive strain, decreasing in magnitude to the balance side (Fig. 5. 1-4).

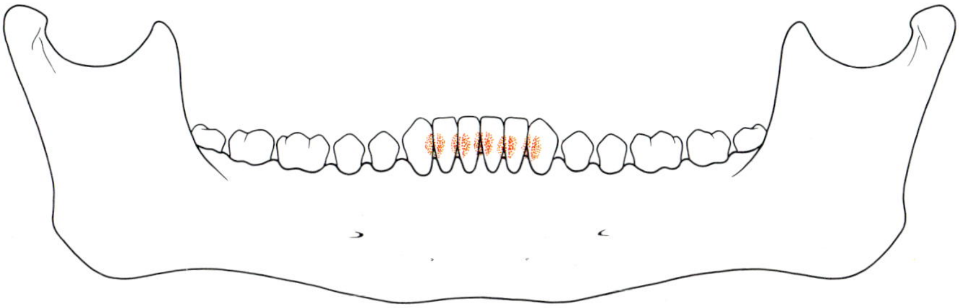

Fig. 5.1-2 Elastic deformation of the mandible during mouth opening, edge-to-edge bite, and maximum centric relation. Distal to the canine region the alveolar process is bent upwards and a fanning out of the teeth occurs; in the anterior tooth region it is stressed by pressure.

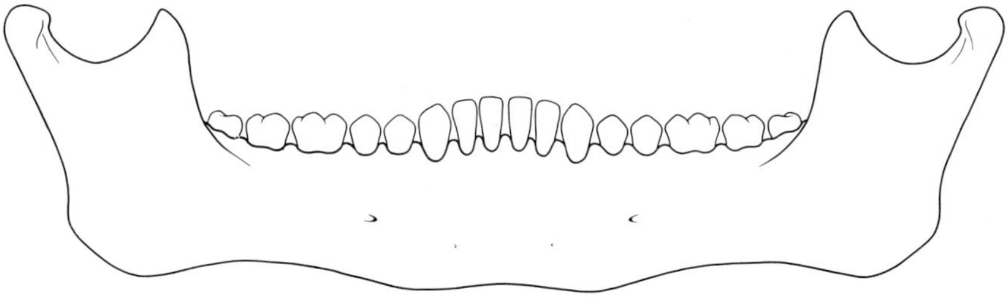

Fig. 5.1-3 In swallowing, in maximum mandibular protrusion, and in all lateral excursions, there is a fanning out of the entire dental arch.

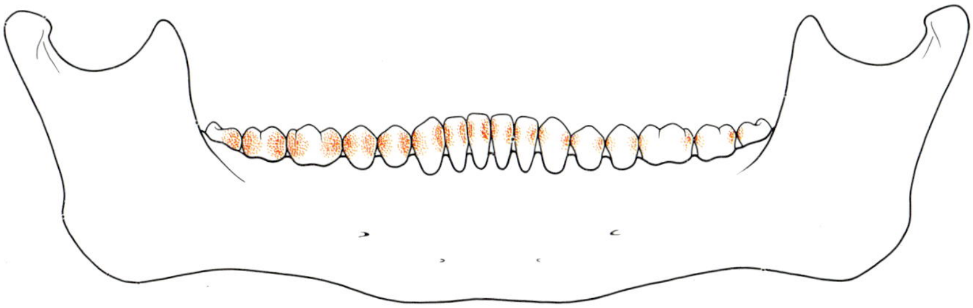

Fig. 5.1-4 The alveolar process is put under stress on the working (chewing) right side, in closing movements the force diminishes as it moves to the opposite side.

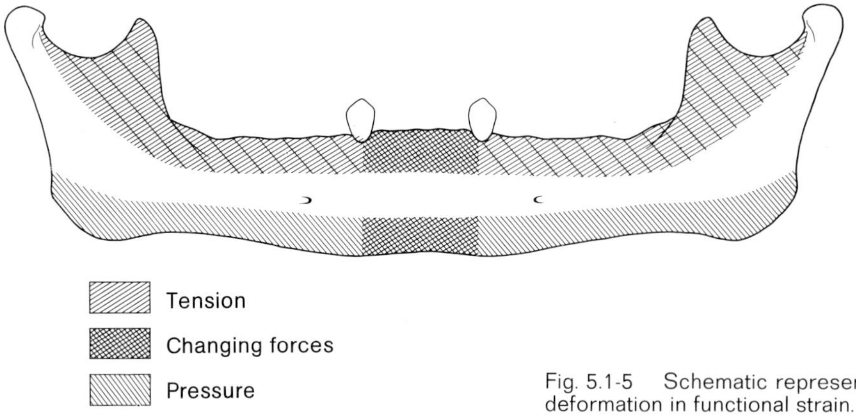

Fig. 5.1-5 Schematic representation of mandibular deformation in functional strain.

Figs. 5.1-6 A to E Osteosynthesis of a mandibular fracture at a mechanically undesirable point:

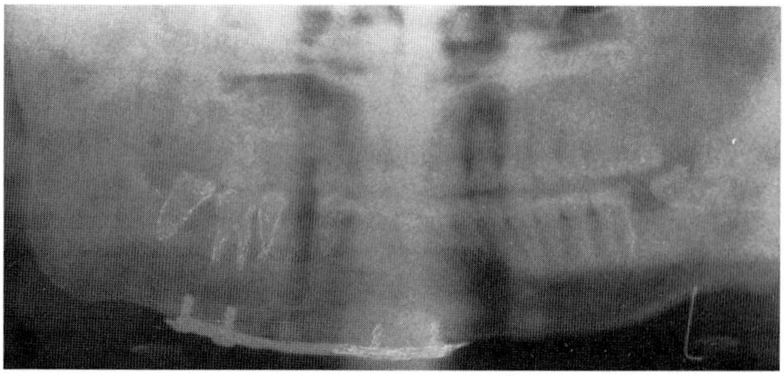

Fig. 5.1-6 A Radiograph.

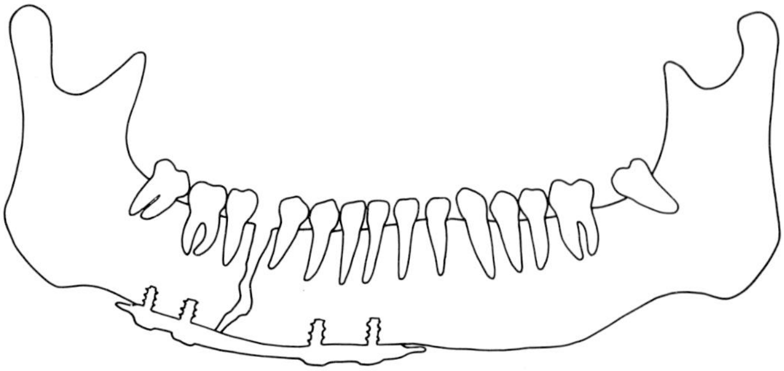

Fig. 5.1-6 B Radiograph, schematically. Note the diastema in the region of the alveolar process.

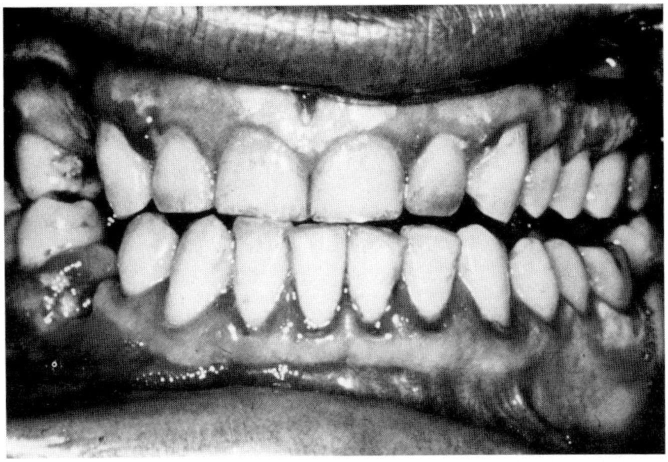

Fig. 5.1-6 C Malocclusion.

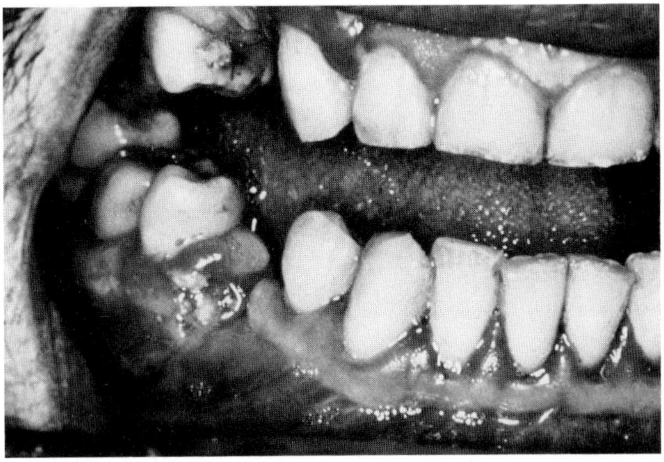

Fig. 5.1-6 D Clearly visible diastema between the first and second right premolar.

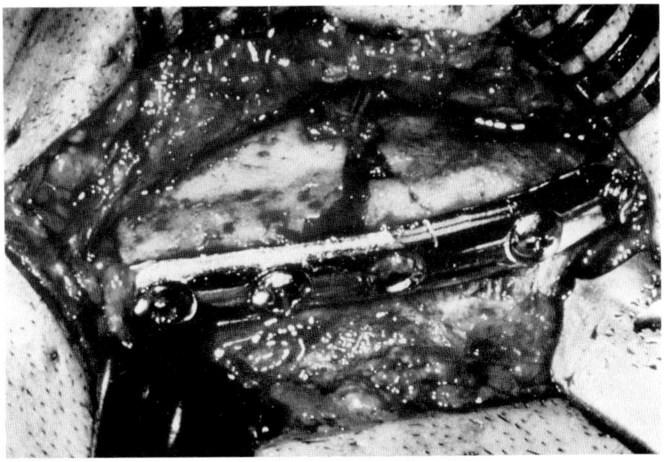

Fig. 5.1-6 E Site after surgical exposure for corrective osteosynthesis. Note the widely gaping fracture site.

Of course the forces which act in the intact mandible act in the broken jaw as well. Here they lead frequently to rather typical displacement of the fragments.

In principle, we may say that alveolar tensile strains are found distal to the canine in all functionally relevant stresses placed on the fractured mandible. The side of the tensile strain changes between the canine abutments for occlusion-dependent functions. In the anterior alveolar regions compression occurs under the same conditions and there are tensile forces at the margin of the chin, so that changing stresses arise between the canines under functional strain (Fig. 5. 1-5).

Recognition of these biomechanical events, which have been largely confirmed by all investigators, is significant in the concept of treatment of mandibular fractures. Accordingly, for example, in fractures in the region distal to the canines the plate should be applied in a craniolingual position. Only at this location can the torsion force components be optimally compensated. For topographical reasons, however, this region is unsuitable for plate osteosynthesis.

The anatomy of the mandible is the source of significant problems associated with osteosynthesis. For example, it is necessary that tooth roots and vessels and nerves running within the bone be considered (*Meyer*, 1976). Among other things, this demands quite specific limitations in size and placement of the device. Stable screw union is possible only at the mandibular margin for this reason.

In treating mandibular fractures with osteosynthesis plates in the horizontal ramus the buccal side of the mandibular margin is especially desirable because of the extensive compact bone layer. For this reason almost all osteosynthesis techniques thus far described are undertaken at this site, although the biomechanics of the body of the mandible make the site an unfavorable one.

If one ignores the biomechanics involved and chooses the most unsuitable site and an unsuitable device, the therapy must fail. An example is provided to illustrate this situation:

A displaced mandibular fracture in the region of the right premolars was fitted with a semitubular plate such as is usually used for treatment of fractures of the shaft of the forearm (Figs. 5. 1-6 A and B). Aside from the minor diastema of the alveolar process caused by the screwing technique establishing a Dynamic Compression Plate—which itself makes its presence known as an occlusal disturbance—formation of the diastema is exacerbated by the play of forces of muscles inserting on the mandible (Figs. 5. 1-6 C and D). Clinical revision of the fracture treated in this way exposed a broadly gaping fracture site (Fig. 5. 1-6 E).

In bone fractures treated without reference to the mechanical situation present, the plane of the fracture cannot take part in the transfer of forces even when compression osteosynthesis was used. The implant itself bears the complete functional strain and thus a fracture or a loosening of the implant may occur, or the bone may fracture at the point where the implant is inserted.

Elimination of tensile forces, as they arise at the level of the teeth when functional strains come into play, is achieved with the usual devices only when additional fixation elements are used to take up tensile forces at the level of the alveolar process. Considerations of this type have been reported by *Snell* and *Dott* (1969), *Muska* (1970), *Spiessl* et al. (1971), *Schargus* and *Schröder* (1976), as well as *Brons* and *Boering* (1977).

Spiessl and his colleagues (1971), in collaboration with the Swiss Association for the Study of Internal Fixation (ASIF) have compensated for the anatomical-functional situation by placement of an additional tension band system in the alveolar region (Fig. 5. 1-7) in addition to the stabilization plate at the margin of the mandible. Only in this way was it possible for them to attain axial stability of the fragments by reducing the tensile forces arising alveolarly. Only this kind of osteosynthesis affords static relationships in the entire region of the fracture line such as are required for primary bone healing. To eliminate the tensile forces in the alveolar region of the fracture site, and additionally to build up a pressure zone at that point, the external compression holes of the plates may be arranged at an angle to the axial direction of the pressure (Fig. 5. 1-8). This permits incorporation of the tension band principle directly into the osteosynthesis plate. Only this type of osteosynthesis plate is able, as an internal device for force transfer, to retain anatomical

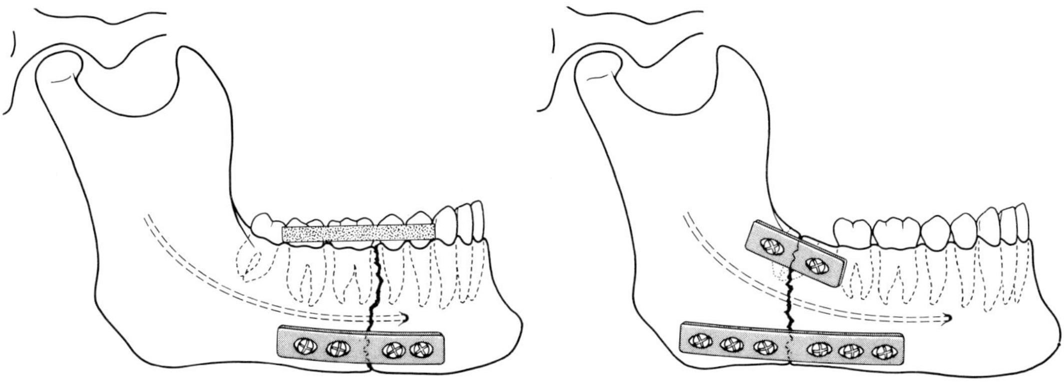

A B

Figs. 5.1-7 A and B Schematic representation of the tension band possibilities proposed by *Spiessl* in the alveolar process region of the mandible.

Fig. 5.1-7 A Tension band arch bar and stabilization plate.

Fig. 5.1-7 B Tension band plate and stabilization plate.

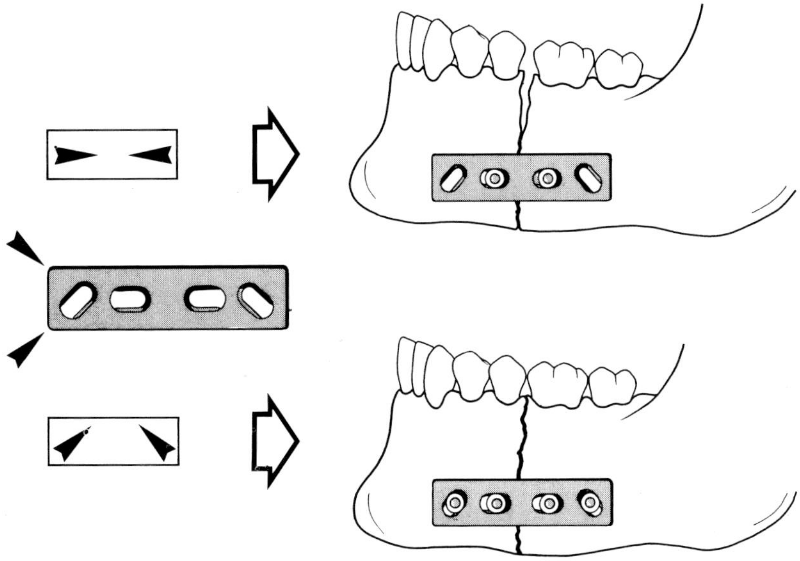

Fig. 5.1-8 Modes of action of the Freiburg tension band plate.

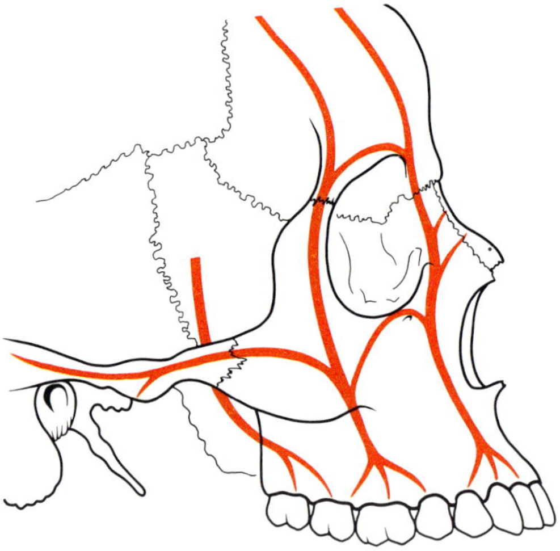

Fig. 5.1-9 Schematic representation of the flow of force in the maxilla, as it arises from distribution of mastication forces.

reduction of the entire fracture surface during exertion of interfragmental pressure.

1.2 Maxilla

The relationships are different in the maxilla. While the mandible is connected via long lever arms to the skull like a parabolically shaped long bone, the maxilla passes into the neurocranium through rigid, connective tissue-filled sutures and forms a single unit with the skull. Bending moments do not arise to the extent that they are found in relation to the mandible because the forces acting on the maxilla, elicited chiefly by chewing pressures, are transferred to the neurocranium via frontal, nasal, zygomatic, and pterygoid pillars (Fig. 5. 1-9). Only in mouth-opening movements, with pulling forces on the masseter muscles which have their attachment on the zygomatic arch, are there alternating forces on the malar sutures or in their immediate vicinity. This means that a fractured zygoma can be displaced caudally through pulling forces, and accordingly that a tension band osteosynthesis must be affixed to the frontozygomatic suture. The fact that the musculature plays hardly any role in the displacement of fractures in the maxilla leads to recognition of the condition that the biomechanics of the maxilla are significantly less problematical here. Only the masseter muscle can elicit relatively large fracture displacement in the zygomatic region.

The force-bearing devices used in the midface must be devised accordingly. They may be much more gracefully shaped than those used in the mandible and act at the level of the frontozygomatic suture against the force exerted by the masseter muscles. Fractures in the Le Fort classification are held in place through craniofacial wire suspension or by means of miniplate osteosynthesis.

While for fixation of malar fractures the interfragmental compression osteosynthesis is preferred, devices fulfill their functions in the remaining parts of the maxilla in adaptation osteosynthesis only. Interosseous wires used here are sufficiently stable, although they have certain disadvantages in contrast with screw devices. Because the bone structures of the midface are extremely thin, drilling alone can cause uncontrollable peak loads and supporting bone elements may be destroyed.

References

Brons, M., and G. Boering (1970)
Fractures of the mandibular body treated by stable internal fixation: A preliminary report. J. oral Surg. 28, 407

Jung, F. (1952)
Die Elastizität der Skeletteile des Gebißsystems. (The elasticity of the bone of the dental system). Stoma (Heidelb.) 5, 74

Koeck, B., and G. Sander (1978)
Über die elastische Deformation der Unterkieferspange. (The elastic deformation of the mandibular body). Dtsch. zahnärztl. Z. 33, 254

Marx, H. (1966)
Die funktionsbedingten elastischen Deformierungen der menschlichen Mandibula. (The functionally derived elastic deformations of the human mandible.) Mainz, Thesis.

Meyer, H. E. (1977)
Ursachen und Verläufe der Frakturen der lateralen Orbita. (Causes and courses of fractures of the lateral orbit). Freiburg, Thesis.

Muska, K. (1970)
Anwendungsmöglichkeit der Hängefixation im zahnlosen Unterkiefer. (Possibilities for use of suspended fixation in the edentulous mandible). Z. ärzt. Fortbild. 64, 1106

Niederdellmann, H., G. Uhlig, and U. Joos (1981)
Das elastische Formverhalten der menschlichen Mandibula unter funktioneller Belastung. (Elastic deformation of the human mandible under functional strain.) Die Quintessenz 32:1113

Pauwels, F. (1950)
Grundriss einer Biomechanik der Frakturheilung. (Outline of the biomechanics of healing of fractures.) Verh. Dtsch. orthop. Ges. 34, 62

Siebert, G. (1978)
Klinisch-experimentelle Untersuchungen zur Auslenkung von Zähnen aufgrund der elastischen Deformierbarkeit der Mandibula. (Clinical experimental investigation on guidance of teeth according to the elastic deformability of the mandible.) Zahnärztl. Welt 11, 543

Snell, J. A., and D. A. Dott (1969)
Internal fixation of certain fractures of the mandible by boneplating. Plast. reconstr. Surg. 43, 281

Spiessl, B., and G. Schargus (1971)
Das Okklusionsproblem bei der funktionsstabilen Osteosynthese des bezahnten Unterkiefers. (The problem of occlusion in functionally stable osteosynthesis of the dentulous mandible). Dtsch. Zahn-, Mund- u. Kieferheilk. 57, 293

Schargus, G., and F. Schröder (1976)
Zuggurtung bei Kieferwinkelfrakturen durch Dreieckverspannung. (Tension banding in fractures of the angle of the mandible through triangular wiring.) Acta Stomatol. Belg. 73, 291

Schumacher, G. H. (1961)
Funktionelle Morphologie der Kaumuskulatur. (Functional morphology of the masticatory musculature.) Leipzig, J. A. Barth

Weber-Thedy, K. W. (1964)
Die Zuggurtungsfunktion der Wurzelhaut oder wie die Toleranzquint die Wurzelhaut bewertet. (The tension band function of the periodontal membrane, or how tolerancequint evaluates the periodontal membrane.) Dtsch. zahnärztl. Z. 19, 426

2. Morphology of Fracture Healing and its Relationship to Biomechanics

Berton A. Rahn

2.1 Mechanical and Biological Conditions after Fracture

A fracture disrupts the continuity of a bone, disturbing the mechanical as well as the biological function. Starting from this initial state, fracture healing is intended to restore the original structure, and thus the function. Knowledge of the mechanical and biological conditions is important for the understanding of the healing process. The pattern of healing is governed, to a fair extent, by the amount of motion in the fracture gap (*Perren* et al., 1969; *Allgöwer* et al., 1971; *Willenegger* et al., 1971; *Müller* and *Perren*, 1972). An essential prerequisite for a rapid and undisturbed healing process is a well functioning blood supply in the fracture region.

The mechanical conditions immediately after fracture are as follows: The fragment end mobility is only limited by the soft tissue envelope. The muscles in the fracture region are contracted, possibly a reflex reaction. These muscle contractions cause an initial, though incomplete, attempt to immobilize the injured area. In addition, the sensation of pain prevents large scale active movements. Force transmission across the fracture plane is possible only to a limited extent. In Figure 5. 2-1, an attempt is made, with the aid of a so-called free body diagram, to analyze the mechanical conditions in the fracture region. A single fragment is considered to be an isolated body, and its reaction under the influence of external forces is investigated. If no forces act on this free body, no displacement and no motion will result. Depending on the location of the fragment, however, a variety of forces will act on it. In most cases, those forces act with long lever arms and displacement will result readily. The forces will act alternately from different directions, and their magnitude varies continuously. As a result, the fragment moves

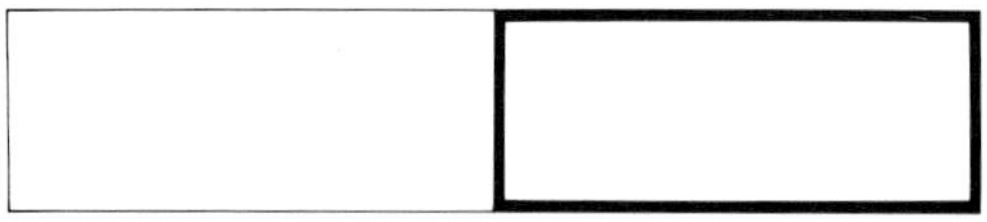

Figs. 5.2-1 A to C Mobility and immobilization of fracture fragments.

Fig. 5.2-1 A The alignment is only maintained as long as no external forces are present.

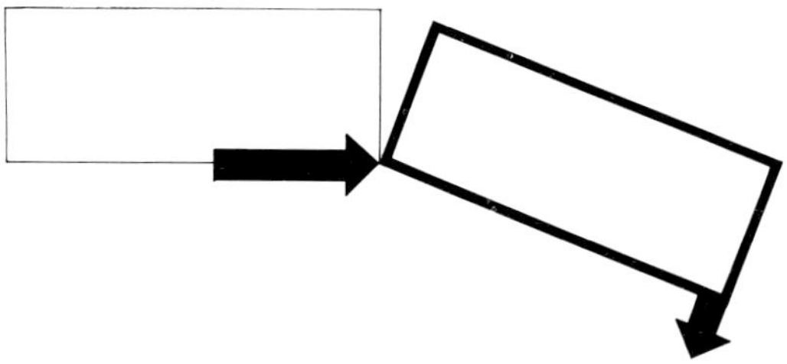

Fig. 5.2.1 B External forces acting with relatively long lever arms easily lead to displacement of the fragment. Intermittent forces of varying magnitude and direction lead thus to a permanent irritation in the fracture gap. This situation is found in spontaneous healing of fractures.

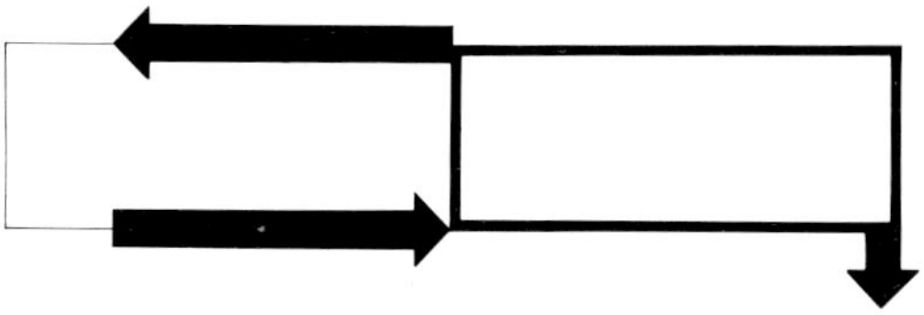

Fig. 5.2-1 C To counteract displacement and to avoid motion in the fracture gap, large forces are necessary. The aligned bone should continue to transmit compression, while the implant must assume the tensional forces.

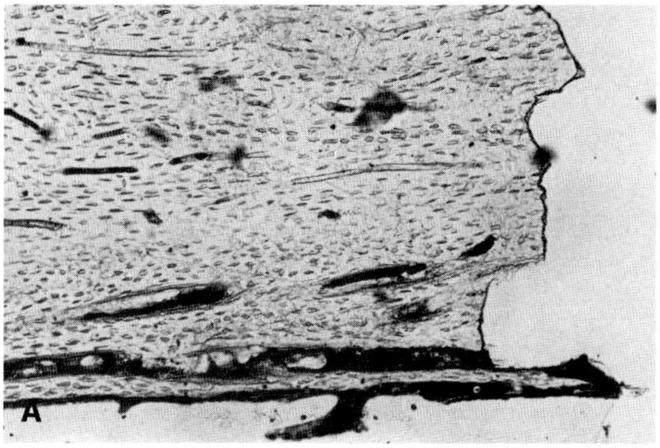

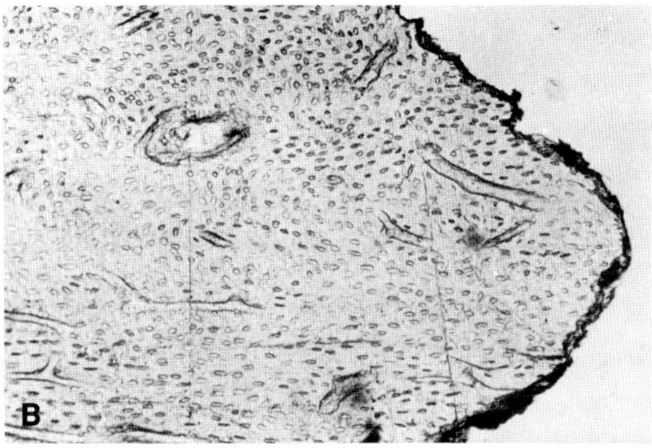

Figs. 5.2-2 A and B Disturbed circulation in the fragments ends.

Fig. 5.2-2 A The blood vessels can be visualized to the very end of the fragment only a few minutes after fracture by the injection of India ink.

Fig. 5.2-2 B One hour after trauma, no ink reaches the extremes of the fragment. A possible cause is thrombosis in the traumatized capillaries.

relative to its environment, especially to other fragments. Thus, a constant disturbance prevails in the fracture gap. To obtain a strain-free fracture gap, relatively high forces are required, because only a small lever arm is available for retention.

The initial biological situation is characterized in the first instance by disturbed circulation. Soft tissues are injured and partially detached from the bone, and large vessels may be destroyed. The vessels within the bone cortex are interrupted at the fragment ends and are closed by blood clotting. During the first hours after trauma, the area of closed vessels increases in size (Figs. 5.2-2 A and B). Border zones at the fragment ends are thus left without blood supply. The pattern of non-perfused regions depends on the possibility for anastomoses in the bone. It may happen that entire fragments, or fragment ends with sharp points, have no circulation. A more or less extensive hematoma will be produced between the fragment ends by the bleeding from interrupted vessels.

2.2 Healing of Bone Defects

Traumatic bone defects which are not related to a fracture generally are not of any major practical significance. When they occur, they are often of iatrogenic origin. The histologic analysis of such healing processes provides valuable information and contributes to the understanding of fracture healing. *Johner* (1972) used an experimental model with a mechanically stable defect zone (Fig. 5. 2-3). He applied drill holes in cortical bone down to a diameter of 0.1 mm and studied the repair process. For small holes up to a diameter of 0.2 mm, i.e., approximately the size of an osteon, he found after one week an osteoid layer on the walls of the drill hole. The inner space later filled with concentric layers of lamellar bone which were deposited at a rate of 1 to 2 microns per day. Thus, for example, a hole with a diameter of 0.1 mm is filled in three to four weeks. For holes larger than 0.2 mm, the filling process also begins at the walls, but at about the same time, a woven bone network is formed which subdivides the space of the defect into smaller compartments. The diameter of these subdivided compartments corresponds approximately to the diameter of osteons. Concentric bone lamellae are deposited in these interstices. This mechanism allows the filling of larger defects at a rate similar to that of smaller holes. The filled region is adapted later to the surrounding bone structure by means of Haversian remodelling. As long as the defect is smaller than 0.6 mm in diameter, the entire wall thick-

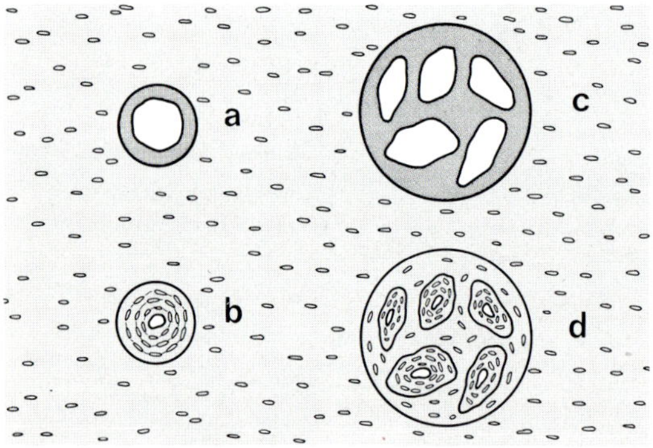

Fig. 5.2-3 Healing pattern of small bone defects. In a small drill hole (0.2 mm) after one week the walls are coated by osteoid (a). After four weeks this defect is filled by concentrically deposited bone lamellae (b). In a larger hole, osteoid and woven bone not only cover the walls but subdivide the defect into smaller spaces (c). After four weeks these smaller spaces are filled by concentrically deposited lamellar bone. Thus, larger defects may be filled at the same speed as small ones (d).
(After *Johner*, 1972, and after *Schenk*, 1973.)

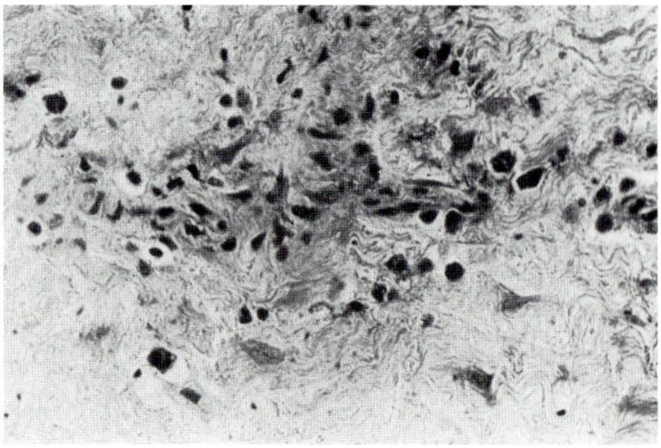

Fig. 5.2-4 Differentiation of connective tissue in the fracture callus. In the fracture gap the hematoma is replaced by granulation tissue, which gradually matures to form connective tissue.

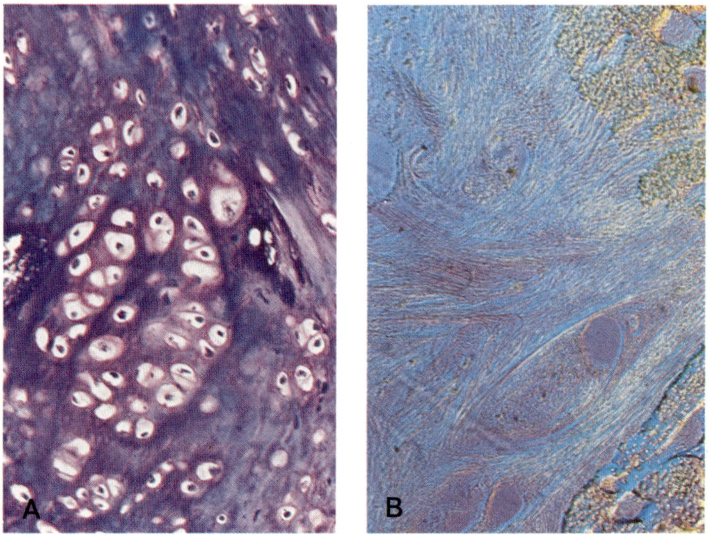

Figs. 5.2-5 A and B Interfragmentary fibrocartilage.

Fig. 5.2-5 A The cartilaginous component is suited to absorb compression.

Fig. 5.2-5 B The collagen fibers have to resist the tensile forces.

ness of a rabbit tibia is filled. For holes larger than 0.6 mm, the filling mechanism is basically the same, except that less than the entire wall thickness becomes filled (*Burstein* et al., 1972; *Johner*, 1972). In these drill holes the bone healing proceeds under the protection of a stable bony frame.

The situation is somewhat different for defects which are created in connection with interrupted continuity of the bone. Such processes are seen, for example, during the lengthening of tubular bones (*Pflüger* et al., 1976; *Rahn* et al., 1978). After an artificial fracture or an osteotomy, the space between the fragment ends is widened continuously with the aid of a distraction device. Immediately after the operation, a hematoma forms between the fragment ends. This hematoma gradually is replaced by granulation tissue which matures into connective tissue. The connective tissue is oriented more or less in the longitudinal axis of the bone, but sometimes also contains structures which are arranged crosswise at an angle of about 45°. Based upon these connective tissue structures, a network of woven bone develops next. This woven bone provides a framework which, as in the filling of large drill holes, allows the formation of lamellar bone in the interstices. This filling process continues until compact bone is obtained.

2.3 Spontaneous Healing of Fractures

2.3.1 Radiological Course

Several radiological findings are characteristic for spontaneous fracture healing. The fragment ends usually become somewhat rounded during the first weeks and the fracture gap becomes wider. After about one week a callus cuff starts to become visible. Its formation begins at a certain distance from the fragment ends and develops towards the fracture gap. This leads to an increase of the bone cross section in the fracture region. Gradually the bony callus arches over from one fragment end to the other until a complete bridge is formed. After this bony bridging the fracture becomes more and more blurred and finally disappears. At the time of bony consolidation the limb starts to take over normal function. However the morphologic healing process is not yet completed at this point but it requires remodelling activities over months and years. Remodelling leads not only to a reopening of the medullary cavity, but also to changes in the entire mass of the callus, until the original tubular shape of the bone is reconstructed.

In special cases, as e.g., in bone fissures or in the case illustrated in Figure 5.2-8, the mobility of the fragments is limited to an extent that an atypical pattern of spontaneous healing occurs. Resorption of the fragment ends is not seen, there is only little or no callus formation and yet one observes the gradual disappearance of the fracture.

2.3.2 Histology

At first the mobility of the fragment ends is still too extreme to permit calcification in the interfragmentary space. The continuous motion even results in resorption of the fragment ends, which become rounded. Initially the interfragmentary region is filled by a hematoma. This is gradually replaced by granulation tissue (Fig. 5.2-4), which further differentiates into connective tissue and, in the region between the fragments, into fibrocartilage (Fig. 5.2-5). The whole shape of the callus cuff is thus preformed by soft tissues. At a distance from the fracture, this callus slowly begins its transformation into fibrous bone (desmal ossification, Fig. 5.2-6). An arch, based on either side of the fracture, is building up slowly. The formation of connective tissue and fibrocartilage already brings about a decrease in the mobility of the fragments, which allows a first mineralization of the callus (Fig. 5.2-7). This leads to an increase of the cross section of the bone (Fig. 5.2-8A), and thus to a longer lever arm to counteract the displacing forces. Thus the demands for the strength of the repair tissues may be reduced. The interfragmentary structures (fibrocartilage) contribute to a damping of motion. The cartilaginous component acts as a kind of hydraulic pressure pad, the fibers absorb tensile forces. The resulting inhibition of movement permits calcification processes in the interfragmentary region as well. The intercellular substance of the cartilage gradually incorporates mineral and can be replaced by bone (chondral ossification, Fig. 5.

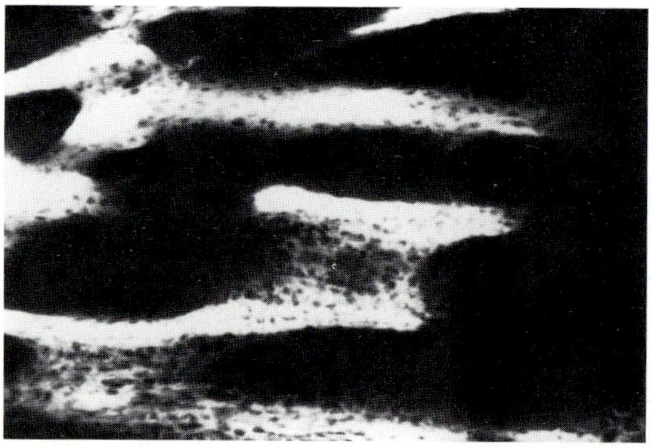

Fig. 5.2-6 Formation of woven bone in the callus. Mineral is incorporated into the connective tissues and woven bone is formed.

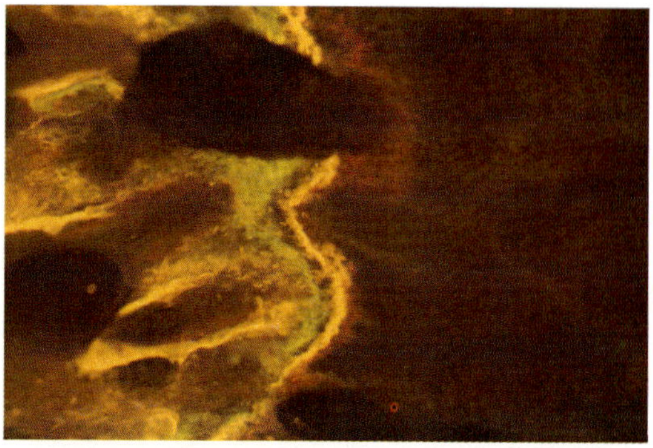

Fig. 5.2-7 Enchondral ossification. A reduction of motion in the fracture area allows mineralization of the cartilage and its replacement by bone. The progress of mineralization is visualized by fluorochrome markers of distinguishable color which were administered at biweekly intervals.

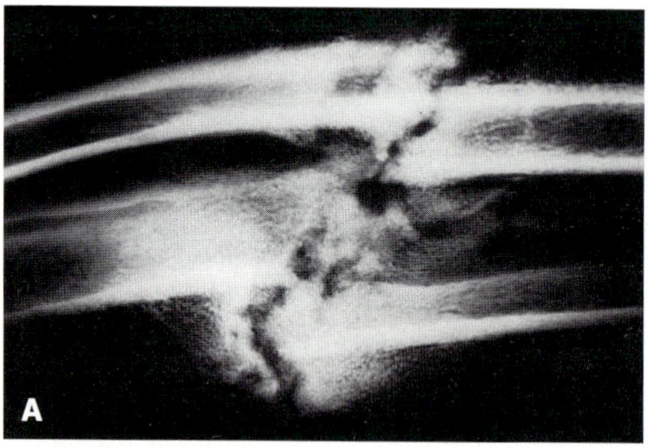

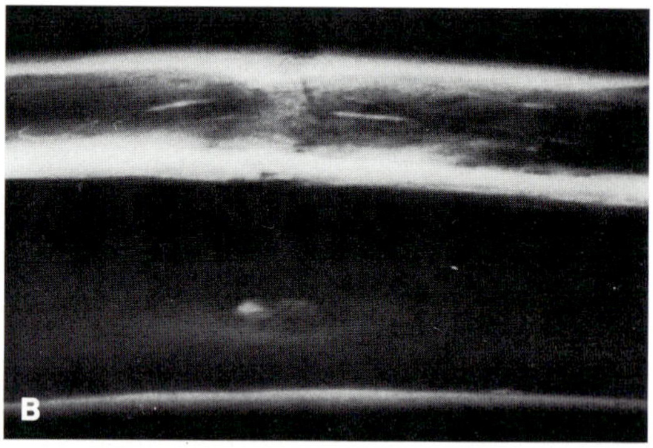

Figs. 5.2-8 A and B Dependence of callus formation on the mechanical conditions.

Fig. 5.2-8 A After a fracture of ulna and radius in the rabbit, under spontaneous healing conditions a large amount of callus is formed.

Fig. 5.2-8 B An isolated fracture of the radius, in the rabbit, shows a different healing pattern. The intact ulna has provided sufficient stability to permit healing with minimal callus formation.

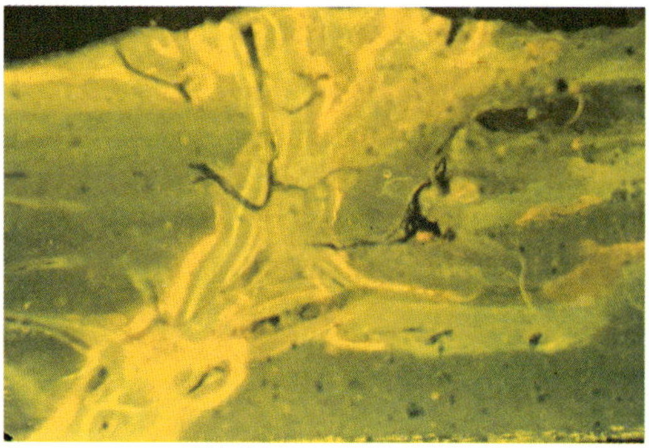

Fig. 5.2-9 Direct lamellar bone formation in spontaneous fracture healing. The absence of interfragmentary motion (see also Fig. 5.2-8 B) allowed the primary deposition of lamellar bone in the fracture gap. The indirect way through fibrocartilage and callus formation was not necessary under these circumstances.

2-7). The narrowing of the interfragmentary space causes a further reduction of the mobility until finally bony bridging has occured. Osteoclastic resorption balanced with osteoblastic bone formation then gradually changes the cancellous callus structure back into a cortical tubular bone. As the new cortices become more compact, the cross-section of the bone is reduced to normal dimensions and a new medullary cavity is formed. The histological process of spontaneous fracture healing is discussed in detail in a monograph by *Coutelier* (1969).
If the mobility of the fragments is small, the "detour" via cartilage and chondral ossification is not necessary. Direct bone formation takes place in the fracture gap, whereby lamellar bone, a highly differentiated type of bone, is formed (Figs. 5.2-8 B and 5.2-9).

2.4 Fracture Healing after Adaptation without Absolute Immobilization

2.4.1 Technical Fundamentals

To avoid malalignment at the end of fracture healing, one tries to align the fragments as accurately as possible. Subsequent treatment aims at maintaining the fragment in an optimal position until the fracture has consolidated. There are numerous techniques for this, including, for example, intramedullary splints (*Rush*, 1957; *Küntscher*, 1962), retention by circumferential wiring or by wire sutures, or external fixation systems which are anchored transcutaneously to the bone. The stabilizing forces provided by these methods of treatment can fulfill their task under resting conditions, but as soon as greater stress acts on the individual fragments, the unavoidable result will be interfragmentary motion. However, the amplitude of these movements is limited by the implants used. These delicate movements have no great effect on the relative position of the fragment ends, but they clearly affect the process of fracture healing.

2.4.2 Radiological Course

During the entire healing process, the appearance after surgical adaptation without absolute immobilisation resembles that of spontaneous fracture healing. The risk of malalignment is largely eliminated and the signs described for spontaneous healing are less pronounced. The limited mobility of the fragment ends leads to some slight resorption. The callus does not need to bear the entire burden of the stabilization and is therefore less distinct. A radiographically visible callus formation, however, is necessary in cases where absolute immobilization is not guaranteed, since this is the only way in which healing can occur. In plate fixation as well it may happen that the stabilization is insufficient. In such a case, too, a callus will be visible which bridges the fracture (*Wieser* and *Allgöwer*, 1962; *Allgöwer*, 1964; *Wieser*, 1964; *Hutzschenreuter* et al., 1969).

2.4.3 Histology

The histologic process also largely corresponds to that of spontaneous fracture healing, but all signs which characterize spontaneous healing—such as resorption of fragment ends, formation of callus and cartilage—are much less pronounced. Figure 5.2-10 shows the healing process in a sheep mandible after wire suturing.

2.5 Fracture Healing after Absolute Stabilization

2.5.1 Technical Fundamentals

The goal in the treatment of fractures with plates and screws is anatomically precise reduction of the fragments and, ideally, their retention in this position. Even under functional load — for example during physiotherapy — the fracture gap remains completely immobilized. Absolute stabilization means that, even microscopically, no relative motion occurs between the fragment ends. Implants cannot be made large enough to resist all the stresses (bending, tension, torsion) permanently. A force transmission by the implant alone would sooner or later lead to fatigue failure of the implant. In plate fixation, therefore, it is preferable to place the implant on the tension side (tension band), while the precisely realigned bone still can take over compression. Technically this is accomplished by placing the plate in such a way that the fragments are elastically compressed against each other. This

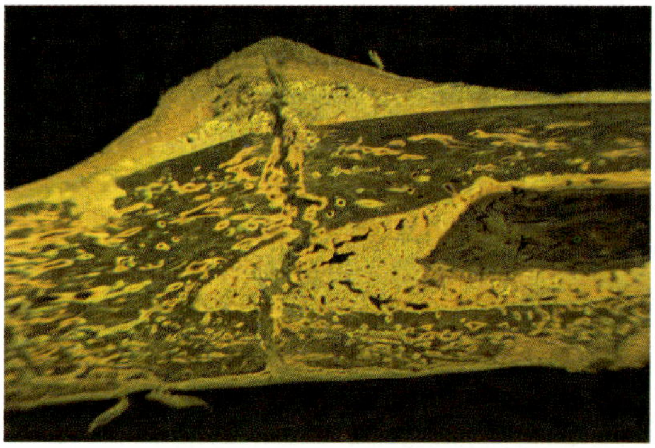

Fig. 5.2-10 Healing via cartilage and callus after interosseous wiring. In this sheep mandible the wire sutures did not offer sufficient stability to avoid interfragmentary motion completely. The alignment however could be maintained to a fair extent and motion was certainly reduced. As in spontaneous healing, callus formation, interfragmentary cartilage and fragment end resorption are characteristic for this situation. Those findings, however, are not as pronounced as during spontaneous healing.

preload of the bone counteracts tension and bending. Interfragmentary compression increases the friction between the fragment ends, and this creates additional stabilization against torsion and shear. If the stress is not excessive, a limb stabilized in this way may therefore be moved like an intact limb. For this reason, a stable internal fixation is especially recommended in those cases in which preservation of mobility is important. This might be the case in TMJ fractures or in older patients where the risk of serious complications would increase with long immobilization.

The application of metal plates to the bone surface affects the force transmission within the bone. Functional stress on the cortex immediately beneath the plate may be reduced to as little as one-third of the normal stress because a large portion of the force is bypassing through the plate.

2.5.2 Radiological Course

The radiological appearance of fracture healing after absolute stabilization differs considerably from the process of spontaneous healing (*Galeazzi*, 1974). Resorption of the fragment ends is absent, and no callus formation is seen during the entire process. The fracture line first becomes blurred and then gradually disappears (Fig. 5.2-11). This pattern was compared by *Danis* (1949) to soldering (soudure autogene). The intense remodelling processes temporarily cause the fracture area to appear less dense.

This healing of a fracture without callus formation, however, is achieved only if immobilization is sufficient. Plates which are too thin and flexible cannot guarantee absolute immobilization (*Hutzschenreuter* et al., 1969). In such a case the fragment ends are resorbed and callus is formed. Some authors (*Geiser*, 1963, 1967; *Küntscher*, 1970) consider fracture healing without callus to be unnatural. They are not aware of the fact that the same healing phenomena as observed after surgical stabilization may occur naturally if the mechanical conditions permit. This may be the case in bone fissures and has been demonstrated in the experiment on the forelimb of the rabbit (Fig. 5.2-8 and 5.2-9).

2.5.3 Histology

Intracortical (Haversian) remodelling is a mechanism that replaces compact cortical bone step by step by new bone of the same structure. In this process, a group of osteoclasts "drills" a tunnel with a diameter of about 0.2 mm in the longitudinal axis of the bone (Fig. 5.2-12). These osteoclasts are followed by vessels and mesenchymal cells, and somewhat farther back, by a front of osteoblasts. These osteoblasts are arranged in a funnel shape; in longitudinal sections their arrangement appears V-shaped and in cross-sections, round. New osteoid is deposited in this canal, which then matures into lamellar bone.

The process of Haversian remodelling can take place directly through the fracture zone if the fragment ends are in close and stable contact. The fractured bone is thus replaced locally by

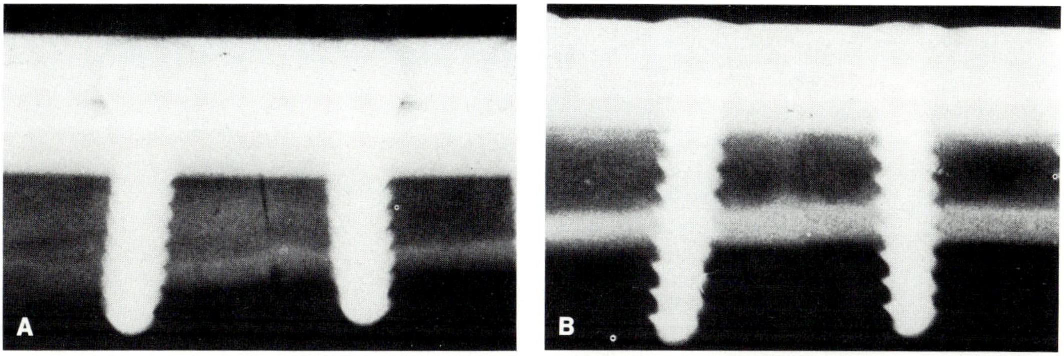

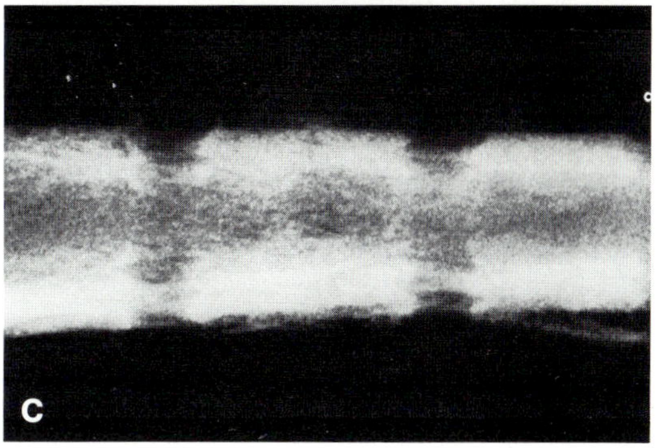

Figs. 5.2-11 A to C Radiological features of primary bone healing. After stable plate fixation of a transversely sectioned rabbit's tibia the healing proceeds without fragment end resorption and without callus formation.

Fig. 5.2-11 A The postoperative film shows the aligned osteotomy clearly.

Fig. 5.2-11 B After five weeks the osteotomy becomes blurred. Callus and fragment end resorption are absent.

Fig. 5.2-11 C Nine weeks postopertively the fragment ends are united to a large extent.

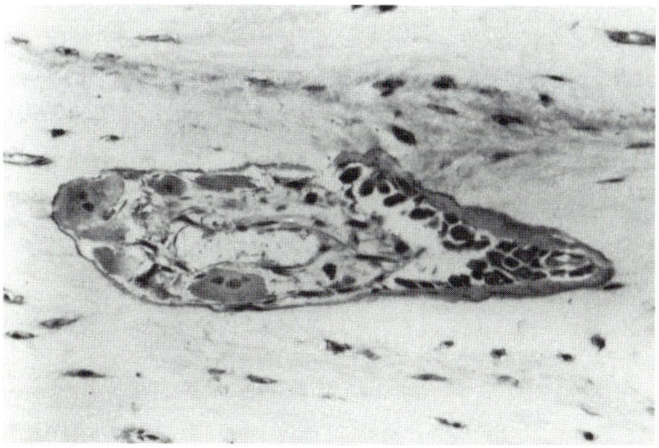

Fig. 5.2-12 Formation of a new osteon. A group of osteoclasts, multinucleated giant cells, "drills" a canal into the cortical bone. This canal is refilled by osteoblasts. This results in an internal remodelling of the cortical bone. (From: *Rahn, B. A.* and *Perren, S. M.*, 1975, Chem. Rundsch. 28: 12).

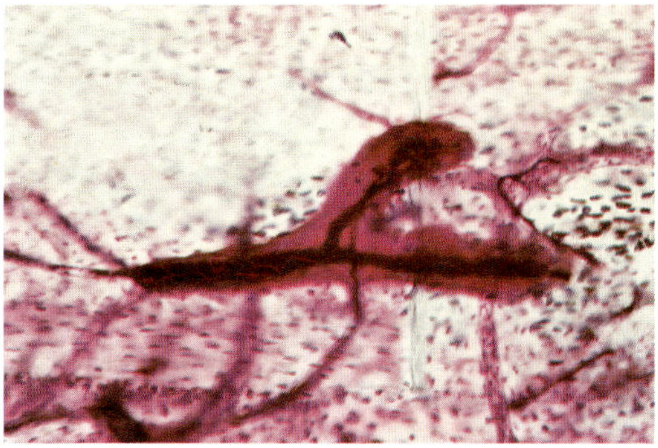

Fig. 5.2-13 Primary healing: Contact healing. An osteon has grown across the immobilized osteotomy line and unites the fragments. The pattern of contact healing can be observed in fractures as well, but smaller contact areas make this finding less frequent. The process of contact healing leads to a direct reconstruction of the original structure. (From: *Rahn, B. A.* et al., 1971).

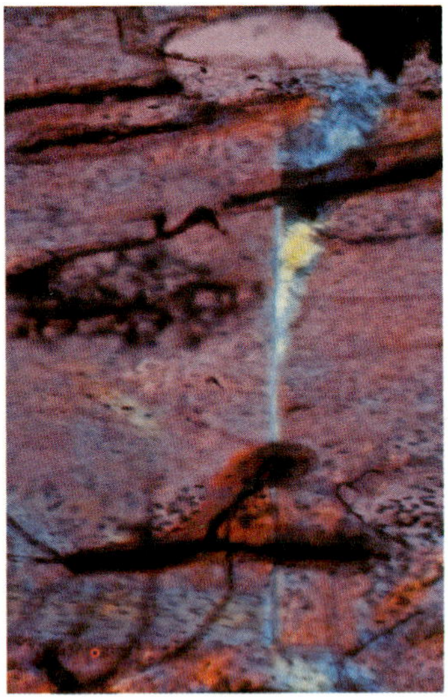

Fig. 5.2-14 Healing of mechanically overloaded areas. Incongruent adaptation of the fragment ends can lead to a high force per unit area and thus to localized overload. If stability is maintained, the zones of irreversible deformation are included in the process of primary healing.

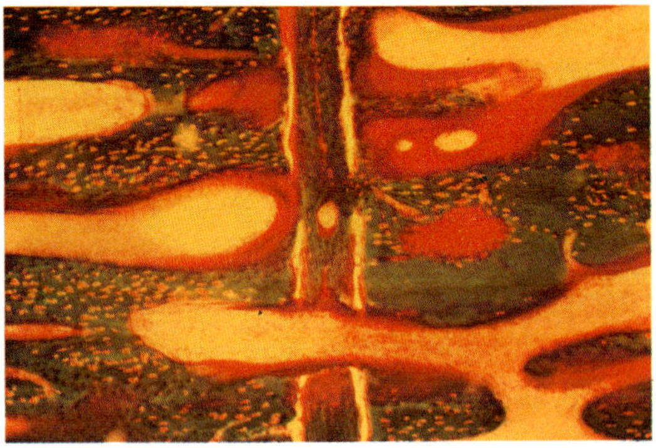

Fig. 5.2-15 Primary healing: Gap healing. Under stable conditions lamellar bone may primarily be deposited in small interfragmentary gaps. The mechanism of intracortical (Haversian) remodelling in a further step leads to longitudinal orientation of the cortical bone structure. (From: *Perren* et al., 1969).

new lamellar bone, which, in its structure, corresponds to a certain extent to the original bone. This process is called contact healing (Fig. 5.2-13). Lack of congruence of the fragment ends can lead to excessive mechanical stress at certain pressure points, resulting in irreversible deformation. If stability is maintained, these zones become involved in the process of contact healing (Fig. 5.2-14).

A second type of healing, termed gap healing, can be observed after stable fixation. A fracture scarcely can be realigned in such a way that contact is produced everywhere. When the plate is applied the interfragmentary compression is not always homogenously distributed. Thus minute gaps may be maintained. Lamellar bone can be deposited directly into these gaps (Fig. 5.2-15) as long as the stability is guaranteed by supporting contact zones in the neighbourhood. This filling process is comparable to the filling of bone defects. By means of Haversian remodelling, such filled defects then are restructured to result in osteons arranged in the longitudinal axis of the bone.

The two patterns, contact healing and gap healing, have been termed primary bone healing (*Schenk* and *Willenegger*, 1963, 1964, 1967; *Rahn* et al., 1971; *Schenk*, 1975) because the healing process leads directly to a restoration of the original structure. Primary bone healing has been demonstrated in various bones (tubular bones, mandible) and in various species, e.g., dog, sheep, rabbit, man (*Schenk* and *Willenegger*, 1963; *Müller*, 1967; *Perren* et al., 1969; *Rahn* et al., 1971; *Luhr*, 1971, 1972; *Prein* et al., 1975; *Niederdellmann* and *Rahn*, 1976). Haversian remodelling starts around the fourth week. In animal experiments Haversian remodelling may render a fracture completely invisible within twelve weeks. Primary bone healing also has been observed in spontaneous fracture healing, in instances where the existing conditions, without any therapeutic assistance, provided sufficient stability.

The reasons for the increased remodelling activity in a fractured and plated bone are not yet completely clear. A direct effect of static compression can be excluded according to the

studies of *Matter* et al. (1974). This investigation has shown that the remodelling pattern seen beneath plates is the same without regard to whether the plates were applied to the bone under tension, under compression or simply in a neutral condition. To what extent the dynamic changes of stress influence the remodelling rate remains to be determined. The disturbance of circulation has certainly its role in triggering remodelling activities (*Gunst* et al., 1979).
Bone is able to adapt its structure to functional demands (*Wolff*, 1892). The use of massive implants leads to a "stress protection" of the bone. A loss of bone substance, a cancellization of the bone cortex, results. Such processes have been observed especially after the application of two plates fixed at right angles to each other. In tubular bones this configuration has led to a distinct weakening of the bone (*Kinzl* et al., 1974).

2.6 Complications

2.6.1 Malalignment

In spontaneous fracture healing, bony union is seldom a problem. Nevertheless, in nature the forces acting on the fragments can sometimes lead to grotesque malalignments. The treatment of fractures is directed at avoiding such situations. From a theoretical point of view, the best method is an anatomically exact reduction and subsequent stable fixation. In practical application, a deviation from this theoretical goal can be accepted, as the results can be functionally satisfactory and the smaller efforts may be an important consideration. In the extremities a slight amount of shortening or small axial deviations often can be tolerated, because the individual is able to compensate to a certain extent. However, degenerative changes in the joints may result as later sequelae. In young individuals with a fracture which has united in a wrong position, the deformity may still be corrected by a remodelling of the bone. In cases of axial deviations, for example, bone is resorbed on the convex side and new bone is deposited on the concave side. Thus, the bone shaft is gradually straightened. There are certain sites, especially in the maxillofacial region, where compensatory processes are not possible and where a malunion has a permanent disturbing effect (e.g., fractures of the orbital floor, fractures in the dentulous jaw). Here, bone remodelling does not provide any improvement of the symptoms.

2.6.2 Nonunion

The pathogenesis of nonunions was the subject of a morphological study by *Müller* et al. (1968) in an experimental model of the dog radius. It appears that nonunions develop because, during the course of fracture healing, the amount of motion in the fracture gap remains too high to allow mineralization of the fibrocartilage. The fibrocartilage persists; it may be torn apart locally and a pseudo-articular space may result. There are different types of nonunions (*Weber* and *Cech*, 1973) which are classified according to their type of reaction. The hypertrophic, well-vascularized nonunions, which form the largest group, are not very difficult to treat. For therapy, it must be kept in mind that the tissue in the space between the fragment ends is callus tissue ready to be transformed into bone and it merely lacks proper immobilization. Therefore this tissue should not be removed for treatment. Merely additional stabilization, e.g. with a plate, is sufficient to restart calcification of the cartilage. The further ossification process and the bony union then take place as in normal fracture healing. A nonreactive, atrophic nonunion creates much greater problems, especially if it is accompanied by infection.

2.6.3 Mechanical Overload of Bone

In a normal plate fixation the ultimate compressive strength of bone is not reached (*Perren* et al., 1969; *Yamada*, 1970). If the fragment ends are incongruent, their contact may be limited to a few points. In this case, the entire force is concentrated at these points. Locally the ultimate compressive strength limit is exceeded and irreversible bone deformation results. Healing of such deformed zones proceeds like normal fracture healing (*Rahn* et al., 1972) (Fig. 5.2-14). If the deformed zone is not separated from the fragment ends and the fracture retains its stability, the Haversian remodelling will proceed through these irreversibly deformed zones. Thus, the pattern of primary bone healing is seen here as well. If portions of deformed bones are disconnected from the main fragments, these loose parts are subjected to motion and, as a consequence, they will be resorbed by osteoclasts.

2.6.4 Infection

In case of infection, the fracture gap contains mainly leucocytes and detritus. At a certain distance from the fragment ends, intense resorption activity can be seen. A few millimeters of the fragment ends are separated from the still intact bone and remain as sequestra at the site of infection. The infection can heal only if these sequestra are either expelled or removed surgically. An infected fracture becomes a problem, particularly if implant material is present in the infected region. Definitive healing of the infection can be achieved only when the foreign material has been removed. *Rittmann* and *Perren* (1974) have shown that, despite an active infection, the implant material can be left in place as long as stability is assured. Thus a bony bridging of the fracture can occur despite the presence of infection and even primary bone healing is possible. After bony consolidation, the implant material can be removed, and the infection can heal.

References

Allgöwer, M. (1964)
Osteosynthese und primäre Knochenheilung. (Osteosynthesis and primary bone healing.) Langenbecks Arch. klin. Chir. 308:423

Allgöwer, M., S. M. Perren, and T. Ruedi (1971)
Biophysikalische Aspekte der normalen und der heilenden Knochenkorticalis. (Biophysical aspects of normal and healing bone cortex.) Langenbecks Arch. klin. Chir. 328:109

Brennwald, J. and S. M. Perren (1972)
Bestimmung der Knochendehnung in vitro und in vivo nach Plattenosteosynthese. (Determination of bone strain in vitro and in vivo following plate osteosynthesis.) Langenbecks Arch. klin. Chir., Suppl. Chir. Forum :39

Burstein, A. H., J. Currey, V. H. Frankel, K. G. Heiple, P. Lunseth, and J. C. Vessely (1972)
Bone strength: The effect of screw holes. J. Bone Jt. Surg. 54 A:1143

Coutelier, L. (1969)
Recherches sur la guérison des fractures. (Study of the healing of fractures.) Brussels, Arscia

Danis, R. (1949)
Theorie et practique de l'osteosynthese. (Theory and practice of osteosynthesis.) Paris, Masson

Galeazzi, G. (1974)
Röntgendiagnostische Befunde bei Osteosynthesen. (Radiographic diagnostic findings in osteosyntheses.) Ther. Umschau 31:722

Geiser, M. (1963)
Beiträge zur Biologie der Knochenbruchheilung. (The biology of healing of bone fractures.) Stuttgart, Enke

Geiser, M. (1967)
Die radiologische Beurteilung der Frakturheilung nach Fixation von Schaftfrakturen mit metallischen Implantaten. (Radiographic evaluation of the healing of fractures following fixation of shaft fractures with metallic implants.) Radiol. clin. biol. 36:65

Gunst, M. A., C. Suter, and B. A. Rahn (1979)
Die Knochendurchblutung nach Plattenosteosynthese. (Blood supply of bone after plate osteosynthesis.) Helv. chir. Acta 46:171

Hutzschenreuter, P., S. M. Perren, and S. Steinemann (1969)
Some effects of rigidity of internal fixation on the healing pattern of osteotomies. Injury 1:77

Johner, R. (1972)
Zur Knochenheilung in Abhängigkeit von der Defektgröße. (Bone healing and its dependence on the defect size.) Helv. chir. Acta 39:409

Kinzl, L., S. M. Perren, and C. Burri (1974)
Veränderungen mechanischer Qualität der unter Druckplatten liegenden Knochenkorticalis. (Changes in mechanical quality of bone cortex beneath pressure plates.) Langenbecks Arch. klin. Chir., Suppl Chir. Forum

Küntscher, G. (1962)
Praxis der Marknagelung. (The practice of medullary nailing.) Stuttgart, Schattauer.

Küntscher, G. (1970)
Das Kallus-Problem. (The callus problem.) Stuttgart, Enke

Luhr, H. G. (1971)
Treatment of mandibular fractures and pseudoarthroses by compression osteosynthesis. Trans. 5th Int. Congr. Plast. Reconstr. Surg., p. 109, Australia, Butterworths

Luhr, H. G. (1972)
Die Kompressionsosteosynthese zur Behandlung von Unterkieferfrakturen. Experimentelle Grundlagen und klinische Erfahrungen. (Compression osteosynthesis for treatment of mandibular fractures. Experimental foundation and clinical experience.) Dtsch. zahnärztl. Z. 27:29

Matter, P., J. Brennwald, and S. M. Perren (1974)
Biologische Reaktion des Knochens auf Osteosyntheseplatten. (Biological reaction of bone to osteosynthesis plates.) Helv. Chir. Acta, Suppl. 12

Müller, J. (1967)
Beitrag zur Primärheilung von Schaftfrakturen beim Menschen. (Primary healing of shaft fractures in man.) Anat. Anz. 120:599

Müller, J., R. Schenk, and H. Willenegger (1968)
Experimentelle Untersuchungen über die Entstehung reaktiver Pseudoarthrosen am Hunderadius. (Experimental investigation of the development of pseudoarthroses in the radius of the dog.) Helv. Chir. Acta 35:301

Müller, M. E. and S. M. Perren (1972)
Callus und primäre Knochenheilung. (Callus and primary bone healing.) Mschr. Unfallheilk. 75:442

Niederdellmann, H. and B. A. Rahn (1976)
Histologische Untersuchungen nach Osteosynthesen am Hundeunterkiefer mit der Freiburger Zuggurtungsplatte. (Histological studies after osteosyntheses of the dog's mandible with the Freiburg tension band plate.) Fortschr. Kiefer- u. Gesichtschir.

Perren, S. M. (1974)
Biomechanik der Frakturheilung. (Biomechanics of healing of fractures.) Orthopädie 3:135

Perren, S. M., A. Huggler, M. Russenberger, M. Allgöwer, R. Mathys, R. Schenk, H. Willenegger, and M. E. Müller (1969)
The reaction of cortical bone to compression. Acta Orthop. Scand., Suppl. 125:17

Pflüger, G., B. A. Rahn, F. Fischerleitner, H. Thoma, and C. Wolner (1976)
Knöcherne Auffüllung des Distraktionsspalts bei Beinverlängerung. (Bony filling of the distraction gap in leg lengthening.) Arch. Orthop. Unfallchir. 86:45

Pflüger, G., F. Fischerleitner, C. Wolner, and B. A. Rahn (1977)
Radiologischer Verlauf bei Beinverlängerung. Klinik und Experimente. (Radiographic course of leg lengthening. Clinical examples and experiments.) Wien. klin. Wschr. 89 (Suppl. 66) :9

Prein, J., B. Spiessl, B. A. Rahn, and S. M. Perren (1975)
Frakturheilung am Unterkiefer nach operativer Versorgung (Fracture healing of the mandible after surgical care.) Fortschr. Kiefer- u. Gesichtschir. 19:17

Rahn, B. A., P. Gallinaro, A. Baltensperger, and S. M. Perren (1971)
Primary bone healing. An experimental study in the rabbit. J. Bone Jt. Surg. 53 A:783

Rahn, B. A., P. Gallinaro, R. K. Schenk, A. Baltensperger, and S. M. Perren (1972)
Compression interfragmentaire et surcharge locale des os (Interfragmentary compression and local overload of bone.) In Boitzy, A.: Osteogenese et compression. Berne, Huber

Rahn, B. A., G. Pflüger, and F. Fischerleitner (1978)
Die Verlängerung von Röhrenknochen. Morphologischer Ablauf. (Lengthening of long bones. Morphological course.) Acta chir. Austriaca 10:9

Rittmann, W. W. and S. M. Perren (1974)
Corticale Knochenheilung nach Osteosynthese und Infektion. (Cortical bone healing following osteosynthesis and infection.) Berlin, Springer

Rush, L. V. (1957)
Atlas der intramedullären Frakturfixation nach Rush. (Atlas of Rush's intramedullary bone fixation.) Munich, Barth

Schenk, R. K. (1973)
Fracture repair : an overview. Proc. 9th Europ. Symp. Calc. Tiss. Vienna, Verlag Wiener Med. Akad.

Schenk, R. and H. Willenegger (1963)
Zum histologischen Bild der sogenannten Primärheilung der Knochenkompacta nach experimentellen Osteotomien am Hund. (The histological appearance of so-called primary healing of compact bone following experimental osteotomy in the dog.) Experientia 20:593

Schenk, R. and H. Willenegger (1964)
Zur Histologie der primären Knochenheilung. (Histology of primary healing of bone.) Langenbecks Arch. klin. Chir. 308:440

Schenk, R. and H. Willenegger (1967)
Morphological findings in primary fracture healing. Symp. Biol. Hung. 7:75

Weber, B. G. and O. Cech (1973)
Pseudoarthrosen. (Pseudoarthroses.) Berne, Huber

Wieser, C. (1964)
Die primäre Knochenheilung und ihre Störung im Röntgenbild. (Primary healing of bone and its interference in the radiograph.) Langenbecks Arch. klin. Chir. 308:435

Wieser, C. and M. Allgöwer (1962)
Die Beurteilung der Knochenheilung nach stabiler Osteosynthese im Röntgenbild. (Radiographic evaluation of bone healing following stable osteosynthesis.) Radiol. Clin. 31:269

Willenegger, H., S. M. Perren, and R. Schenk (1971)
Primäre und sekundäre Knochenbruchheilung. (Primary and secondary healing of bone fractures.) Chirurg 42:252

Wolff, J. (1892)
Das Gesetz der Transformation der Knochen. (The law of transformation of bones.) Berlin, Hirschwald

Yamada, H. (1970)
Strength of biological materials. Baltimore, Williams and Wilkins.

Chapter 6

Appliances for Immobilization

Norbert Schwenzer and Wolfgang Steinhilber

1. Fundamentals

Wire ligatures, arch bars and splints are aids in the treatment of jaw fractures; they are applied to the teeth, alveolar processes, and skeletal parts of the face or cranium. Their function is the fixation of injured skeletal parts among one another and to uninjured portions, as well as the immobilization of fractured or loosened teeth. For example, the injured mandible is attached to the uninjured maxilla and midface, the injured midface to the forehead, or the mandible and midface, if both are involved, to the cranium.
The oldest devices for this job are extraoral bandages, also known as craniofacial bandages. These have been known since the time of *Hippocrates*. The bandages and head supports recommended then were made of cloth or leather. Specific forms of these bandages are the "funda maxillae" and the "capistrum simplex" and "duplex".
The next step was the development of combined extra- and intraoral appliances. With these, the teeth or the alveolar process of the fractured mandible were enveloped by a metal or rubber device and attached by means of bandages, screws, brackets, or springs to the chin or to a pressure pad located beneath the chin. For fractures of the maxilla and middle third of the face, intraoral devices also were extended between the lips and attached to the calvarium by means of bandages.

The application of tooth-supported appliances of various types to the maxilla and mandible and immobilization of the mandible by intermaxillary fixation are the customary form of treatment, used most frequently today for fractures of the dentulous mandible. In addition a great variety of intraoral devices are available for the partially dentulous or edentulous jaw.
A splint must provide stable attachment to the teeth or to the cranium—while doing minimal damage to the enamel, tooth-supporting structures, soft tissues, and bones—as well as affording good immobilization of the injured portions of the mandible and midface. The splint should be as inconspicuous as possible i.e., made of a minimal amount of material, and, by allowing easy access to its elements, be amenable to easy care. These requirements are satisfied to different degrees by the appliances to be discussed.

2. Classification of Splints

Based on the purposes of splinting, we distinguish between emergency appliances, definitive splints, and aids to functional treatment.
The **emergency appliance** is a temporary device intended to bridge the interval until definitive treatment is performed; during this time further damage from secondary displacement of fragments, friction of the fragments, or wound infection is minimized.
The **definitive splint** has the role of stabilizing and immobilizing the fractured jaw segments during the entire time of treatment until bone consolidation takes place.

The **aids to functional treatment** should bring about partial immobilization of the fracture and permit residual motion, but only within certain limits and in a specific direction (e.g., elastic bands, orthodontic appliances).
According to the **site of application**, we distinguish between intraoral, extraoral, and intra-extraoral appliances.
Intraoral splints are attached to the teeth or alveolar processes. They have been used for a long time for treatment of mandibular fractures when a sufficient number of teeth are present. In fractures in the middle third of the face, they are used in combination with surgical procedures. This group of splints includes custom-made occlusal dentures and base plates for partial dentulous and edentulous jaws.
Extraoral appliances, in the form of support bandages (head gear, chin cup), should be regarded merely as emergency measures or simple temporary measures. With these one cannot achieve anything approaching immobilization.
Intra-extraoral appliances are suitable for support after surgery if the fixation achieved is insufficient, and also if surgical procedures cannot be carried out because of severe generalized disease.
Based on the **material** used, we distinguish among metal splints, acrylic splints, wire-acrylic arch bars, as well as additional devices consisting of plaster casts, cloth, or leather.
Metal appliances are made in the form of wire and wire ligature devices and of arch bars consisting of ready-made materials which are on hand. Open cap splints and cap splints made of metal should be made in the laboratory from impressions and models.
Acrylic appliances include open cap splints and cap splints of acrylic, which are fabricated in the laboratory and are attached with wire ligatures, acrylic, or cement. The largest group of these appliances consists of prosthetic splints (occlusal dentures) for partially dentulous jaws and base plates for edentulous jaws.
Wire-acrylic devices are arch bars and wire appliances coated with acrylic. The continuous-loop wire (*Stout*, 1943; *Obwegeser*, 1952) and the wire-acrylic arch bar (*Schuchardt*, 1956) are usually coated with cold-curing acrylic after being placed in the mouth. The enamel should be treated with a fluoride preparation beforehand. All wire-acrylic appliances, however, can also be fabricated in advance in the laboratory and can be inserted in the mouth after being coated with acrylic.
Based on the technique, we distinguish between appliances which are applied directly and those made in advance in the laboratory and applied indirectly.
Direct appliances include all single- and continuous-wire appliances, arch bars (*Sauer*, 1889), and wire-acrylic arch bars (*Schuchardt*, 1956). Their advantage is the immediate definitive treatment of the patient.
Indirect appliances are made in advance in the laboratory on a model, from an impression taken of the patient.
Their advantage is that less work has to be done on the patient; the disadvantage is the dependence on the laboratory and the resulting time delay.

3. Technique of Application

3.1 Interdental Wiring

Indications. On the one hand, this method is used for emergency devices for temporary fixation and immobilization, for example, for patients with multiple trauma, if other forms of treatment are unavailable, and during transport. On the other hand, these devices are also employed for definitive care when an adequate number of teeth is present to achieve a stable bite.
The wire ligatures can be used singly, next to or above one another, and also as continuous wire ligatures. We use them frequently for loosened teeth in the deciduous and mixed dentition.
Advantages. Only steel wire and a few instruments are needed. Application always takes place directly in the mouth.
Disadvantages. Because of their limited stability, they are unsuited for monomaxillary fixation. Periodontal damage may occur.

Technique:
Direct interdental wiring (*Gilmer*, 1887) is the simplest form of ligature. In the maxilla and man-

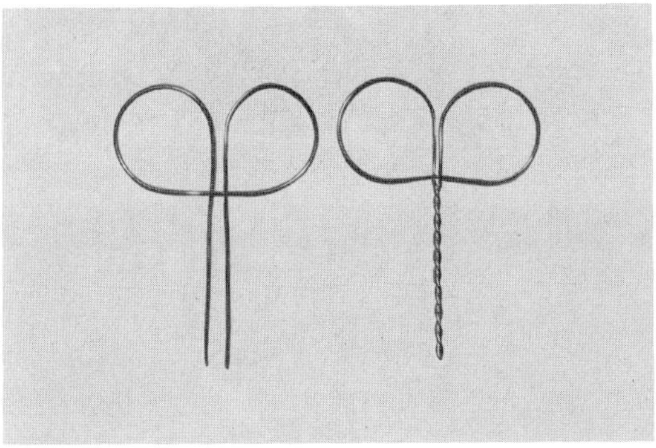

Fig. 6-1 *Ernst*'s ligature. Placement of the ligature wire.

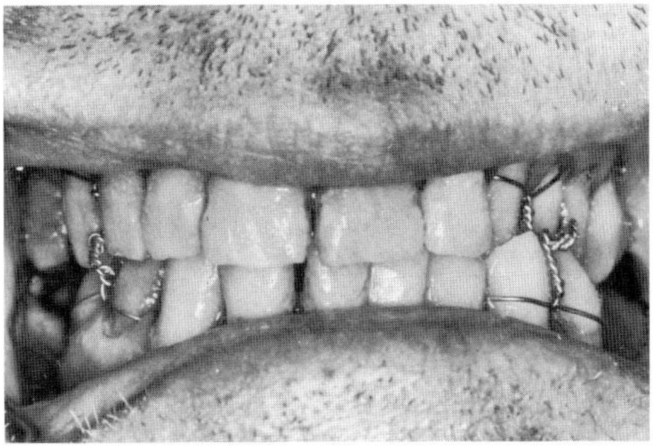

Fig. 6-2 Temporary immobilization of the mandible with *Ernst* ligatures.

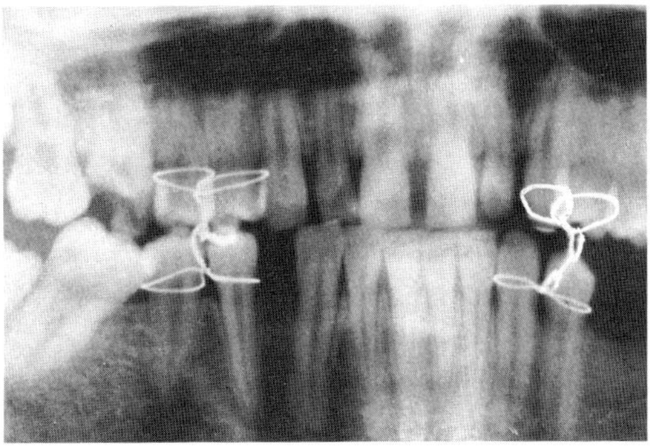

Fig. 6-3 Orthopantomogram. *Ernst* ligatures for temporary immobilization of the mandible.

dible, single wire ligatures are applied with soft steel wire. For intermaxillary fixation, the maxillary wires are wound together with the mandibular wires (see Fig. 8. 2-23). *Hering* (1960) coats the ends of the ligatures with cold-curing acrylic (see Fig. 8. 2-24).

Ernst's **wire** (1927, 1932). Soft, 0.4 mm diameter wire is guided around two adjacent teeth in such a way that both ends extend buccally in the same interdental space between the two teeth and the buccal cross wire is grasped by the two ends of the wire (Figs. 6-1 to 3).

For temporary immobilization of the mandible in fractures outside the dental arch and in fractures and contusions of the TMJ, an Ernst ligature in each half of the jaw is sufficient; the ends of the ligature wires, which lie opposite each other in the maxilla and mandible, are twisted together.

For temporary stabilization of a fracture within the dental arch, three Ernst wires are required; one each for two teeth on either side of the fracture and the third, around the teeth adjoining the fracture, applied after reduction. The purpose of this procedure is protection of the teeth adjacent to the fracture.

The *Kazanjian* **button** (1933) already has been described under emergency devices (see p. 112 and Fig. 4-16).

Interdental eyelet wiring (*Eby*, 1920; *Ivy*, 1922) also includes two adjoining teeth on each side (see also pp. 260 f. and Fig. 8. 2-28).

During tightening of the ligature, the eyelet is drawn into the interdental space. This compli-

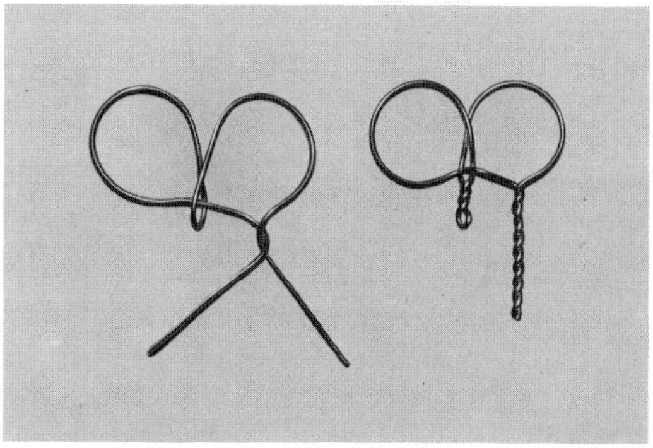

Fig. 6-4 Eyelet wire. The buccal wire does not pass through the eyelet, but between the interdental wires. During tightening of the ligature, the eyelet is not pulled into the interdental space.

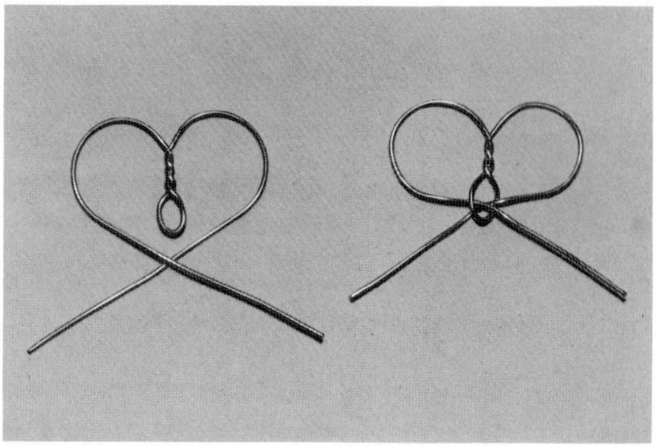

Fig. 6-5 Modified eyelet wire.

cates the application of intermaxillary tie wires. Therefore it is preferable to draw the buccal wire between the interdental wires rather than through the eyelet (Fig. 6-4). Figure 6-5 shows a further modification. *Williams* (1968) applies a second loop for the buccal wire, in addition to the eyelet for the tie wires (see Fig. 8.2-30).

Continuous or multiple-loop wiring (*Stout*, 1943; *Obwegeser*, 1952) is carried out with soft steel wire, 0.4 to 0.5 mm thick. The eyelet wiring is extended over the entire dental arch (Fig. 6-6 A; see also Figs. 8.2-26 and 27). By means of a coating with cold-curing acrylic, improved stability can be achieved (Fig. 6-6 B).

The **cable arch wire** (*Risdon*, 1929) consists of 1 mm thick soft steel wire which is applied to the last tooth of the dental arch on each side. The twisted ends are adapted to the dental arch, twisted together in the middle, and fastened to the remaining teeth by single ligatures of 0.35 mm steel wire (see Fig. 8.2-31). Coating with cold-curing acrylic may be used.

3.2 Arch Bar Wiring

Half-round, oval, round, or flat wire is bent at the labial surface of the dental arch to fit the shape of the necks of the teeth, is attached to the teeth with single ligatures, and may contain supporting elements (hooks or eyelets) for elastic bands or tie wires. The most commonly used devices are *Sauer*'s (1889) arch bar (Fig. 6-7 A), *Hauptmeyer*'s (1924) arch bar (Fig. 6-7 B), the profile arch bar of *Schlampp* (1942, Fig. 6-7 C), and the prefabricated arch bar (*Jelenko, Winter, Erich, Niro*, Fig. 6-7 D).

Indication. Readily adaptable prepared device for fractures in the dentulous jaw.

Advantages. Only ligature wires need to be kept on hand, and only few instruments are needed. Free-hand adaptation and application of the appliance is possible.

Disadvantages. Danger of slipping off to the tooth cervix. Damage to enamel and periodontium can occur. Wires may need to be tightened from time to time.

Technique. The wire is pre-bent to fit the gingival seam (this is more easily done on a model) and attached to each tooth with two single ligatures. The twisted portions of the single ligatures, which are adjacent to each other, can remain about 5 mm long and can be bent apically. In this way, small hooks are formed for the attachment of elastic bands or tie wires, if no suitable supporting structures have been applied to the splint.

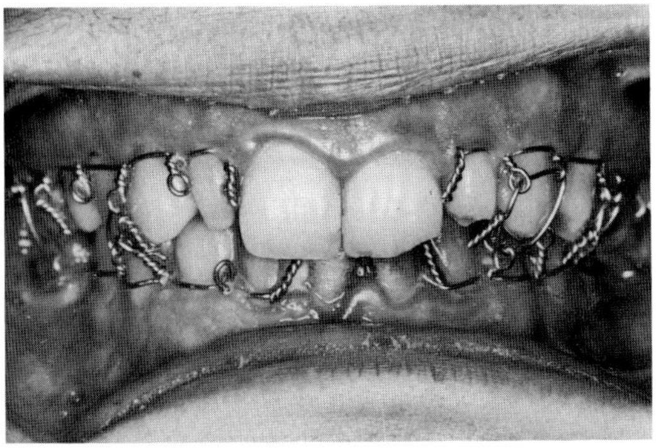

Fig. 6-6 A Continuous loop wiring *(Stout-Obwegeser)*.

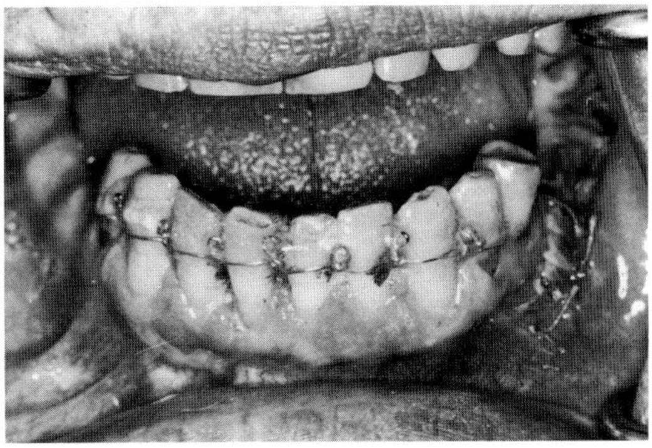

Fig. 6-6 B Continuous loop wiring with acrylic coating.

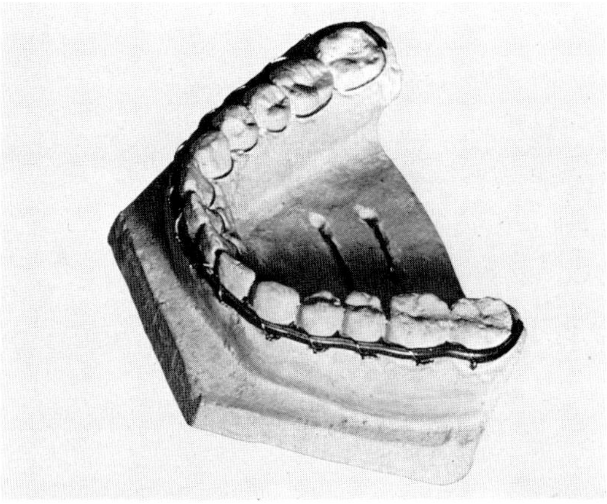

Fig. 6-7 A *Sauer*'s arch bar.

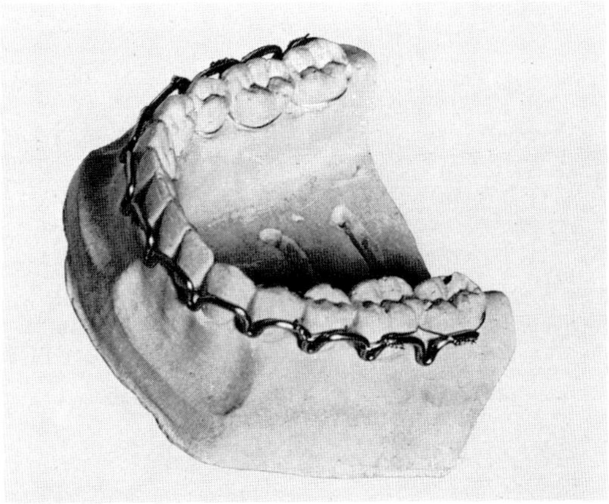

Fig. 6-7 B *Hauptmeyer*'s arch bar.

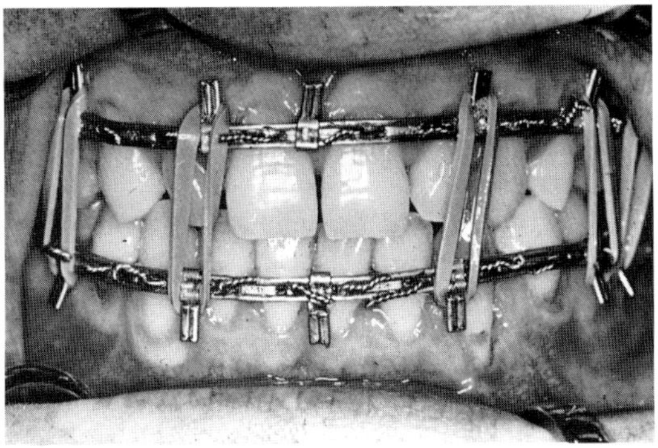

Fig. 6-7 C Profile arch bar (*Schlampp*, 1942).

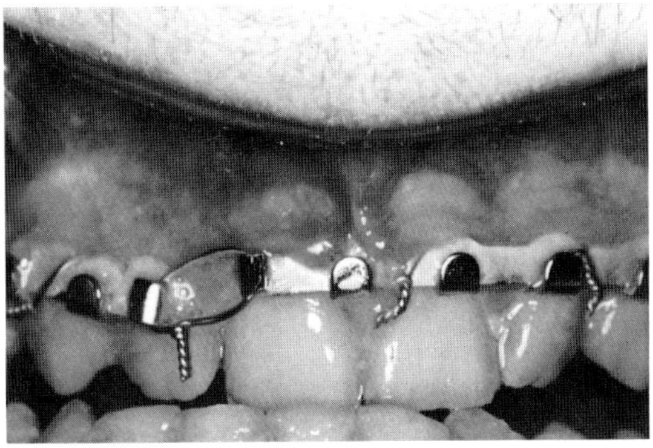

Fig. 6-7 D Niro arch bar.

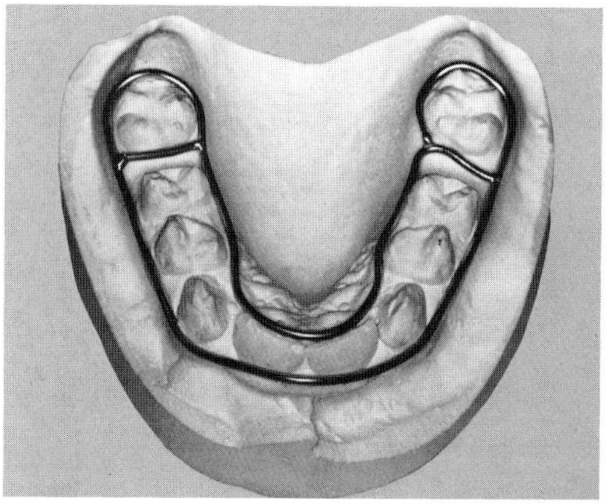

Fig. 6-8 Circumferential arch bar (*Hammond*, 1874).

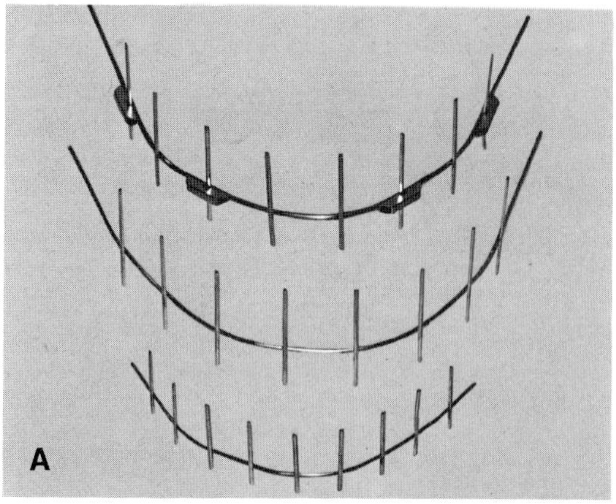

Figs. 6-9 A to C Wire-acrylic arch bar (*Schuchardt*, 1956).

Fig. 6-9 A Prefabricated arch bars.
Top: Arch bar with cannulas for the maxilla, for maxillary fractures.
Middle: Arch bar for maxilla and mandible, for mandibular fractures.
Bottom: Arch bar for deciduous dentition.

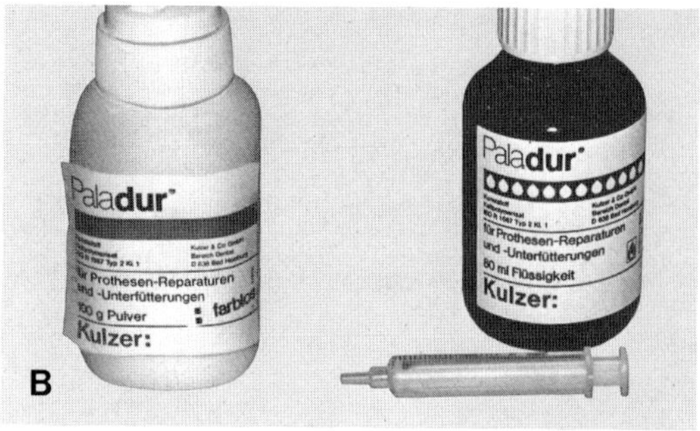

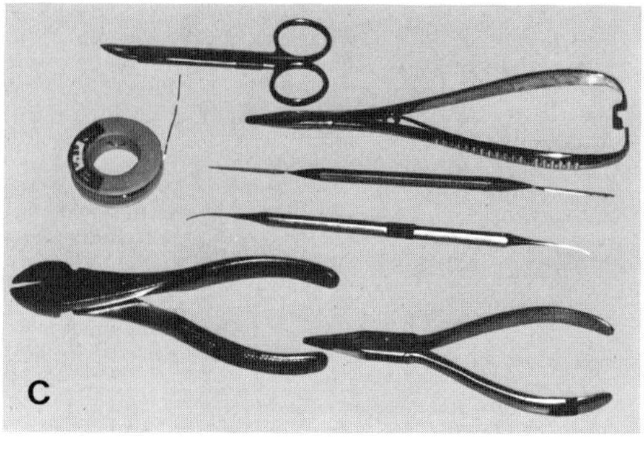

Figs. 6-9 B and C Instruments for splinting.

3.3 Circumferential Arch Bar (*Hammond*, 1874)

Description. The difference from the device described above is that a thinner wire, usually round, is placed around the entire dental arch on the vestibular and palatal sides. The rows of wires are connected, in some locations, by bars extending over the dental arch (Fig. 6-8).
Indication. Device for fractures in the partial edentulous arch.
Advantages. Improved stability in the partial edentulous arch compared to the arch bar. Fewer single ligatures are required.
Disadvantages. The arch bar must be made in the laboratory from a model.

3.4 Wire-Acrylic Arch Bar (*Schuchardt*, 1956)

Description. The splint consists of a half-round, 2 mm thick soft wire arch with 6 to 8 perpendicular cross wires, 1.4 mm thick, which are fastened to the connecting bar wire at a distance of 1.5 cm. One side of a cross wire serves as a future support for elastic bands and tie wires; the other side is used only during insertion of the arch bar as an occlusal stabilizing element for avoiding slippage to the gingival margin.
For the treatment of maxillary fractures, both sides of the arch bar include square tubes designed to accommodate extraoral connecting bars or suspension wires. In addition, an eyelet can be applied at the center for fixation of extension devices. The arch bar is made commercially;* it is also available in a smaller form for the deciduous dentition (Fig. 6-9 A). In addition, 0.35 mm soft steel (V4AS) wire (one ligature per tooth) as well as cold-curing acrylic are needed (Fig. 6-9 B).
Indications. The arch bar is suitable for all fractures in the dentulous or partially dentulous maxilla and mandible, and for immobilization of loosened teeth. In addition, it can be used in all orthodontic operations.
Advantages. The prefabricated arch bar permits direct splinting of all types of fracture without the use of a model. Periodontal damage cannot occur, for the arch bar, when properly applied, never rests on the gingival margin, unlike most other types of arch bars.

Technique (Fig. 6-10):
Basically, first the maxillary arch bar and then the mandibular bar is applied.
First, the bar is fitted to the dental arch. With complete dentition, it should extend on both sides to the second molar. In case of a deficient number of teeth, the third molars should be included as supporting elements. The splint is bent in such a way that the middle cross wire lies between the central incisors. The occlusal ends of the cross wires are then bent toward the occlusal surfaces with flat-nosed pliers in such a way that they can be positioned on the interdental spaces in the premolar region and in the fissures in the molar region; in this way, slipping of the splint to the gingival margin is prevented. In this process, the arch bar is made to lie at the level of the dental equator. The occlusal hooks are then shortened so that they do not protrude the occlusal surfaces of the crowns. The ends of the cross wires which extend to the vestibular side sometimes must also be shortened so that they will not cause ulceration in the vestibule. The cut ends of the cross wires are then smoothed by grinding. After adaptation of the bar to the dental arch, the ligatures are placed around each individual tooth.
If plaster models are available, the arch bar can be bent to fit the model.
The wire ligatures are guided in such a way that the wire runs below the wire arch on the mesial side and above it distally. The ends of the wires are twisted together with a ligature forceps or a hemostat and shortened to a length of about 5 mm. Then they are bent to fit the arch bar.
Besides simple guiding of the wire, it is also possible, especially with cone-shaped teeth, to wind the distal end of the wire around the arch bar and then to twist it together with the mesial portion. In such cases, a cross ligature or a double ligature is preferable (see Fig. 8.2-4).
It has proved satisfactory first to attach the bar on both sides in the premolar region and then to tie in the arch bar from the center in the distal direction. When this has been done, the bar is stabilized with acrylic. Prior to this, it is advisable to touch up the dried teeth with a fluoride com-

* Manufacturer: Renfert, D-7700 Singen/Hohentwiel, Germany.

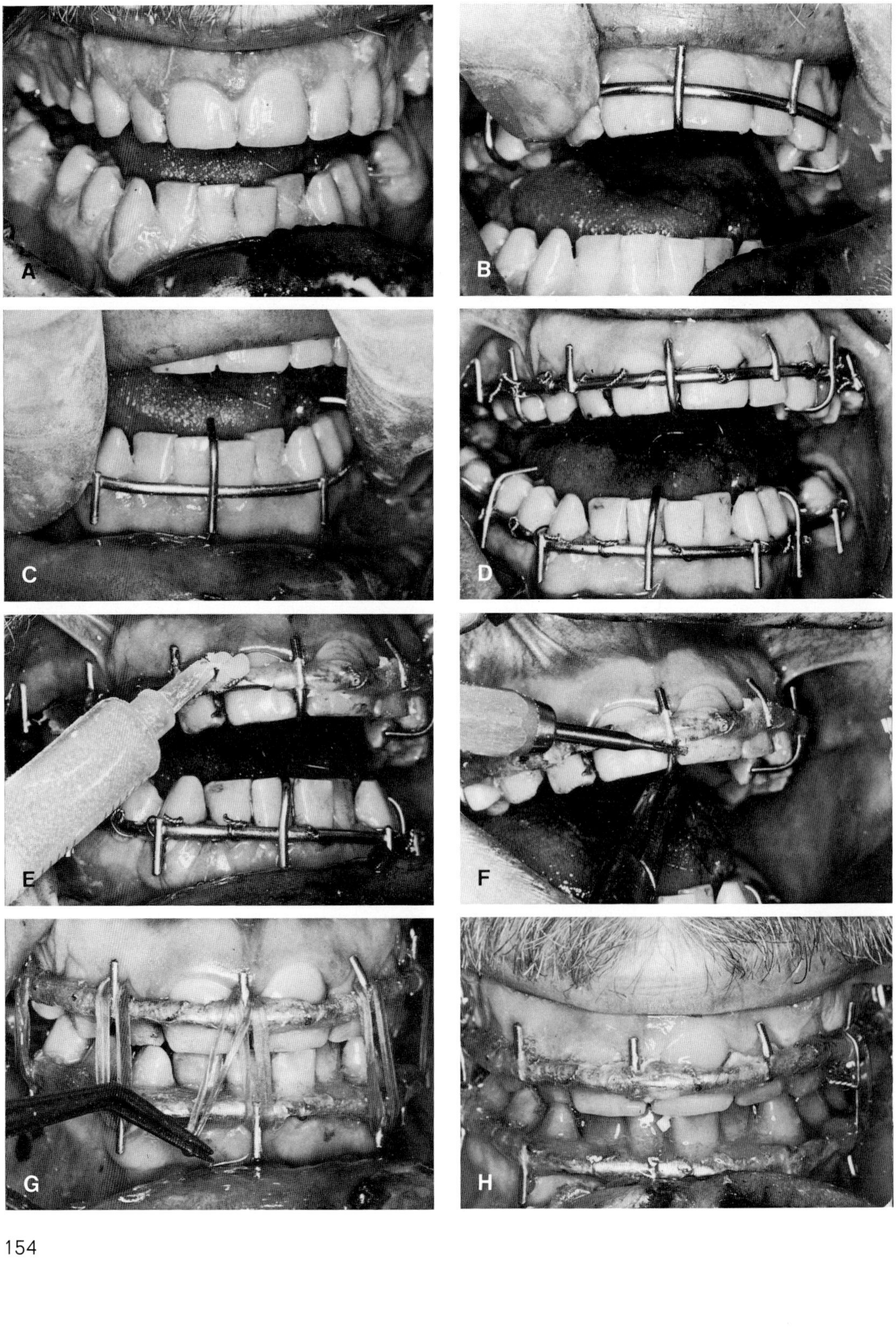
A
B
C
D
E
F
G
H

pound for prevention of caries (*Krüger* and *Chrissatis*, 1971).

After repeated examination of the wire ends, which may have to be tightened once again with a flat-nosed pliers, the ligatures and the open spaces between the teeth and the arch bar are filled in with acrylic. Thus the appliance is absolutely stabilized at the same time, so that subsequent bending is no longer possible. The gingival margin remains free, so that adequate cleansing is possible. It has proved convenient to apply the acrylic with a disposable syringe. When the acrylic has hardened, the hooks toward the occlusal side are severed with pliers or with a fissure bur. The ends are smoothed by grinding. At the same time, sharp edges on the acrylic can be smoothed. After the maxillary arch bar has been attached by this method, the mandibular bar is applied.

In cases of mandibular fractures, the procedure may be different, depending on whether the fracture is outside or within the dental arch. For fractures outside the dental arch, i.e., fractures of the condylar process or of the ascending ramus, an uninterrupted arch bar can be applied to the mandible. The procedure is that described above. After both appliances are in place, the mandible is reduced, the goal being the restoration of the centric occlusion. This can be done manually, so that after proper occlusion is achieved, intermaxillary fixation with wire ligatures (soft steel wire, 0.35 mm) is carried out. If immediate reduction is impossible, progressive reduction must be undertaken with the aid of elastic bands which are attached to the corresponding hooks of the maxillary and mandibular arch bars.

In fractures within the dental arch, it is necessary, when direct manual reduction and immediate bridging of the fracture by means of the arch bar do not succeed or are only partially successful, to apply a divided arch bar. The dividing site usually corresponds to the fracture site. It is advisable to let the adjacent parts overlap. After adjustment of the occlusion with elastic bands or manually, the parts of the arch bar are joined with wire and acrylic, and thus the fracture site is rigidly bridged.

In case of a slight displacement, the coating with acrylic in the vicinity of the fracture site can be omitted initially. After centric occlusion has been achieved, the arch bar is stabilized with acrylic in the appropriate section.

It is quite possible to divide the bar at the fracture site afterwards and, after improving the occlusion, to restore the acrylic connection.

In edentulous jaws, the gaps can be bridged with acrylic saddles. The acrylic bridges can be applied directly in the mouth as well as on the model (see p. 158).

Removal of Wire-Acrylic Arch Bar

After healing of the fracture has occured, the appliances can be removed relatively quickly and easily. The arch bar is severed at the center with pliers, causing the acrylic to separate, and the arch bar is cut apart. Then the arch bar is bent outward and, after cutting off the wire ligatures on the buccal side, is rolled away from the dental arch from the mesial toward the distal side.

Figs. 6-10 A to H Application of a wire-acrylic arch bar.

Fig. 6-10 A Malocclusion.

Fig. 6-10 B Fitting of the arch bar to the maxilla.

Fig. 6-10 C Fitting of the arch bar to the mandible.

Fig. 6-10 D Arch bars tied in place with ligatures (0.35 mm). Cross wires which are bent toward the occlusal surface prevent slipping of the splint to the gingiva.

Fig. 6-10 E Application of cold-curing acrylic with a disposable syringe.

Fig. 6-10 F Severing of the occlusal ends of the cross wires with the fissure bur.

Fig. 6-10 G Adjustment of the occlusion with elastic bands.

Fig. 6-10 H Intermaxillary fixation with tie wires which must still be applied in the incisor region.

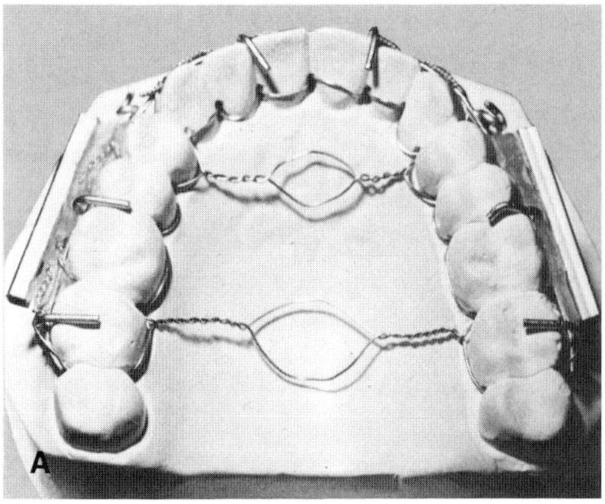

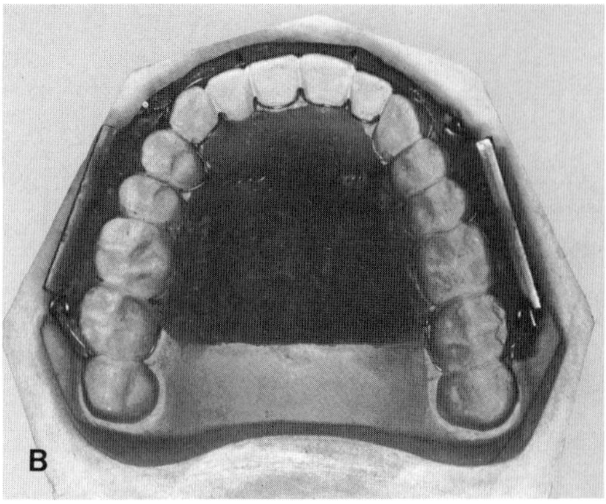

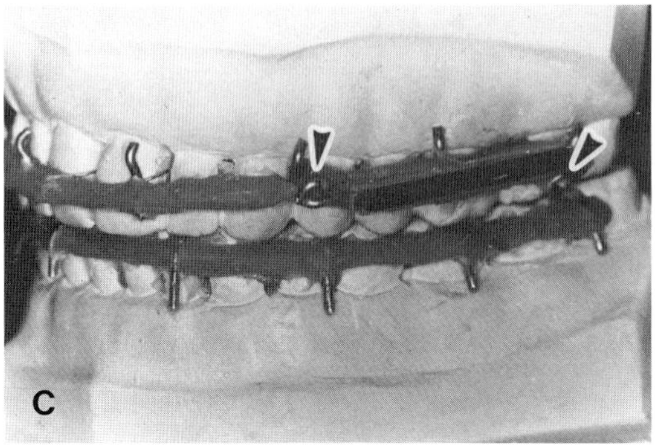

Figs. 6-11 A to C Wire-acrylic arch bar with square tubes and palatal plate.

Fig. 6-11 A Transmaxillary wires across the palate.

Fig. 6-11 B Completed palatal plate.

Fig. 6-11 C Completed device. The square tubes will receive the side bars of the *Kingsley* splint. In addition, two loops are provided for fixation of the wire suspension (arrows).

Modification of the Wire-Acrylic Arch Bar for Maxillary Fractures

With multiple fractures of the maxilla, especially with sagittal fractures, it is necessary to use additional palatal reinforcement of the wire-acrylic arch bar according to the method reported by *Schwenzer* (1961). Here too, it is possible to carry out the stabilization either directly in the mouth or on the model. To effect palatal reinforcement, one applies one additional wire ligature each, with a diameter of 0.4 cm, which crosses the palate in the region of the first premolars and the first molars. These two wire ligatures which extend across the palate can be used for reduction of sagittal fractures which are accompanied by widening of the maxilla if the ends of the ligatures are twisted together. They are then reinforced with a palatal plate of cold-curing acrylic (Fig. 6-11 A and B). In the edentulous spaces the palatal plate combines with the vestibular acrylic coating of the attached arch bar to provide improved stability. Between the acrylic and the palatal mucosa, one can insert either a layer of gauze saturated with an ointment or a thin gutta percha plate. The heat created during the setting process is decreased by applying wet, cold compresses.

When the appliance is fabricated by the indirect process, the palatal plate of cold-curing acrylic is made on the model after sawing apart and rejoining the two halves of the jaw in the correct position. In this case, reinforcement with crosswise wire ligatures is not necessary.

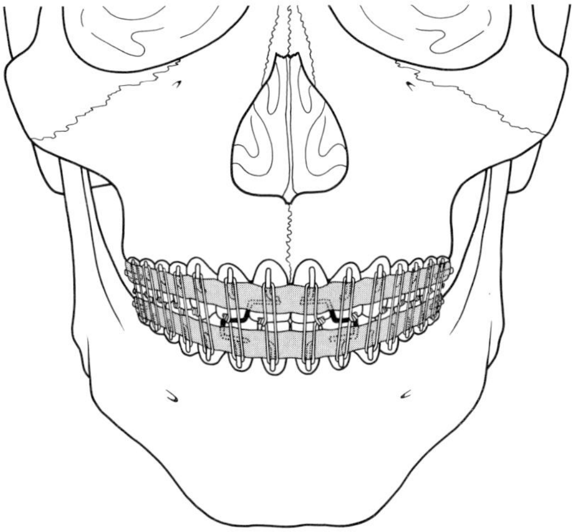

Fig. 6-12 Acrylic open-cap splint (*Schrudde*, 1953).

For fractures in the middle third of the face, the maxilla, provided with a wire-acrylic arch bar, must be attached to the forehead; this is usually accomplished by means of internal skeletal fixation (see Chapter 10), and requires application of anchors on the maxillary splint.
In the simplest case, a loop at the level of the second premolar on each side of the bar wire, through which the suspension wires are passed, is sufficient. A better method consists of two loops or square tubes on each side of the arch bar, so that the traction forces of the suspension wires are distributed (Fig. 6-11 C).

3.5 Other Acrylic-Coated Appliances

Description. These include a group of devices which are either applied in the mouth and coated with acrylic or fabricated in the laboratory and only need to be fastened in the mouth with individual ligatures.
Indication. Same as wire-acrylic arch bar described above.
Advantages. The acrylic coating generally improves the stability of the appliances. Periodontal damage is avoided, since these devices do not come in contact with the gingiva. If the splint is made in advance in the laboratory, the time required for insertion is short, and no monomer reaches the enamel.

Disadvantages. If the splint is made in advance, it is necessary to take an impression, which, however, can be limited to the labial and buccal surfaces of the teeth.

Technique:
Direct interdental wiring with acrylic coating (*Hering*, 1960).
As in the *Gilmer* method (1887), each tooth receives a single ligature. The ends of the ligature wires, which are twisted together, are shortened to a length of 2 cm. Then cold-curing acrylic is applied to the vestibular surfaces of the tooth crowns, enclosing the ligatures. The acrylic is shaped into a ribbon-like vestibular splint. The ends of the wires which extend from the acrylic are twisted together into rosettes. They serve as holding elements for the tie wires or elastic bands (see Fig. 8.2-24).
Prefabricated arch bars can be coated with acrylic in a similar way (*Hofmann*, 1958).
The **acrylic open cap splint** (*Schrudde*, 1953) is made in the laboratory. On the model, the gingival seam is covered with wax into which wires designed to receive the intermaxillary tie wires or elastic bands are fused. In addition, wires are passed through interdental spaces and possible edentulous spaces; these wires connect the oral and vestibular portions of the splint. After applying the gingival wax covering and the wires, cold-curing acrylic is added to the buccal

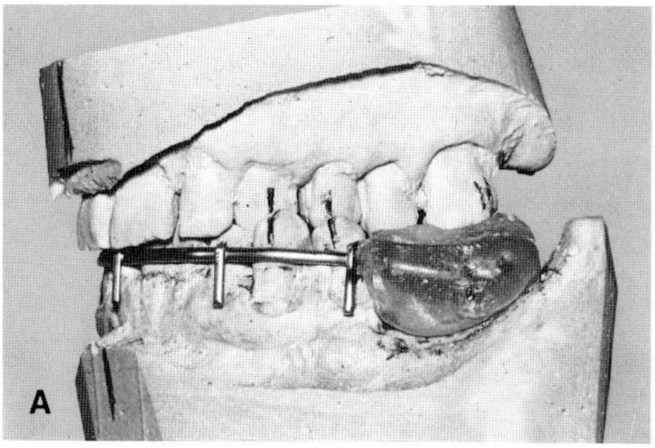

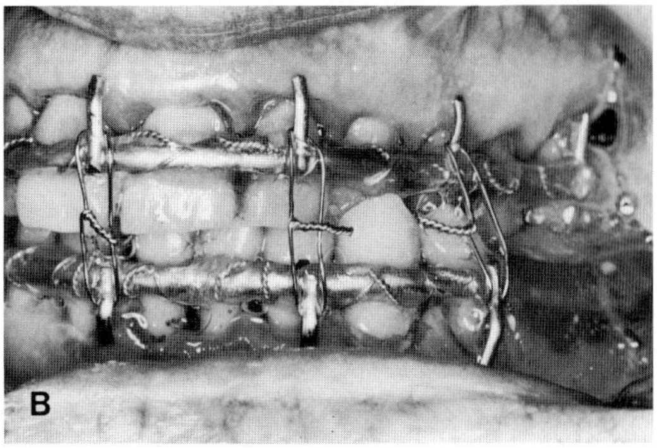

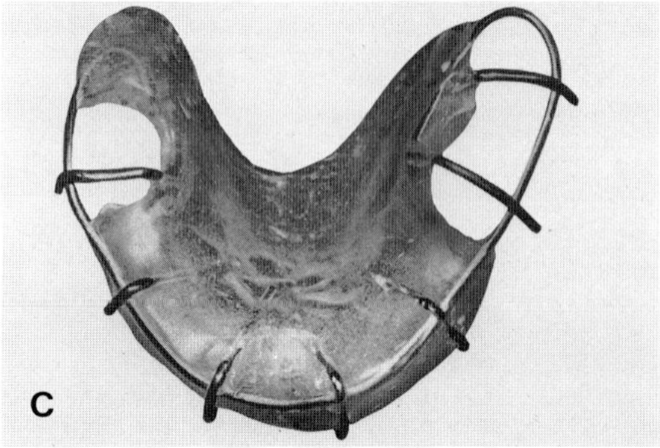

Figs. 6-13 A to C Arch bar with saddle.

Fig. 6-13 A Mandibular appliance prepared on the model.

Fig. 6-13 B Arch bar applied to the mandible.

Fig. 6-13 C Arch bar with palatal plate for the maxilla.

and oral crown surfaces, except on the occlusal surfaces. After the acrylic hardens, the splint is removed from the model, completed, shaped, and polished. The finished splint is mounted with a non-viscous cold-curing acrylic (Fig. 6-12).

3.6 Arch Bar with Prosthesis Saddles

Description. Arch bar prefabricated in the laboratory and provided with a prosthetic saddle for edentulous jaw segments. The splint is attached with single ligatures to the available teeth.

Indication. Device for jaw fractures, and for immobilization after orthodontic surgery in the partial dentulous maxilla and mandible.

Advantages. Weight placed on edentulous jaw segments results in an even distribution, over the entire alveolar process, of the forces that arise during immobilization. In dentulous segments, the advantages are those of the wire-acrylic arch bar.

Disadvantages. Portions of the splint supported by mucosa tend to become soiled; they are not accessible for cleansing, and self-cleansing is not possible. Danger of pressure points if attached tightly.

Technique. Fabrication in the laboratory after impression (Fig. 6-13). In dentulous segments, the splint is attached with single ligatures to all available teeth. The free-end saddle is attached to the mandible by a circumferential wire (*Krüger* and *Rivas*, 1966; see also Fig. 8.4-1), and to the maxilla by circumzygomatic wiring. For avoidance of pressure points, a lining of black gutta percha is desirable.

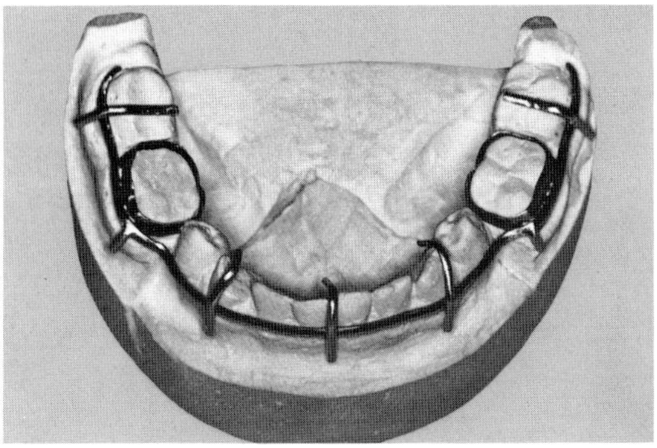

Fig. 6-14 Arch bar with soldered ring bands, prepared according to results from the model manipulation.

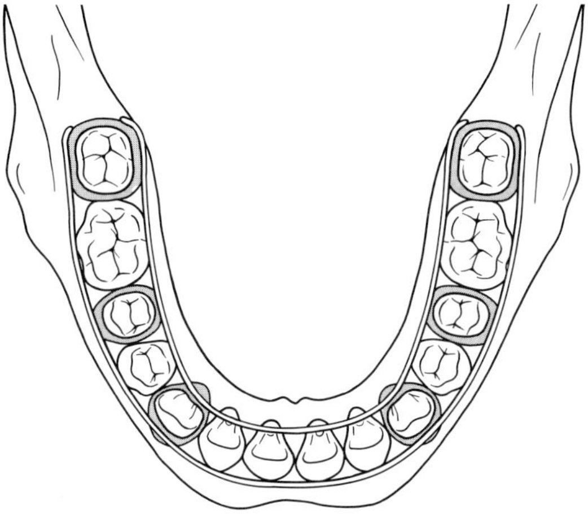

Fig. 6-15 Ring band arch bar (*Greve*, 1950).

3.7 Banded Dental-Arch Wire Appliance

Description. Metal ring-shaped bands which are placed around individual teeth or all teeth, and are connected with an arch bar by means of buccal tubes, screws, or soldering (Fig. 6-14). Described in detail are: the banded arch wire splint according to *Angle* (1905; see Fig. 8.2-7) with the screw on the lingual side, and that of *Schröder* (1911; see Fig. 8.2-8) with the screw on the buccal side, and the banded splint according to *Schlampp* (1942; see Fig. 8.2-9) and *Greve* (1950; Fig. 6-15).
Indication. In partially dentulous jaws after jaw fractures and with orthodontic surgery in the body of the mandible or in individual segments of the alveolar process. As space maintainer in fractures involving loss of bone (*Wassmund*, 1927).
Advantages. Soldered bands improve the support of a splint in partially edentulous jaws and in a fragment which has few teeth. If screws are used, tension or pressure can be applied to jaw segments, teeth, or groups of teeth.
Disadvantages. Greater expense in fabrication of the splint and in its application to the patient. Banded individual teeth can receive too much stress (*Weiskopf*, 1969).

Technique. An impression is taken and a model is made. Bands are fitted in the mouth and then transferred to the model. After completion in the laboratory, ligatures are placed intraorally and the appliance is mounted.

3.8 Open Cap Splint, Cast Metal Splint

Description. Splint of metal or acrylic, which adheres like a band to the buccal and lingual surfaces of all teeth and is attached with ligatures or with cement (Figs. 6-16 and 17).
Indication. Device for all fractures in dentulous jaws. Suitable for long-term splinting, i.e., for delayed healing of a fracture, in fractures due to gunshots or with defects, for alveolar process fractures and loosened teeth.
Advantages. Good stability when fit is good. The splint is inconspicuous if it is made as a delicate metal splint.
Disadvantages. Great technical expenditure. Much time is required for preparation and insertion. Removal is difficult, especially for metal splints.

Technique. Exact impression is taken. Master model for fabrication of the metal splint as a model casting. Attachment of the open cap splint in the mouth by means of cement or acrylic. For ease of insertion, the vestibular bar can be severed and reconnected by means of a ligature or screw. The considerably more delicate cast metal splint is tied with wire ligatures (cf. also chapter 8, pp. 251 f.).

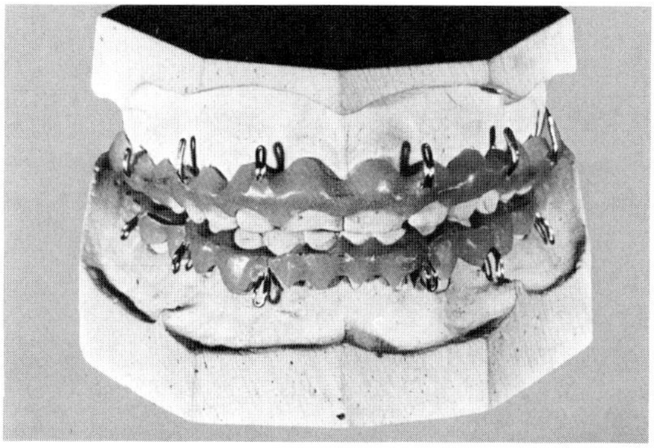

Fig. 6-16 Acrylic open cap splint, with hooks for immobilization.

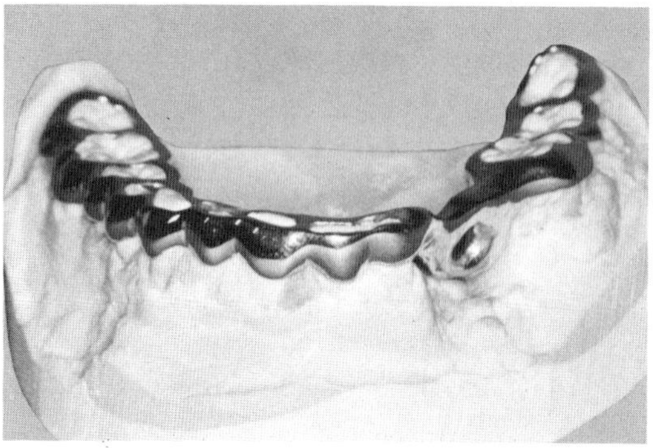

Fig. 6-17 A Metal open cap splint for mandibular defect fracture.

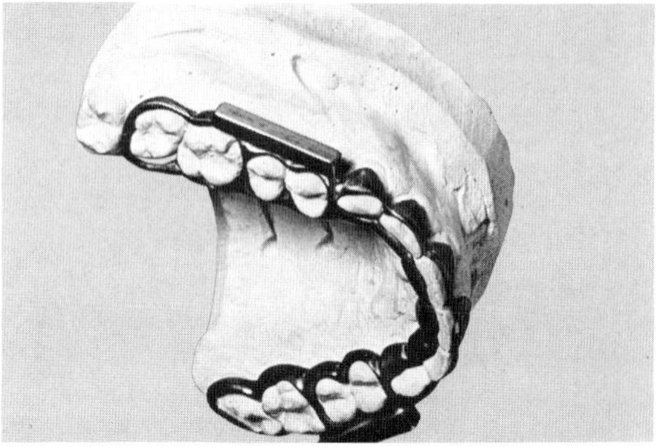

Fig. 6-17 B Open cap splint for the maxilla, with square tubes for attachment of extraoral side bars.

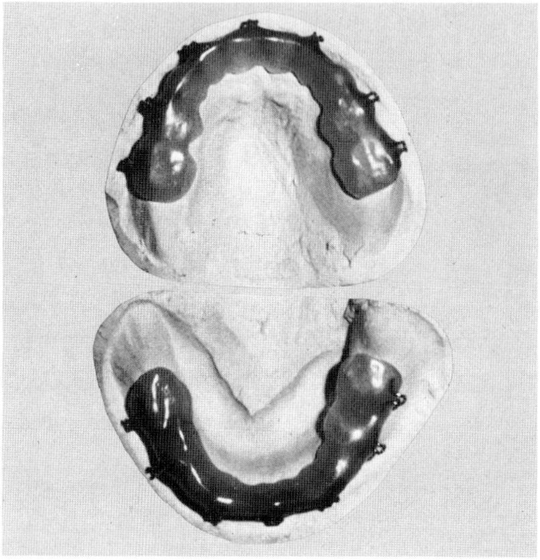

Fig. 6-18 Cap splints for maxilla and mandible, for mandibular fracture in deciduous dentition.

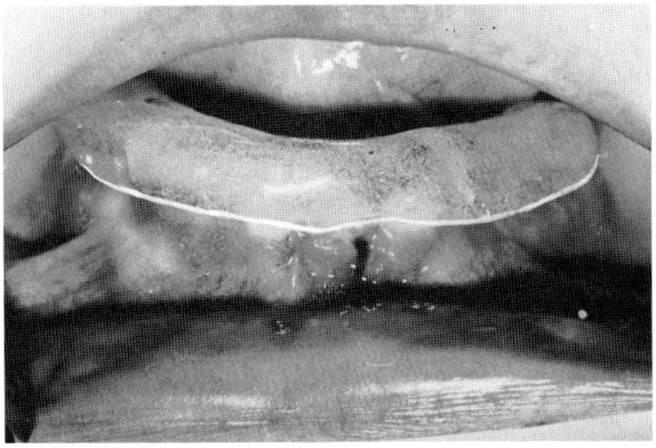

Fig. 6-19 Cap splint of cold-curing acrylic, fabricated in the mouth and inserted with circumferential wiring, for mandibular fracture in a one-year-old child.

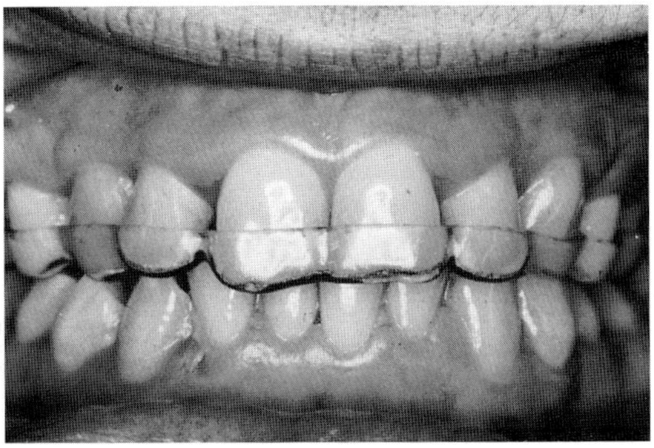

Fig. 6-20 Miniplast splint (*Drum*, 1966) for follow-up-treatment.

3.9 Cap Splint

Description. Splint made of metal or acrylic, covering the entire surfaces of all teeth (Fig. 6-18; see also Fig. 8.2-16).
Indication. Device for all fractures in dentulous jaws. For the deciduous dentition (Fig. 6-18) if insertion of an arch bar is impossible.
Advantages. Great stability.
Disadvantages. For metal cap splints, great technical expenditure and time-consuming procedure. In case of displacement, difficulties are encountered in exact reduction when the splint is attached. No means for adjusting the occlusion, and no control over occlusion.

Technique. Exact impression is taken. Master model for model casting. Fixation in mouth with cement. Sometimes, supplementary suspension in the maxilla or circumferential wiring in the mandible is necessary.

3.9.1 Cap Splint of Cold-Curing Acrylic

For mandibular fractures in infants and small children, a simple acrylic pressure pad on the teeth and alveolar process in the form of a cap splint is sufficient. Cold-curing acrylic in a soft form is shaped into a roll, inserted in the mouth, and pressed on carefully. When heating begins, the acrylic is taken out and should be left to finish hardening outside the mouth. After shaping and polishing, the splint is attached to the mandible by means of circumferential wires (Fig. 6-19).
Pfeifer (1959) described an acrylic cap splint which covers only the teeth and is also fabricated in the mouth of cold-curing acrylic and inserted with cement or acrylic. The gingival margin remains free. This cap splint is especially suitable for fixation of loosened teeth or of teeth of the deciduous and mixed dentition which are fractured in the root region.

3.9.2 Miniplast Splint (*Drum*, 1966)

The miniplast splint, made of acrylic, is a special form of cap splint. It is formed on the model by a thermal vacuum technique, with pressurized air (**Erkopress**®). Its many applications in traumatology include loosened teeth, fractures of the alveolar process, or reimplantations. It provides stabilization of the teeth to one another. Following operations of maxillary prognathism and osteotomies in the alveolar process, it provides uniform distribution of biting and masticatory stresses over the entire dental arch. For delayed bleeding, extractions in hemophiliacs, and for palatal surgery, this provides an ideal dressing pad (Fig. 6-20).

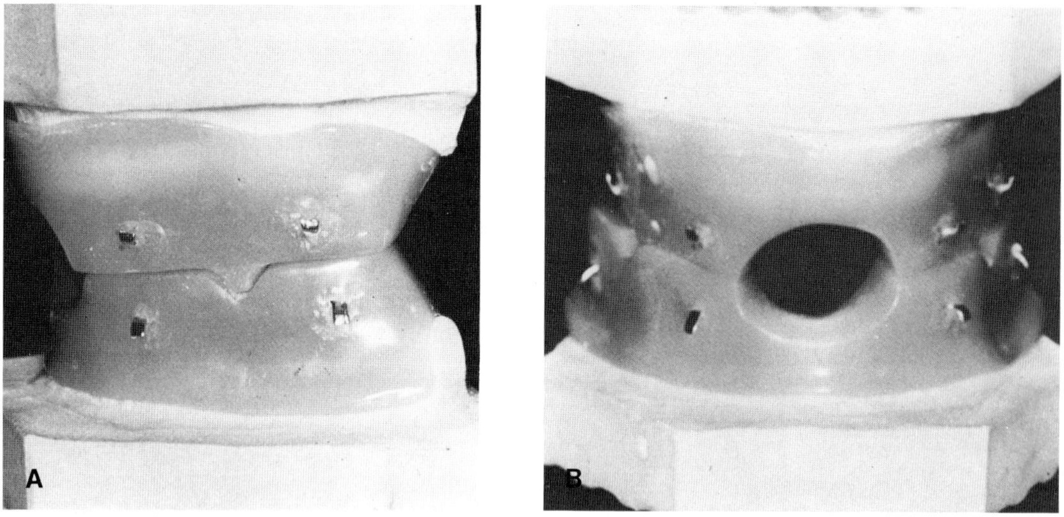

Figs. 6-21 A and B *Gunning* splints.
Fig. 6-21 A Lateral prongs in the bite wall for bite fixation.
Fig. 6-21 B Frontal space for intake of nourishment.

3.10 Prosthetic Splints (Base Plates, Occlusal Dentures)

Description. Occlusal dentures with bite rims of acrylic and base plates as devised by *Gunning* (1866/67, Fig. 6-21), or the patient's dentures with auxiliary devices (Fig. 6-22) are put to use as splints.
Indication. Device for all fractures of the jaws and facial skeleton in the edentulous or nearly edentulous maxilla or mandible.
Advantages. The prosthetic splint represents the only means for stabilizing and immobilizing edentulous jaws by conservative measures.
Disadvantages. The rigid insertion of a large denture base promotes friction of the mucosa. The accumulation of detritus leads to the risk of infection. Sites of perforation of the mucosa by the suspension wires may become infected. Suspension wires may cut into the bone.

Technique. An impression is made including a bite impression, if possible. Fabrication in the laboratory; the bite rims in the front are removed in part so that a space is preserved for food intake. Some front teeth may be removed from dentures.
In the maxilla, internal fixation of the splint by suspension to the frontal bone or zygomatic arch is possible. External fixation is accomplished by means of a *Kingsley* splint (1880) attached to a plaster head cap. Prosthetic splints of the mandible must be fixed by circumferential wiring.
It is advisable to line prosthetic splints with black gutta percha so that pressure points on the mucosa are avoided.
For edentulous patients who have no dentures, it is possible to fabricate a maxillary dressing pad by the **direct procedure**; this is helpful for fixation of the middle third of the face.
For this purpose, a disposable impression tray is shortened at the edges in such a way that it does not cut into the vestibule and is filled with cold-curing acrylic. Before the acrylic sets, the tray is pressed to the maxilla and is removed shortly before the acrylic hardens. After shaping of the maxillary plate fabricated in this way, it can be attached to the suspension wires (Fig. 6-23). It has been found useful as well to line the splint made in this way with gutta percha, so that pressure points are avoided.

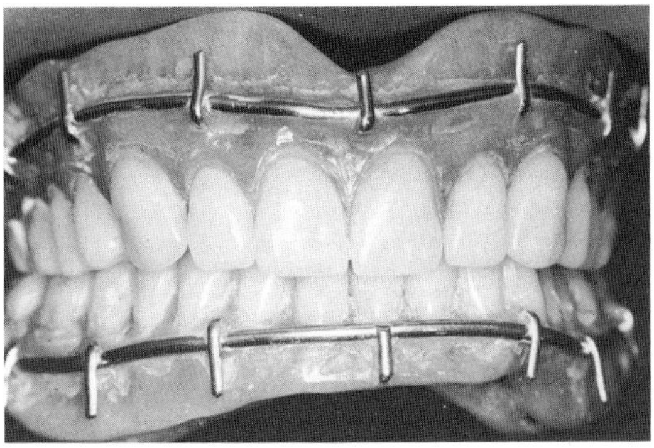

Fig. 6-22 Maxillary and mandibular prostheses, prepared to be inserted as a splint.

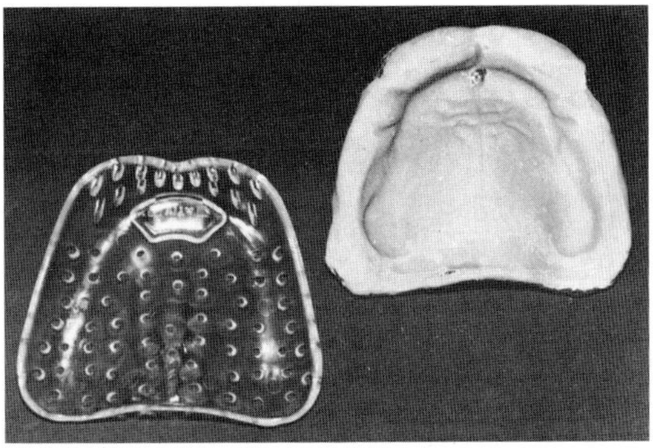

Fig. 6-23 Direct fabrication of a base plate in an edentulous maxilla.
Left: Disposable impression tray which is coated with cold-curing acrylic and fitted in the mouth. Shortly before hardening of the acrylic, the tray is removed and shaped with the bur. The plate, not yet prepared, is on the right.

3.11 Mandibular Lingual Splint *(Hofer, 1939)*

Description. In the completely or partially dentulous mandible, an acrylic plate is fitted to the lingual side, similar to a partial denture, and has drill holes at the level of each interdental space; the drill holes are connected by grooves. Ligature wires are guided around the individual teeth through the drill holes (see Fig. 8.2-11).
Indication. Mandibular fractures in the presence of a deep bite.

3.12 Sectional Splints

Description. Sectional splints consist of buccal and oral portions which are connected as if by a hinge. The buccal part is divided in the middle. Both parts can be unfolded. After insertion of the splint, they are closed and locked by a screw or a wire. Undercut regions can thus be utilized for retention. Practical sectional splints were described by *Kersting* (1904), *Stout* (1943), *Wirth* (1955), and *Neuner* (1957; see Figs. 8.2-12 to 15). Sectional splints can be removed for cleaning and then reinserted.

Indication. If the splint has to be worn for a very long time, e.g., if healing of a fracture is delayed, or for alveolar fractures.

3.13 Monoblock, Activator

Description. A device adopted from orthodontics, for functional treatment and follow-up treatment of fractures of the mandibular condylar process (*Reichenbach*, 1957, 1958). It does not provide immobilization of the mandible, but guides the movements of the mandible in a specific way and fixes the position of the mandible when the mouth is closed.
Indication. Functional treatment of fractures of the mandibular condylar process.
Advantages. By means of proper guidance of the mandible, correction of lateral deviations and relief of stress on the temporomandibular joint. Regular insertion and removal of the device provides a form of prevention of ankylosis because of the necessary wide opening of the mouth.

Technique. Impressions and wax bite are taken,

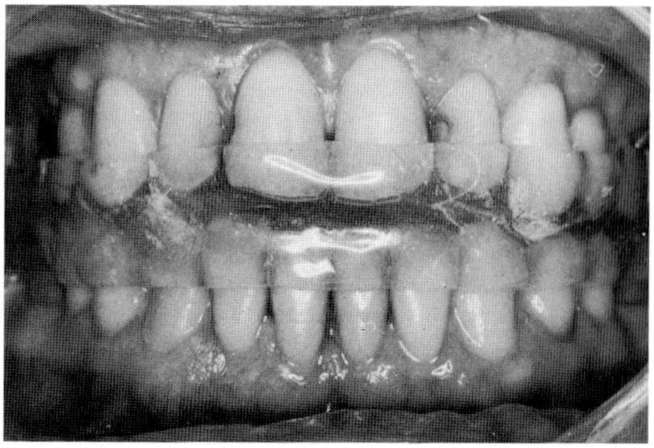

Fig. 6-24 Monoblock for fracture of mandibular condylar process; not yet milled.

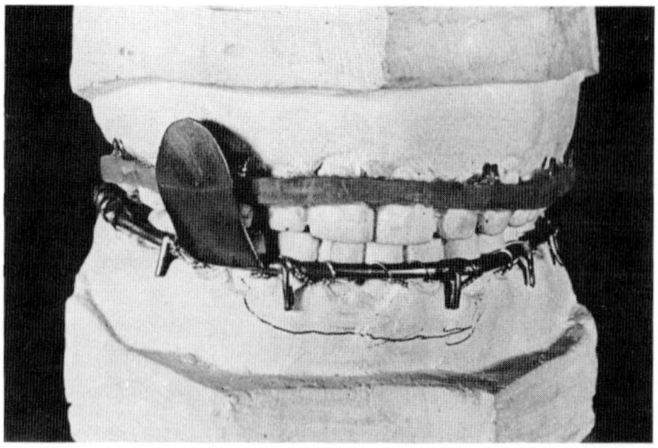

Fig. 6-25 Inclined plane applied to the mandibular splint for correction of lateral deviation of the mandible.

After fabrication in the laboratory (Fig. 6-24), the desired pattern of motion for the mandible is milled in. If the bite impression causes difficulties, the maxillary and mandibular parts can be fabricated separately and combined in the mouth in the desired position of the mandible by means of cold-curing acrylic (*Krüger*, 1971).

3.14 Sliding Splints and Inclined Planes

Description. These are auxiliary elements which are applied to a great variety of splints and have the task, for springtype immobilization of the mandible or after release of the immobilization, of guiding the mandible and preventing lateral deviations (*Sauer*, 1887; Fig. 6-25; *Schröder*, 1911).

Indication. Fractures of the mandibular condylar process with severe limitation of mobility. Resected mandible.

Disadvantages. Sliding splints in the mouth are very cumbersome. Danger of intraoral injury. Therefore they are usually replaced nowadays with elastic bands or the monoblock.

3.15 Kingsley Splint ("Hirschgeweih")

Description. Metal side bars, fitted into square tubes on the maxillary splint or maxillary denture are directed outward through the angle of the mouth and parallel to the buccal surface in the dorsal direction (Fig. 6-26 A) and attached to a plaster head cap by means of elastic bands (*Kingsley*, 1890; *Bimstein*, 1911; *Schröder*, 1911; *Wassmund*, 1927) or by means of rigid plaster connecting bars (*Kapovits*, 1959; Fig. 6-26 B).

Indication. Fractures in the middle third of the face, with dentulous or edentulous maxilla. Nowadays, internal skeletal fixation is used in most cases.

Advantages. Conservative treatment of fractures in the middle third of the face without surgical intervention. For injuries of the elderly. If surgery is contraindicated because of multiple trauma or systemic disease.

Disadvantages. Less stability than with internal skeletal fixation. Bulky appliance.

Technique. The splint on the maxilla can be a metal open-cap splint or a wire-acrylic arch bar with a palatal plate and laterally soldered square tubes which receive the side bars (Figs. 6-26 A, 27 A and B). In the edentulous or nearly edentulous maxilla, one uses an occlusal denture or a base plate, or the patient's denture armed with buccal tubes. After insertion of the splint or base plate, the side bars are fitted. The head cap is made of plaster (see below), and attachments to anchor the appliance for cranial fixa-

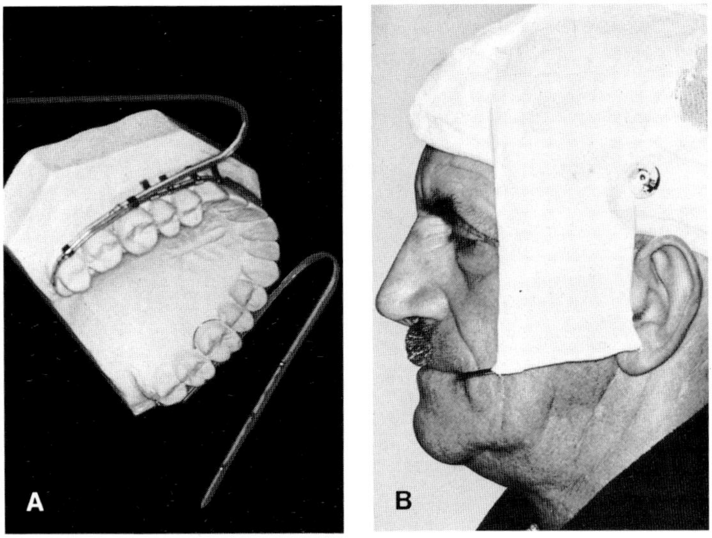

Figs. 6-26 A and B Kingsley splint for the maxilla.

Fig. 6-26 A Arch bar with square tubes and side bars prepared on the model.

Fig. 6-26 B Side bars with lateral plaster bars attached to the plaster head cap.

tion are incorporated. Fixation of the side bars takes place by way of elastic bands or with lateral plaster bars (Figs. 6-26 B and 6-27 C).

3.16 Plaster Head Cap with Extension Bar

Description. A rigid bar (*Stenzel*, 1902) or spring-supported bar (*Rehrmann*, 1935) is applied to a plaster head cap; it exerts continuous traction on fractured parts of the middle third of the face or the mandible by way of rigid or spring-supported auxiliary elements.
Indication. Extension and stabilization of fractures in the middle third of the face in combination with internal skeletal fixation or *Kingsley* splint (Figs. 6-27 to 6-29), especially if, in cases of concomitant bilateral fractures of the condylar process, the dorsal support by way of intermaxillary fixation to the mandible is lacking (Fig. 6-28). The *Stenzel* bar is used chiefly for fixation of a maxilla reduced by means of a traction apparatus (see below and chapter 10). For functional treatment of bilateral condyle fractures in children, *Rehrmann* and *Schettler* (1966) proposed the use of spring traction hooks which are applied to the edge of the chin and permit movement of the mandible.
Disadvantages. Cumbersome appliance.

Technique. Cut or braid and pin back the hair; place tubular gauze bandage (**Stülpa®**) over it. Then several plaster bandages are placed circularly around the head, with cross-shaped reinforcements placed between them by means of windings of the plaster bandage across the apex and longitudinally over the sagittal suture. A strong metal bar with a plate soldered to it for retention is incorporated starting from the center of the apex, after the first few turns. Before the last circular winding of the bandage, the tubular gauze bandage is folded back over the plaster bandages so that a smooth lower edge is formed. Stress should be applied to the bar only after several hours of drying time.
In case of central or centrolateral fractures in the middle third of the face, the *Stenzel* bar is guided over the center of the forehead to the center of the upper lip so that the maxilla can be extended forward and fixed in place (Figs. 6-27 C and 6-28). In case of fractures with crushing of the zygoma, the bar is directed laterally and a small zygomatic hook is attached to it for continuous traction (Fig. 6-29).

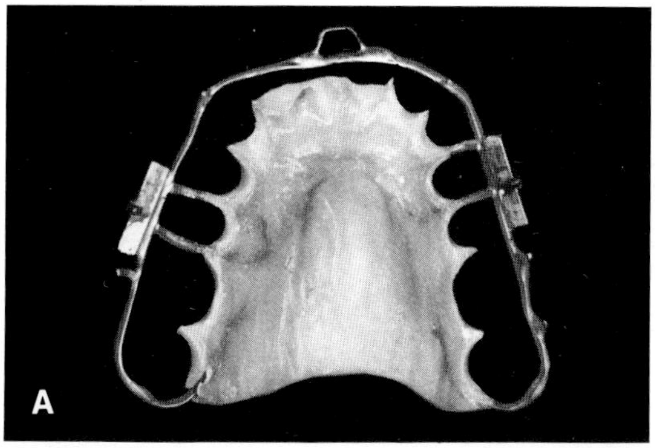

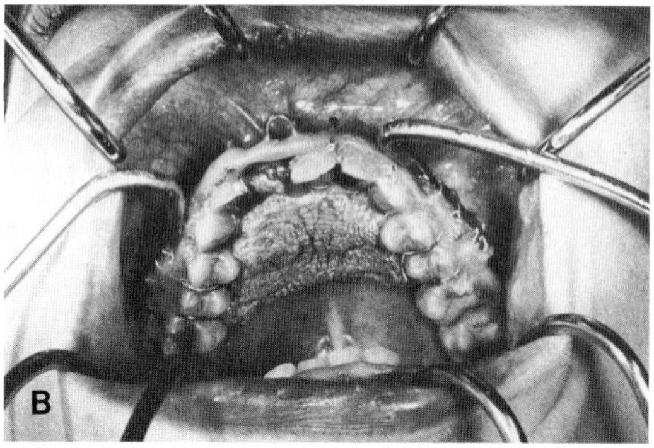

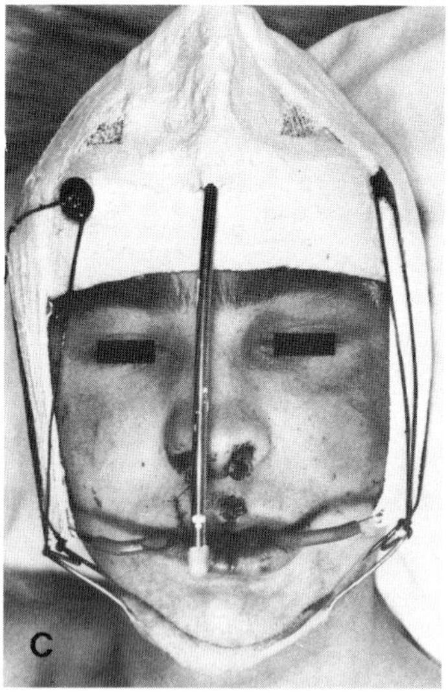

Figs. 6-27 A to C Intra-extraoral appliance with plaster head cap, *Stenzel* bar and chin cap for fracture in the middle third of the face.

Fig. 6-27 A Prepared arch bar with palatal plate, square tubes and frontal loop.

Fig. 6-27 B Arch bar inserted and side bars in place.

Fig. 6-27 C Completed bandage with *Stenzel* bar and chin cup and bilateral plaster bars.

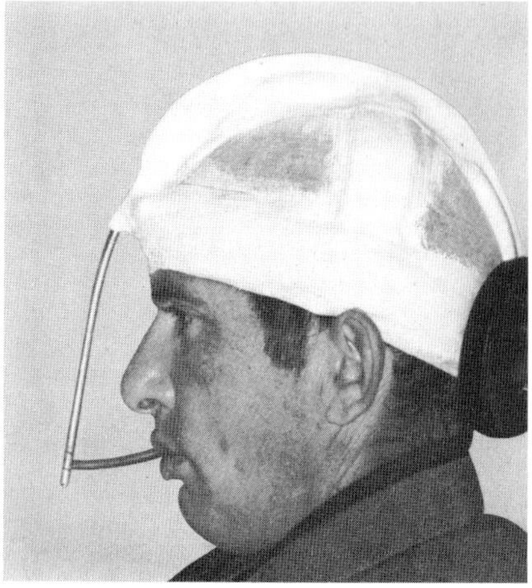

Fig. 6-28 Plaster head cap with *Stenzel* bar, for fracture in middle third of the face combined with bilateral fracture of the condylar process. The fracture in the middle third of the face is immobilized by means of internal wiring and intermaxillary fixation. Since dorsal support by way of the mandibular joints is lacking, the maxilla and mandible must be held in the correct position by fixation to the *Stenzel* bar.

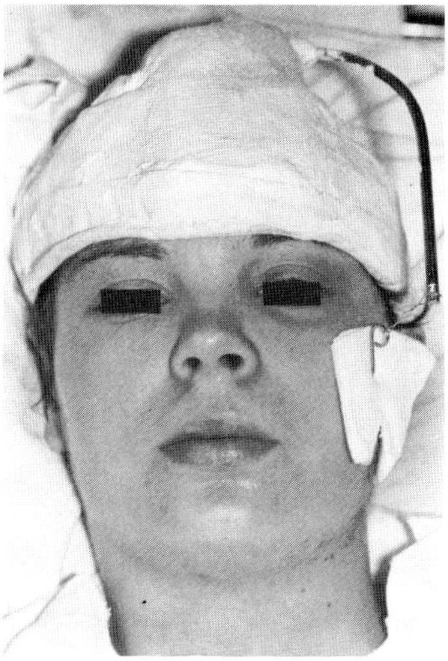

Fig. 6-29 *Stenzel* bar, applied laterally to the plaster head cap for zygomatic traction.

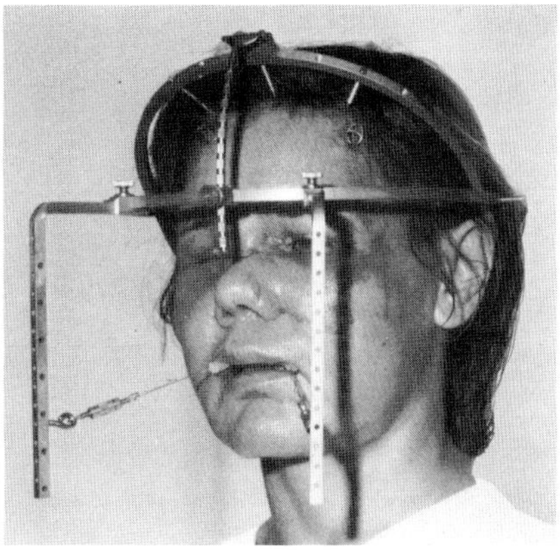

Fig. 6-30 Halo frame.

The spring bar proposed by *Rehrmann* (1935) supports a hook which, inserted in the region of the symphysis, draws the mandible forward (see vol. 2, chapter 14).

Extension of the Middle Third of the Face

The retracted middle third of the face can be reduced by means of a traction apparatus if manipulation does not permit immediate reduction. One has to make certain that the stress chosen is not too great (up to 1 kg) and that the extension is applied only during short time intervals (see chapter 10).

3.17 Halo Frame

Description. The halo frame is a steel or titanium ring that is screwed to the skull cap for fixation. The device is based on the principle of the adjustment frame used in neurosurgery for stereotactic operations. Traction and fixation elements can be attached to the ring, which surrounds the entire skull in the manner of a halo.

Indication. In principle, the halo frame can be used wherever the plaster headcap is appropriate, especially, therefore, in multiple fractures of the midface.

Advantages. Chiefly, stability and variability. With the aid of the halo frame, one can extend in specific regions without interfering with the mandible. Adjustments may be made easily in specific regions.

Disadvantage. The clumsiness of the device and its martial appearance. It should be noted, however, that patients are not seriously inconvenienced by the device despite its appearance.

Technique. The halo frame may be fixed in place with the use of local anesthesia. The skin of the head need not be shaved, but the relevant sections of the skull must be scrubbed thoroughly with a disinfectant solution. In general, 4 or 5 screws are used to fix the halo frame, 2 in the occipital region and 2 or three in the anterior temporal region (Fig. 6-30). The screws, twisted in place through the frame, must be placed directly in the bone; it is desirable to pierce the scalp with small incisions at the site of each screw. The head frame should be placed so that it has some contact with the skull. Secure seating of the screws must be checked at regular intervals.

3.18 Nasal Splint

Description. Plaster bandage applied across the bridge of the nose, extending from the forehead to the tip of the nose (Fig. 6-31). Also applicable as adhesive plaster bandage.

Indication. Fractures of nasal bone, fractures

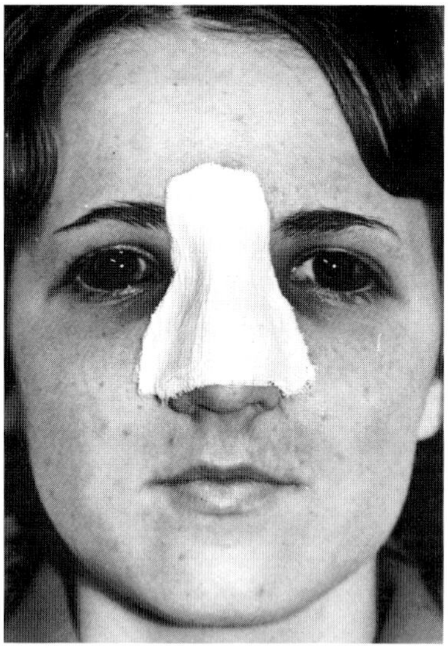

Fig. 6-31 Plaster nasal splint.

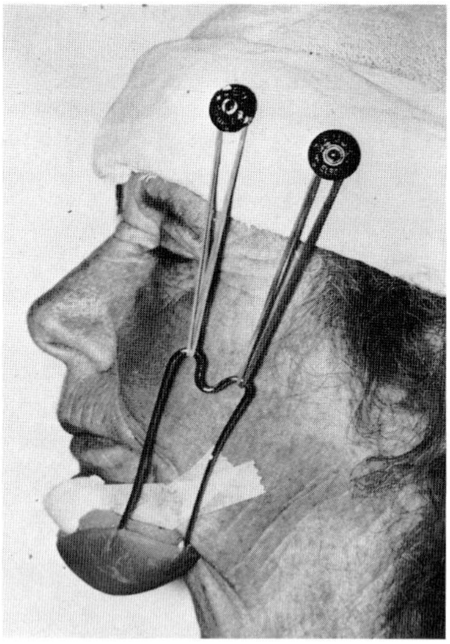

Fig. 6-32 Chin cup, fastened to the head cap by elastic bands.

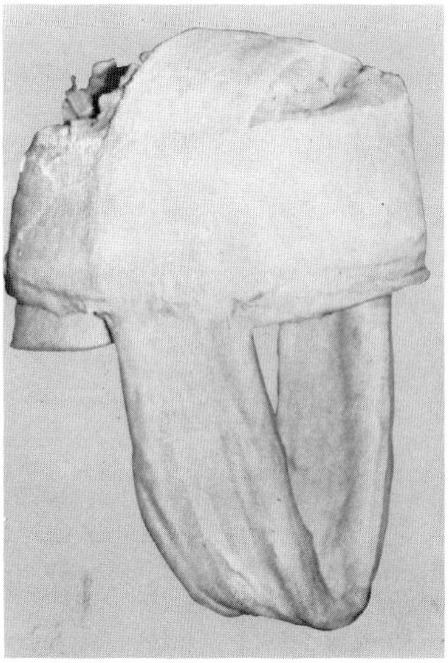

Fig. 6-33 Plaster head-chin bandage as an emergency bandage.

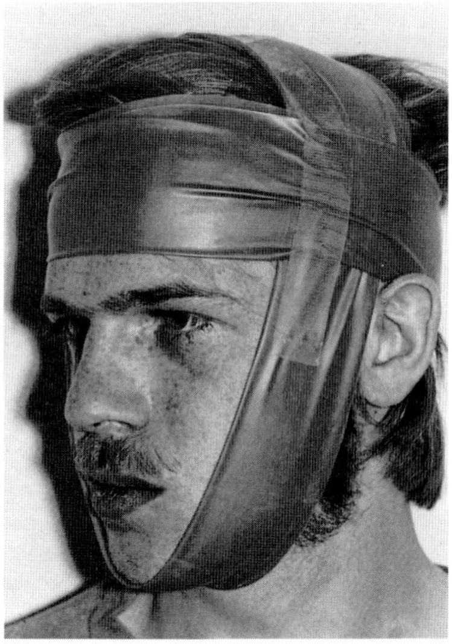

Fig. 6-34 Head bandage of rubber dam elastic (emergency bandage).

in the middle third of the face with detachment of the nasal bones, osteotomy of nasal bones, surgery on nasal septum.

Advantages. Support of nasal skeleton, usually combined with rubber-reinforced foam tamponade of the anterior nasal passages.

Disadvantages. The smaller the nasal plaster-of-paris bandage, the longer it adheres firmly. Nasal casts extending over the forehead are lifted off due to facial motions.

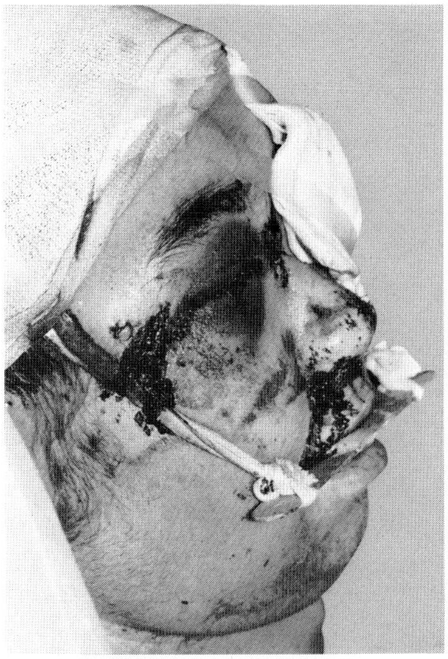

Fig. 6-35 Emergency bandage for fractures in the middle third of the face, made of tubular gauze bandage (Stülpa®) and wooden spatula.

Technique. A plaster bandage 6 or 8 cm wide is cut into small triangular pieces. The triangles are moistened in succession and applied to the bridge of the nose. The plaster bandage adheres well to defatted skin or to a small paper-adhesive dressing. It can be fixed in addition by means of strips of adhesive tape.

3.19 Chin Cup

Description. Mold-shaped acrylic plate with wire bars which are attached with elastic bands to a plaster head cap (Fig. 6-32).
Indication. Emergency bandage, temporary immobilization of fractures of the mandibular condylar process in older patients. Only limited immobilization of the mandible is achieved.

Technique. For a well-fitting chin cup, it is necessary to take impressions and to fabricate it on the model. Metal-eye buttons are attached to the plaster head bandage as retainers for the elastic bands (Fig. 6-32).

3.20 Head Bandages

Description. Head bandages made of gauze, elastic bandages, tubular gauze bandages or rubber dam elastic.
Indication. Emergency bandages for use during transport.

Technique. A bandage dressing is applied with two windings, one passes over the forehead, brow, and back of the head and the second over the mandible, brow, and apex. For padding dressing gauze can be placed underneath (Fig. 6-33). The bandage consisting of rubber dam strips is applied in a similar way (Fig. 6-34).
As an emergency bandage for fractures in the middle third of the face, with a highly mobile maxilla, one uses a tubular gauze head bandage in which the ends, after being pulled through, are tied not below the mandible, but with a wooden spatula. The spatula presses the upper teeth upward and is prevented from slipping by application of cold-curing acrylic (Fig. 6-35).

References

Angle, E. H. (1905)
Angle's System zur Gradrichtung und Festhaltung unregelmäßig gestellter Zähne und zur Behandlung von Kieferbrüchen. (Angle's system for straightening and retaining irregularly placed teeth and for the treatment of fractures of the jaw.) 4th Ed., Berlin S. S. White

Bimstein, J. (1911)
Kieferbrüche und Orthodontie. (Jaw fractures and orthodontics.) Korresp. bl. Zahnärzte (Berlin) 40: 13. Quoted by Schröder, H. (1911)

Drum, W. (1966)
Die Drum-Miniplast-Schiene. (The Drum Miniplast splint.) Dtsch. zahnärztl. Z. 21: 109

Eby, J. D. (1920)
Principles of orthodontics in the treatment of maxillofacial injuries. Int. J. Orthodont. 6: 273

Ernst, F. (1927)
Die zahnärztliche Behandlung der Unterkieferbrüche. (Treatment of mandibular fractures.) In Kirschner, M., and O. Nordmann "Die Chirurgie" (Surgery.) Vol. 4/I, p. 842 Berlin-Wien, Urban & Schwarzenberg

Ernst, F. (1932)
Die Schienenverbände bei Ober- und Unterkieferbrüchen. (Splints in fractures of the maxilla and the mandible.) In Bruhn, C., A. Kantorowicz, and C. Partsch: Handbuch der Zahnheilkunde. (Handbook of dentistry.) vol. 1, 4th ed., p. 115, München, Bergmann

Gilmer, T. L. (1887)
A case of fracture of the lower jaw with remarks on treatment. Arch. Dent. 4: 388

Greve, K. (1950)
Die Behandlung der Kieferfrakturen. (Treatment of jaw fractures.) In Port-Euler: Lehrbuch der Zahnheilkunde. (Textbook of dentistry.) vol. 5, p. 694, München, J. F. Bergmann

Gunning, T. B. (1866/67)
The treatment of fractures of the lower jaw by interdental splints. N. Y. med. J. 3: 433, and 4: 11, and 274

Hammond, G. E. (1874)
Die Behandlung von Kieferfrakturen. (The treatment of jaw fractures.) Dtsch. Vjschr. Zahnheilk. 14: 197

Hauptmeyer, F. (1924)
Die Behandlung der Brüche des Unter- und Oberkiefers mittels Zahnschienen. (The treatment of fractures of the mandible and the maxilla with tooth splints.) In: Partsch, C., Chr. Bruhn, and A Kantorowicz; Handbuch der Zahnheilkunde. (Handbook of dentistry.) vol. 1, 2nd ed. p. 103, München, J. F. Bergmann

Hering, H.-J. (1960)
Eine einfache Methode der Kieferbruchschienung mit Hilfe von schnellhärtendem Kunststoff. (A simple method for splinting jaw fractures with cold-curing acrylic.) Dtsch. Zahnärztebl. 14: 742

Hofer, O. (1939)
Neuere Erkenntnisse in der Zahn-, Mund- und Kieferchirurgie. Über Frakturen der Kiefer. (Newer knowledge in oral surgery. Fractures of the jaws.) Zbl. Zahn- Mund- Kieferheilk. 4: 327

Hofmann, M. (1958)
Ein Beitrag zur direkten/freihändigen Versorgung von Kieferfrakturen unter Anwendung einer Metallhohlband-Palavitschiene. (The direct free-handed treatment of jaw fractures with a hollow metal rod/Palavit splint.) Dtsch. zahnärztl. Z. 13: 9

Ivy, R. H. (1922)
Observations of fractures of the mandible. J. Amer. med. Ass. 79: 295

Kapovits, M. (1959)
Die Behandlung von Oberkieferfrakturen durch Fixierung mit Draht-Palavitverbänden, Kopfgips und Verschraubung. (The treatment of fractures of the maxilla by fixation with wire-acrylic arch bars, plaster head caps, and screw placement.) Fortschr. Kiefer- u. Gesichtschir. 5: 323

Kazanjian, V. H. (1933)
Treatment of automobile injuries of the face and jaws. J. Amer. dent. Ass. 20: 757

Kersting, G. (1904)
Behandlung von Unterkieferbrüchen. Dtsch. med. Wschr. 30: 390

Kingsley, N. W. (1880)
A treatise on oral deformities. London, H. K. Lewis

Krüger, E. (1971)
Kombinierte Extensions- und Aktivatorbehandlung zur funktionellen Therapie doppelseitiger Kiefergelenkfrakturen bei Kindern. (Combined extension and activator treatment in the functional therapy of bilateral temporomandibular joint fractures in children.) Dtsch. zahnärztl. Z. 26: 875

Krüger, E., and S. Chrissafis (1971)
Kariesprophylaxe durch lokale Anwendung von Aminfluoriden bei der Versorgung am Kieferbruchpatienten mit der Drahtkunststoffschiene nach Schuchardt. (Caries prevention by local application of amine fluoride in the treatment of jaw fracture patients with the Schuchardt wire-acrylic arch bar.) Dtsch. zahnärztl. Z. 26: 1227

Krüger, E., and L. A. Rivas (1960)
Modifikationen der Drahtkunststoffschiene nach Schuchardt. (Modifications of the Schuchardt wire-acrylic arch bar.) Dtsch. zahnärztl. Z. 21: 685

Neuner, O. (1957)
Vereinfachte Schienungstechnik zur Behandlung von Unterkieferfrakturen. (Simplified splinting technique for the treatment of mandibular fractures.) Dtsch. zahnärztl. Z. 12: 726

Obwegeser, H. (1952)
Über eine einfache Methode der freihändigen Drahtverschienung von Kieferbrüchen. (A simple method for free-handed wire ligation of jaw fractures.) Öst. Z. Stomat. 49: 652

Rehrmann, A. (1935)
Die doppelte Kinnfraktur und ihre Behandlung. (The double fracture of the chin and its treatment.) Dtsch. Zahn-, Mund- u. Kieferheilk. 2: 122

Rehrmann, A., and D. Schettler (1966)
Die Behandlung der doppelseitigen Kiefergelenkfrakturen bei Säuglingen und Kleinkindern mit der Reposition und elastischen Fixation nach Rehrmann. (Treatment of bilateral fractures of the temporomandibular joint in infants and toddlers through reposition and elastic fixation according to the Rehrmann technique.) Dtsch. zahnärztl. Z. 21: 777

Reichenbach, E. (1957)
Verletzungen der Kiefer- und Gesichtsknochen und der benachbarten Weichteile. (Injuries of the jaw and facial bones and adjacent soft tissue.) In Häupl, K., W. Meyer, and K. Schuchardt: "Die Zahn-, Mund- und Kieferheilkunde", (Dentistry.) vol. 3/I, p. 639, München – Berlin, Urban & Schwarzenberg

Reichenbach, E. (1958)
Probleme der Frakturbehandlung beim wachsenden Schädel. (Problems in the treatment of fractures in the growing skull.) Fortschr. Kiefer- u. Gesichtschir. 4: 213

Risdon, F. (1929)
The treatment of fractures of the jaws. Canad. med. Ass. J. 20: 260

Sauer, C.
Quoted by Schnoor, G. (1887): Professor Sauer's Anwendung der schiefen Ebene nach Fortnahme des rechtseitigen Teiles des Unterkiefers vom Gelenkkopf incl. bis zum ersten Prämolar. (Professor Sauer's use of the inclined plane after removal of the right side of the mandible from the condyle to and including the first premolar.) Dtsch. Mschr. Zahnheilk. 5: 217

Sauer, C. (1889)
Notverband bei Kieferbrüchen mit Eisendraht. (Emergency splinting for jaw fractures, with iron wire.) Dtsch. Mschr. Zahnheilk. 7: 381

Schlampp, H. (1942)
Die Versorgung der Kieferbrüche und der Kieferschußbrüche nach dem Profilschienensystem. (Care of jaw fractures and gun shot jaw fractures with the profile splint system.) Dtsch. Zahn-, Mund- u. Kieferheilk. 9: 89

Schröder, H. (1911)
Handbuch der zahnärztlich-chirurgischen Verbände und Prothesen. (Handbook of oral surgical splints and prostheses.) Berlin, H. Meusser

Schrudde, J. (1953)
Die Behandlung von Kieferbrüchen mit Schienenverbänden aus Palavit. (Treatment of jaw fractures with Palavit splints.) Zahnärztl. Welt 8: 424

Schuchardt, K. (1956)
Ein Vorschlag zur Verbesserung der Drahtschienenverbände. (A proposal for the improvement of arch bar technique.) Dtsch. Zahn-, Mund- u. Kieferheilk. 24: 39

Schwenzer, N. (1961)
Die freihändige Versorgung von Oberkieferfrakturen unter Verwendung der Drahtbogen-Kunststoffschiene nach Schuchardt. (Freehanded care of fractures of the maxilla with the use of the Schuchardt wire-acrylic arch bar.) Dtsch. Zahn-, Mund- u. Kieferheilk. 36: 274

Stenzel (1902)
Demonstration eines Extensionsverbandes für gewisse Brüche des Unterkiefers. (Demonstration of an extension appliance for certain fractures of the mandible.) Verh. Dtsch. Ges. Chir. 31: 83

Stout, R. A. (1943)
Intermaxillary wiring and intermaxillary elastic traction and fixation. In: Manual of standard practice of plastic and maxillo-facial surgery. Military surgical manuals I, p. 272, Philadelphia – London, W. B. Saunders

Wassmund, M. (1927)
Frakturen und Luxationen des Gesichtsschädels. (Fractures and dislocations of the facial skull.) Berlin, H. Meusser

Weiskopf, J. (1969)
Die Frakturen des Unterkiefers und ihre orthopädische Behandlung. (Mandibular fractures and their orthopedic management.) In Reichenbach, E.: Traumatologie im Kiefer-Gesichtsbereich. (Maxillofacial traumatology.) p. 217, München, J. A. Barth

Wirth, F. (1955)
Eine kombinierte Kunststoff-Draht-Kieferbruchschiene. (A combined wire-acrylic splint.) Zahnärztl. Rdsch. 64: 425

Chapter 7

Fractures and Luxation of Teeth* and the Alveolar Process

Jacques A. Baart and Willem A. M. van der Kwast

1. Introduction

Lesions of the teeth* are among the most common features of traumatic injuries of the face. As a matter of fact it is difficult to give statistically justifiable percentages of the incidence of lesions of the anterior teeth, as these percentages are bound to differ with the social differences among the various countries. It has to be assumed, moreover, that a number of such lesions remain undiscovered because radiological examination, which might indicate root fractures, was omitted in some studies.

Yet, to give some factual information of the incidence of anterior lesions, it may be noted that *Schützmannsky* (1963) found lesions of the permanent teeth in 10.5 % and of the deciduous teeth in 18.9 % of 25,074 children examined. Maxillary central incisors are damaged about 10 times as frequently as their mandibular counterparts. Lesions of the canines and premolars hardly play any role. The principal causes of trauma are injuries sustained during play, athletic activities or traffic accidents. Anterior tooth injuries due to moped and car accidents are usually found in patients about the age of 20 years. High-risk groups are epileptics and drug addicts as well as patients intubated for anesthesia under laryngoscopic control. In a number of cases, dental lesions are part of a more extensive pattern of injury. In particular, midfacial fractures can involve dental injuries, often in combination with lesions of the alveolar process. In this context it should be noted that dental lesions can be so conspicuous that especially fractures of the maxilla easily may be overlooked.

It is obvious that dental lesions are more likely to occur as the teeth are in a more exposed position. Children with marked protrusion of the maxillary anteriors and an atrophic upper lip run a high risk of frontal dental injuries (*Dorenbos*, 1972; Fig. 7-1).

1.1 Prevention of Traumatic Dentoalveolar Lesions

The maxim that anyone who knows the causes of a disease is in possession of the key to its

* Teeth are identified in this book in accordance with the tooth numbering system of the F.D.I.
For permanent teeth, the numbering system is as follows:

maxillary right	maxillary left
18 17 16 15 14 13 12 11	21 22 23 24 25 26 27 28
48 47 46 45 44 43 42 41	31 32 33 34 35 36 37 38
mandibular right	mandibular left

The first numeral designates the quadrant: 1 identifies the right maxillary quadrant, 2 the left maxillary, 3 the left mandibular and 4 the right mandibular quadrant. The second numeral identifies the specific tooth, thus: 1 is the central incisor, 2 the lateral incisor, 3 the canine, 4 the first premolar, 5 the second premolar, and 6, 7, and 8 the first, second and third molars, respectively. Examples: 13 is the right maxillary canine, 36 the left mandibular first molar.

For deciduous teeth, the numbering system is as follows:

maxillary right	maxillary left
55 54 53 52 51	61 62 63 64 65
85 84 83 82 81	71 72 73 74 75
mandibular right	mandibular left

The quadrants are numbered 5 through 8 for the deciduous dentition; the deciduous molars are identified as 4 and 5. Thus, for example, 51 identifies the right maxillary central incisor and 75 the left mandibular second deciduous molar.

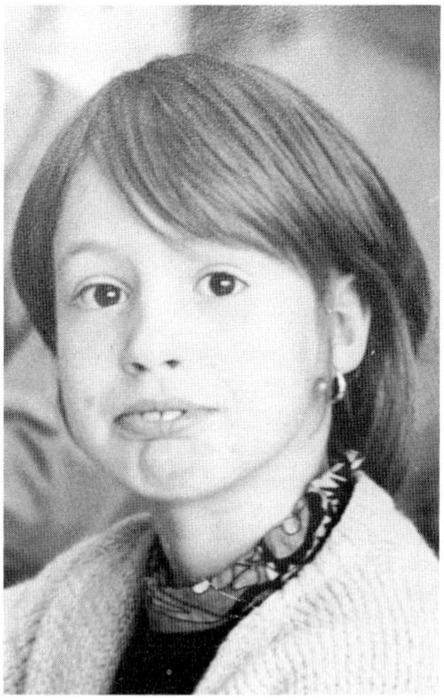

Fig. 7-1 A 9-year-old girl with an open lip bite resulting from marked protrusion of the maxillary anterior teeth.

prevention or treatment is only partly true with regard to traumatic dentoalveolar lesions. The exploratory life of a toddler, who proceeds by trial and error, entails many falls, after all. An over-restrictive attitude inspired by the desire to prevent dentoalveolar injuries, however, could seriously inhibit the child's psychomotoric development. Furthermore, anterior dental lesions as a result of aggressive behavior or drunkenness are inevitable. Nonetheless, several methods are suitable for prevention of dental lesions.

The first approach is that of advice and information. It can be pointed out to parents that children who drink water with their mouths on the tap run the risk of fracturing a front tooth. Schools can be advised to have rubber tiles laid beneath jungle gyms in the playground. An anti-slip layer on the floor around swimming pools can contribute to the prevention of facial injuries. The same applies to safety belts and helmets worn in traffic.

A second, more active form of prevention is based on alteration of dental factors. In young patients with marked protrusion, the sagittal overbite can be reduced with the aid of orthodontic appliances until adequate labial occlusion is achieved.

The third possibility of prevention lies in protection of the face or dental arches. Mouth protectors have been in use for a long time in contact sports, and no pugilist is likely to enter the ring without such protection. In team sports involving direct bodily contact, the use of intraoral or extraoral mouth protectors is advisable. Ice hockey, football and field hockey are team sports in which dentoalveolar injuries account for a large percentage of the lesions sustained. Helmets or mouth protectors also can be used in high-risk groups, as is already done in children suffering from frequent epileptic seizures.

1.2 Classification

Dental lesions may consist of injuries to the solid structures, with or without invasion of the pulp cavity and with or without periodontal damage. Distinction also should be made between fractures and luxations of the teeth.

The literature presents several classifications. However, a classification is meaningful only if it indicates a relation to therapeutic or prognostic consequences, or both.

In 1973 the World Health Organization published the "Application of the International Classification of Diseases to Dentistry and Stomatology." This classification, like that of *Ellis* and

Davey (1970) is based on anatomy as well as on therapy does not specify the mode of therapy.

A serviceable classification based on that of the WHO is the following:

a) Crown fracture
   1. enamel cracks
   2. uncomplicated crown fracture
   3. complicated crown fracture
b) Root fracture
c) Luxation
   1. concussion
   2. subluxation
   3. intrusion (luxation)
   4. extrusion (luxation)
   5. lateral luxation
   6. exarticulation
d) Fracture of the alveolar process.

Muller and *Taatz* (1965) noted that it is important to distinguish between extra-alveolar and intra-alveolar fractures. The former are in fact identical to crown fractures. With periodontal diseases, however, root fractures can also be extra-alveolar. Axial fractures are of clinical significance inasmuch as it is essentially impossible to save the tooth involved.
The intra-alveolar fractures can be classified as those near the gingiva and those near the apex. This division is of importance in connection with the vitality of the pulp. The prognosis in terms of pulp vitality really depends on two factors: the width of the fracture space and the risk of pulp infection. The latter increases as the fracture line is nearer the gingival margin.

In the prognostic evaluation of dental luxations, a distinction should be made among:

1. luxation of the tooth without dislocation (first degree);
2. luxation of the tooth with dislocation (second degree);
3. luxation with exarticulation of the tooth from the alveolus (third degree).

First degree and second degree luxations have a similar prognosis in terms of preservation of the tooth.

1.3 Examination of Dental Lesions

The traumatized patient often appears in a disordered, confused condition. Young patients with dental lesions, moreover, often weep and are uncooperative. Blood-tinged saliva escapes from the mouth and consequently the situation is unclear but requires careful and systematic investigation.
The history provides information about time, place and cause of the accident. The interval between accident and treatment is of importance, not only for the type of therapy but also for the prognosis. A pulp which has long been exposed as a result of a frontal injury, for example, requires different treatment than a recent, complicated crown fracture. When a tooth has been knocked out, the prognosis largely depends on the duration of the extraoral period.
One should also obtain information about the events between the accident and arrival at the hospital. Is there retrograde amnesia, nausea, vomiting? Are there indications of cerebral concussion? In the case of exarticulation, it is important to know how the exarticulated tooth was transported. The patient's general health and medical history as well as his dental history (orthodontic measures?) are other important data. Finally, the patient is asked to describe pain and other symptoms.
The accident site indicates whether tetanus prophylaxis is required. Anterior injuries in infants are unusual but can have been caused by a fall from a commode. The presence of extensive soft tissue lesions (frenulum) or fractures of the ribs and limbs, however, should raise the suspicion of the battered child syndrome.
The incidence of dentoalveolar injuries increases as the infant begins to walk and explore. Such injuries in school-age children often result from falls in the street or the playground. Crown fractures are common in these cases, and one of the factors which explains this is the absolute or relative protrusion of the maxillary anterior teeth at this age.
Once the history has been taken, extraoral and intraoral examinations are made, beginning with tests to determine the sensibility of the lips and cheeks. The mandibular condyles are palpated

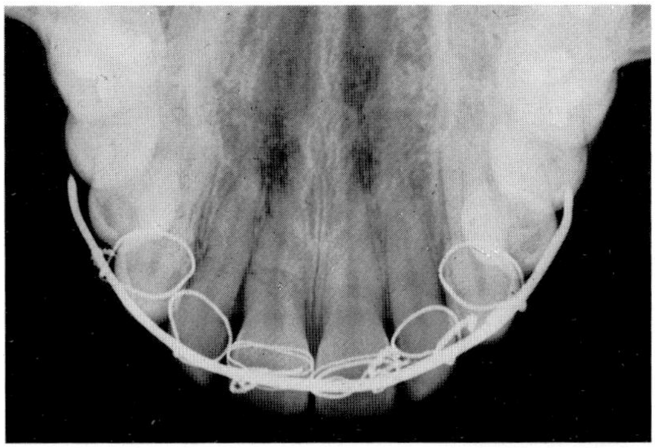

Fig. 7-2 Occlusal radiograph immediately after splinting. The root fracture of 11 is shown as an ellipse.

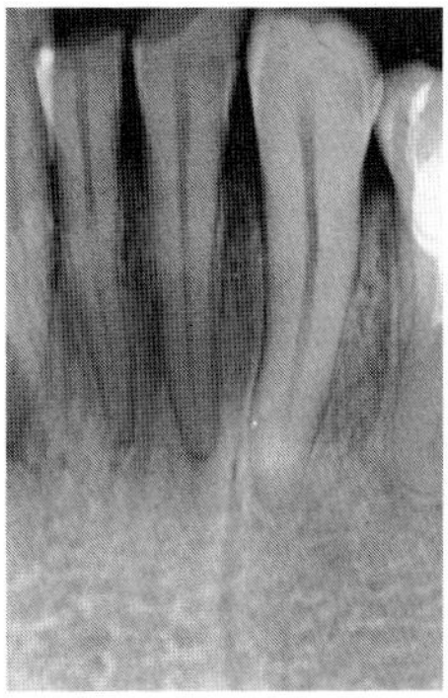

Fig. 7-3 Sharply defined broadening of the periodontal space due to luxation of 31, 32.

during mandibular movement; the lower margin of the mandible and the zygomatic bone are examined. Extraoral wounds are carefully inspected for glass fragments and dirt.

Intraoral examination involves inspection of the teeth, with emphasis on their color; a pink color indicates a recent pulp infarction and a grey color a nonvital pulp. The mucosa is checked for hematomas and abrasions; it is to be borne in mind that lingual hematomas are more suspect of mandibular fracture than buccal or labial hematomas. A hematoma of the upper lip, often associated with lesions of the labial mucosa, may be indicative of intraalveolar fractures and is therefore an indication for radiological examination.

Lesions of the mucosa of the alveolar process may indicate a fracture of the alveolar process, even in the absence of clinical or radiological evidence. Palpation is more likely to reveal fractures of the alveolar process than radiological examination.

Pulp vitality testing immediately after the accident is of limited importance. A negative reaction to thermal and electrical stimuli is not necessarily conclusive of pulp necrosis. The pulp may be in a state which could be described as shock, and not recover for days, weeks or even months. This condition is caused by reversible edema of the myelin sheaths of the sensory nerves. Vitality tests regain some reliability only after 4 to 6 months. Particularly with very young patients, an expectant attitude with regard to pulp trephination is imperative, although radiographic examination is advisable. Immediately after the accident, teeth with an intra-alveolar fracture are generally more likely to show a positive reaction than luxated teeth.

An exact diagnosis of intra-alveolar fractures and dental luxations can be made only on the basis of radiological findings. Not only can fractures and luxations thus be evaluated, but an impression also can be gained of the stage of development of the tooth. Moreover, the distance between the pulp chamber and enamel can be determined, and the lips and other soft tissues can be examined for the presence of foreign bodies, including fragments of enamel.

A periapical radiograph often is not sufficient for evaluation of fractures of the alveolar process because these fractures can be localized relatively far from the root apices. Here a film in occlusal projection may be useful. An oblique root fracture is visible on the film as an ellipse (Fig. 7-2). It is sometimes necessary to use several films at different angles for adequate evaluation.

In the event of dental luxation, the radiograph shows a sharply defined widening of the periodontal space as a result of the involvement of the anchoring apparatus (Fig. 7-3). The degree of luxation cannot be determined exclusively on the basis of a radiograph.

To avoid blurring due to movement, and an unnecessarily large skin dose, it is advisable to combine a fast film with a short exposure time and high kilovoltage. In the examination of unconscious patients with lost exarticulated teeth, it is advisable to make plane radiographs of the abdomen and thorax to determine that no teeth have been aspirated or swallowed.

2. Lesions of Deciduous Teeth

Lesions of deciduous teeth pose their specific problems; they are encountered in the youngest group of patients, often accompanied by very anxious and sometimes guilt-ridden parents. The patients' youth imposes unmistakable limitations on therapy, but it is precisely in this group of patients that spontaneous recovery from injury is frequently observed: wounds in young children usually heal quickly and without sequelae, and this is true of soft tissues as well as of skeletal parts.

Lesions of the teeth in children under six years of age are usually taken lightly. After all, the deciduous teeth have a limited life-span and will be replaced by permanent teeth. In actual practice this means that lesions of deciduous teeth are often treated by extraction, particularly if the patient is over three years of age. In all cases of injury to the deciduous teeth, however, the question of the possible consequences for the permanent teeth should be raised. It is an established fact that traumatic lesions of the deciduous teeth can give rise to irreversible damage of the permanent teeth. The difficulty, however, lies in the fact that in most cases it is impossible to predict with any certainty whether (and if so, how) damage of the permanent teeth will become manifest. Only after eruption of the permanent teeth can one adequately evaluate the effect of lesions of the deciduous teeth on the state of the permanent teeth. That is why it is hazardous—from a forensic point of view as well—to take lesions of the deciduous teeth too lightly.

Lesions of the deciduous teeth can so unfavorably influence the permanent dentition that expensive orthodontic or prosthetic measures may be required even years later. It is important therefore to inform the parents of the uncertain long-term prognosis, and for reasons of legal liability as well. Depending on the circumstances of the accident, advice against signing a release proffered by an insurance company can be exceedingly useful and valuable.

An impression of the possible causes of lesions of deciduous teeth is presented in a publication by *Mehnert* (1974). In 45 children he elicited the following causes: a fall on the floor or in the street, playground or swimming pool in 15 cases; a blow from a playmate in 2; a fall from a bench or couch in 2; a knock against the edge of a table or bed in 3; and one child was hit by a stone thrown at him. It is interesting to learn from this publication that heteroanamnestic data were inconclusive in many cases. This may indicate reluctance of parents based on guilt-feelings.

2.1 Fractures of Deciduous Teeth

Fractures of the crown (Fig. 7-4) or roots (or both) of deciduous teeth are extremely rare; luxations or avulsions are usually involved. This has been ascribed to the fact that the juvenile alveolar bone is resilient, and that blunt injuries are involved in most cases. Moreover it is maintained that, consequent to increasing root resorption, the lever action of the crown in relation to the root is too weak to effect a fracture.

2.2 Luxations of Deciduous Teeth

Luxations of deciduous teeth are quite common and can be encountered in a wide variety of forms. For example, there may be total luxation of a deciduous tooth: the tooth has been knocked out and the alveolus is empty. An alternative possibility is extrusion of a deciduous tooth: the tooth is dislodged as a result of violence, but some contact with adjacent structures persists. In other cases the opposite situation may present itself when the tooth is knocked into the jaw by violence; this is sometimes described as intrusive luxation.

Subluxation of deciduous teeth also is quite common: the teeth are merely knocked loose to some extent.

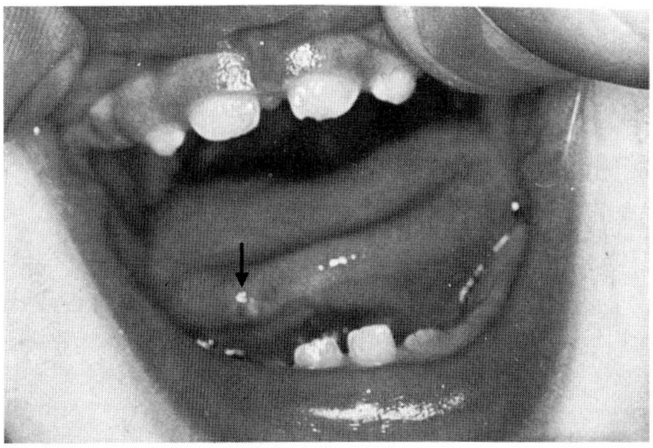

Fig. 7-4 Enamel fracture of the left deciduous incisor. Note the enamel fragment impacted in the tongue.

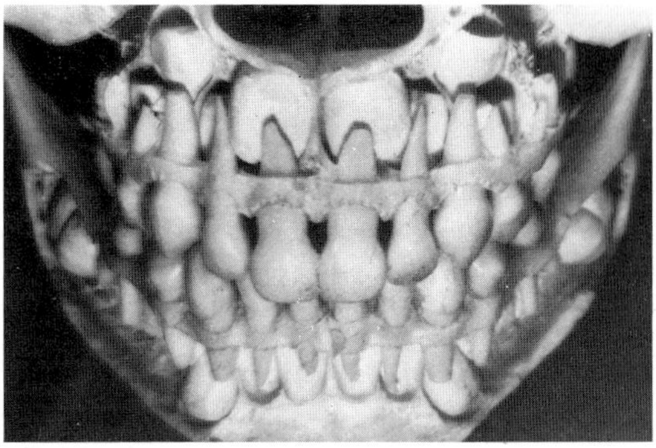

Fig. 7-5 The buds of the permanent incisors are localized palatally to the deciduous incisors. Intrusive luxation of the deciduous incisor will not cause dislocation of its successor. (Courtesy of Prof. Dr. *F. P. G. M. van der Linden*. Development of the human dentition. Harper & Row, 1976.)

2.3 Consequences for the Permanent Teeth

An important question is whether, and how, lesions of deciduous teeth can lead to damage of permanent teeth. It is a serious mistake to assume that untoward consequences are eliminated with the change of dentition. On the contrary: in many cases it is unfortunately necessary to account for permanent consequences. It should be borne in mind that it is often impossible to evaluate exactly the extent to which and the way in which the permanent teeth will suffer damage as a result of lesions of deciduous teeth. Even very careful radiography fails to provide adequate information in this respect. Data from the literature (e.g., *Mehnert*, 1974) show that damage to the permanent teeth may be anticipated in one-third of such occurrences. An important factor in this context is the patient's age at the time of the accident. At the age of one year, the primordium of the permanent maxillary incisor is localized far towards the palate and the formation of solid structures (enamel and dentin) has progressed to about half the crown. At this age, therefore, it is improbable that a traumatic injury causing intrusion of a deciduous tooth could affect the primordium of the permanent incisor, for the deciduous tooth is more likely to be displaced labial to the permanent primordium without directly damaging it. Any damage inflicted on the primordium at this age is likely to be limited to the enamel-forming structure on the labial side of the crown; the primordium, however, retains its position.

The formation of the entire permanent crown is not complete until age 3. Meanwhile, the primordium has come to be located more labially. In this phase the primordium of the permanent maxillary incisor is localized immediately palatal and cranial to the apex of the root of the deciduous incisor (Fig. 7-5). At age 5, finally, the permanent incisor is localized immediately above the already partly resorbed root of the deciduous incisor. It is evident from this description that the risk of displacement of the primordia of the permanent teeth and malformation of the roots increases with increasing age. In fact, this risk is fairly considerable immediately before the deciduous tooth is lost.

These are the principal consequences for the permanent teeth after lesions of the deciduous teeth. The least dramatic consequence is interference with the development of the enamel of the permanent tooth in the form of either hypoplasia or hypocalcification. Hypoplasia occurs when enamel formation is imperfect or interrupted as a result of damage to the ameloblasts. Hypocalcification occurs as a result of

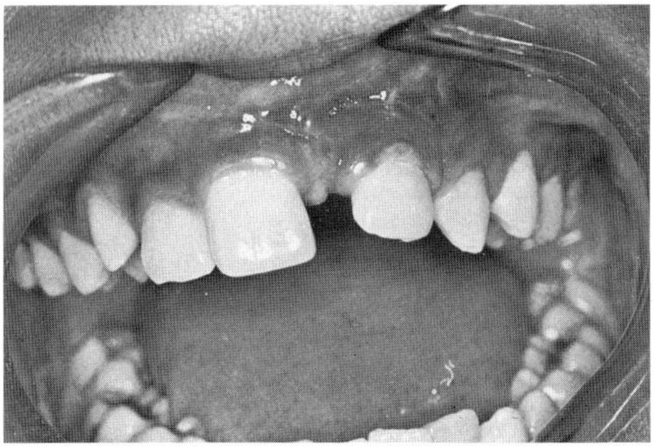

Fig. 7-6 A At age 13, tooth 21 has not yet erupted.

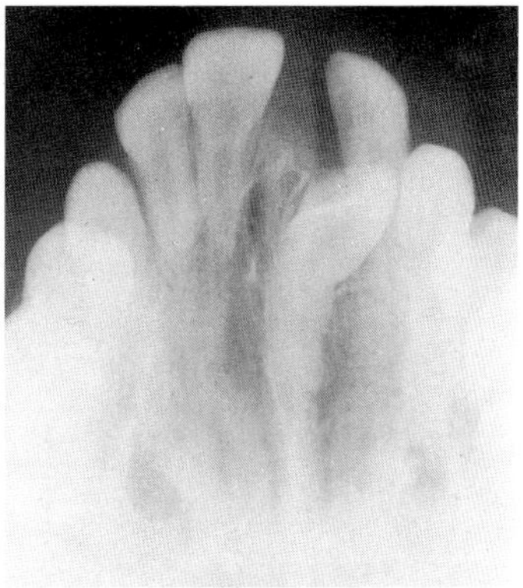

Fig. 7-6 B The occlusal radiograph shows a dilaceration of 21, probably from an intrusive luxation of the deciduous predecessor.

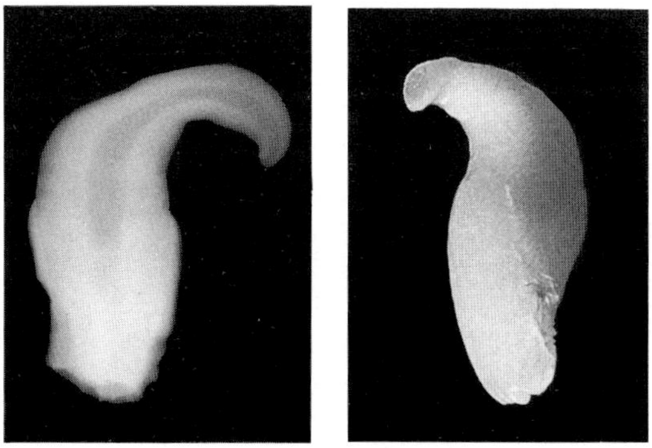

Figs. 7-6 C and D Radiograph and photo of the removed 21.

disturbed maturation of the enamel matrix; this is believed to result from an inflammatory reaction caused by tissue damage. In the case of hypocalcification, the color of the tooth can range from white to yellow, and the enamel surface need not necessarily show any defect. The dark-yellow discoloration can result in part from an intraosseous hemorrhage in the alveolar process, caused by an intruding deciduous tooth. As a result of such a hemorrhage, hemosiderin can be incorporated in the enamel to be formed and the discoloration results. Hypoplasia can be visible on radiographs as radiolucency, but hypocalcification need not produce radiologically visible changes.
Another possibility is a disturbance in the formation of the root of the permanent tooth, which consequently remains incomplete; pathological calcification or degeneration of pulp can then occur in the pulp cavity. Yet another possibility is displacement of the bud of the permanent tooth, causing it to erupt into the wrong position, i.e., usually too far towards the palate; in such cases subsequent orthodontic treatment is required to correct the 'abnormal' position.
Dilaceration also can occur, in which case crown and root are not in line. This malformation develops when violence causes displacement of the already calcified part of the tooth in relation to the uncalcified part (Fig. 7-6). Dilaceration becomes clinically manifest by non-eruption of the tooth. Further examination in such cases often reveals a bone-hard swelling which is palpable labial to the non-erupted tooth. Radiologically, dilaceration is not always readily detectable, particularly if the curvature lies in the sagittal plane. In some cases the tooth seems to be broken at the junction between crown and root. A lateral nasal radiograph (with the

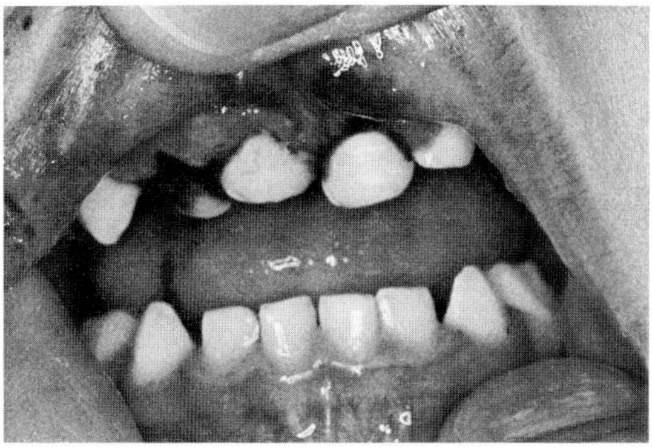

Fig. 7-7 A Luxation of deciduous teeth.

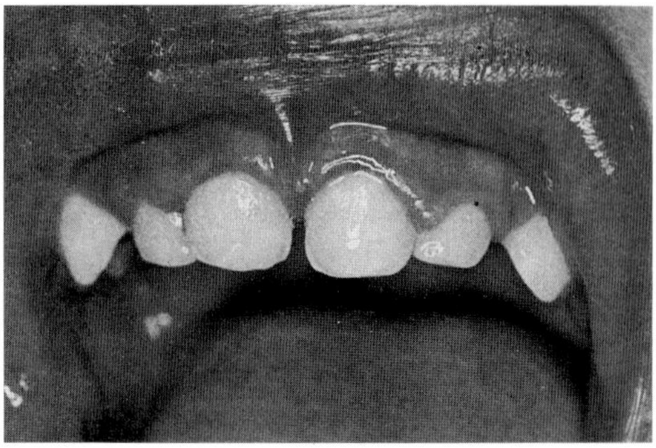

Fig. 7-7 B Intraoral features 2 weeks after the injury show excellent healing without treatment.

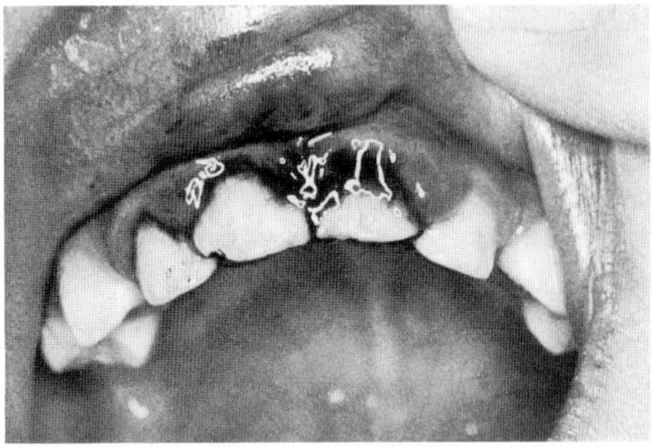

Fig. 7-8 A Intrusion of deciduous maxillary central incisors.

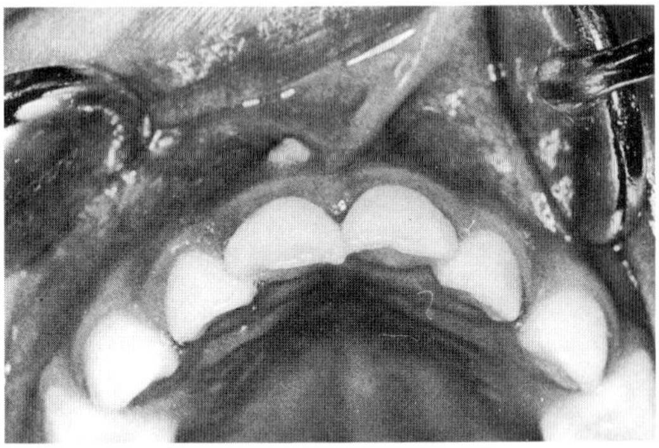

Fig. 7-8 B Intraoral features 6 months after the injury show a fistula of the right central incisor.

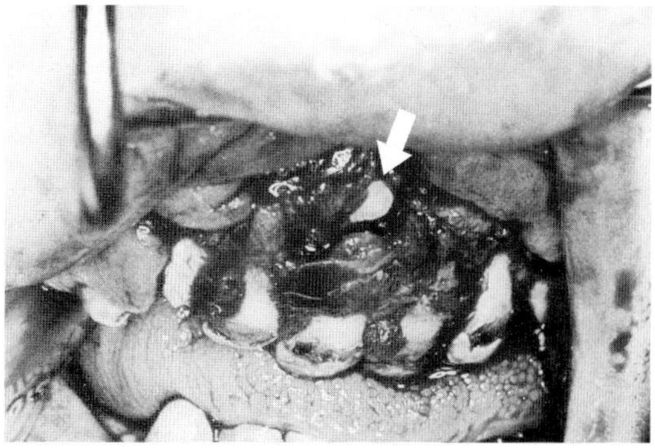

Fig. 7-9 A Lateral luxation of all deciduous incisors as a result of injury. 11 is exposed. Extraction of the deciduous teeth is indicated in this patient.

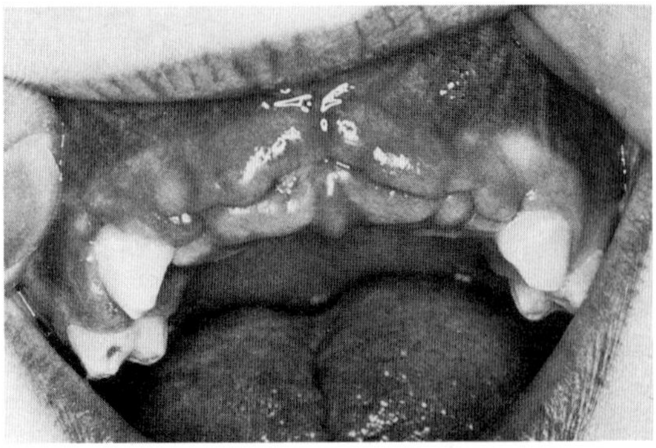

Fig. 7-9 B Intraoral features 1 month after the injury.

aid of an occlusal radiograph) can be conclusive in such instances.
Finally, the formation of the root of the permanent tooth can be delayed, so that its eruption occurs too late.
As already pointed out, one cannot predict which of the above possibilities will present itself after a traumatic injury to the deciduous teeth. In any case, the possibility of an earlier traumatic injury should always be considered in the frequent examples in which eruption occurs in the wrong position or is delayed.

2.4 Therapy

The treatment of lesions of the deciduous teeth poses some general problems. For example, a child is usually not very responsive after an accident, and in many cases this precludes more extensive treatment. Another difficulty which interferes with any treatment aimed at preservation of a tooth involved is the shape of the deciduous teeth. The use of fixation devices is markedly impeded by the short, conical shape of the deciduous teeth.
Regardless of the method chosen in the treatment of lesions of the deciduous teeth, the most important point is to save as much of the permanent teeth as possible. Generally, this is best ensured by treatment which is as simple as possible.
For fractures of the deciduous teeth, extraction is really always the treatment of choice, particularly if there is a crown fracture with exposed pulp. Only in teeth in which root formation has been completed, in which the apical foramen is small and root resorption has not yet started, can root canal treatment be considered. Such a situation, however, is extremely rare.
A root fracture of a deciduous tooth is also a clear indication for extraction. It is to be borne in mind that attempts to remove the apical root fragment are best omitted here because they are more likely to be harmful than beneficial in connection with the permanent dentition. Iatrogenic lesions of the permanent dentition can result from such attempts.
Reimplantation with subsequent fixation should never be attempted after complete extrusion of a deciduous tooth. Extrusions usually take place when the root already shows advanced resorption. The permanent tooth bud already is so far advanced that reduction of the gap in the dentition no longer can be expected. Orthodontic measures such as the use of space maintainers therefore can be omitted.
In the frequent cases of luxation with intrusion, the question arises whether active treatment is indicated. Intruded teeth are best left where they are; spontaneous re-eruption often follows within a few months (Figs. 7-7 and 8).
Small periodontal wounds which may be associated with intrusion of a tooth also are best left untreated: they heal without complications in a few days. It is advisable, however, to instruct the parents to have the child use a disinfectant mouthwash to prevent infection. In obviously complicated cases, antibiotic medication is indicated.
If the injury involves several teeth, with corresponding bone lesions, the risk of damage to the buds of the permanent teeth is greater. In these cases, which involve intrusion of several deciduous teeth, repositioning of the teeth followed by fixation is suggested. Fixation is best achieved with the aid of a cold-curing acrylic with which the entire dental arch is bandaged.
Accidents frequently cause subluxation of one or several teeth which are more or less loosened. If the affected children are three or four years old, attempts at simple fixation can be made. If the teeth are only slightly loosened, active treatment can be omitted and it is sufficient to instruct the parents to make sure that the tooth (teeth) involved is spared as much as possible. If the child is older than four years and if the tooth is significantly loosened as a result of luxation, extraction again is the best solution (Fig. 7-9).
Whatever the injury to the deciduous teeth and whatever the treatment chosen, there is always a possibility of damage to the permanent dentition, and the parents always should be made aware of this possibility.

3. Lesions of Permanent Teeth

3.1 Crown Fractures in the Permanent Dentition

Many different types of crown fractures have been distinguished, with a wide variety of combinations of enamel, dentin, pulp and cementum: e.g. enamel fracture, enamel-dentin fracture without pulp exposure and enamel-dentin-(cementum) fracture with pulp exposure (*Schwenzer* and *Steinhilber*, 1974). The three most common types—infraction, uncomplicated and complicated crown fractures—will be discussed here.

3.1.1 Enamel Cracks

Cracks are incomplete enamel fractures without loss of dental tissue. Such cracks are often overlooked, although they are quite common. They also occur in the absence of any facial injury. They are caused by direct violence on the labial aspect of the maxillary incisors and are often combined with luxations. These cracks can be traced easily by exposing the labial aspect to a beam of light thrown parallel to the longitudinal axis of the tooth. Cracks alone require no therapy, but vitality should be tested with the aid of a pulp tester. *Rock* (1974) reported that pulps in teeth which show no crown fracture but have been exposed to violence have a relatively low chance of survival, perhaps owing to periapical rupture of the pulp tissue. According to *Ellis* and *Davey* (1970), traumatized teeth without fracture run a greater risk of pulp damage than fractured teeth because the energy which causes the fracture is not transmitted to pulp and adjacent tissues. The cracks can occasionally cause 'leaks' in the dentin and irritation of the odontoblast processes at the amelodentinal junction. If the pain does not disappear spontaneously as a result of deposition of secondary dentin, prosthetic measures will have to be considered.

The prognosis of crown cracks is excellent unless luxation has occurred simultaneously.

3.1.2 Uncomplicated Crown Fractures

Uncomplicated crown fractures are confined to the enamel only or involve enamel and dentin, but without exposure of the pulp. An enamel fracture occurs almost exclusively at the mesial or distal corner of an incisor (Fig. 7-10). After a blow on the chin, the mandibular incisors may be knocked against their maxillary counterparts in end-to-end contact, and a labial fragment of enamel can snap off (Fig. 7-11). By scratching the fractured surface with a probe, it can be established whether the amelodentinal junction has been passed.

Enamel fractures are treated by grinding sharp fragments down to smoothness, followed by application of fluoride solution to the fracture surface. Vitality must be tested at regular intervals. In the case of amelodentinal fractures without pulp exposure, the patient often indicates pain spontaneously. The dentin is tender to the touch and an increased response to cold and heat can be observed (Fig. 7-12).

Very careful exploration of the dentin with a slender endodontic reamer may reveal a small perforation to the pulp: the so-called pinpoint exposure (one should beware of causing such a perforation while exploring; this risk is particularly grave at sites at which the pulp beneath it gives the dentin a pink hue).

Intraoral examination should be completed by a vitality test and radiography. The radiograph can be used to evaluate the size of the pulp chamber, the thickness of the layer of dentin and the stage of root development.

In the treatment of amelodentinal fractures it should be remembered that some dentin tubules have been cut tangentially and that their surface is larger as the patient is younger. The treatment of choice in uncomplicated crown fractures consists of protection of dentin and pulp from thermal, mechanical and bacterial influences.

Application of calcium hydroxide to the cut tubules has a favorable effect on the pulp and lends adequate protection. Calcium hydroxide has the advantage over zinc oxide-eugenol in that it does not affect odontoblast activity (*Epstein* 1962). Because this indirect pulp cap is insufficiently proof against mechanical effects, the layer of calcium hydroxide should be pro-

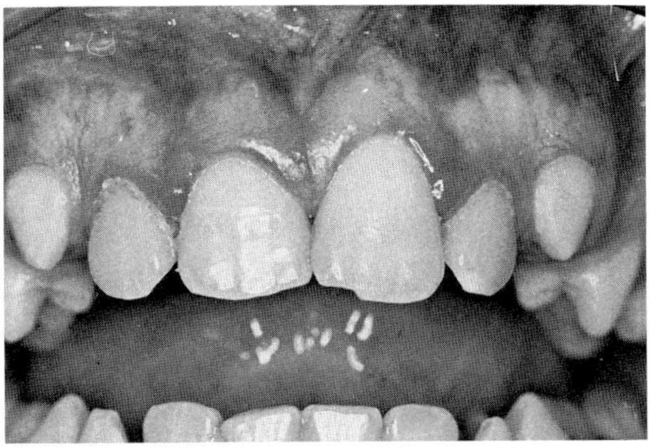

Fig. 7-10 Enamel fracture of 11, 21.

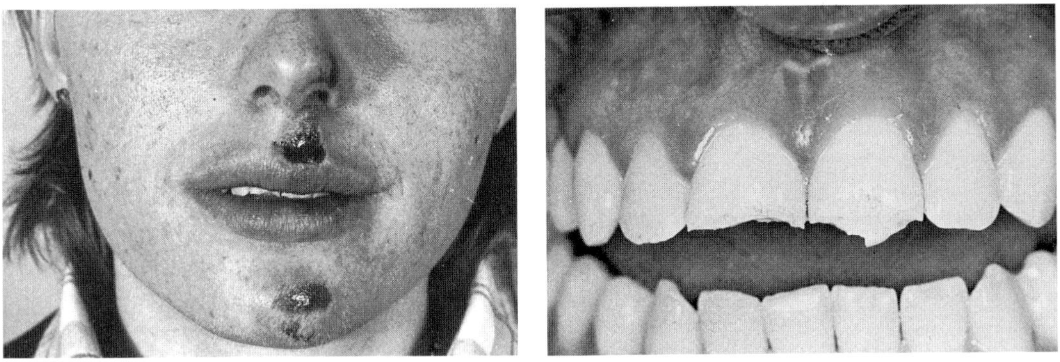

Figs. 7-11 A and B A blow on the chin caused an enamel fracture of 11, 21.

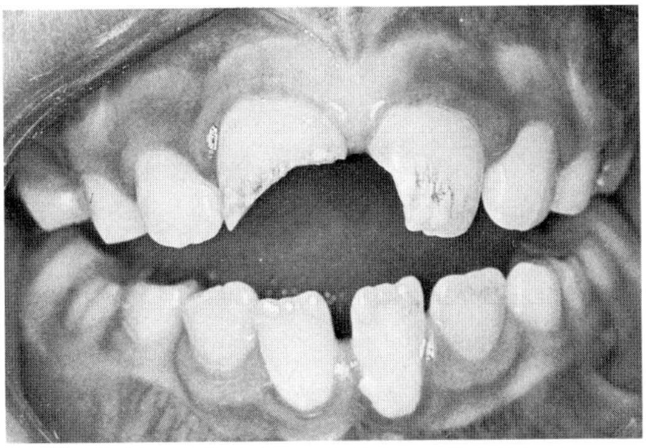

Fig. 7-12 Amelodentinal fractures 11, 21. The patient spontaneously indicates pain. No exposure of pulp tissue.

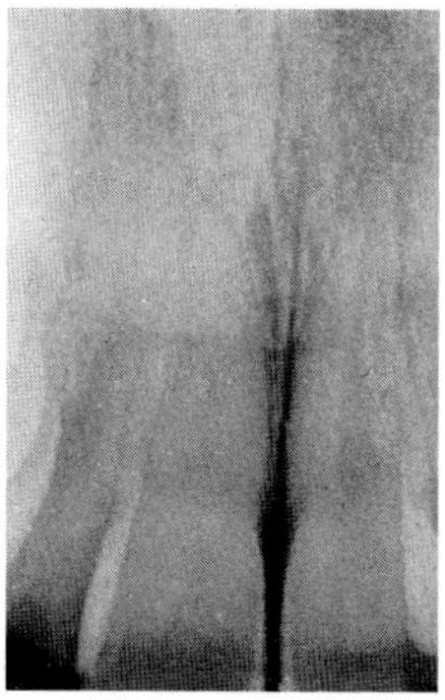

Fig. 7-13 Obliteration of the root canal due to secondary dentin apposition after uncomplicated crown fracture of 11.

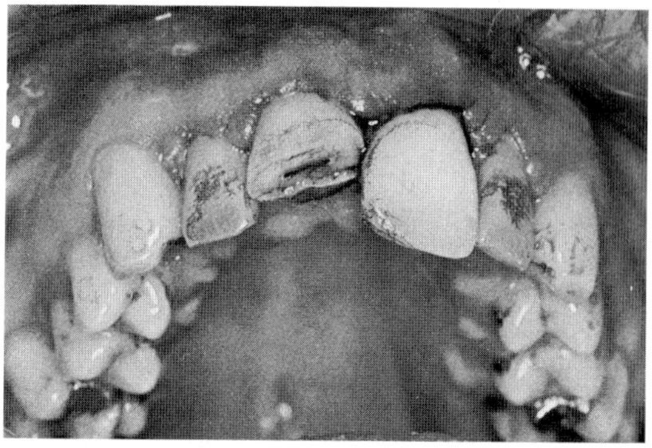

Fig. 7-14 Complicated crown fracture of 11 and subluxation of 21. The pulp of 11 is exposed, and blood flows from the gingival sulcus of 21.

tected—either by means of a strong cement such as zinc oxyphoxphate, or by a temporary metal or acrylic crown. The latter has the advantage of preventing migration of adjacent teeth because it restores the points of contact.

After about six weeks, secondary dentin has formed against the roof of the pulp chamber and the final restoration can be effected with restorative materials or fitting of a jacket crown.

The prognosis of uncomplicated crown fractures is very good. According to *Rock* (1974), the pulp remains vital in about 80% of uncomplicated crown fractures. We must add to this that a negative reaction to a thermal or electrical pulp test can be caused by obliteration of the pulp chamber or deposition of secondary dentin (Fig. 7-13).

3.1.3 Complicated Crown Fractures

A patient with a facial injury which has caused one or several complicated crown fractures is bound to seek medical advice very quickly because an exposed pulp is very painful. At intraoral examination, dentin and pulp prove to be very tender to the touch (Fig. 7-14). A capillary hemorrhage from the crown pulp is observed. Radiography is necessary so that the appropriate therapy may be planned.

Therapy

Treatment of young patients should be aimed at ensuring an optimal chance of completion of root formation. With older patients however, vital extirpation of the pulp under local anesthesia can be carried out.

In all cases of complicated crown fracture it must be assumed that the pulp is infected and that direct capping with calcium hydroxide will result in pulp degeneration. In young patients, the contents of the root canal must be kept vital to assure completion of root formation and to make possible adequate subsequent endodontic therapy. Pulpotomy (vital amputation) is the therapy of choice here.

The procedure is as follows: local anesthesia is given and the tooth is isolated with the aid of a rubber dam. If this seems impossible owing to insufficient crown height, one may consider first the application of a temporary crown without occlusal surface, or an orthodontic band. The tooth is then disinfected, and further treatment is carried out as aseptically as possible. The pulp chamber is opened with a round bur, and the crown pulp is amputated with a sharp, flat excavator without exerting traction on the remaining pulp tissue. Next, an attempt is made to arrest the bleeding from the crown pulp with the aid of sterile cotton plugs. To protect the remaining pulp, a thin mixture of calcium hydroxide is applied without pressure. A layer

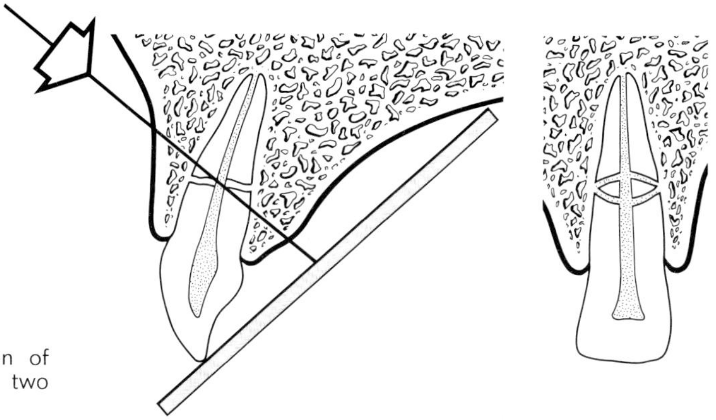

Fig. 7-15 Radiographic demonstration of simple root fracture represented by two curved lines on the film, like an ellipse.

of zinc oxide-eugenol is applied to this, and finally a firm temporary or definitive protection is placed in position. After about six weeks, radiography reveals a dentin bridge over the residual pulp. The vital amputation can be considered successful if no pain develops and root formation is completed. Failures are recorded in about 7 to 28 % of cases (*Andreasen* 1972). After closure of the apex, the pulpotomy should be followed by conventional endodontic treatment; otherwise there is a grave risk of obliteration and calcification of the pulp, which would greatly impede the subsequent placement of an adequate restoration.

3.2 Root Fractures in the Permanent Dentition

Root fractures are much more common in the permanent than in the deciduous dentition. The length of the clinical crown and the firmness of the alveolar bone are factors of importance in this respect. Combined crown-and-root fractures are rare; however, root fractures are often associated with fractures of the labial aspect of the alveolar process.

Root fractures may be classified as high or low fractures and those through the middle one-third of the root. Complicated crown fractures, with the fracture line through the cementum intra-alveolarly, are regarded as cervical or high root fractures.

It should also be mentioned that traumatized teeth without symptoms or radiological changes may have sustained cementum fracture from torsion. Their healing takes place via osteocementum, and is more rapid as the tooth is better immobilized. *Taatz* and *Stiefel* (1964) advise therefore that all traumatized teeth should be splinted.

3.2.1 History and Examination in Root Fractures

The history often demonstrates that root fractures are not associated with pain. Displacement and some slight extrusion often are observed. Teeth with low or apical root fractures are likely to show little or no increase in mobility. If digital pressure is exerted on either side of the alveolar process while the traumatized tooth is moved with the other hand, one can quickly establish whether a root fracture or luxation is involved. Vital teeth nearly always show axis tenderness. Vitality is verified with the aid of a pulp tester. A fracture will or will not be conspicuous, depending on the course of the fracture line and the direction of the central beam from the X-ray tube.

In dubious cases it is advisable to make a second radiograph from a different angle. A simple root fracture is often represented by two curved fracture lines on the dental film; together these form an ellipse (Fig. 7-15; see also Fig. 7-2).

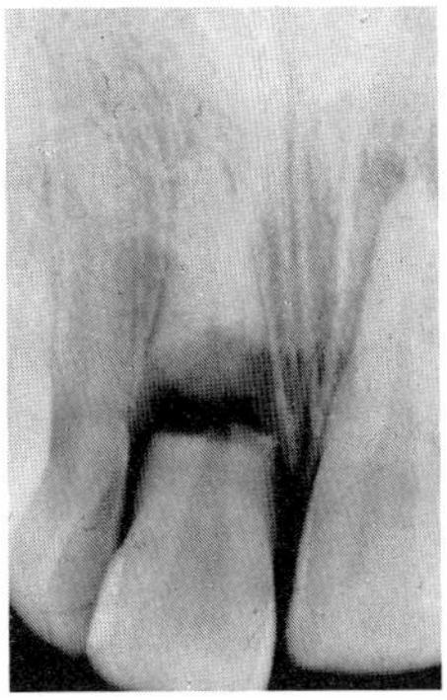

Fig. 7-16 Root fracture 11 through the middle third of the root.

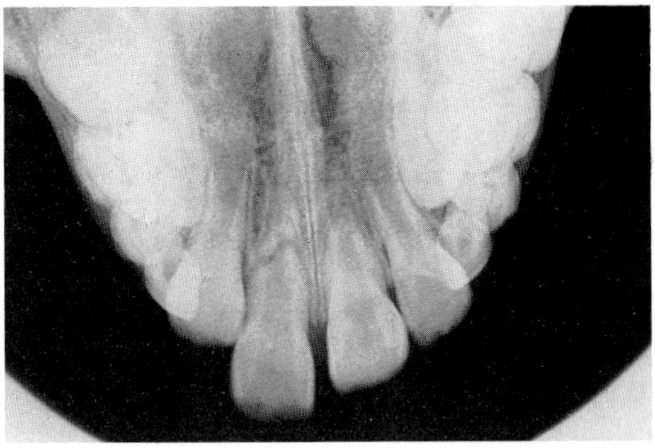

Fig. 7-17 Apical root fracture of an incomplete 11. The center of resistance in a young patient is situated lower than in an adult and the apex is more fragile.

These lines represent the course of the fracture on the labial and the palatal or lingual aspect, respectively. Apart from the course of the fracture line, the degree of dislocation of the coronal part and the stage of development of the root should receive attention.
It is a striking fact that most root fractures extend through the middle one-third of the root. The impact of violence on the labial aspect causes rotation of the tooth because of the center of resistance, which lies halfway the length of the root. Most root fractures, therefore, are localized at this level (Fig. 7-16). An impact of sharp violence which does not give the tooth time to rotate, is likely to cause a root fracture through the coronal part. Apical fractures (Fig. 7-17) are rare; those which occur usually involve the mandibular anterior teeth, propably because these have fragile apices.

3.2.2 Therapy of Root Fractures

The treatment of root fractures is in principle the same in all cases and resembles that of fractures of the limbs; this means that reduction, fixation and immobilization are imperative in all circumstances. Despite the analogy to bone fractures, dental root fractures can hardly be expected to show *restitutio ad integrum* when they heal; the regenerative powers of the tooth are insufficient for complete restitution.

Only where a coronal root fracture communicates with the gingival sulcus is consolidation improbable, so that the crown must be removed. In all other cases the fracture is reduced and repositioning is verified radiologically, if possible (Fig. 7-18). The tooth then is immobilized for eight weeks with a rigid splint. Types of splint and methods of splinting have been discussed in detail in Chapter 6. It has been demonstrated that any type of splint will do if it is sufficiently rigid and remains *in situ* sufficiently long. Some intrusive pressure on the fractured tooth or teeth is desirable.
Vitality is tested at regular intervals and consolidation is followed radiologically. *Andreasen* (1971) reported 55 % incidence of pulp necrosis. It is quite apparent that this necrosis develops mainly in coronal fractures with significant dislocation. The survival of the pulp is believed to depend on the possibility of decompression and restoration of the circulation. In luxated teeth, these necessary factors are not available.
The best chance for lasting success generally may be anticipated for fractures through the lower or the middle third of the root.
In his excellent textbook on traumatic injuries of the teeth, *Andreasen* (1972) proposed a radiological and histological classification of the healing of root fractures. He distinguishes the following four types:

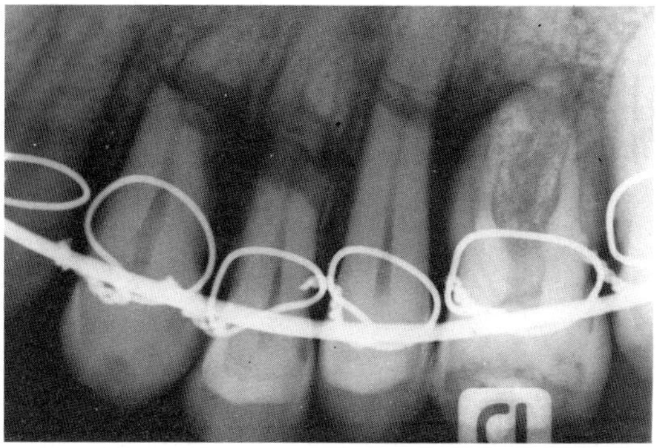

Fig. 7-18 Root fractures 2 3, 2 4, 2 5. Radiograph immediately after splinting. Reduction insufficient.

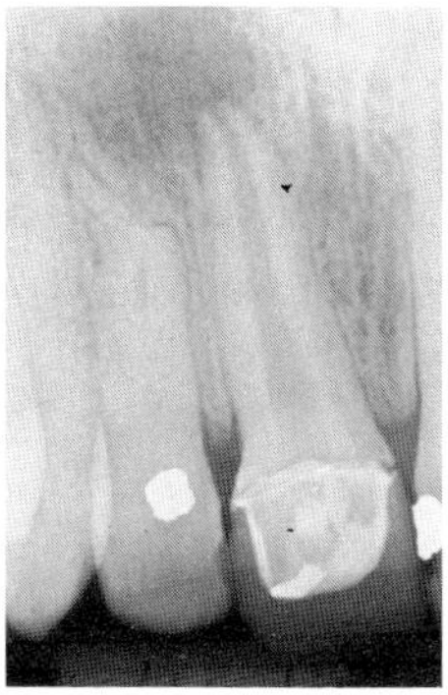

Fig. 7-19 Later stage of root fracture 1 2. Healing with obliteration of root canal and interposition of calcified tissue.

1. Interposition of calcified tissue.
   The fracture space is hardly visible radiologically and the fragments are in close contact without peripheral rounding of the fracture. There is no clinical evidence of abnormal mobility or pain on percussion.
   The tooth shows a vital response. The calcified tissue interposed in the fracture space histologically is highly cellular dentin and, toward the periodontal space, cement-like tissue.
   In a later stage, dental radiographs often show obliteration of the pulp in the coronal fragment (Fig. 7-19).
2. Interposition of connective tissue.
   The dental radiograph shows peripheral rounding of the fracture fragments and a radiolucent fracture line persists. Clinically the tooth is not mobile unless the fracture line is located exactly subgingivally.
   The tooth usually shows a vital response. Histologically, the fracture fragments are covered with cementum and strands of connective tissue extend through the fracture. In surgery, this fracture healing would be described as syndesmosis.
3. Interposition of bone and connective tissue.
   Radiological examination reveals a bridge of bone between the fragments and, contrary to categories (1) and (2), the periodontal membrane extends around each fragment.
   The tooth shows a vital response and is not mobile. This type of healing is usually observed in teeth which are in a phase of eruption. The coronal fragment continues to erupt, while the apical part remains *in situ.*
4. Interposition of granulation tissue.
   Radiological examination discloses broadening of the fracture space, which is radiolucent. The tooth is mobile, slightly extruded, and often painful at percussion. The pulp has a nonvital response and in some instances a fistula is present. Histological examination reveals granulation tissue between the fragments.
   The coronal part of the pulp is necrotic, while the apical part may still be vital.
   In root fractures close to the cervix, communication with the gingival sulcus can be the cause of necrosis and inflammation. As a rule, however, the pulp is ruptured as a result of the dislocation and revascularization consequently does not occur.

Only the last mentioned type requires further treatment, by methods which depend on the fracture site and the patient's age and wishes. First of all, it is possible to extract the entire tooth, with subsequent orthodontic or prosthodontic treatment. If the fracture line is located close to the root cervix, removal of the coronal fragment can be contemplated (as is done also

Figs. 7-20 A to D Orthodontic extrusion of 2 1.

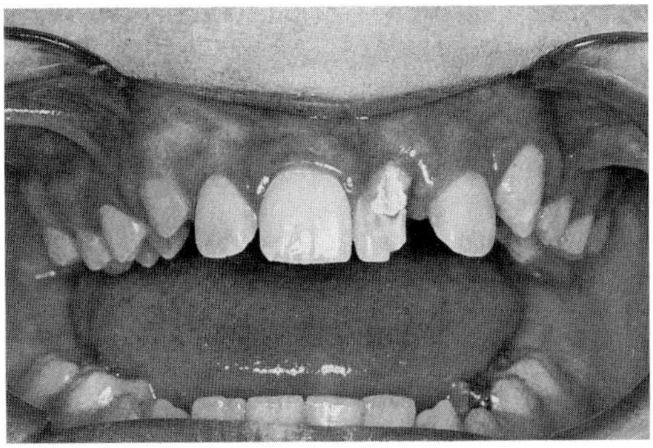

Fig. 7-20 A Unfavorable fracture of the crown including a cervical part of the root.

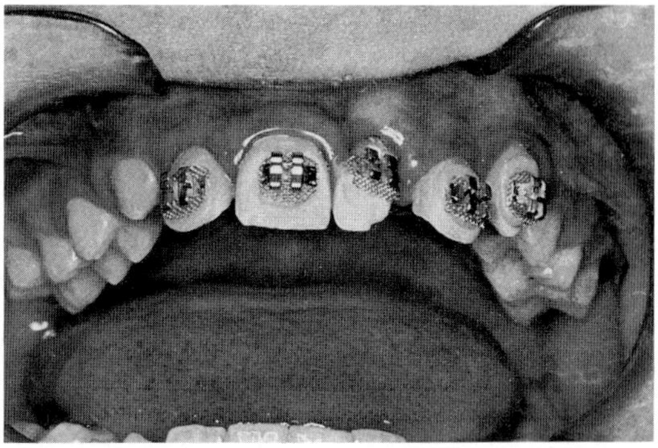

Fig. 7-20 B After endodontic treatment, orthodontic extrusion is performed.

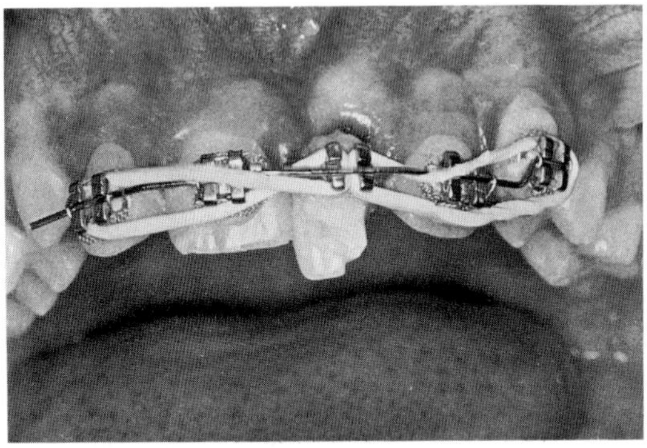

Fig. 7-20 C Orthodontic extrusion is completed.

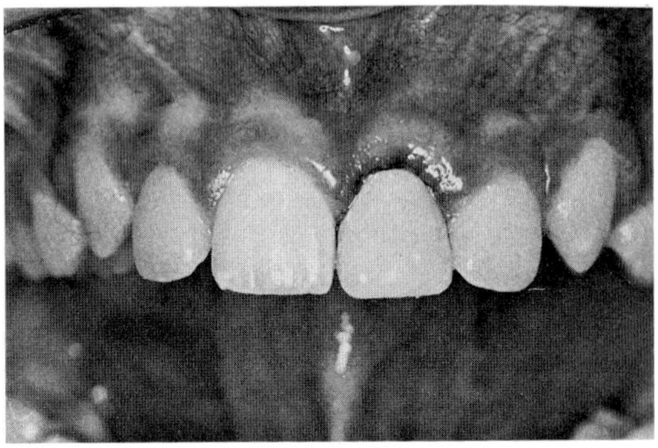

Fig. 7-20 D A temporary jacket crown has been placed.

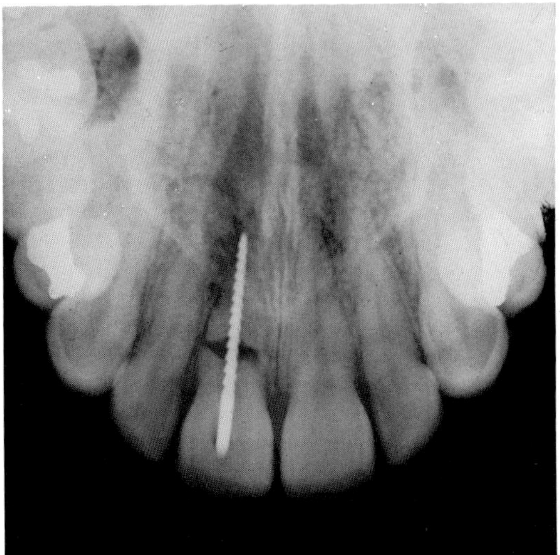

Fig. 7-21 Intraradicular splint of 1 1 after root fracture.

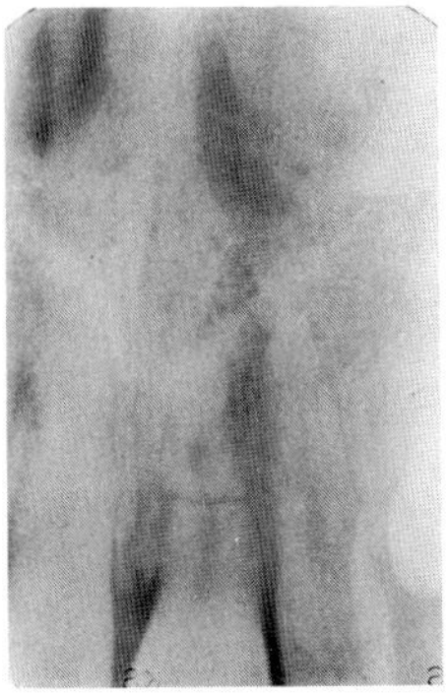

Fig. 7-22 A Root fracture of 21.

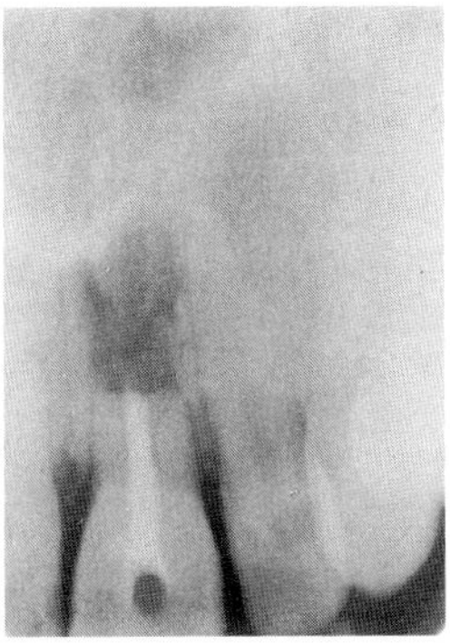

Fig. 7-22 B The aftertreatment consisted of endodontic therapy and removal of the apical fragment.

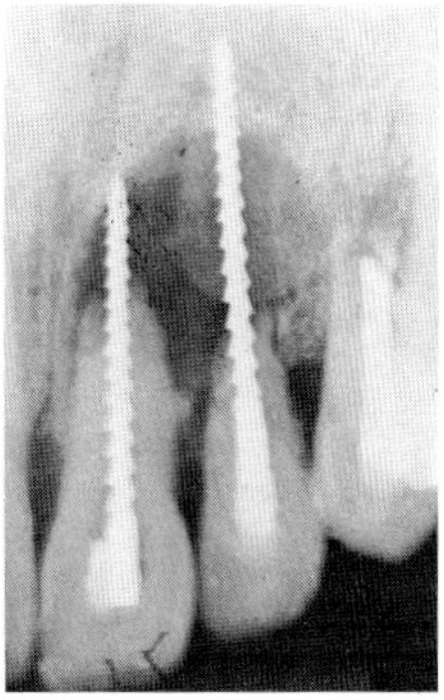

Fig. 7-23 Fixation of the coronal fragments with the aid of intraosseous pins. Radiographs 5 years after injury.

in complicated root fractures in communication with the gingival sulcus), with subsequent endodontic treatment. Next, gingivectomy or extrusion by orthodontic means can be carried out in preparation for definitive restoration. Gingivectomy gives an only modest esthetic result, but orthodontic extrusion, after endodontic treatment (Fig. 7-20), is a good alternative if the root length is sufficient (*Heitherway*, 1973).
If the coronal fragment is to be spared, endodontic therapy with intraradicular splinting is indicated (Fig. 7-21). A silver or gutta percha point may be placed first if the apical fragment is sufficiently large and then a gold-platinum pin is cemented.
With short apical fragments, separate endodontic therapy can be omitted. In spite of such a rigid intraradicular splint, bony interposition of tissue usually does not occur, although it is possible (*Lamers*, 1971).
When pulp necrosis has developed because of dislocation of the coronal fragment and when the fracture surface is close to the apex, the apical fragment still can be vital. Here endodontic therapy can be provided exclusively to the coronal part, while the apical part is subsequently removed, if necessary, in the manner of an apicoectomy (Fig. 7-22). According to *Andreasen* (1971), the latter two methods have not proven very successful.
When, after removal of the apical fragment, the tooth proves to be mobile, a long pin of gold-platinum alloy can be inserted through the root canal of the coronal fragment into the bone (Fig. 7-23). This method seems fairly successful (*Andreasen*, 1971). Apart from the complication of pulp necrosis, internal and external root resorption can occur in exceptional cases.
In **summary**, it can be said that vitality tests and radiography play an important role in determining the prognosis for root fractures. If there are no symptoms, if the tooth shows a (vague) vital response and if there is radiological evidence of consolidation, no therapy need be instituted.
Therapeutic intervention is indicated in the presence of obviously increased mobility, pain, non vital pulp, and a broadened and inflamed fracture space.
After removal of the coronal and apical fragments, orthodontic or prosthetic treatment is required. After removal of only the coronal fragment, orthodontic extrusion is preferred to gingivectomy.
Intraradicular splinting is a third possibility. A final alternative is to treat only the canal of the coronal fragment, while removing the apical fragment. If the coronal fragment is very mobile, a rigid pin can be inserted through the tooth into the alveolar bone in the manner of an implant.

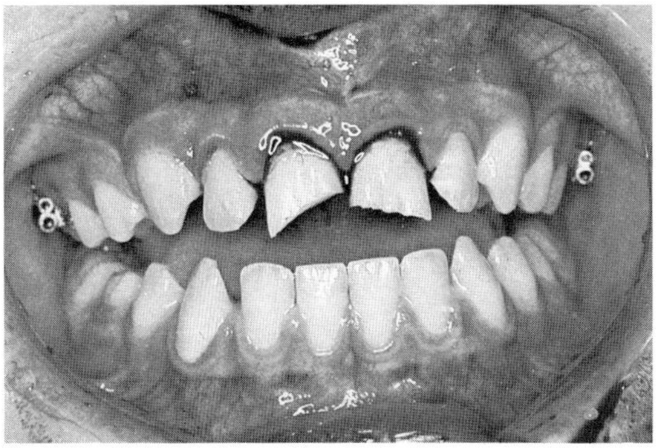

Fig. 7-24 Complicated crown fracture of 11, 21 with subluxation of both teeth. Very slight mobility and bleeding from the gingival sulcus.

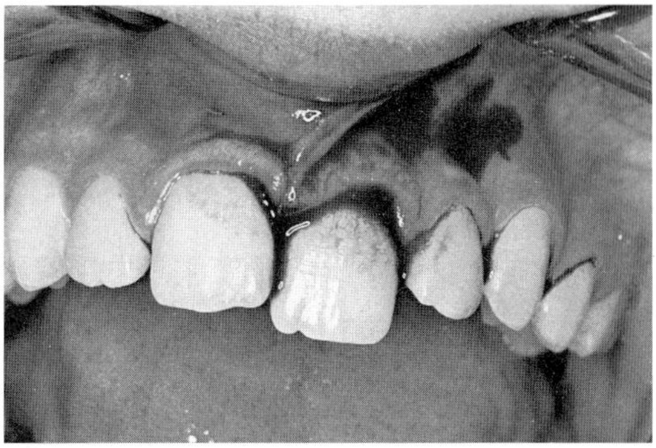

Fig. 7-25 Extrusion of 2 1. Bleeding from gingival sulcus; the tooth has partially left its alveolus.

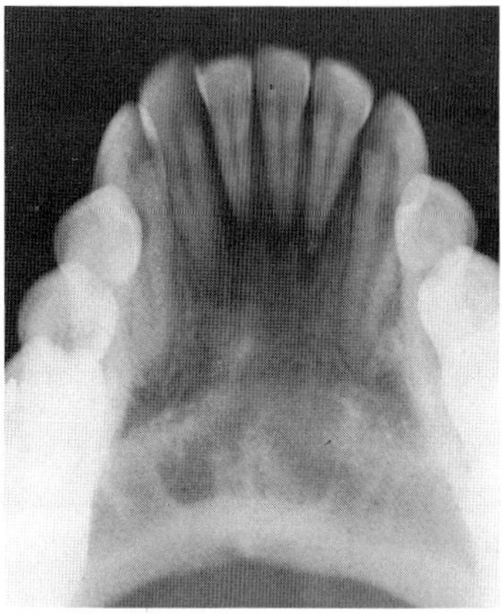

Fig. 7-26 Occlusal radiograph of mandibular anteriors after extrusive luxation of 4 1, 3 1, 3 2. The sockets are partly empty.

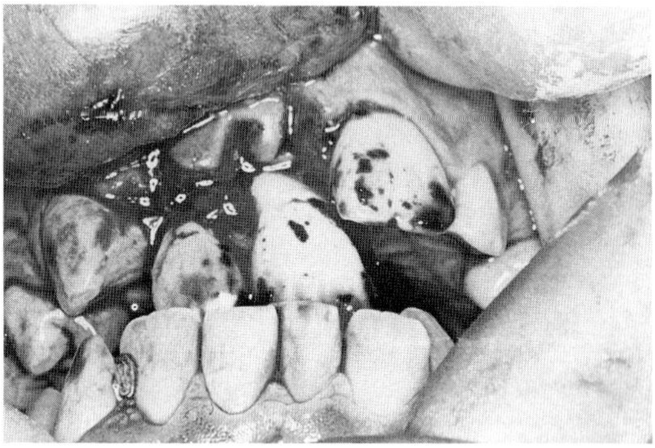

Fig. 7-27 Lateral luxation of 1 2, 1 1. Both teeth show extrusion and palatal dislocation. Occlusion is disturbed.

3.3 Luxations in the Permanent Dentition

Luxations are classified into six types, depending on the mobility and the direction of displacement, as described on page 175. If there is no longer any contact between tooth and alveolus, the term exarticulation applies; other terms used in such cases are total extrusive luxation or avulsion. This type of luxation will be discussed in the next section.

The luxation is usually caused by the impact of a blunt object. In many such events, several teeth are injured simultaneously. The adult dentition differs from the deciduous teeth in that intrusion rarely occurs. Luxation of permanent teeth often is associated with infraction, root fracture or an uncomplicated coronal fracture.

3.3.1 Diagnosis

In the case of **concussion** there is slight damage to the periodontal membrane. The tooth shows no abnormal mobility but is painful on percussion as a result of hemorrhage and edema in the periodontal space. The tooth shows a positive reaction to faradic current and sometimes some extrusion. The radiograph is uncharacteristic.

Subluxation likewise involves no displacement; at best some extrusion. Hemorrhage in the gingival sulcus is often observed, with painful percussion and slight mobility (Fig. 7-24). Sensibility is intact and the radiograph shows a broadened periodontal space.

Intrusion is characterized by displacement of the tooth in the alveolar process. Mobility frequently is not increased, and the tooth shows a non-vital response. Intrusion of teeth with long roots can lead to fracture of the floor of the nose or even of the bottom of the maxillary sinus. The most conspicuous symptom in such cases is epistaxis (*Schwenzer* and *Steinhilber*, 1974). Although intrusive luxation is rare in the permanent dentition, it does require special attention because it entails the risk of loss of several teeth. The dental radiograph usually does not show the periodontal space because the tooth is in infraposition.

In the case of **extrusion** the tooth partly leaves the alveolus and is loosened (Fig. 7-25). Percussion or palpation are not painful; the response to the vitality test is negative. The radiograph shows a broadened periodontal space or a partly empty alveolus, according to the degree of extrusion (Fig. 7-26).

Lateral luxation usually involves displacement palatally (Fig. 7-27). Mobility is increased and there is some extrusion. The labial wall of the alveolar process often is fractured, and rupture of the mucosa may be present. Vitality has been lost and occlusion is disturbed.

3.3.2 Therapy

Concussion is the only form of luxation which requires no treatment. Vitality testing and instruction to the patient suffice. The tooth should be favored when eating, and such habits as thumb-sucking and nail-biting should be avoided. Vitality usually is intact, but the tooth may show yellow discoloration as a result of pulp obliteration.

In intrusive luxation—as in intrusion of deciduous teeth—an expectant attitude can be adopted. Once the degree of intrusion has been established with accuracy, the prognosis is discussed with the patient (and the parents, if present). Vitality is usually lost (*Andreasen* 1972); perhaps the tooth cannot extrude again and becomes ankylosed as a result of calcification of the periodontal ligament or progressive external root resorption. Internal resorption, too, is occasionally observed, discoloration of the crown can occur, and the periodontium can be affected. Involvement of the marginal alveolar bone and root resorption can develop so quickly that deep pockets result and loss of adjacent teeth is threatened. Extraction of the intruded teeth then is required.

Another complication, particularly in juvenile patients, is delayed eruption of a tooth as a result of ankylosis; this involves a threat of infraocclusion of the tooth. Surgical removal of the tooth ought to be considered, because orthodontic treatment is no longer possible and postponement of extraction leads to unnecessary loss of height of the alveolar process. For this reason, *Eschler* (1972) recommends waiting for possible extrusion of the intruded tooth for two months. If no eruption occurs, orthodontic extrusion becomes necessary.

Subluxations, extrusions and lateral luxations require a similar type of therapy, which should always focus on creating possibilities for restoration of the periodontium. In the case of subluxation with only slight mobility and hardly any loss of blood from the gingival sulcus, therapy can be omitted.

A luxation can be reduced manually under local anesthesia, but this is difficult when much blood has collected between the tooth and its socket. Here intrusion should be attempted when splinting; if necessary, an acrylic plate can be used. The repositioning is verified radiologically, if possible, whereupon fixation and immobilization can commence.

Many authors express preference for a particular method of splinting. In comparative studies, *Andreasen* and *Hjorting-Hansen* (1966) and *Jacobson* and *Zachrisson* (1975) reported that they were unable to demonstrate differences between the results obtained by three different methods. The impression is that the efficacy of splinting depends on the accuracy with which it is carried out. The three principal

Figs. 7-28 A to F Fabrication of an metal arch bar.

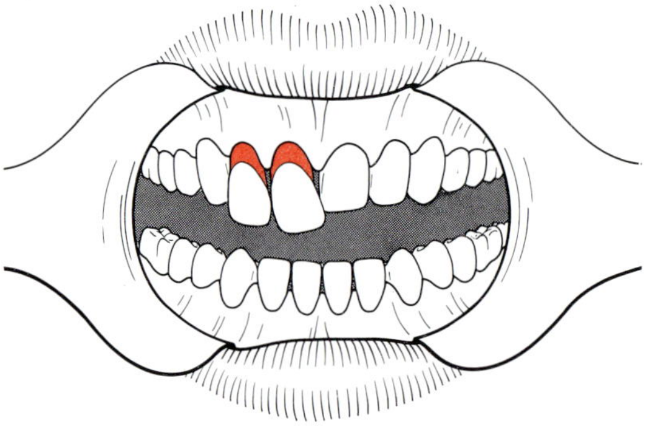

Figs. 7-28 A Appearance after injury: luxation of 1 2, 1 1.

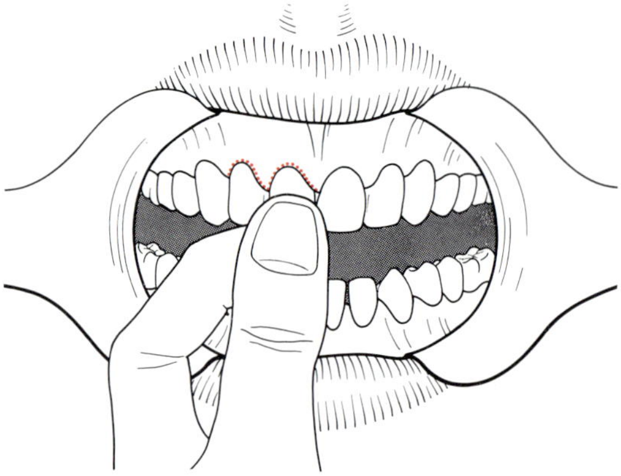

Fig. 7-28 B Manual repositioning after local anesthesia.

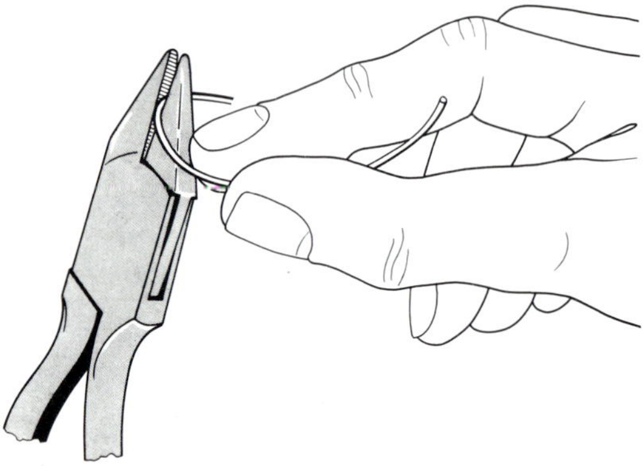

Fig. 7-28 C Shaping of the semicircular arch bar.

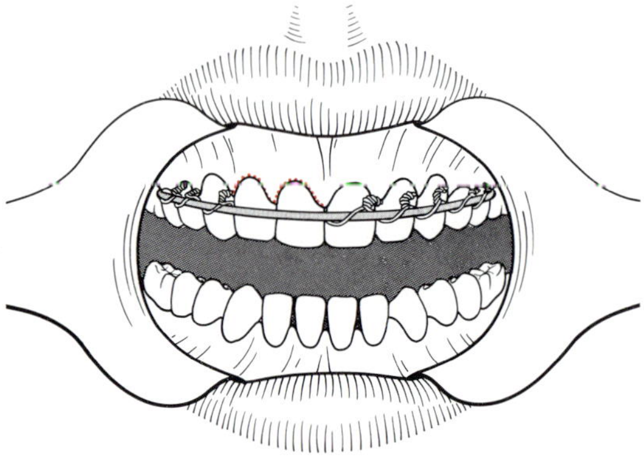

Fig. 7-28 D Splinting of all the nontraumatized teeth with ligatures apically of the cingulum.

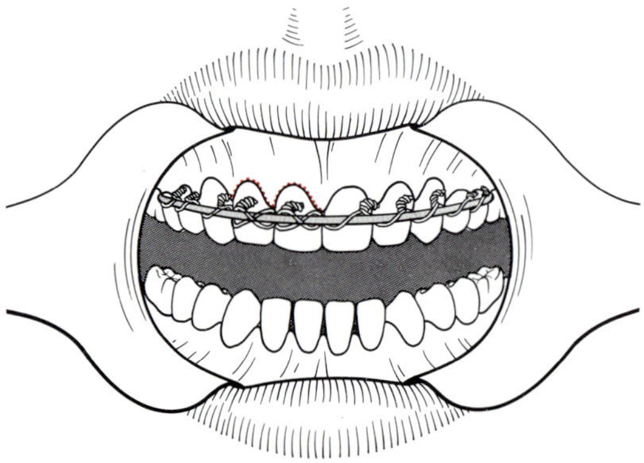

Fig. 7-28 E Fixation of the injured 12, 11. Ligatures incisally of the cingulum.

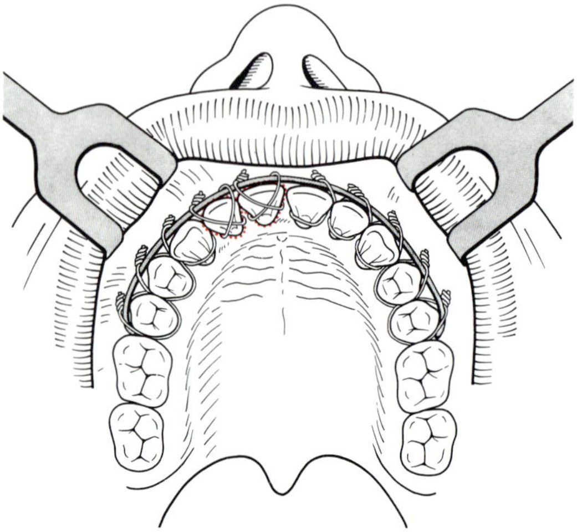

Fig. 7-28 F Occlusal view with cross-ligatures around 1 2, 1 1, both incisally of the cingulum.

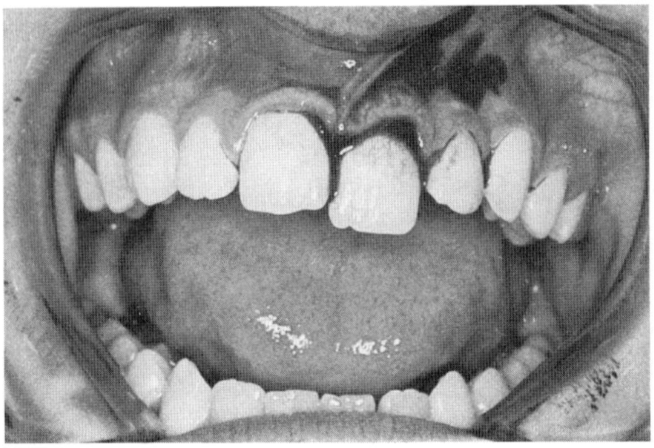

Fig. 7-29 A Extrusion of 2 1.

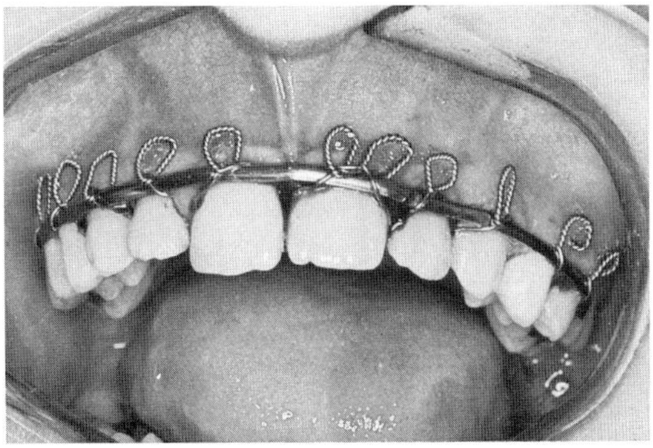

Fig. 7-29 B Metal arch bar for fixation of the extruded 2 1. A cross ligature used for the traumatized tooth rests palatally on the cingulum.

criteria to be fulfilled by any method of splinting are the following:

1. quick splinting should be possible;
2. fixation without damage to tooth or gingiva should be possible;
3. the splints should be sufficiently rigid.

These criteria are fulfilled by three methods which will be discussed briefly.

1. Metal arch bar

A semicircular arch bar is bent with the aid of bending pliers until it contacts at the level of the interdental papillae with all the teeth to be splinted. At least two intact teeth on each side of the injured teeth are included in the splint. The arch bar is fixed against the teeth with stainless steel wire ligatures (0.3 or 0.4 mm diameter). The wires are tightened and cut off, the ends being tugged behind the splint (interdentally). The injured teeth are then so splinted that some slight intrusive force is exerted. This can be achieved with cross ligatures (0.3 mm) or with a ligature in which the palatal or lingual wire lies incisally to the cingulum (Figs. 7-28 and 7-29). This method can be improved greatly by using cold-curing acrylic. A metal arch bar cannot be used without difficulty in a shedding dentition or in non-cooperative patients.

2. Acrylic splint

An acrylic splint has some advantages over a metal arch bar. It can be used on an interrupted dental arch, does not damage the periodontium and can be used reasonably well even in uncooperative patients. A disadvantage lies in the long interval between accident and immobilization (regardless of whether an intraorally or extraorally made splint is used (Figs. 7-30 and 7-31). *Kristoferitsch* (1974) describes a good, inventive method in which two thin acrylic plates are pressed together with a metal wire reinforcement between them. Sufficient occlusal and incisal acrylic is removed so that the original occlusion is maintained. *Anke* (1973) recommends cementing the acrylic splint made extraorally with silicate cement. *Andreasen* (1972) and *Simpson* et al. (1974) describe intraorally prepared acrylic splints, cemented with carboxylate and zinc oxyphosphate cement, respectively.

3. Composite splint and orthodontic brackets

In another manner of splinting, use is made of the etching technique. A few methods and examples will be treated here:

a) The luxated tooth can be fixed to the neighboring teeth by means of "composite". The labial surfaces are cleaned well and are etched in the usual way. The injured tooth is fixed by having the patient bite on a cotton wad. Subsequently the "composite resin" is applied (Fig. 7-32).
The disadvantage of this method is that the

Figs. 7-30 A to D Fabrication of an acrylic splint in a shedding dentition.

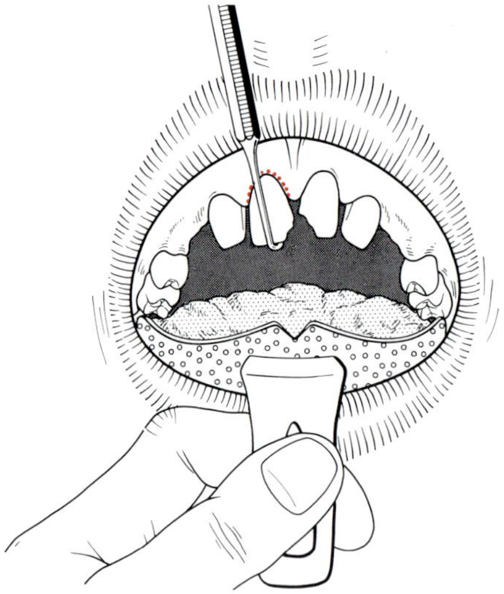

Fig. 30 A Impression and use of a modifield dental probe.

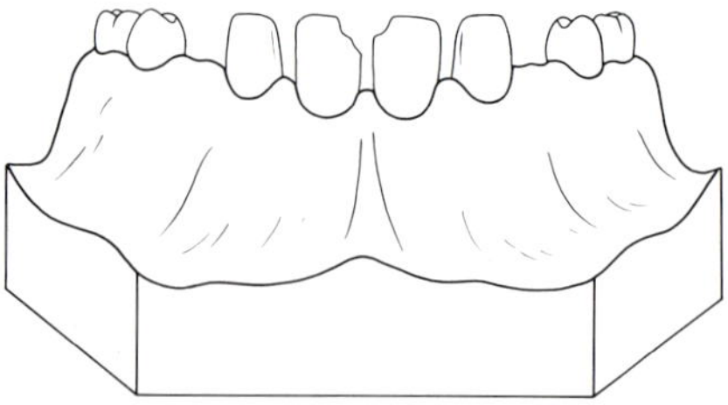

Fig. 30 B Model in white plaster.

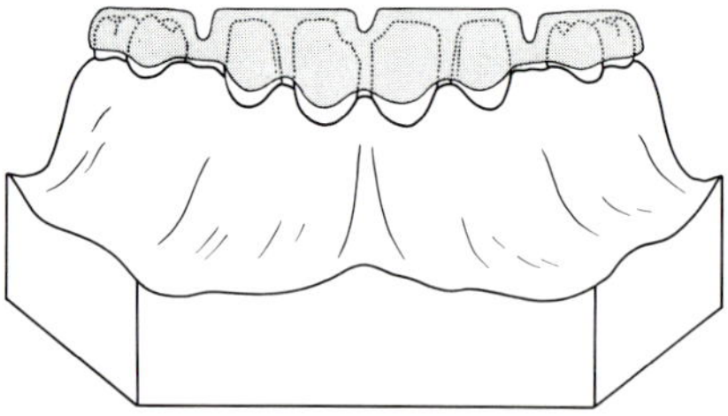

Fig. 30 C Plaster model with finished acrylic splint.

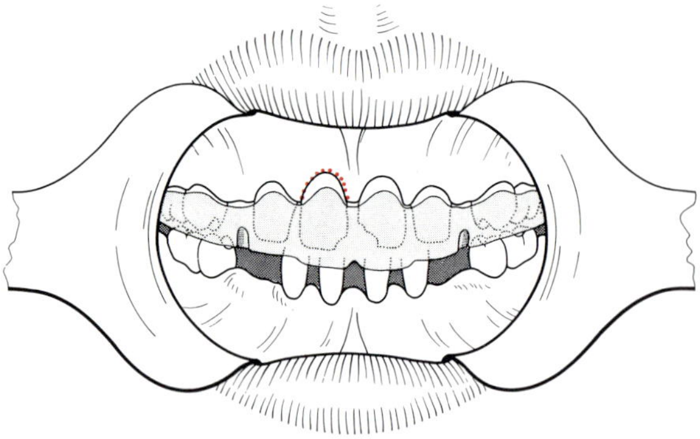

Fig. 30 D Intraoral appearance after cementing the splint.

material does not stick under the influence of articulation. The method is quick, which is an advantage with non-cooperative patients.

b) In a second method, a wire is fastened directly to the labial surfaces by means of composite.
This method is quick and very useful with non-cooperative patients. As opposed to the method in which no wire is used, the advantage here is that several teeth can easily be included in the splint (Fig. 7-33). However, the splint becomes loose easily, probably as a result of small fissures in the material which arise while the composite is hardening, since the wire cannot be fixed well.

c) Finally, there is a method in which the etching technique and the use of orthodontic brackets is combined. It is advisable to place the brackets as much as possible in one line, for otherwise the fixation will not be stable.
The brackets are etched on the affected tooth and at least 2 neighboring teeth. Thereafter a rectangular orthodontic wire is bent and if necessary is hardened.
Finally the arch is fixed in the brackets (Fig. 7-34).

Regardless the method used, the fixation is maintained for four to six weeks. Oral hygiene, splint stability and vitality of the injured teeth (if possible) are tested at regular intervals.

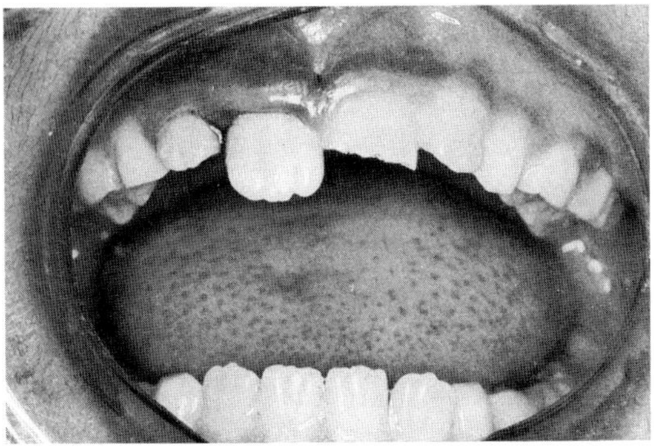

Fig. 7-31 A Subluxation of 11 and uncomplicated crown fracture of 21 in a shedding dentition.

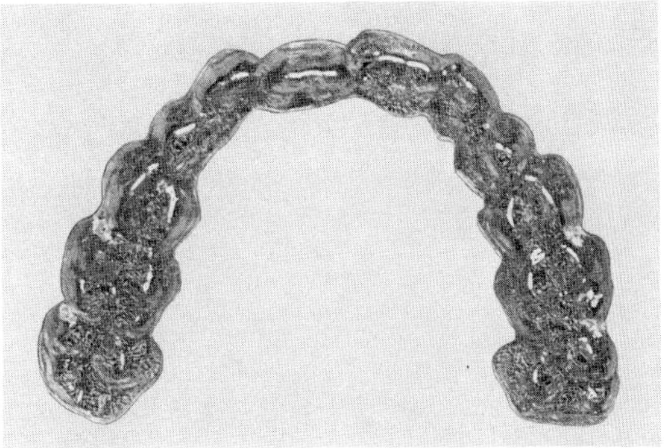

Fig. 7-31 B Acrylic splint.

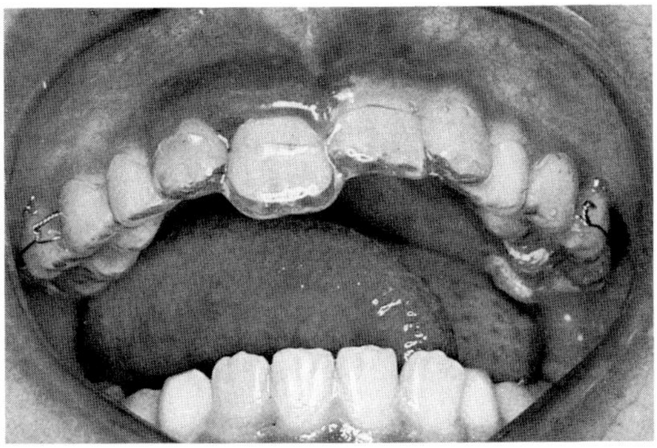

Fig. 7-31 C Splint in place. The exposed dentin of 21 is covered with a layer of Ca $(OH)_2$.

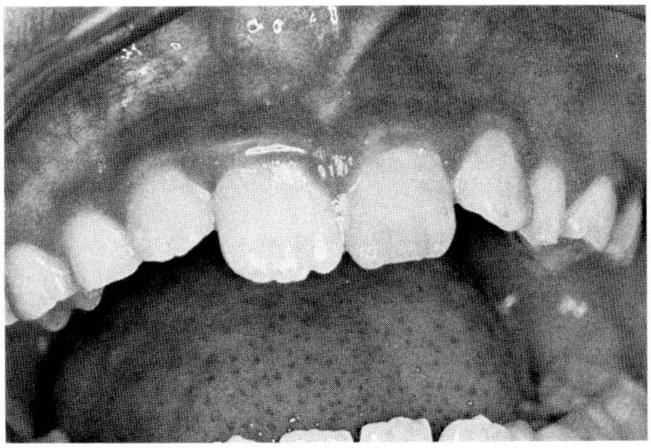

Fig. 7-31 D Restoration of 21 with a composite filling material.

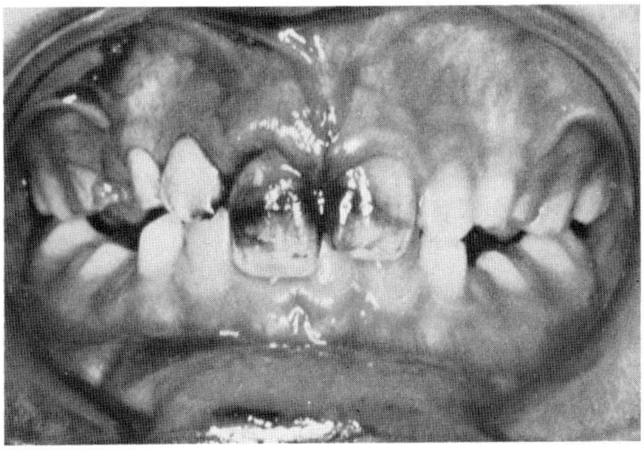

Fig. 7-32 A A young patient with a luxated 11.

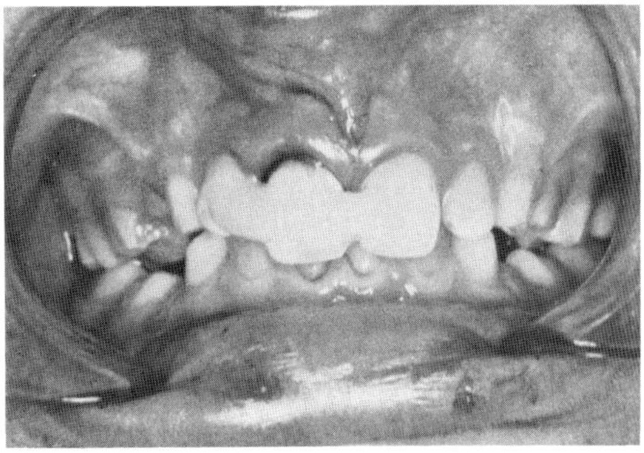

Fig. 7-32 B By means of composite material which is applied to the enamel after etching, the injured tooth is fixed to both neighboring teeth. A metal splint is not used.

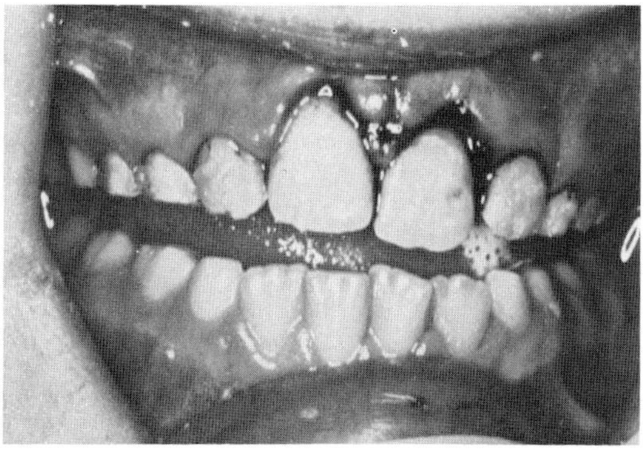

Fig. 7-33 A A patient with a luxated 21.

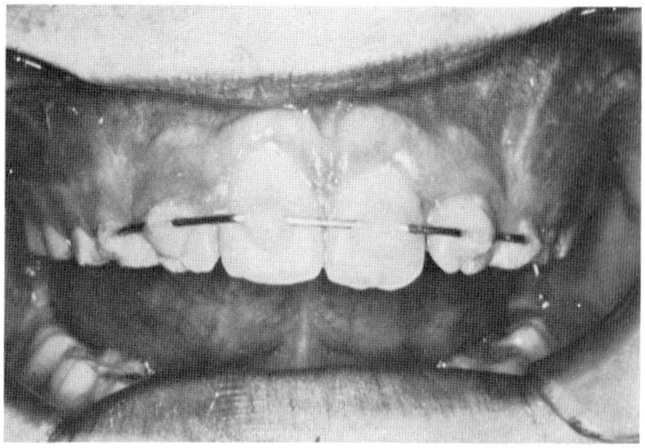

Fig. 7-33 B An arch bar is bent from a rectangular orthodontic wire. After etching the labial enamel surfaces, the splint is fixed by means of composite material.

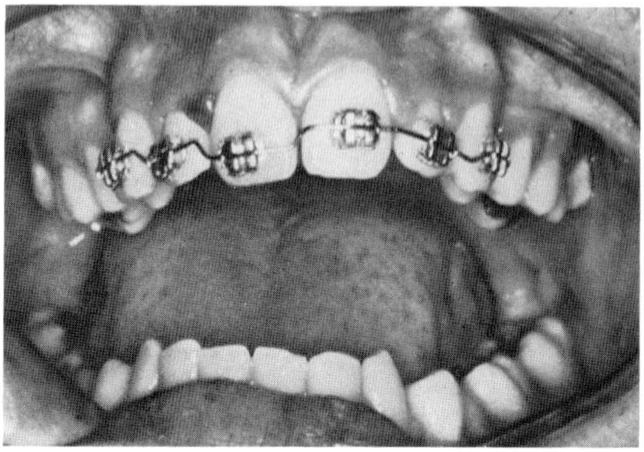

Fig. 7-34 A The exarticulated 1 1 is replanted. An orthodontic bracket is applied to the neighboring teeth and the affected tooth by means of the etch technique. A rectangular orthodontic wire is bent to fit properly in the brackets and thereafter it is fixated.

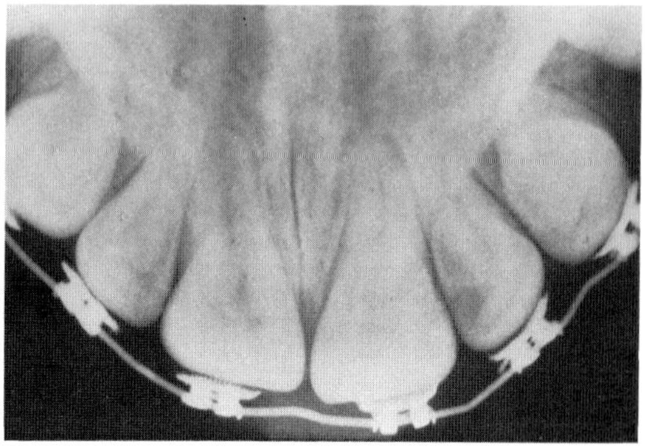

Fig. 7-34 B An occlusal radiograph shows a successful repositioning of the 1 1.

3.3.3 Prognosis

The prognosis of subluxations, extrusions and lateral luxations largely depends on the regenerative power of the pulp tissue and periodontium. Pulp survival chances are best in young patients with as yet incomplete root formation after slight displacement.

Pulp necrosis develops in 24 to 59 % of the luxated teeth, in 50 % of the extrusions and 25 % of the subluxations (*Andreasen*, 1972). Pulp necrosis can be diagnosed only on the basis of vitality tests and clinical and radiological findings.

If the root canal contents are necrotic, endodontic treatment is required; for completed roots, this poses no special problems. In young patients with a wide root canal lumen, conventional endodontic canal treatment is bound to fail. In such cases three approaches are possible.

The first focuses on further completion of the root, and treatment consists of extirpation only of the necrotic tissue. In some cases, the final 3 to 4 mm pulp tissue remains vital and can ensure completion of the apex after pulpotomy.

The second approach calls for application of a very thick gutta percha point, of which the

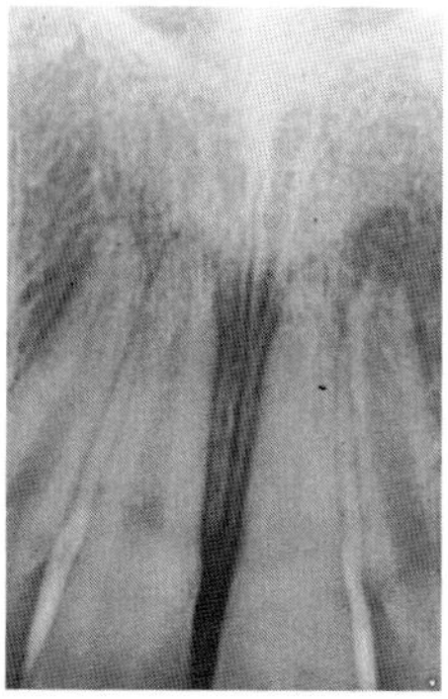

Fig. 7-35 Obliteration of the root canal of 21 two years after extrusive luxation.

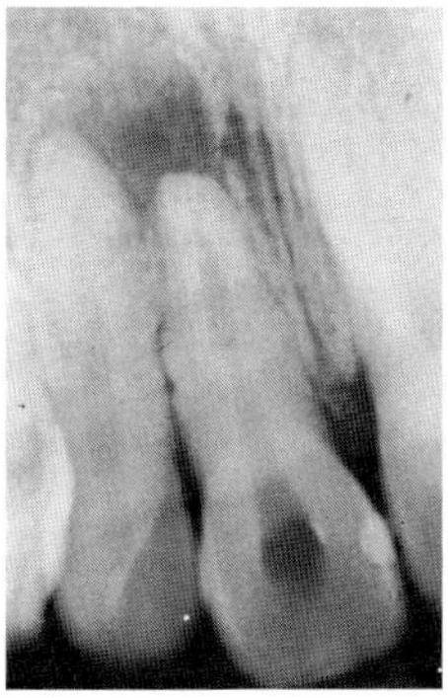

Fig. 7-36 Internal and external root resorption and central osteitis of 11 after extrusive luxation.

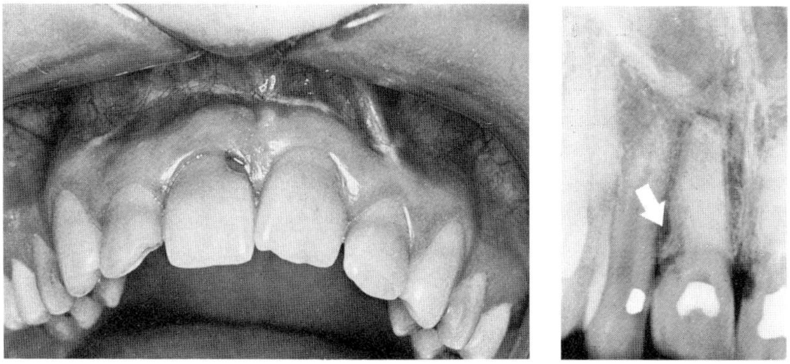

Figs. 7-37 A and B Progressive external root resorption with ankylosis after luxation of 1 1. Clinical and radiological features 4 years after the injury.

outer layer has been softened with chloroform.

The third approach involves filling of the canal and apicoectomy. In combination with an orthograde gutta percha point, a retrograde filling can be inserted; alternatively the large gutta percha point can be condensed apically with a warm hand instrument (*Andreasen*, 1972). Apart from pulp necrosis, pulp obliteration occurs in about 25 % of cases of luxation (Fig. 7-35). The first symptoms are yellow discoloration of the crown and gradual diminution of vitality. Obliteration occasionally is associated with pulp necrosis, in which case extirpation of pulp tissue is nearly impossible. Given a combination of pain and incipient pulp obliteration, endodontic treatment is indicated.
Apart from obliteration, internal root resorption can occur, in which case endodontic treatment likewise is indicated (Fig. 7-36).
In general, the regenerative power of the periodontium is limited, and consequently complications are not infrequent after luxations. Moreover, complications can develop which depend on the degree of luxation, the condition of the periodontium and the rigidity of the splint. Mucosal ruptures and fractures of the alveolar process also have an unfavorable effect on the

prognosis. Progressive root resorption, with or without ankylosis (Fig. 7-37), is observed in 6 to 11 % of the luxated teeth, but less often after subluxation than after extrusion (*Andreasen*, 1972). *Birkedal-Hansen* (1973) demonstrates on the basis of animal experiments that subluxation histologically causes external root resorption and ankylosis.

The clinical, radiological, histological and therapeutic aspects of external root resorption will be discussed further in the next section.

Unlike intrusion, subluxation and extrusive luxation rarely inflicts permanent damage in the periodontium. The post-traumatic marginal bone loss is compensated by remodelling (*Andreasen* 1972).

3.4 Exarticulations in the Permanent Dentition

In dealing with patients whose teeth have been knocked out, history-taking as well as extraoral and intraoral examination should be done with care but quickly and objectively so that therapy, if required, can be instituted as soon as possible. It is of importance to know how long ago the exarticulation (avulsion or total extrusive luxation) occurred, where the accident happened, and how the tooth was kept in the meantime. Physical examination focuses especially on the presence of fractures of the alveolar process or the jaw. In addition, efforts should be made to identifiy lesions of the lips and other soft tissues. Finally the tooth, kept in physiological saline, is cautiously examined for caries, bone remnants and the width of the apical foramen, without damaging the periodontal membrane. A radiograph is taken to exclude fractures of adjacent teeth or the alveolar process.

Exarticulations are modestly represented among frontal injuries and are slightly more often observed in deciduous than in permanent dentition. In many cases the maxillary incisors are involved, and the accident is due to obtuse violence sustained in a fall or a fight.

3.4.1 Indications for and Contraindications to Replantation

When planning treatment of exarticulations, one should consider whether there are contraindications to replantation. The literature advises to omit replantation when the anterior teeth in the maxilla are crowded, in the case of a pronounced Angle Class II, in very young patients, and in the case of exarticulation associated with complicated fractures and periodontally weak dentitions.

A long extraoral period also constitutes a contraindication. Once it is decided that an exarticulated tooth should not be replanted, the situation is the same as that of lost exarticulated teeth or replanted teeth lost soon after replantation.

The decision to fill the resulting diastema with some prosthetic appliance is more readily made for older patients than for children or adolescents. In adults, rapid migration of adjacent teeth is less likely and extrusion of antagonists less rapid than in juvenile patients; a space-maintainer is consequently less necessary. For very young patients an expectant attitude should be assumed because the mesial drift of erupting adjacent teeth often largely closes the diastema spontaneously. In this context it should be noted that although this attitude has the advantage of obviating the need for orthodontic treatment at the age of 6 or 8, it has the disadvantage, however, that the contralateral central incisor moves to exactly a midline position, which is not very acceptable cosmetically (Fig. 7-38).

Diastema closure in the maxilla implies a shortening of the arch length. In a dentition with Angle Class I occlusion, extraction of a mandibular incisor then should be considered.

To ensure an optimal cosmetic result, a diastema should be closed exclusively from the distal side (*Sergl* and *Stodt*, 1970; Fig. 7-39). In Angle Class II patients, a lost incisor can be replaced with a premolar to be extracted in the context of the orthodontic treatment (*Schmuth*, 1967; *Van der Linden*, 1972).

In nearly all cases of exarticulation there is a good indication for replantation and fixation. Replantation sometimes serves only to keep open an expected diastema (*Hotz*, 1958) or to postpone orthodontic treatment. In the case of comminuted fractures of the dental socket with exarticulation of the tooth, replantation can be useful for reconstruction of the alveolar process and the soft tissues, but in these cases the prognosis of the replanted teeth is poor (*Eschler*, 1972). Replantation of an exarticulated tooth in

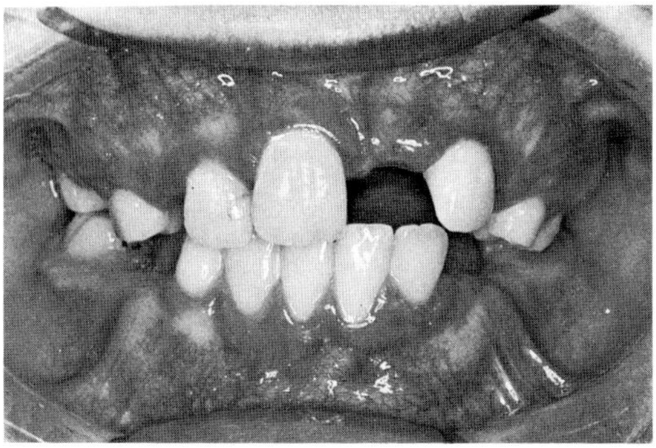

Fig. 7-38 A 21 was lost due to an injury.

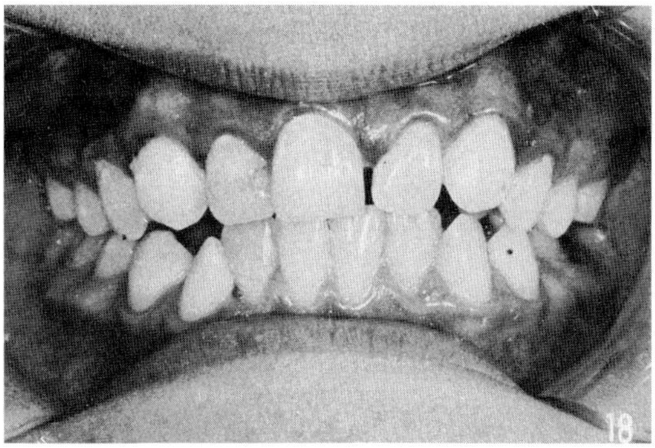

Fig. 7-38 B As a result of movement from right and left, the diastema largely closed without orthodontic treatment. 22 is to be given a jacket crown. Note: Midline in upper front to be shifted. (Courtesy of Dr. *J. Bodegom*).

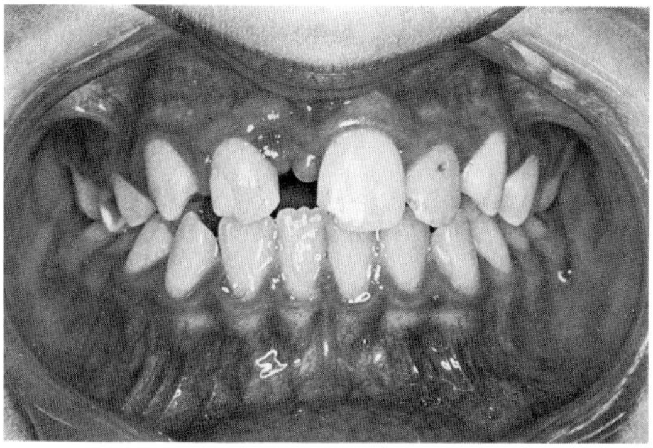

Fig. 7-39 A As a result of a facial injury, 11 was lost and the periodontium of 12 was weakened.

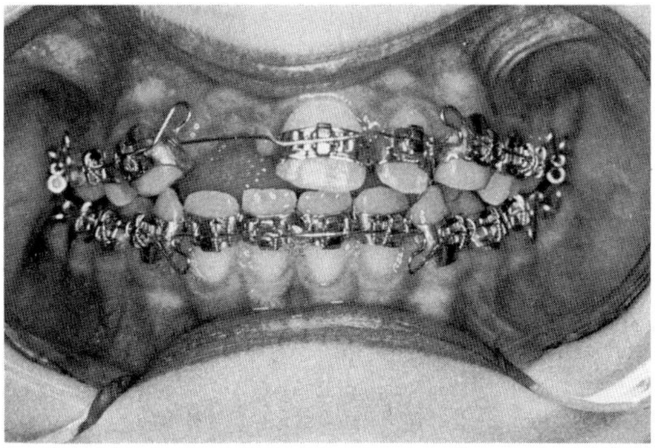

Fig. 7 39 B Orthodontic treatment after extraction of 12.

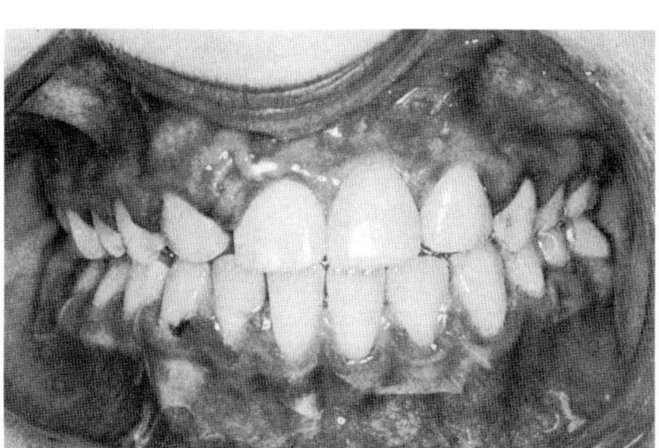

Fig. 7-39 C Intraoral features at the start of the retention period. 21 has moved through the midline to the position of 11; 22 has been given a temporary jacket crown. Note the midline. (Courtesy of Dr. *T. Tijdeman*).

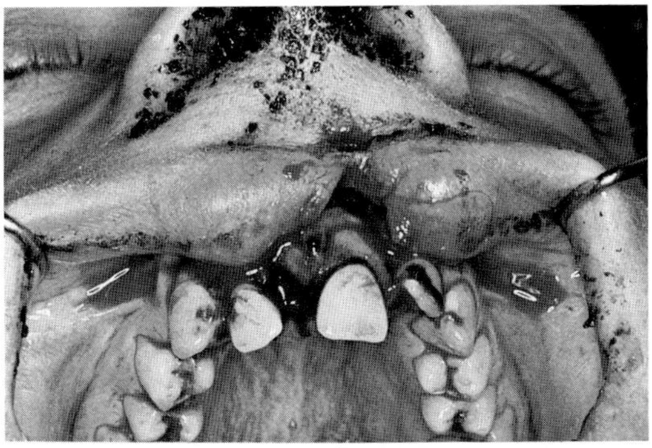

Fig. 7-40 A Luxation of 12 and 21, and exarticulation of 11.

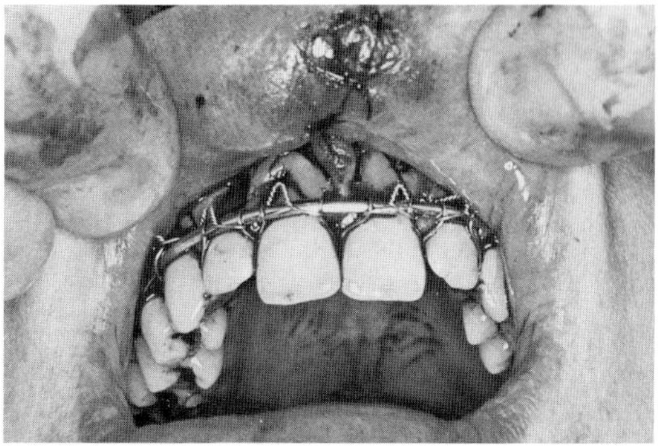

Fig. 7-40 B Intraoral features immediately after replantation of 11 with the splint in situ.

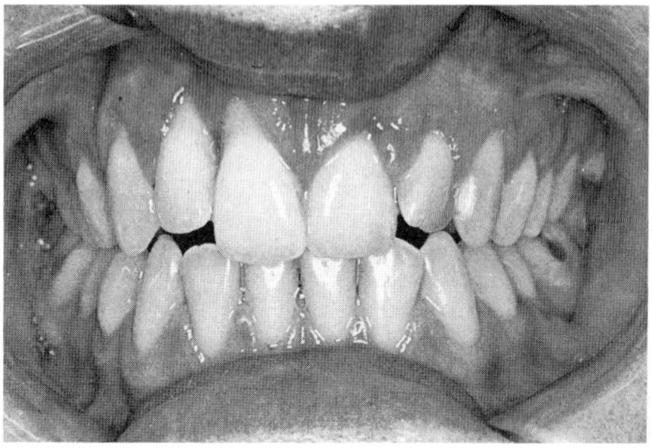

Fig. 7-40 C 5 weeks after the injury.

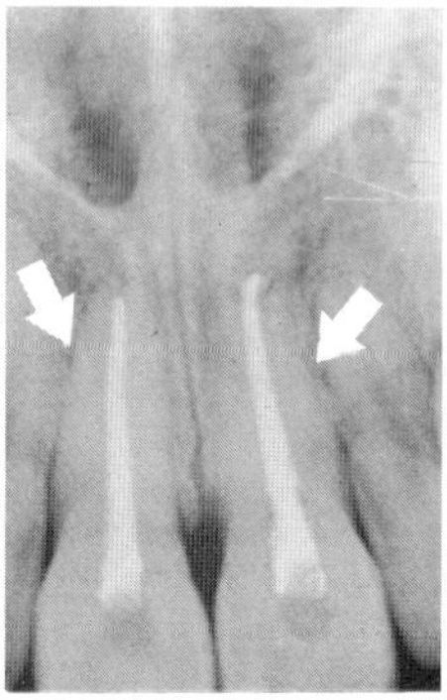

Fig. 7-41 Radiological features of surface resorption on 1 1, 2 1 six months after exarticulation.

the fracture line of a mandibular fracture sometimes ensures more stable reduction, and also has a fair prognosis (*Lu*, 1973).

3.4.2 Therapy

In the past there have been several different theories about the treatment of exarticulations because of the uncertain prognosis of replantation. Today, there is great uniformity in procedure. In the treatment of exarticulations, any activity which postpones replantation or can damage the vital periodontal membrane is to be avoided.

The exarticulated tooth is placed carefully in a saline solution and cleansed. Contacts between root surface and instruments, gauze, etc., are minimized. The socket is rinsed with physiological saline to remove the coagulum and foreign bodies (if any). Curettage is never carried out.

The tooth is then replanted under local anesthesia, and fixation is effected with the aid of an arch bar or an acrylic splint (Fig. 7-40). A radiograph is taken to verify the replantation and tetanus prophylaxis is provided if necessary. Some authors recommend that endodontic treatment be carried out during the 'extraoral' period (*Mierau* and *Naujoks*, 1966), combined if necessary with apicoectomy to enhance the chance of success of the repositioning (*Boering*, 1959; *Hovinga* 1968; *Ellis* and *Davey*, 1970; *Schwenzer* and *Steinhilber*, 1974).

Others prefer retrograde endodontic therapy in order to save time (*Eschler*, 1972). *Tolmeijer* (1975) recommends postoperative antibiotic medication, but *Andreasen* and *Hjørting-Hansen* (1966 a) demonstrate that antibiotics have no favorable effect on the resorption pattern and acceptance of the replant.

In a small series of cases, *Skieller* (1960) demonstrated that vitality returns in about 50 % of replanted teeth with an open apex, and in about 25 % of completed teeth. It therefore seems advisable not to sacrifice vitality in advance in all cases. Extraoral endodontic therapy entails a risk of damage to the periodontal membrane, moreover, so that replantation is unnecessarily postponed.

In our opinion it is advisable to perform endodontic treatment some weeks after splinting.

After about six weeks the splint is removed and the tooth is examined radiologically and tested for vitality. For at least a year, the patient should return at regular intervals so that pulp problems can be managed quickly and resorption recognized.

3.4.3 Prognosis

The prognosis of a replantation depends on several factors:

1. interval between accident and replantation
2. method of storing the exarticulated tooth
3. the patient's age
4. degree of damage to the tooth
5. condition of the socket
6. root length
7. degree of functional stress (*Tolmeijer*, 1975)

Andreasen and *Hjørting-Hansen* (1966 a) demonstrate that the extraoral period is of particulary great importance for the prognosis. A replanted tooth can remain *in situ* for an average of 5 to 10 years, but a few are lost within weeks or months. There are reports of replanted teeth which are still functioning well after 20 years or more (*Andreasen*, 1972; *Dind*, 1974).

As already mentioned, pulp revascularization is rare after replantation of exarticulated teeth with completed roots. The gingiva makes a good recovery after replantation, although it is not unusual to find a gingival sulcus of slightly increased depth. The principal problem in replantations, however, is root resorption, which occurs in 80 to 96 % of cases (*Hovinga*, 1968; *Andreasen*, 1972).

Radiologically as well as histologically, three types of external root resorption are distinguished after replantation; these three types are also observed after luxation of teeth (*Andreasen* and *Hjørting-Hausen*, 1966 b; *Birkedal-Hansen*, 1973).

After successful replantation, the young connective tissue is replaced within 2 weeks by collagen fibers in the ruptured periodontal membrane. When healing is disturbed, the membrane is replaced by granulation tissue and progressive resorption of the hard dental tissues and the alveolar bone commences.

In **non-progressive surface resorption**, radiologically and microscopically normal healing of the periodontium is observed. At some sites there is histological evidence of superficial lacunar resorption without an inflammatory component. The lacunae are found filled with new cement or cementoid tissue. The dental radiograph shows a normal periodontium with a few small superficial resorptions (Fig. 7-41). The tooth has a normal position and sounds normal on percussion. In view of the self-limiting character of the superficial resorption, no therapy need be instituted. In 90 % of all teeth replanted within 20 minutes, no radiological evidence of resorption is found and replantation can be described as successful. However, progressive root resorption is observed in nearly all teeth replanted after 2 hours or more.

The second type of external root resorption is **replacement resorption** or **ankylosis**. The radiograph shows progressive resorption of the root within a year, and replacement by bone without radiolucent lacunae (Fig. 7-42). The periodontal membrane has disappeared. Replacement of dentin by alveolar bone already indicates that ankylosis is bound to develop. This is clinically apparent from a high percussion sound and the infraposition of ankylosed teeth in juvenile patients (Fig. 7-43). Replacement resorption is progressive, and does not start until after a few months. Finally, the entire root disappears and the tooth is lost.

There is no established therapy of progressive replacement resorption. However, early extraction should be considered (as in persistent in-

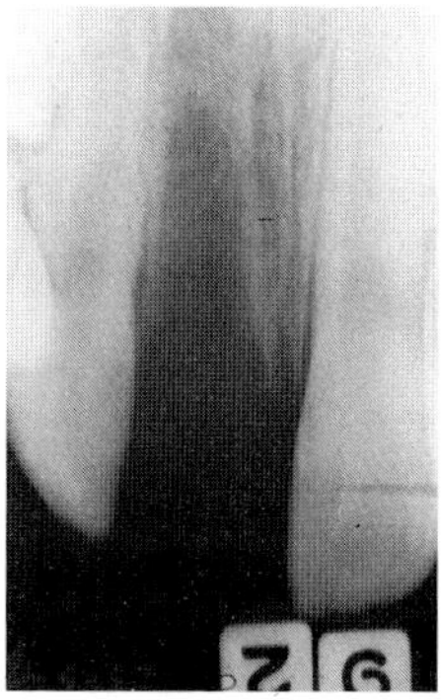

Fig. 7-42 A Exarticulation of 11.

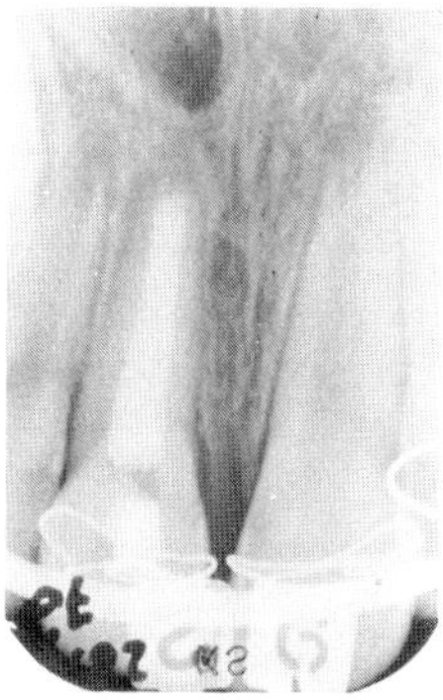

Fig. 7-42 B Features after replantation.

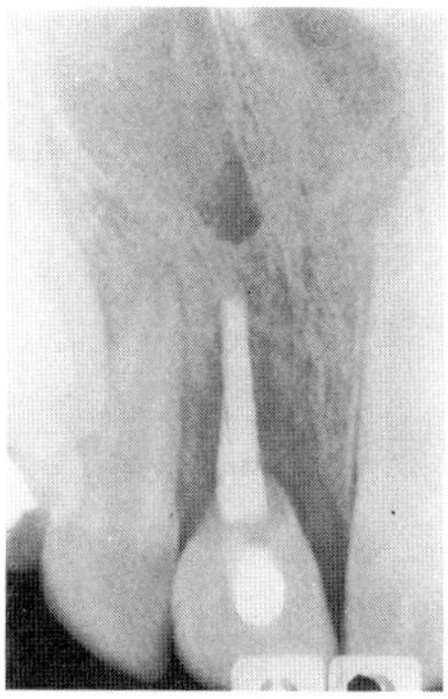

Fig. 7-42 C Replacement resorption after one year.

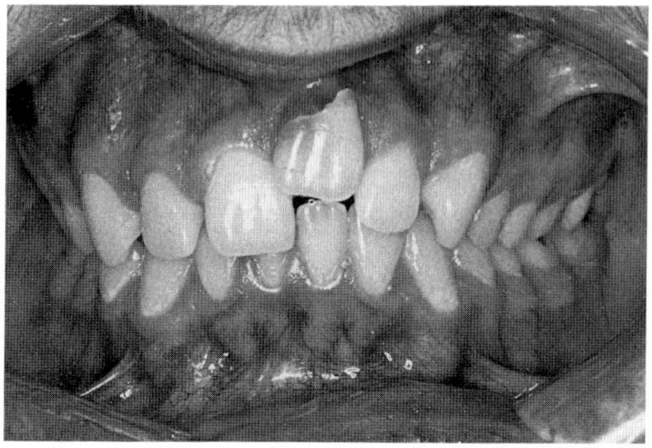

Fig. 7-43 Replacement resorption and ankylosis after exarticulation of 21 in a young patient, resulting in infra-position later.

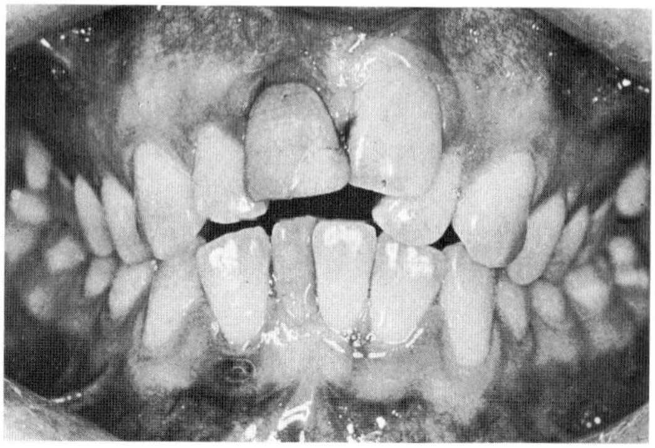

Fig. 7-44 Infra-position of 11, 21 which were knocked out 6 years previously.

trusions) if ankylosis is accompanied by imminent infraposition (Fig. 7-44). If extraction is postponed, local growth of the alveolar process is retarded and consequently it becomes difficult to make a cosmetically satisfactory prosthesis. Histological examination reveals organization of the clot in the periodontal space, followed by replacement of the granulation tissue by bony trabeculae. In this way, bone ankylosis is established with the tooth and the dentin becomes part of the osseous system and is gradually replaced by bone.

The third and most progressive type is **inflammatory resorption**, which is radiologically characterized by rapid lacunar resorption with large radiolucencies (Fig. 7-45). Resorption can begin a few weeks after replantation and the entire root may disappear within a few months. In juvenile patients, in particular, the process is strikingly progressive.

Clinical experience shows that teeth with inflammatory resorption quickly loosen and become painful to percussion. Histological examination reveals regions of resorption in cement and dentin, with inflammatory changes of the periodontal membrane.

The pathogenesis of inflammatory resorption is still unsettled. *Andreasen* and *Hjørting-*

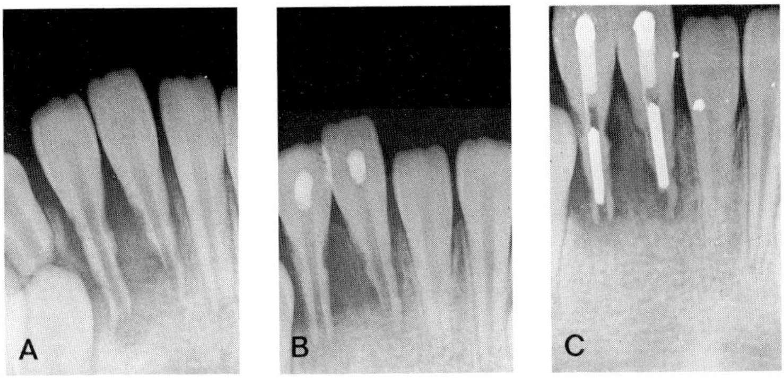

Fig. 7-45 A Inflammatory resorption at 4 2, 4 1 after exarticulation in a young patient. Intraoral radiographs of the teeth 9 weeks after the injury.

Fig. 7-45 B Treatment consisted of removal of the necrotic tissue inside the root canals and filling with Dycal® base.

Fig. 7-45 C One year later the resorption has stopped and two silver posts have been cemented.

Hansen (1966a, 1966b) ascribe this resorption to inflammatory influences arising from the necrotic pulp after surface resorption of the replanted tooth. The fact that inflammatory resorption is often associated with a necrotic pulp and periapical radiolucency supports *Andreasen*'s view.

In juvenile patients in whom the dentin tubules are wide and the (necrotic) pulp is large, rapid infection of the periodontal membrane can occur. This would partly explain the rate of resorption in young patients.

Arguments against *Andreasen*'s hypothesis, however, can be found in data published by *Birkedal-Hansen* (1973) on inflammatory resorption with vital pulp, observed after subluxation. Inflammatory resorption also can occur in teeth given adequate endodontic therapy before onset of resorption. The rate at which resorption destroys the root in young patients also can be explained on the basis of the small amount of mature root dentin. *Andreasen* (1971) recommends that endodontic therapy be given as quickly as possible with calcium hydroxide to fill the root canal; his initial results are encouraging. It can be stated in conclusion that after replantation, only the pulp of young teeth has a chance of revascularization. Independent of the condition of the pulp, root resorption can occur; this is the more significant if the extraoral period is longer. Self-limiting surface resorption exerts no influence on the prognosis for the tooth.

Replacement resorption often gives rise to ankylosis, and causes infraposition of teeth in the process of eruption. Here early extraction is required to ensure a cosmetically satisfactory prosthesis. Inflammatory resorption begins as surface resorption but then takes a very progressive course, possibly as a result of autolytic components from the necrotic pulp. If it is detected in time, resorption can be stopped by endodontic therapy.

4. Fractures of the Alveolar Process

Although several types of fracture of the alveolar process are distinguished, only two types are of importance in this context: fractures of the labial part of the socket (partial fracture of the alveolar process) and fractures of the entire alveolar process with or without communication with the socket.

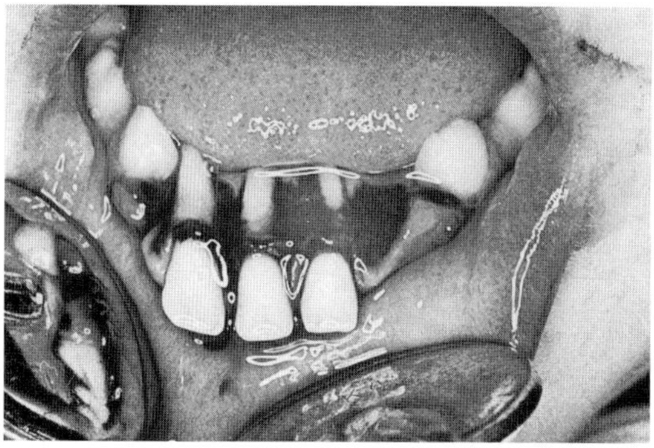

Fig. 7-46 Partial fracture of the alveolar process with simultaneous luxation of 42, 41, 31 and exarticulation of 32.

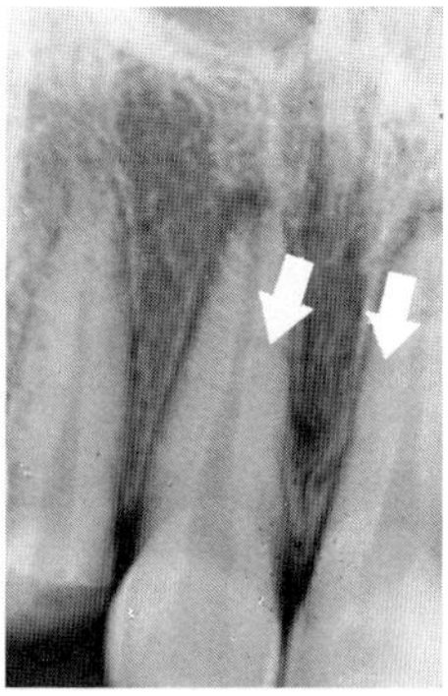

Fig. 7-47 Partial fracture of the alveolar process with involvement of 11, 12. The fracture in the labial cortex is visible and appears as a root fracture of the two maxillary central incisors.

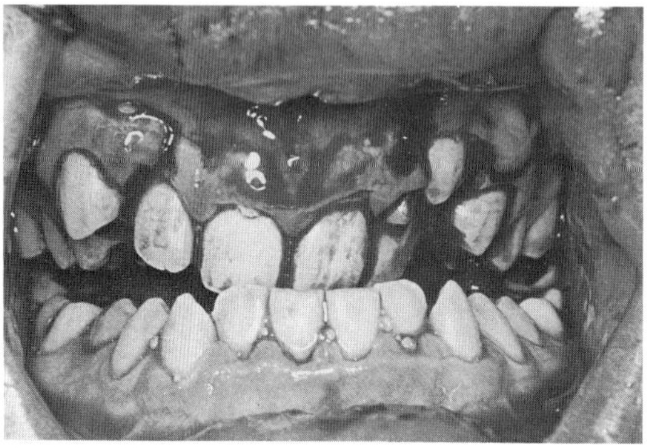

Fig. 7-48 A Partial fracture of the alveolar process with involvement of 12, 11, 21, 22.

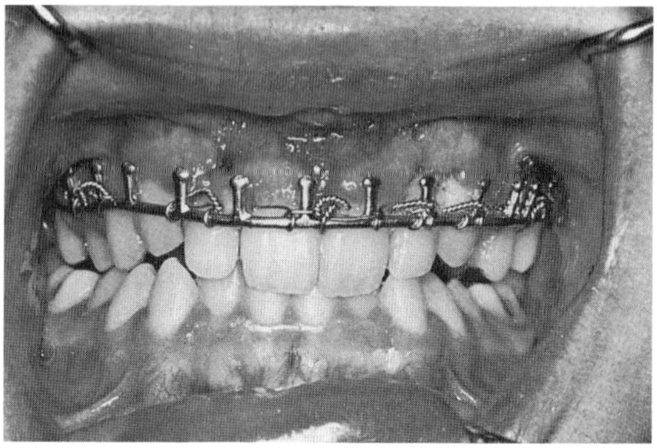

Fig. 7-48 B Intraoral appearance immediately after splinting.

4.1 Partial Fractures of the Alveolar Process

Fractures of the labial part of the alveolar process are often seen in combination with lateral luxation or exarticulation resulting from fights or car accidents. Extraoral examination should focus especially on indications of maxillofacial fractures. Intraoral examination reveals displacement of a few teeth and gingival laceration (Fig. 7-46). On palpation of a tooth, the entire labial cortex proves to be mobile.

In some cases the fracture line is readily palpable and the apices of a few teeth fenestrate the labial cortex. Occlusion is often disturbed and the teeth show a negative reaction to faradic current (Fig. 7-47). An intraoral radiograph by no means always reveals the fracture line, unless marked dislocation exists. A lateral cranial film sometimes shows a shoulder in the labial cortical plate above the apices of the teeth.

Because partial fractures of the alveolar process often are associated with luxations or exarticulations, therapy focuses primarily on reposition of the teeth involved. At the same time, the fractured fragment is repositioned in the alveolar process by means of digital pressure. If the apices penetrate the cortex, an attempt should be made to reposition the fragment, including the teeth, by apical pressure on the labial side and palatine pressure behind

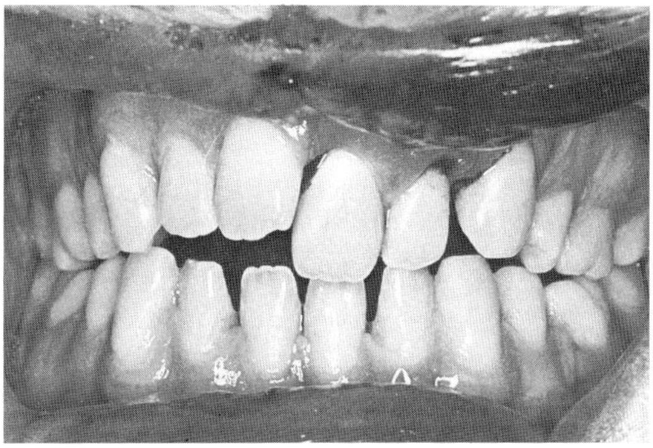

Fig. 7-49 Total fracture of the alveolar process at 2 1, 2 2.

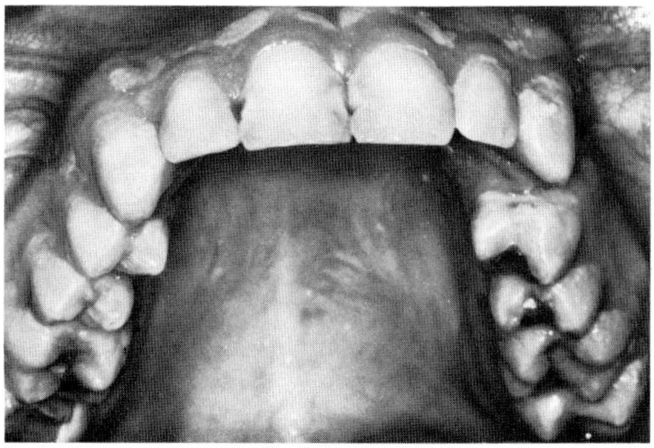

Fig. 7-50 A Palatally displaced fracture of the alveolar process at 2 4, 2 5, 2 6, 2 7.

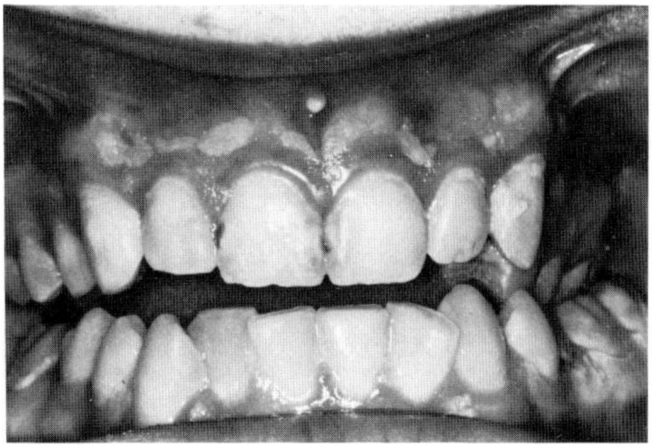

Fig. 7-50 B Disturbance of occlusion.

(*Andreasen,* 1972). Surgical removal of the apices, however, is rarely necessary to ensure adequate reduction. Moreover, this increases the risk of necrosis of the gingiva, or sequestration. Comminuted fractures should be carefully cleansed and loose bone splinters should be removed. The gingiva and the mucosa then are sutured, and the teeth involved can be fixed to the residual dentition with the aid of a rigid splint (Fig. 7-48). Osteosyntheses or pressure plates against the alveolar process are not indicated. The patient is asked to report regularly for sensitivity tests and early diagnosis of periapical inflammations, if any. The splint is removed after about six weeks.

The prognosis of partial fractures of the alveolar process is excellent, although sequestration may occur occasionally. The prognosis of the teeth involved depends on the type and degree of luxation. Pulp necrosis and external root resorption are observed frequently. If the vascularization remains intact or is restored, the pulp can obliterate.

4.2 Total Fractures of the Alveolar Process

These are much less common than partial fractures. They occur almost exclusively in the maxilla, and clinically bear a close resemblance to

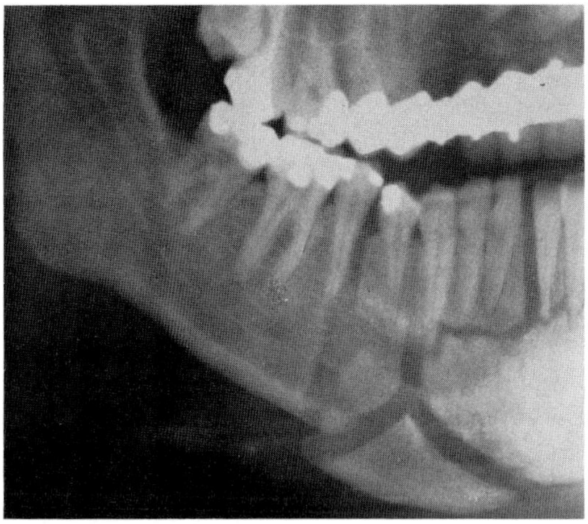

Fig. 7-51 Fracture of the alveolar process at 44, 43, 42, 41 combined with fracture of the body of the mandible.

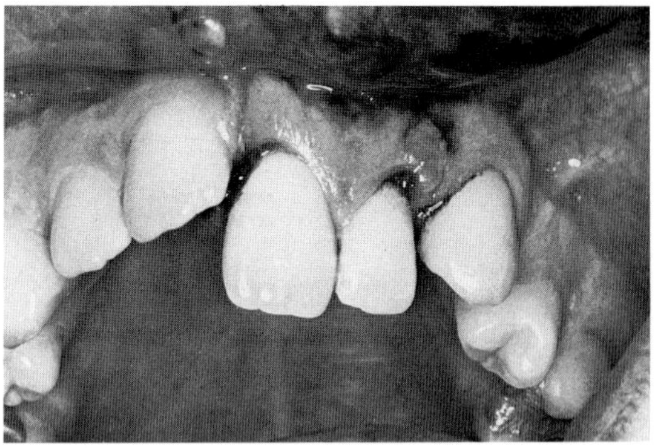

Fig. 7-52 A Total fracture of the alveolar process at 21, 22.

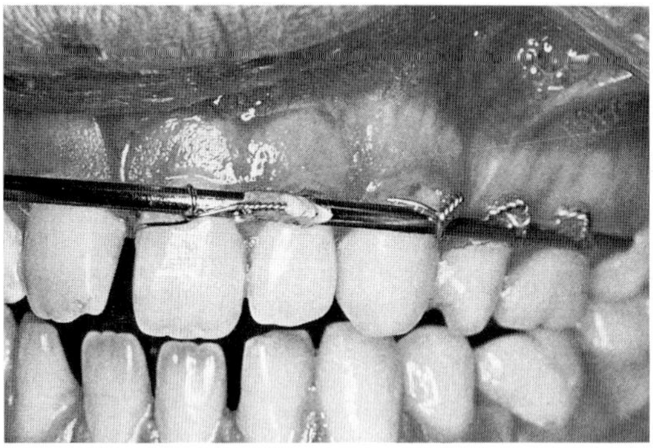

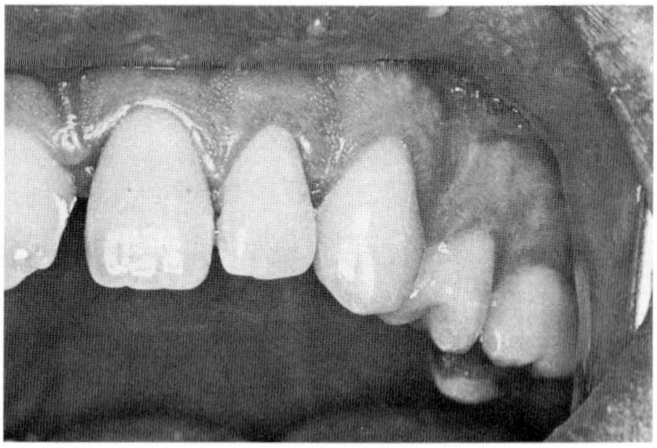

Figs. 7-52 B and C Intraoral appearance after splinting, and 9 weeks after the injury.

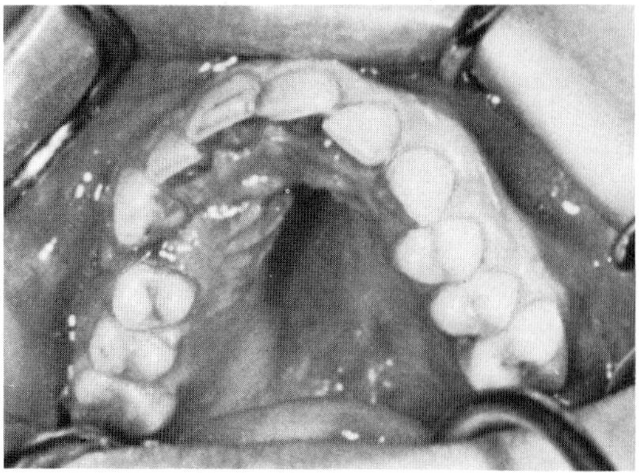

Fig. 7-53 A Palatally displaced fracture of the alveolar process at 17, 16, 15, 14.

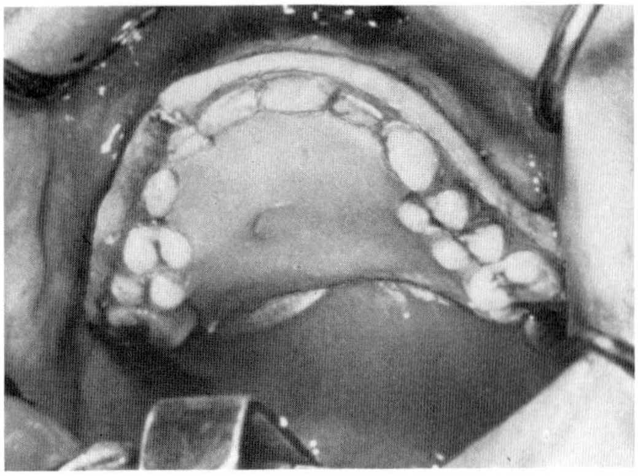

Fig. 7-53 B Appearance after splinting with wire-acrylic arch bar and palatal acrylic plate.

LeFort I fractures. Total fractures of the alveolar process are rarely associated with luxation of teeth, unless the fracture line extends precisely through the apex of the frontal teeth. In such cases extrusions are observed.

Intraoral examination reveals a dislocated upper anterior segment with labial and possibly palatal hematomas and lacerations (Fig. 7-49) or a palatally displaced fracture of the alveolar process in the premolar and molar region (Fig. 7-50). We have seen a fracture of the alveolar process in the premolar region immediately beneath the zygomatic arch as a result of a facial injury. The premolar-molar region was in supraposition as a result of early extractions in the mandible. In this patient, rupture of the antral mucosa was manifest by hemosinus and unilateral epistaxis.

Fractures of the mandibular alveolar process may be combined with fractures of the body of the mandible (Fig. 7-51).

It is not difficult to diagnose total fractures of the alveolar process if, at palpation of a tooth, an entire fragment proves to be mobile or luxated. An occlusal radiograph usually clearly reveals the fracture line and supplies information on root fractures or extrusive luxations of teeth, if any.

In these cases, too, treatment consists of suturing of the lacerations, followed by reduction of the fracture and fixation with a rigid splint for 6 to 8 weeks (Fig. 7-52). Palatally displaced fractures of the maxillary premolar and molar region require an additional palatal acrylic plate (Fig. 7-53). Strong contacts between maxilla and mandible during occlusion or articulation should be avoided or ground down. The fracture reduction should be verified radiologically.

Recovery is usually uneventful, although pulp necrosis occurs frequently. Sequestration and progressive root resorption are rare.

5. Dental Lesions as a Complication in Injuries of the Jaw

Fractures of the jaw can be associated with lesions of teeth. Depending on the nature of these lesions, fracture healing can be influenced. It is therefore important always to establish whether (and, if so, how) teeth are involved in the tissue damage. Particularly in the mandible, disturbed 'fracture healing' not infrequently proves to be caused by infection arising from the teeth. These complications can be expected less frequently in the maxilla.

In the mandible, dental lesions related to mandibular fractures are observed in particular at the site of the canine and the third molar, which may or may not be impacted.

When an intact tooth is located in the fracture line, it is impossible to predict whether complications are to be expected. It used to be a widely advocated view that such teeth always had to be extracted; today, however, this view is too radical.

Several possibilities exist. For example, the fracture line can extend exactly along the alveolus, as a result of which the cementum of the root can become necrotic. In such instances the periodontium cannot be expected to become reattached to the root, and consequently the tooth cannot be saved in the long run, often because of the formation of deep pockets. That a fracture line extends in this way can be established not only radiologically, but also by probing the tooth adjacent to the fracture. If this probing meets no resistance whatever (i.e., if a smooth root surface is found), fracture healing without complications should not always be expected.

There is no definite rule of thumb for these situations. When anterior teeth are involved, a waiting attitude is advisable. For more distal teeth, the decision to resort to extraction is less difficult. Teeth with a single root are less likely to cause complications than multirooted teeth.

When fractured teeth are located in the fracture line of the jaw, their extraction is imperative (Figs. 7-54 and -55). Here it is a virtual certainty that vitality will be lost, whereupon the organism will deal with the tooth in question as it deals with a sequestrum.

Consistent preventive extraction of teeth in the fracture line has some unmistakable disadvantages. It is questionable, for example, whether a normal coagulum will form in the socket. Moreover, stabilization of a fracture is unfavorably influenced by extraction of teeth. Finally, subsequent prosthetic care can pose problems, particularly with anterior teeth and premolars.

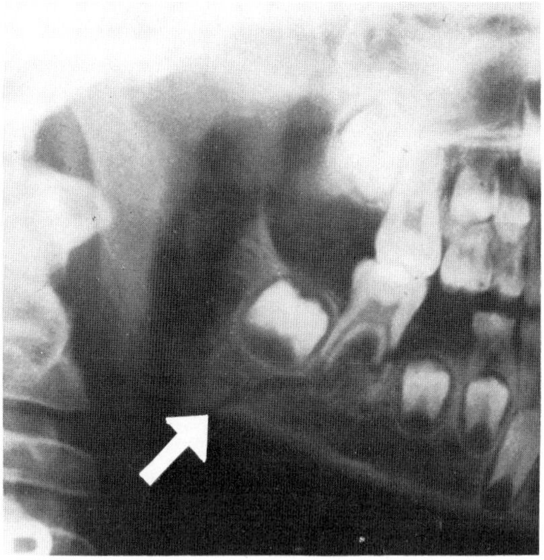

Fig. 7-54 Mandibular fracture at the molar region. 46 is in the fracture line and has a fracture of the mesial root

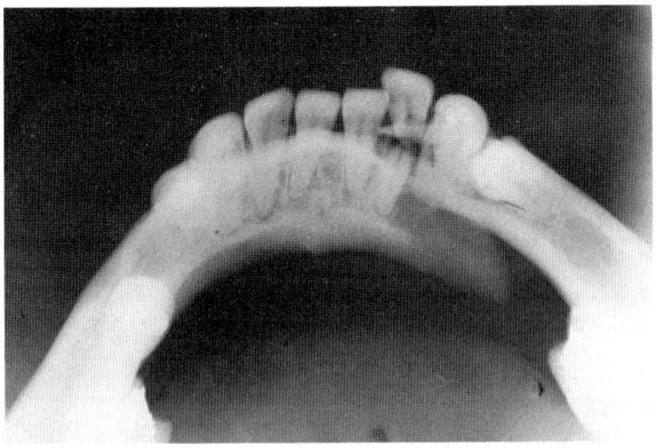

Fig. 7-55 Mandibular fracture and fracture of the root of 31, which is in the fracture line.

To summarize:

1. Intact teeth in the fracture line should be left *in situ* whenever possible. Complications will be an exception when antibiotics are given and when repositioning and fixation of the fracture is done as quickly as possible.
2. Teeth which obviously were not vital prior to the injury should be extracted consistently, and the same applies to root remnants.
3. Unlike teeth with fractures at the level of the root, teeth with fractures at the level of the crown always can be saved.
4. The condition of the alveolus and the periodontium is decisive for uneventful fracture healing. Optimal healing is dubious when there is extensive periodontial damage resulting in the formation of a deep pocket; primary extraction is preferred in this situation.
5. A risk must be taken in certain instances. If, for example, a devitalized second molar is the only tooth situated distal to the fracture line in the mandible, it should be left *in situ* with a view to occlusion and prevention of cranial displacement of the proximal fragment, and also with a view to simplification of fracture treatment. In these cases, however, such a tooth should be extracted after about five weeks because of the risk of pseudarthrosis.

References

Andreasen, J. O. (1971)
Treatment of fractured and avulsed teeth. J. Dent. Child. 38: 29

Andreasen, J. O. (1972)
Traumatic injuries of the teeth. Copenhagen, Munksgaard

Andreasen, J. O., and E. Hjørting-Hansen (1966 a)
Replantation of teeth. I. Radiographic and clinical study of 110 human teeth replanted after accidental loss. Acta odont. Scand. 24: 263

Andreasen, J. O., and E. Hjørting-Hansen (1966 b)
Replantation of teeth. II. Histological study of 22 replanted anterior teeth in humans. Acta odont. scand. 24: 287

Anke, B. (1973)
Drum-Schiene zur Fixierung traumatisierter Frontzähne. (The Drum Miniplast splint for fixation of injured teeth.) Quintessenz 24: 5/31, Ref. 4819

Birkedahl-Hansen, H. (1973)
External root resorption caused by luxation of rat molars. Scand. J. dent. Res. 81: 47

Boering, G. (1959)
De uitgeslagen tand. (The exarticulated tooth.) Ned. T. Tandheelk. 66: 403

Dind, E. (1974)
A propos de la durée des réimplantations. (The prognosis of replanted teeth.) Schweiz. Mschr. Zahnheilk. 84: 770

Dorenbos, J. (1972)
Algemeen tandheelkundige en orthodontische aspekten bij traumata van fronttanden. (Dental and orthodontic aspects of traumatic injuries of the anterior teeth.) Ned. T. Tandheelk. 79: 398

Ellis, R. G., and K. W. Davey (1970)
The classification and treatment of injuries of teeth of children. Ed. 5. Chicago, Yearbook Med. Publ. Co.

Epstein, L. I. (1962)
Traumatic injuries to anterior teeth in children. Oral Surg. 15: 334

Eschler, J. (1972)
Die Verletzungen der Frontzähne bei Jugendlichen. (Injuries of the anterior teeth in children.) Heidelberg, A. Hüthig

Heitherway, G. S. (1973)
Combined endodontic-orthodontic treatment of transverse root fractures in the region of the alveolar crest. Oral Surg. 36: 404

Hotz, R. (1958)
Die Bedeutung, Beurteilung und Behandlung beim Trauma im Frontzahngebiet vom Standpunkt des Kieferorthopäden. (Orthodontic judgement and treatment of injuries of the anterior teeth.) Dtsch. zahnärztl. Z. 13: 401

Hovinga, J. (1968)
Replantatie en transplantatie van tanden. (Replantation and transplantation of teeth.) Goes, Oosterbaan & Le Cointre N. V.

Jacobson, I., and B. U. Zachrisson (1975)
Repair characteristics of root fractures in permanent anterior teeth. Scand. J. dent. Res. 83: 355

Lamers, A. C. (1971)
De intraradiculaire spalk bij dwarse wortelfracturen. (Intraradicular splinting of root fractures.) Ned. T Tandheelk. 78: 313

Linden, F. P. G. M. van der (1972)
De orthodontische behandeling van een geval met agenesie van een premolaar en verlies door trauma van een centrale incisief in dezelfde bovenkaakhelft. (Orthodontic treatment in a patient with agenesis of a premolar and loss of a central incisor due to trauma in the maxilla on the same side.) Ned. T. Tandheelk. 79: 436

Lu, M. (1973)
Replantation of avulsed anterior teeth in patients with jaw fractures. Plast. reconstr. Surg. 51: 377

Mehnert, H. (1974)
Untersuchungen über die Auswirkungen von Milchzahnverletzungen auf das bleibende Gebiß. (Examinations on the effect of injuries of the deciduous teeth on the permanent dentition.) Öst. Z. Stomat. 11: 407

Mierau, H. D., and R. Naujoks (1966)
Traumatische Zahnschäden. (Injuries of the teeth.) Fortschr. Kiefer- u. Gesichtschir. 15: 206

Müller, W., and H. Taatz (1965)
Therapie and Spätergebnisse der Alveolarfortsatzfrakturen im Säuglings- und Kleinkindesalter. (Treatment and late results of fractures of the alveolar process in children.) Dtsch. zahnärztl. Z. 20: 1190

Rock, W. P., P. H. Gordon, L. A. Friend, and M. C. Grundy (1974)
The relationship between trauma and pulp death in incisor teeth. Brit. dent. J. 136: 236

Schmuth, G. P. F. (1967)
Die Behandlung des traumatischen Zahnverlustes durch kieferorthopädische Maßnahmen. (Orthodontic treatment of loss of teeth due to trauma.) Zahnärztl. Welt 68: 15

Schützmannsky, G. (1963)
Unfallverletzungen an jugendlichen Zähnen. (Traumatic injuries of juvenile teeth.) Dtsch. Stomat. 13: 914

Schwenzer, N., and W. Steinhilber (1974)
Allgemeine Frakturenlehre. (Guidelines of treatment of fractures.) Zahnärztl. Prax. 25: 9

Sergl, H. G., and W. Stodt (1970)
Experimental investigation of the aesthetic effect of various tooth positions after loss of an incisor tooth. Trans. Europ. Orthodont. Soc., 46. Congress, Hamburg

Simpson, T. H., G. W. Harrington, and E. Natkin (1974)
A splinting method for replantation of teeth in a noncontiguous arch. Oral Surg. 38: 104

Skieller, V. (1960)
The prognosis for young teeth loosened after mechanical injuries. Acta odont. Scand. 10: 171

Taatz, H., and A. Stiefel (1964)
Zur Histologie der Zementrissfrakturen. (Histologic features of cement avulsion.) Dtsch. zahnärztl. Z. 19: 281

Tolmeijer, J. A. (1975)
Geluxeerde en uitgeslagen tanden. (Luxation and exarticulation of teeth.) Ned. Tijdschr. Geneesk. 119: 949

World Health Organization (1973)
Application of the international classification of diseases to Dentistry and Stomatology. ICD-DA, Geneva, W. H. O.

Zachrisson, B. U., and I. Jacobson (1975)
Long-term prognosis of 66 permanent anterior teeth with root fracture. Scand. J. dent. Res. 83: 345

Chapter 8

Mandibular Fractures

1. Classification, Diagnosis, and Fundamentals of Treatment

Eberhard Krüger

1.1 Classification

There are many possible ways of categorizing mandibular fractures (*Wassmund*, 1927; *Reichenbach*, 1957; *Thoma*, 1958; *Kazanjian* and *Converse*, 1959; *Dingman*, 1964; *Rowe* and *Killey*, 1968; *Weiskopf*, 1969; *Krüger*, 1974). In the following, only the most common principles of categorization have been listed:

A. Relation to the external environment:
  a) Simple fractures without laceration of skin and mucosa,
  b) Compound fractures with communication to the external environment via a soft tissue wound of the skin or mucosa or through the periodontal membrane of a tooth.

B. Types of fractures:
  a) Incomplete fractures: infractions, fissures;
  b) Greenstick fractures with an undamaged periosteum (subperiosteal fractures) in children;
  c) Complete fractures
  d) Comminuted fractures with numerous fragments, after gunshot injuries or serious industrial accidents.

C. Dentition of the jaw with reference to the use of splints:
  a) Sufficiently dentulous jaw,
  b) Edentulous or insufficiently dentulous jaw,
  c) Primary and mixed dentition.

D. Localization:
  a) Fractures of the symphysis region between the canines,
  b) Fractures of the canine region,
  c) Fractures of the body of the mandible between the canine and the angle of the mandible,
  d) Fractures of the angle of the mandible in the third molar region,
  e) Fractures of the mandibular ramus between the angle of the mandible and the sigmoid notch,
  f) Fractures of the coronoid process,
  g) Fractures of the condylar process.

Dingman and *Natvig* (1964) provide the percentages of the frequency of the various localizations (Fig. 8.1-1); fractures of the symphyses and of the canine region are joined in one group; in addition fractures of the alveolar process are considered. Other statistics, by *Hagan* and *Huelke* (1961), *Schuchardt* et al. (1966), *Müller* (1969), as well as *Larsen* and *Nielsen* (1976) yield similar results with minor deviations.

Fractures of the symphysis region appear medially or paramedially. In children, the symphysis of the mandible constitutes a particularly weak spot (*Wassmund*, 1927). Fractures on the axis line therefore usually appear only in children. In adults, on the other hand, the symphysis is especially strong, and thus the line of the fracture is usually situated paramedially. The cause is either direct application of force to the chin or stress from both sides, with fracture in the region of the chin (Fig. 8. 1-2). The displacement is usually minor in medial fractures of the symphysis region because the symmetrically effective muscular forces neutralize each other reciprocally. The masseter muscle, which is dominant in relation to the internal pterygoid muscle, effects a slight tipping of the alveolar

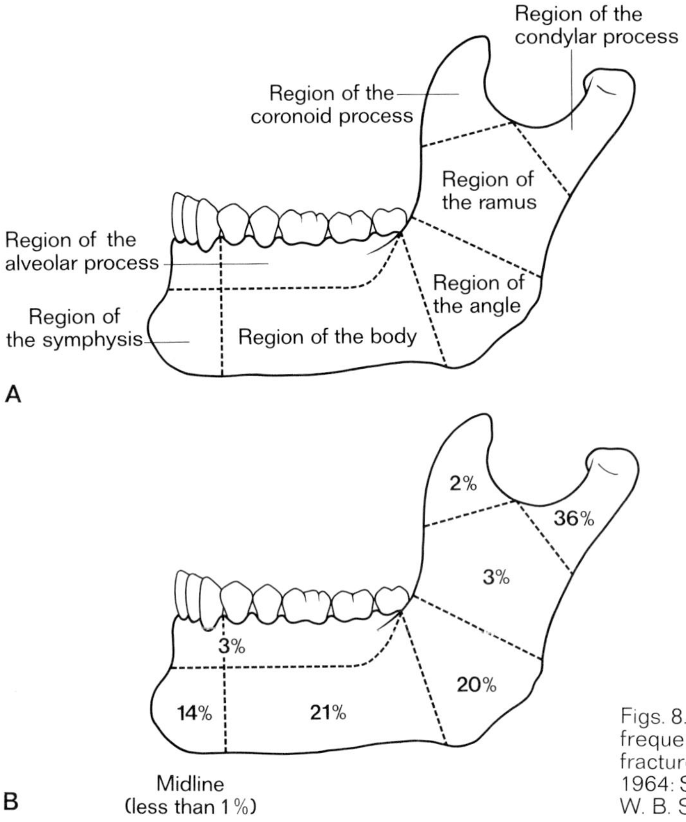

Figs. 8. 1-1 A and B   Statistics concerning the frequency of the varoius sites of mandibular fractures. (From: Dingman, R. O. and P. Natvig, 1964: Surgery of facial fractures. Philadelphia, W. B. Saunders Co.)

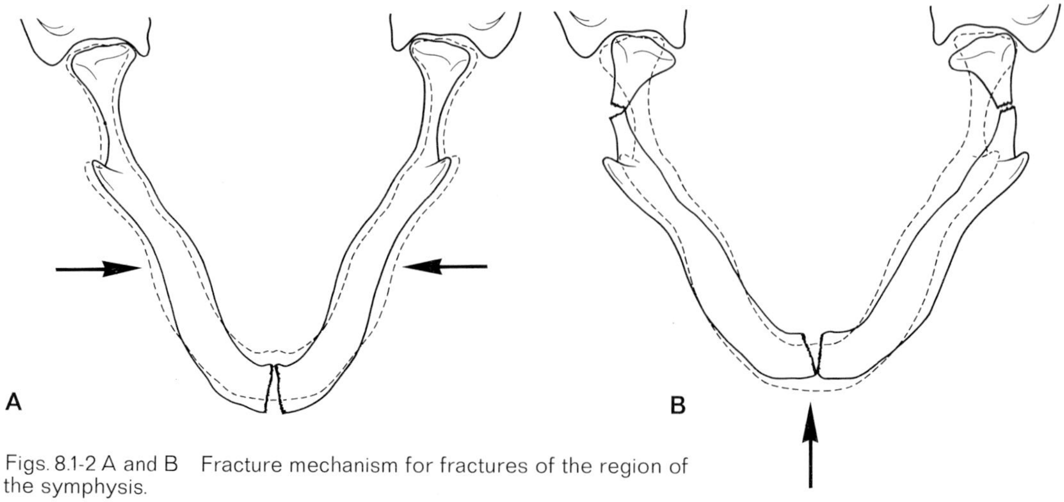

Figs. 8.1-2 A and B   Fracture mechanism for fractures of the region of the symphysis.

Fig. 8.1-2 A   Indirect fracture from lateral force effects.

Fig. 8.1-2 B   Direct fracture from force acting from the front, with simultaneous bilateral fracture of the condylar neck.

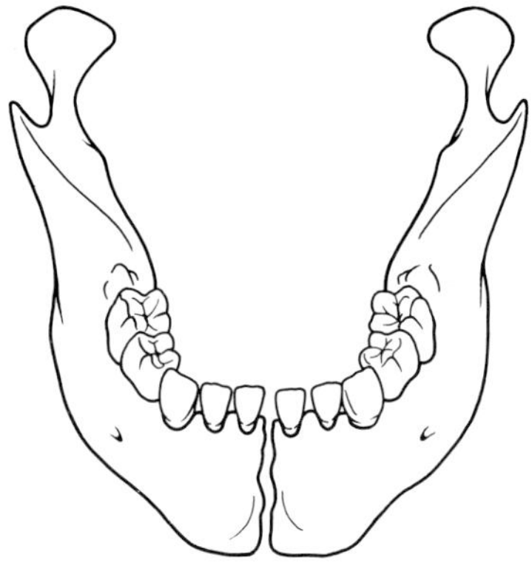

Fig. 8.1-3 Fracture of the symphysis in a child's mandible.

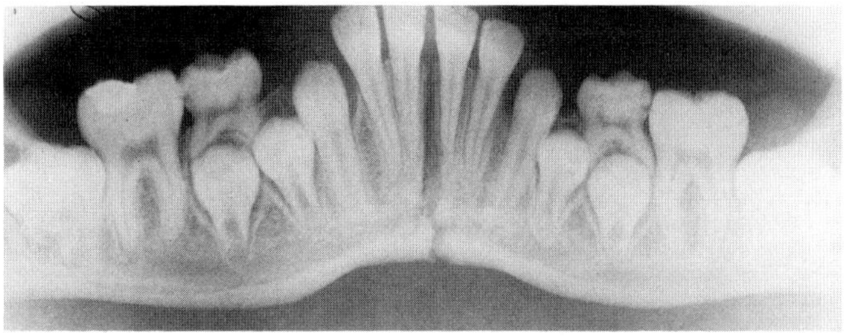

Fig. 8.1-4 Radiograph of a fracture of the symphysis in a 10-year-old girl. There was a simultaneous bilateral fracture of the condylar neck.

process in a lingual direction; this is hardly perceptible in the region of the dental arch. In a radiograph, however, a slight gaping of the fracture can be observed on the mandibular inferior border (Figs. 8.1-3 and 8.1-4).

Paramedial fractures are usually more displaced. The geniohyoid, digastric, and genioglossus muscles pull the large mandibular fragment downward.

Fractures of the canine region extend in the dentulous mandible through the medial or distal periodontal membrane of the canine. The relatively long canine root is a static weak point in the mandible (*Wassmund,* 1927). Fractures in the canine region usually occur as bending fractures, resulting from indirect, and more rarely, direct, force (Fig. 8.2-5). Occasionally, shear fractures appear (Fig. 8.2-6).

Displacements principally result from the mouth-opening suprahyoid muscles, which pull the large fragment downwards. The small fragment is usually tipped with the teeth toward the inside (masseter muscle, pterygoid muscle). Either the large or the small fragment, depending on the kind of force effect and the situation of the fracture, is shifted in an oral direction (Figs. 8.1-7 and 8.1-8).

Fractures of the body of the mandible in the premolar and molar regions are direct or indirect bending fractures (Fig. 8.1-9).

Displacement arises principally with transverse fractures and after diagonal fractures which ascend in a mesial direction. The small fragment here is displaced toward the inside by the mouth-closing musculature and the lateral pterygoid muscle, while the mouth-opening musculature

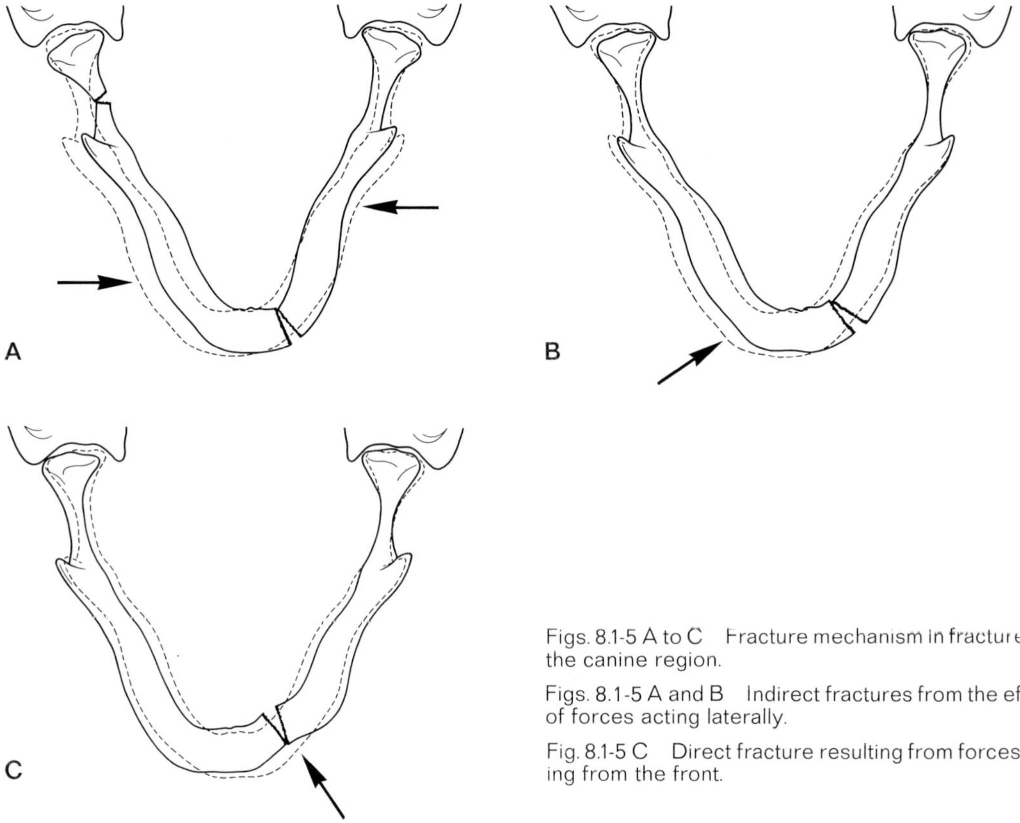

Figs. 8.1-5 A to C Fracture mechanism in fractures of the canine region.

Figs. 8.1-5 A and B Indirect fractures from the effect of forces acting laterally.

Fig. 8.1-5 C Direct fracture resulting from forces acting from the front.

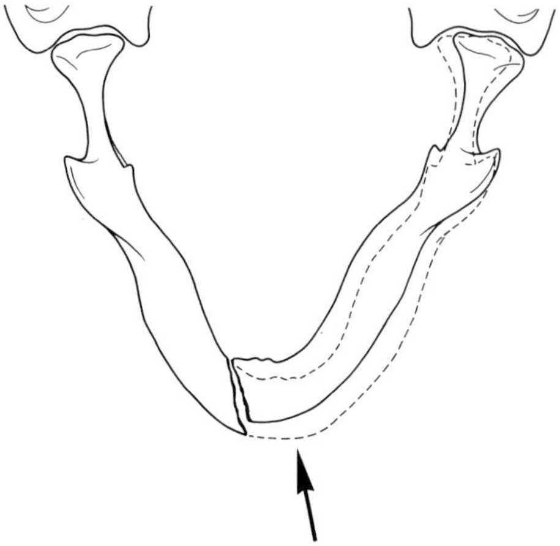

Fig. 8.1-6 Fracture mechanism of a shear fracture in the canine region.

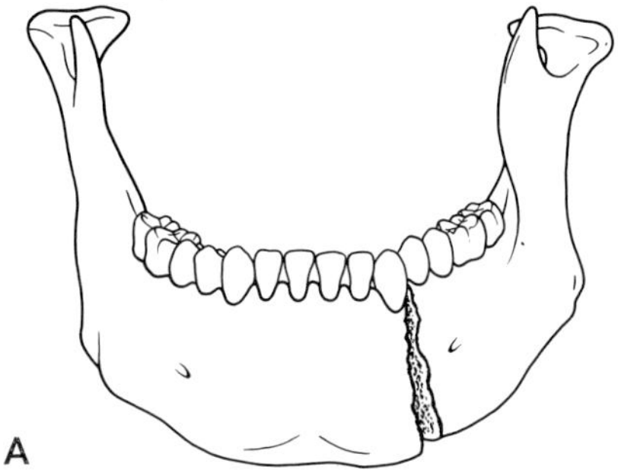

A

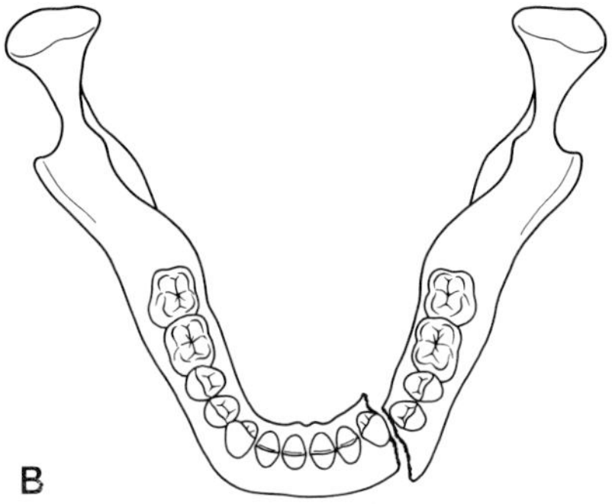

B

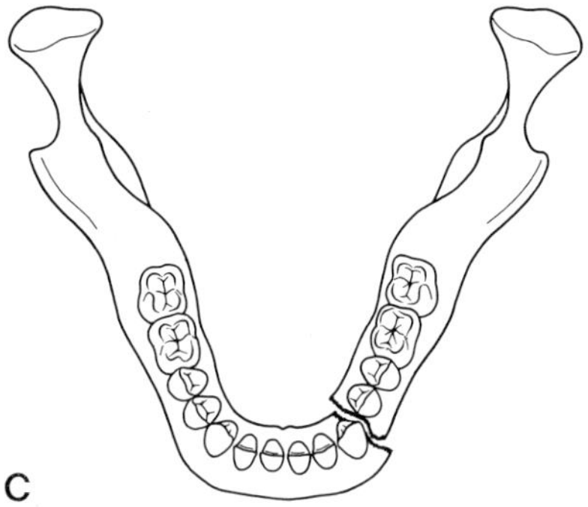

C

Figs. 8.1-7 A to C Fractures in the canine region.

Fig. 8.1-7 A The small fragment is displaced upwards and tilted internally. The large fragment is pulled down by the mouth-opening muscles.

Fig. 8.1-7 B The large fragment is displaced inwardly.

Fig. 8.1-7 C The small fragment is displaced inwardly.

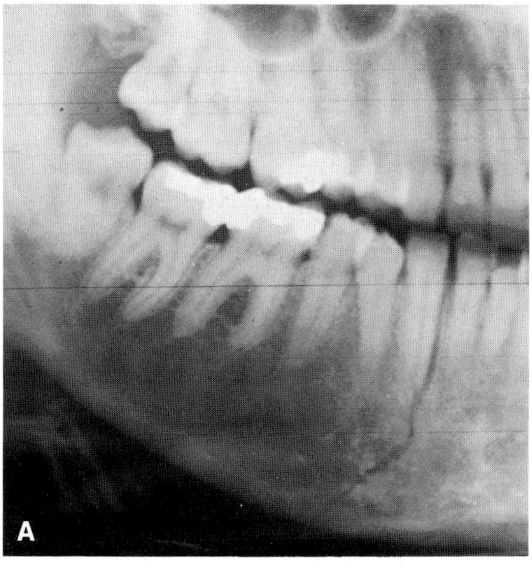

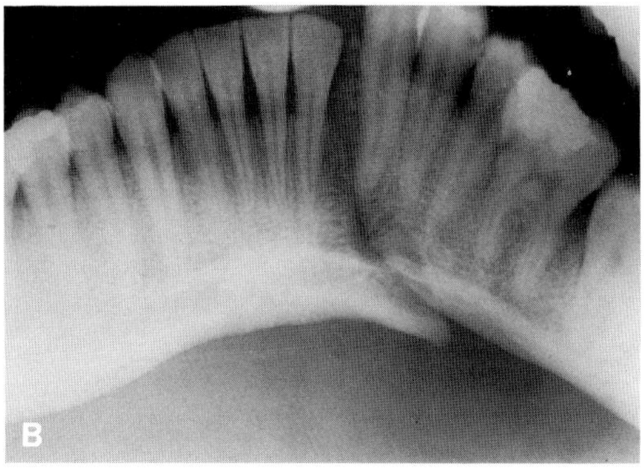

Fig. 8. 1-8 A Radiograph of a slightly displaced fracture anterior to 4 3.

Fig. 8.1-8 B Radiograph of a more significantly displaced fracture anterior to 3 3. The small fragment is displaced cranially; the large fragment dorsally.

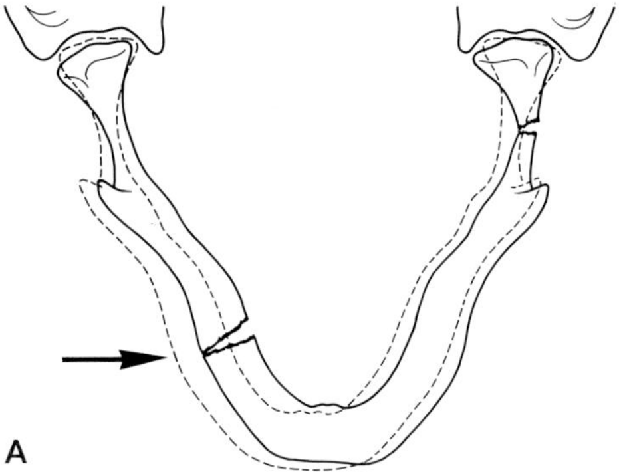

A

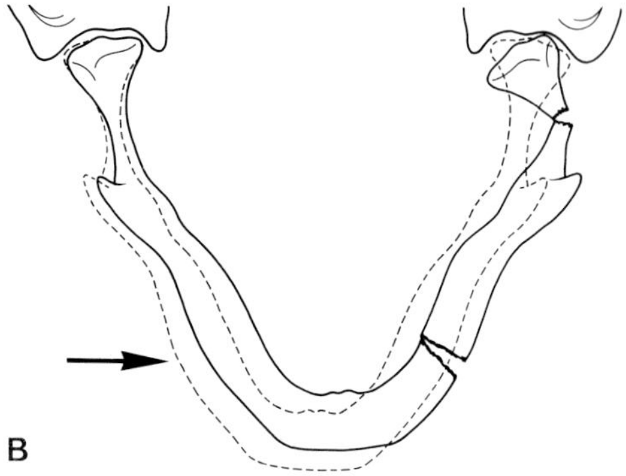

B

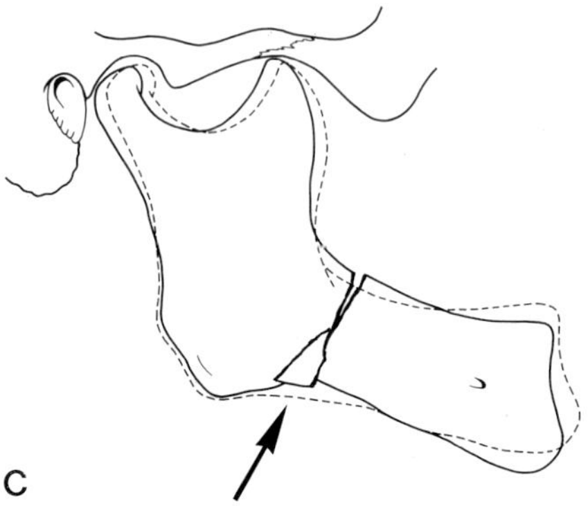

C

Figs. 8.1-9 A to C Fracture mechanism in fractures of the posterior tooth region.

Fig. 8.1-9 A Direct fracture from force acting from the side.

Fig. 8.1-9 B Indirect fracture from force acting from the opposite side, with simultaneous fracture of the condylar neck.

Fig. 8.1-9 C Direct fracture from force acting from the border of the mandible.

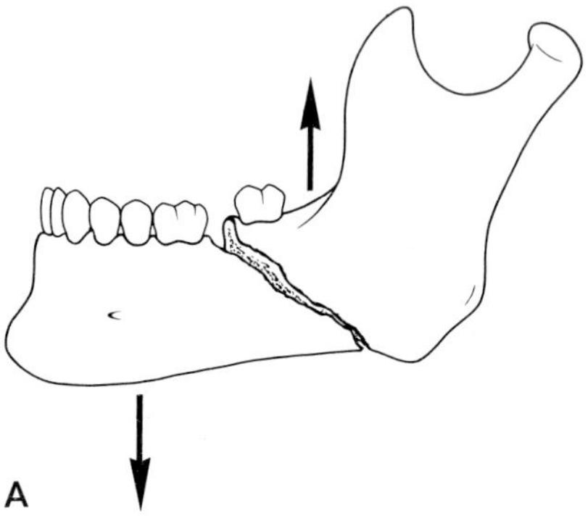

A

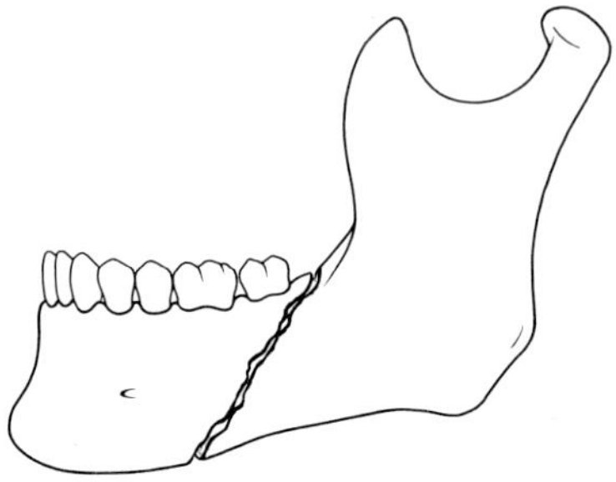

B

Figs. 8.1-10 A and B Oblique fractures in the posterior tooth region.

Fig. 8.1-10 A When the line of the fracture rises mesially, displacement is possible. The small fragment tends to move upward, the large fragment downward.

Fig. 8.1-10 B When the line of the fracture rises distally, the fragments support each other so that no vertical displacement is possible.

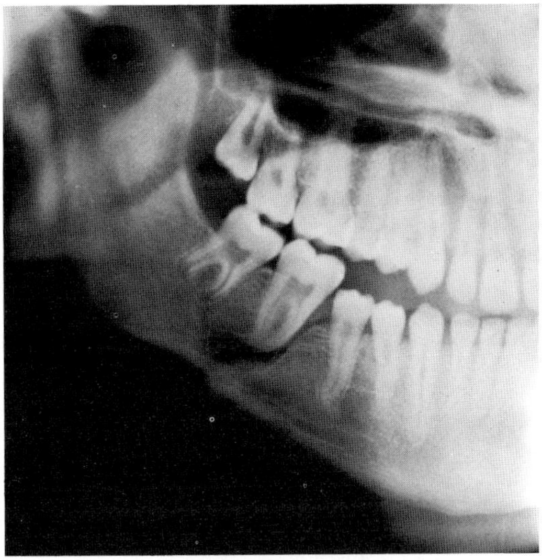

Fig. 8.1-11 A Radiograph following a mesially ascending fracture between 46 and 45. Displacement of the small fragment upward and the large fragment downward.

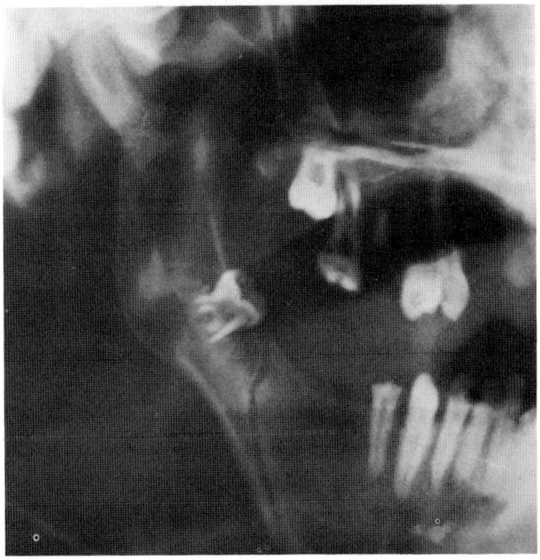

Fig. 8.1-11 B Radiograph of a distally ascending fracture on the right side of the mandible. No displacement of the fragments. Simultaneous fracture of the condylar neck.

and the lateral pterygoid muscle on the opposite side pull the large fragment downward and outward (Figs. 8. 1-10 A and 8. 1-11 A). When there is contraction of the fragments, the type of force effect determines which fragment is situated on the outside and which on the inside. Vertical deviations are not possible with diagonal fractures ascending in a distal direction if the fracture surfaces of the fragments are in contact and thus support each other (Figs. 8. 1-10 B and 8. 1-11 B).

Fractures of the angle of the mandible occur as direct or indirect bending fractures (Fig. 8. 1-12). Here, too, as in the canine region, there is a mandibular weak point (*Wassmund*, 1927). In this vulnerable region, which is particularly susceptible to the effects of force, the compact body of the mandible becomes the thin ascending ramus.

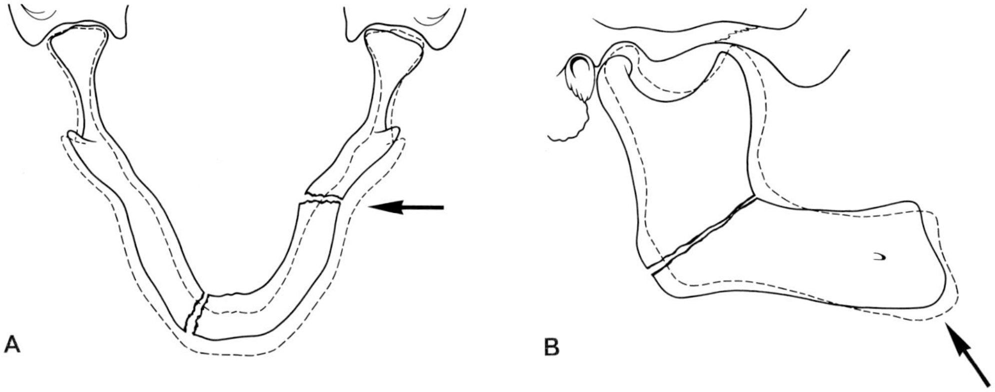

Figs. 8.1-12 A and B Fracture mechanism in fractures of the angle of the mandible.

Fig. 8.1-12 A Direct fracture from force acting on the angle of the mandible, with simultaneous indirect fracture in the canine region on the opposite side.

Fig. 8.1-12 B Indirect fracture from force acting on the chin.

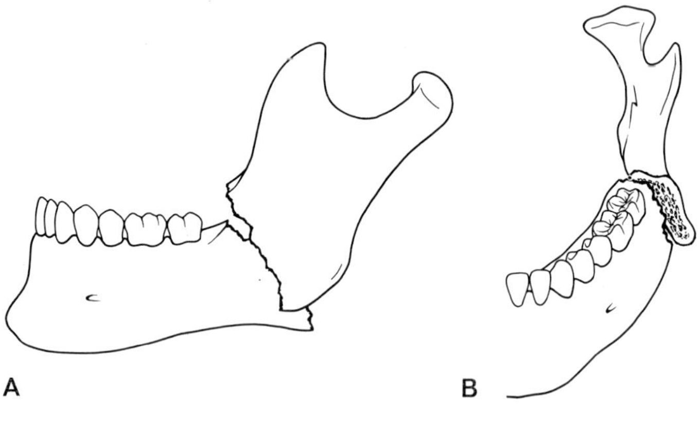

Figs. 8.1-13 A and B Fractures in the angle of the mandible.

Fig. 8.1-13 A Displacement of the smaller fragment downward.

Fig. 8.1-13 B Lateral displacement of the smaller fragment.

This region is frequently weakened by a partially or completely impacted wisdom tooth.

There is no displacement if the periosteum and the musculature (masseter muscle, internal pterygoid muscle) are intact. When the muscles are torn, the small fragment shifts out of place outward (masseter muscle) and upward (temporalis muscle; Figs. 8.1-13 and 8.1-14). In the course of this, muscle tissue can become clamped between the ends of the fracture.

Fractures of the ramus of the mandible are uncommon. They appear as vertical and horizontal fractures. The **vertical fracture**, which extends from the angle of the mandible to the sigmoid notch, is a shear fracture. The angle of the mandible is affected from below, and the glenoid fossa acts as an abutment (Fig. 8.1-15). Displacement is usually minor (Fig. 8.1-16).

The horizontal fracture is a compression fracture, with a diagonal displacement if force was applied to the angle of the mandible (Fig. 8.1-17). The upward displacement with the pivot in the temporomandibular joint (TMJ) arises from the temporalis muscle and the medial displacement from the lateral pterygoid muscle (Figs. 8.1-18 and 8.1-19).

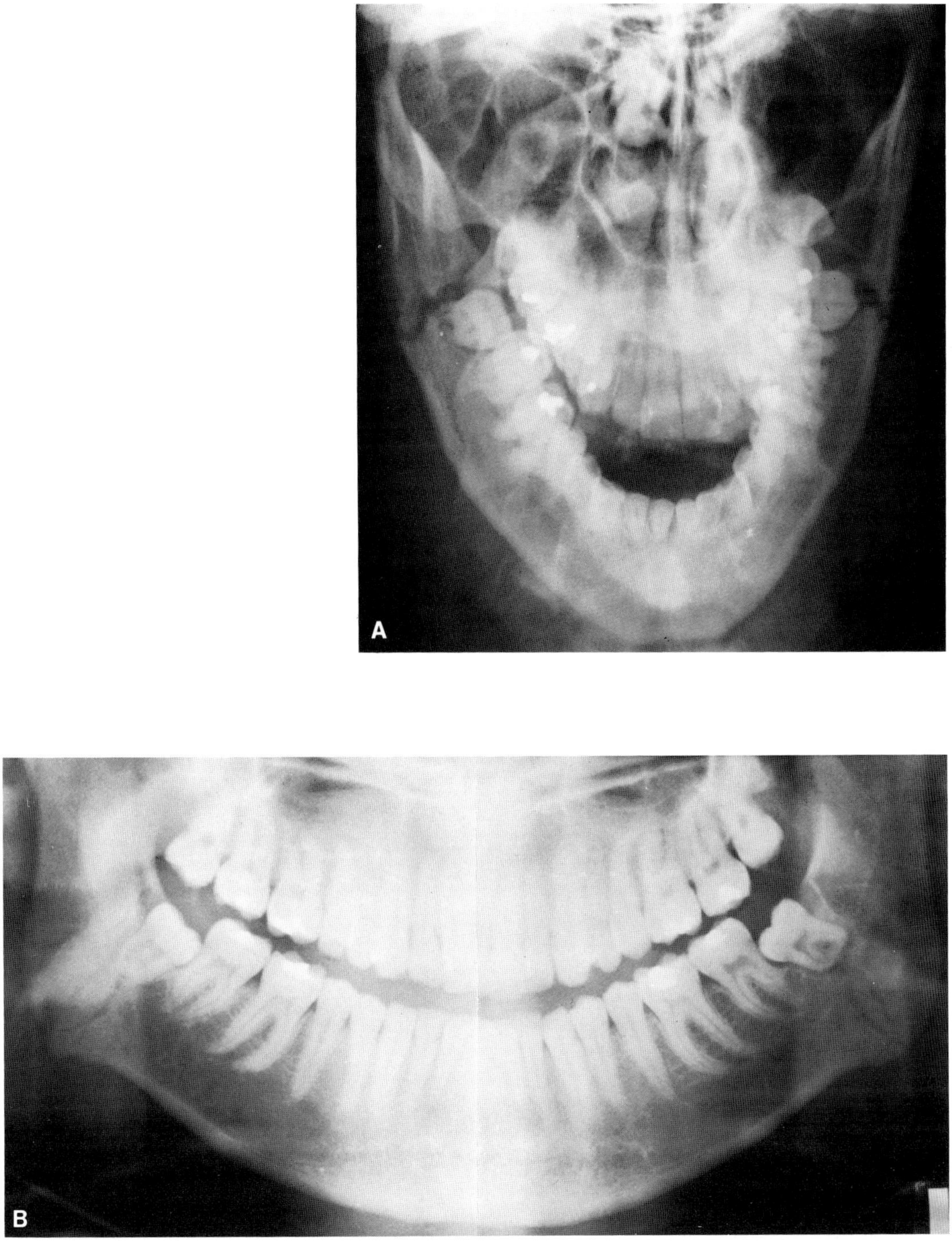

Figs. 8.1-14 A and B Radiographs of a bilateral, slightly displaced fracture of the angle of the mandible. The third molars are in the fracture line.

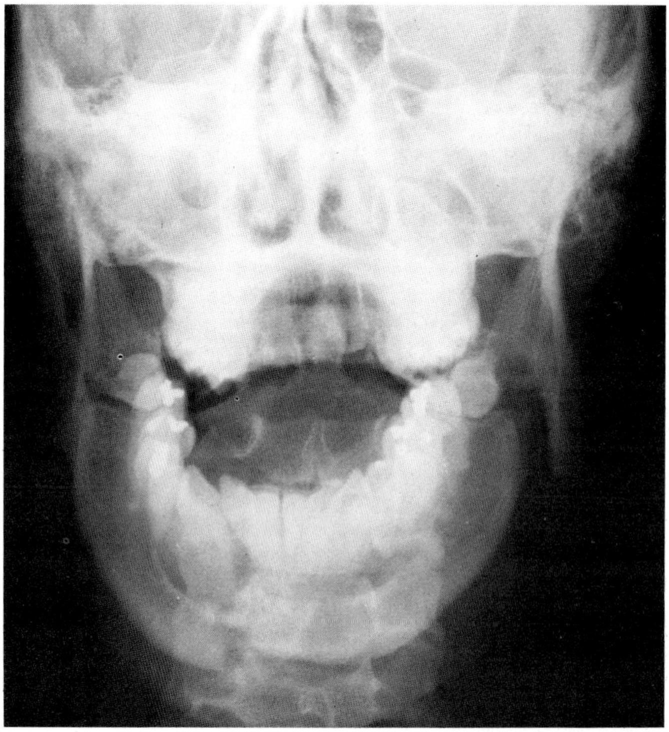

Fig. 8.1-14 C Radiograph of a bilateral fracture of the angle of the mandible with thc third molars in the fracture line. There is a stronger displacement laterally on the left side. In addition, a fracture of the right canine region is present.

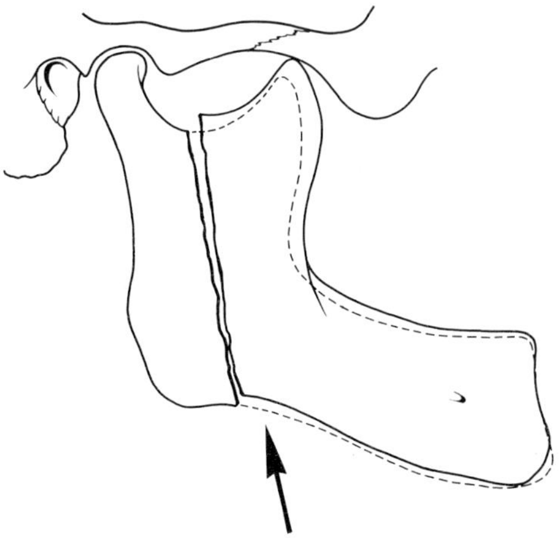

Fig. 8.1-15 Fracture mechanism of a vertical shear fracture in the ascending ramus, through force acting from below.

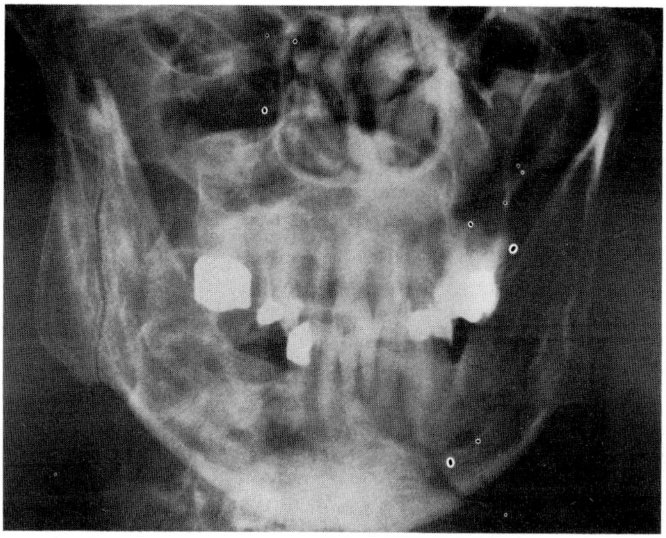

Fig. 8.1-16 Radiograph of a vertical fracture of the right ascending ramus with simultaneous fracture in the left canine region.

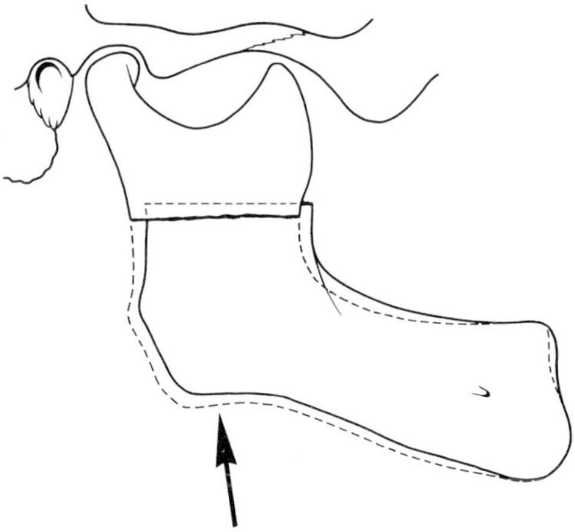

Fig. 8.1-17 Fracture mechanism of a horizontal fracture of the ascending ramus, through force acting from below.

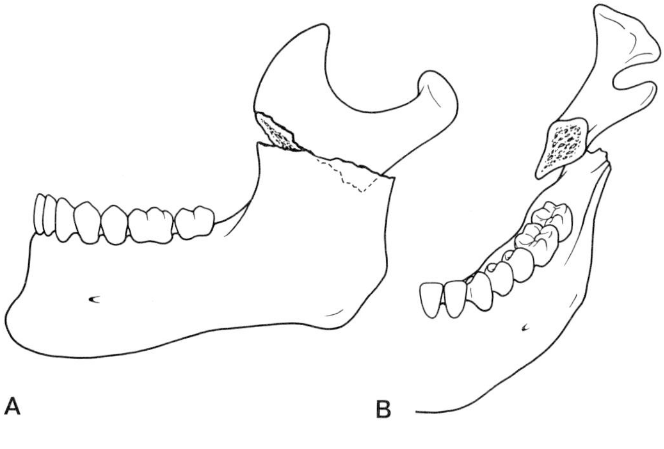

Figs. 8.1-18 A and B Horizontal fractures of the ascending ramus.

Fig. 8.1-18 A Displacement of the small fragment upward through the temporalis muscle.

Fig. 8.1-18 B Displacement of the small fragment medially through action of the lateral pterygoid muscle.

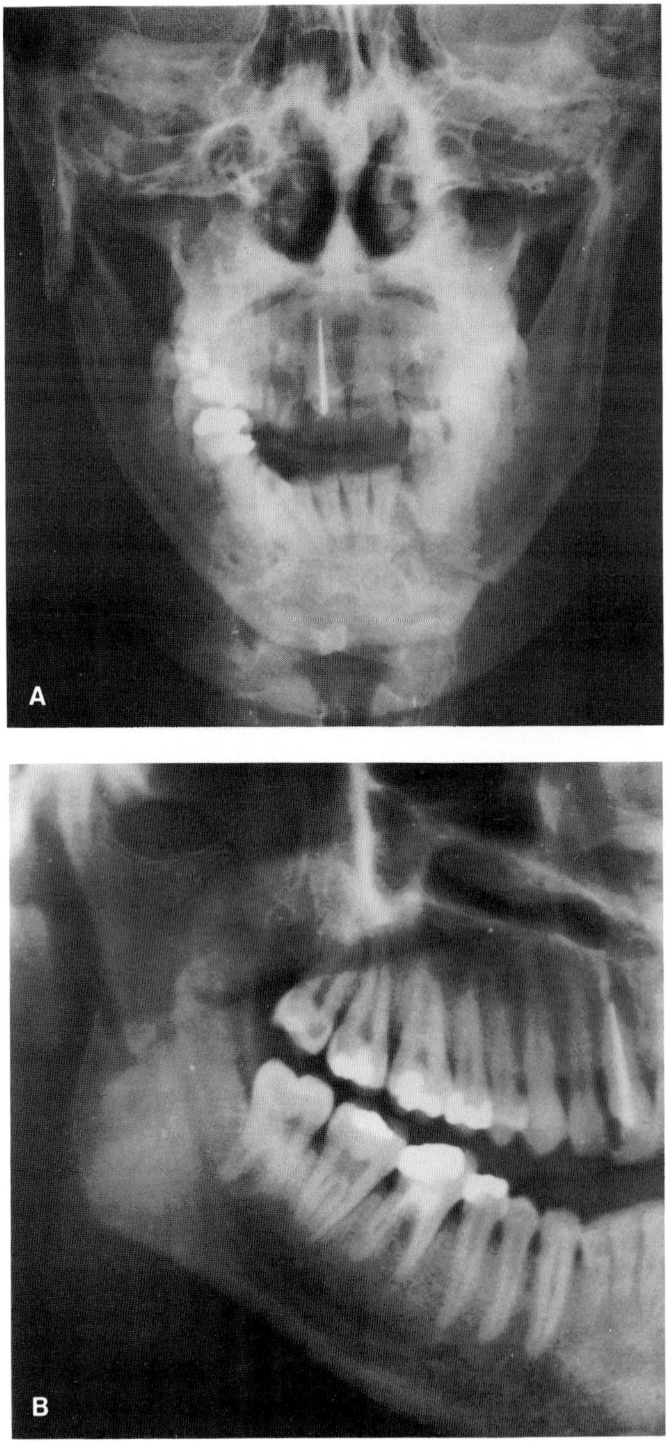

Figs. 8.1-19 A and B Radiographs of a horizontal fracture of the right ascending ramus, with simultaneous fracture in the left canine region.

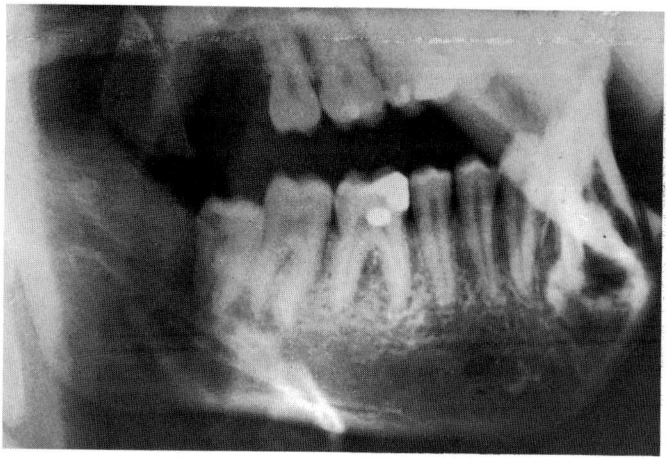

Fig. 8.1-20 Radiograph of a fracture of the coronoid process.

Fractures of the coronoid process (Fig. 8. 1-20) are similarly rare, but are most likely to appear in connection with fractures of the cheek bone or the mandible. *Schröder* and *Wassmund* (1927), and also *Reichenbach* (1957) at first wanted to see isolated fractures of the coronoid process interpreted as avulsion fractures. *Dechaume* et al. (1957), *Weiskopf* (1957) and later, *Reichenbach* and *Müller* (1964 and 1966) held that this mechanism of formation was suspect. They are of the opinion that traumatic fractures occur exclusively in combination with other fractures. When there is a simultaneous cheek bone fracture, then it is a case of a direct bending fracture of the coronoid process. What is involved in conjunction with other mandibular fractures, is either an indirect bending fracture from blows to the malar arch, to the pterygoid process and/or to the maxillary tuberosity, or a shear fracture after a fracture of the condylar process from force applied from the front and impact of the coronoid process against the cranical base.

Fractures of the condylar process are discussed in a separate chapter because of the particular problems associated with them.

All mandibular fractures occur as simple, double, or compound fractures. Furthermore, they can be combined with fractures of the midfacial region.

1.2 Diagnosis

Diagnostic measures should be performed very carefully, in order that the patient does not suffer any unnecessary pain. The goal of the clinical examination is to obtain an idea of where fracture sites may be located, so that a targeted radiographic examination can follow. It is not always necessary to apply all the diagnostic procedures because many fractures can be identified simply by inspection.

The patient experiences **pain** in the region of the fracture, particularly with mandibular movement when he tries to eat and when the doctor examines him. The pain arises from movements of the fracture ends, on the one hand by pulling on the inferior alveolar nerve and on the other by irritation of the periosteum and the adjacent soft tissue. A particular symptom of a fracture is **compression pain.** This arises if the mandible is pressed together on the longitudinal axis. In the course of this, the patient feels pain at the fracture site. In the case of fractures between the mandibular foramen and the mental foramen, the pulling or tearing of the mandibular nerve can cause **anesthesia** in the region of the lower lip and chin, i.e., in the area of the mental nerve innervation.

A fracture hematoma is usually present at the fracture site in fresh mandibular fractures and is obvious as an irregular tight swelling (Fig. 8. 1-20). As with a perimandibular abscess, the

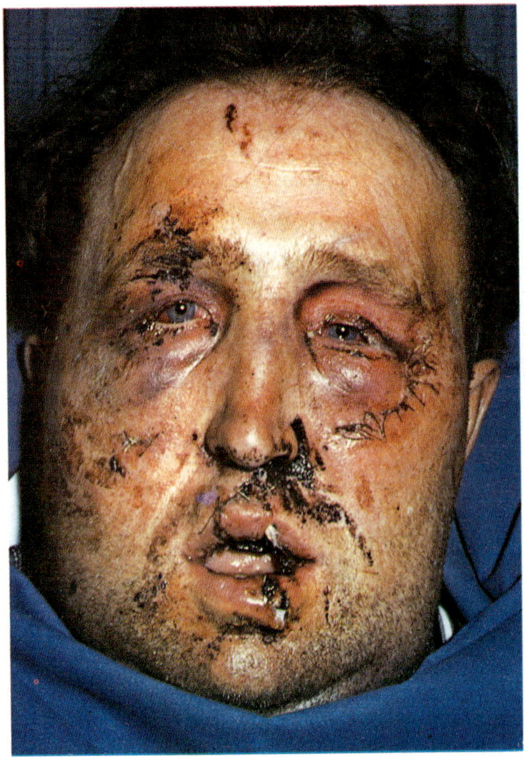

Fig. 8.1-21 Fracture line hematomas in midface and mandibular fractures.

mandibular interior border is ill-defined in the vicinity of the hematoma. It is not rare to find the adjacent skin and mucosa infiltrated with blood from the hemorrhage. With compound fractures, where the fracture communicates with the external environment by a soft tissue wound, the hematoma can drain somewhat. The swelling, which is then less, stems primarily from the wound edema.

A disturbance of the occlusion is usually found with displaced fractures if dentulous fragments have been displaced. There are differentiations made between lateral and vertical shifts and between anterior and distal displacements of the broken mandibular fragments. Bilateral subcondylar fractures with upward and backward telescoping of the rami result in an open bite in the anterior region. Displaced fractures within the dental arch cause the formation of a shoulder (Fig. 8. 1-22) and the gingiva is usually torn at the fracture site.

Abnormal mobility of the fracture ends is easy to ascertain with displaced fractures within the dental arch. A light tapping on the dental arch with a tongue depressor is frequently sufficient to show that the arches are mobile in relation to each other. Sometimes the patient can feel a **crepitation** (grating, cracking, or grinding sound) when the fragments are moved.

Even if there is no hematoma, disturbance of occlusion or formation of shoulders, a fracture still can be present. If the history indicates there may be a fracture without the examination providing any evidence to support it, then the mandible is palpated, first carefully and then if there is no pain, more forcefully.

Certain processes are recommended for testing abnormal mobility and compression pain (*Grimm*, 1969; *Reichenbach*, 1967; *Spiessl* and *Schroll*, 1972):

Tests for abnormal mobility through opposing movement with both hands:

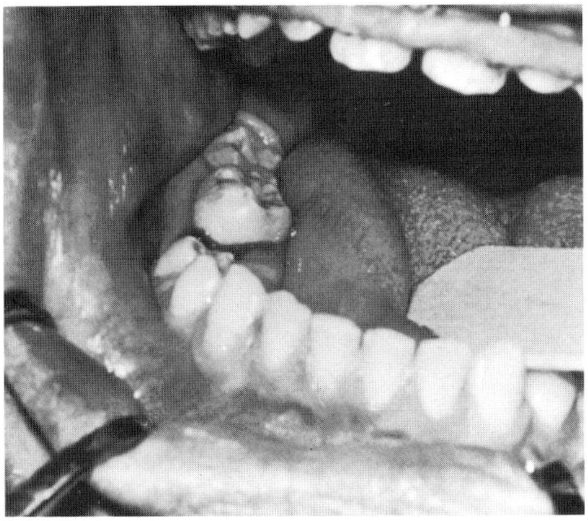

Fig. 8.1-22 A Shoulder formation in the dental arch in a fracture between 46 and 45.

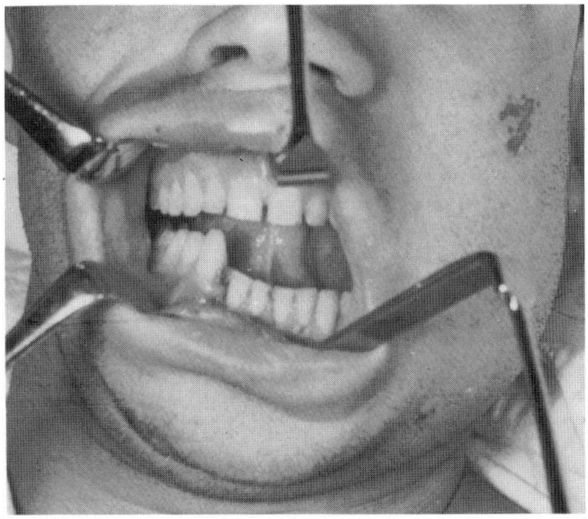

Fig. 8.1-22 B Shoulder formation in the dental arch in a fracture between 43 and 42. Fracture line hematoma in the region of the left cheek in a fracture of the angle of the mandible.

anterior region: index finger on the occlusal surfaces of the premolars, thumb on the mandibular border (Fig. 8. 1-23 A);

buccal region: index finger on the occlusal surfaces of the last molar and on the incisal edges of the anterior teeth, and the thumb on the mandibular border (Fig. 8. 1-23 B);

region of the angle of the mandible: index finger of one hand on the anterior margin of the ramus of the mandible, index finger of the other hand on the occlusal surface of the first molar and thumb on the mandibular border (Fig. 8. 1-23 C);

Test for compression pain with fractures in the subcondylar region and in the ramus: pressure against the chin with the mouth slightly opened (Fig. 8. 1-23 D).

This procedure should be applied only if the examination has yielded no unequivocally clear results, and then only very gently, becoming more forceful only when there is no pain. If these tests are negative, it can be assumed with great probability that no mandibular fracture is present.

The site of the fracture often can be localized on the basis of the clinical examination. The clinical finding must always, however, be supported radiologically.

The radiological examination provides exact representation of all fracture sites and of the relationship between the fracture and the surrounding area. Every fracture site must be represented in two perpendicular planes, so that any possible displacement is certain to be included. For the buccal regions and the rami, one plane is usually represented from the posterior-anterior view of the mandible. For depiction of the second plane, oblique lateral views of the body or ramus of the mandible or of the condyle (*Parma*) as well as a panoramic radiographic view (Panorex, Orthopanthomograph) are helpful; the anterior region is represented in two planes by a panoramic intraoral radiograph and an occlusal view. The teeth adjacent to the fracture are best portrayed with dental films.

The question of whether a tooth is situated at a fracture site is most reliably answered with the help of a dental film: the fracture line extends in such cases through the periodontal membrane (Fig. 8. 1-24).

If the radiological representation is not successful, e.g., with displaced fragments which have shifted over one another, then attempts can be made to answer this question through clinical examination during the treatment of the fracture.

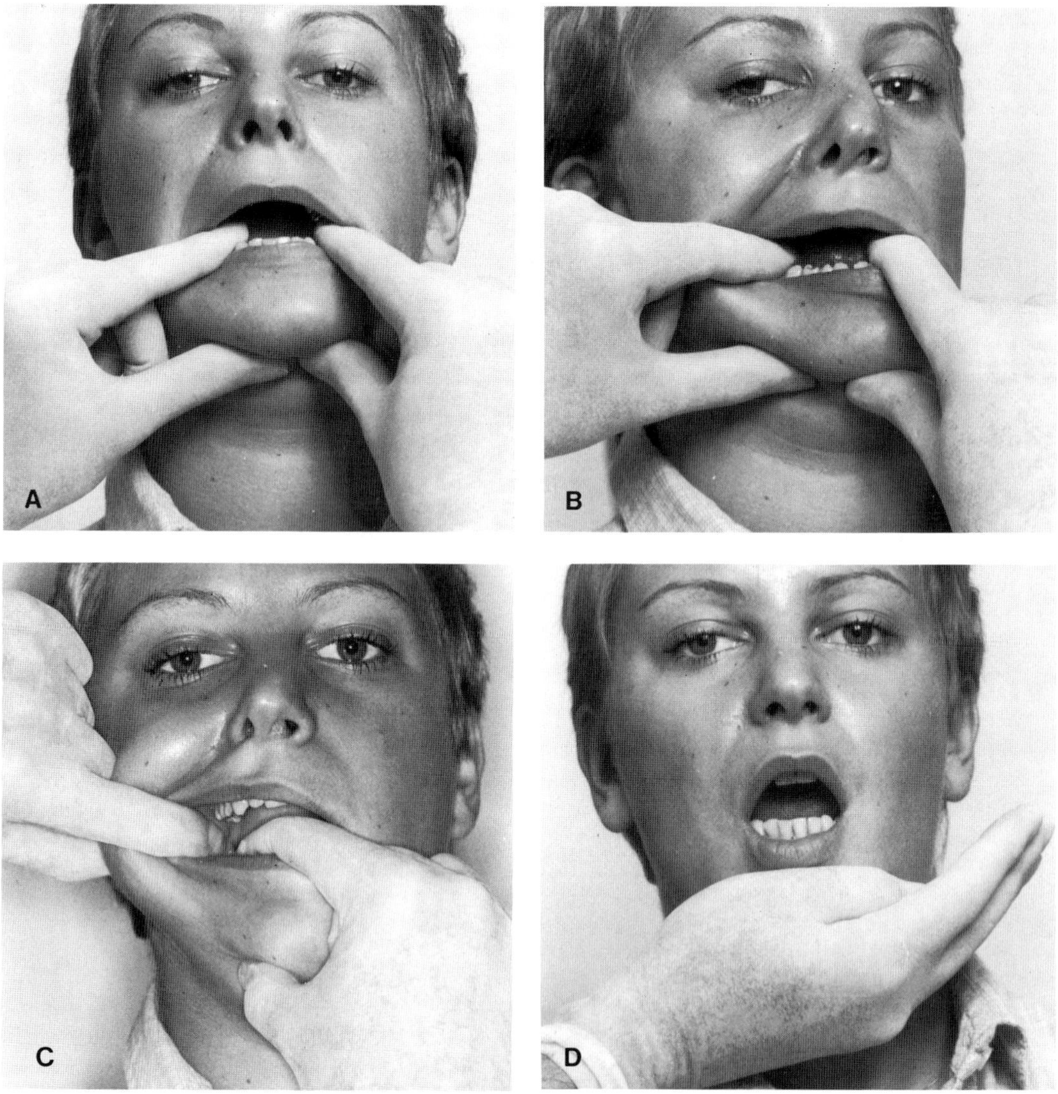

Figs. 8.1-23 A to D Confirming the abnormal mobility and the compression pain when there is suspicion of mandibular fracture.

Fig. 8.1-23 A In the anterior region.

Fig. 8.1-23 B In the buccal region.

Fig. 8.1-23 C In the region of the angle of the mandible.

Fig. 8.1-23 D Testing for compression pain through pressure on the chin with the mouth slightly open.

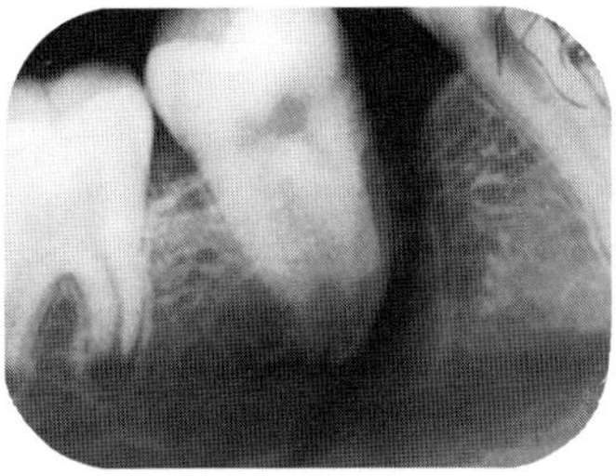

Fig. 8.1-24 Radiograph showing 46 in the fracture line.

When the ends of the fracture are pulled apart, which is possible only with a lacerated gingiva or after surgical exposure, the exposed root of a tooth situated in the fracture can be recognized. After evaluation of the radiographs, it may prove necessary to take further exposures.

1.3 Fundamentals of Treatment

The goal of treatment must be to bring the ends of the fracture into their anatomically correct position with as much precision as possible and to make sure, by means of appropriate fixation, that bony consolidation can take place in this position. To be sure, even without therapeutic measures, most cases will result in a bony healing; this takes, however, a significantly longer period of time and not infrequently ends with an incorrect positioning of the fracture ends. Only when there is extreme fragment mobility—e.g., with a wide fracture (longitudinal displacement with distraction) or with interposition of soft tissue—will bony healing not ensue and a pseudarthrosis result.

If the ends of the fracture are not too greatly mobile, spontaneous healing of the fracture usually occurs. As a result of the mobility, there are initially some manifestations of resorption at the ends of the fracture, whereby the gap of the fracture becomes wider. Within the second week there is the formation of a callus cuff in the area surrounding the fracture and of fibrous cartilage in the interfragmentary region. Thus, the mobility is limited, which is a prerequisite for the desmoid ossification of the callus cuff, and the chondral ossification of the gap which now takes place. After bone has completely bridged the fracture gap, remodelling into lamellar bone with differentiation into spongy and compact bone takes place under functional strain.

The extent of the resorptive processes, as well as the callus and cartilage formation, depends on the degree of fragment mobility (Tab. I). The less this is, the more discrete is the tissue reaction in the fracture. If there is no fragment mobility present at all, and if the gap of the fracture is not wider than 1 mm, e.g., with infractions or with functionally stable fixation through plates and screws, then callus and cartilage formation is completely lacking. Instead, there is a direct bridging by lamellar bone (Haversian remodelling). This process is designated primary bone fracture healing, and is thus differentiated from the secondary bone fracture healing which is characterized by the intermediate formation of callus and fibrous cartilage.

An awareness of these healing processes is important for planning therapy. Fractures with only slightly mobile fracture ends will heal without therapeutic measures. Fractures with highly mobile fragments require fixation. This can ensue indirectly with a splint or directly through osteosynthesis.

Indirect fixation achieves immobilization of the fracture fragments by means of a **splint** attached to the teeth or jaw, which bridges the site of the fracture and thus serves the function of the plaster cast in the treatment of fractures of extremities. The splint is usually effective in the vicinity of the body of the mandible. With a monomaxillary device, therefore, only

Table I

Fragment mobility	Healing process	Formation of callus and fibrous cartilage	Susceptibility to infection
Extensive	Pseudarthrosis	Exists, but no sort of ossification	+++++
Medium Slight Minimum	Secondary healing	Extensive Medium Slight	+++ ++ +
∅ (Rigid fixation, stable under functional strain)	Primary healing	∅	(+)

the fractures of that region are included. With fractures of the angle and ramus of the mandible, therefore, immobilization of the mandible in relation to the maxilla is necessary in addition (**intermaxillary fixation**). The maxilla also must be splinted. In this situation, the small fragment is not gripped by the splint. In many cases, this does not disturb the healing of the fracture; occasionally, however, particularly with extensive displacement, an osteosynthesis, e.g., through interosseous wiring, is required for adaptation of the fragments. An intermaxillary fixation also is usually necessary for multiple fractures in the body of the mandible and in fractures in the molar region where the splint does not have enough support for the small fragment.

Intraoral splints are attached to the teeth in the dentulous jaw. In the edentulous or sparsely dentulous jaw, plates similar to prostheses are used as splint elements and fixed in the mandible by circumferential wiring (*Black; Gilmer*, 1881; *Gordon*, 1937; *Ivy* and *Curtis*, 1938; *Parker*, 1942; *Thoma*, 1958; and others) and in the maxilla with circumzygomatic and internal wiring (*Adams*, 1956; *Lelsney*, 1953; *Thoma*, 1943, 1958; *Hayward*, 1962; *Krüger*, 1964; and others).

Some further possibilities for indirect fixation are **skeletal pin fixation** (*Anderson*, 1936; *Converse* and *Waknitz*, 1942; *Waldron* et al., 1943; *Converse*, 1943; *Winter*, 1943; *Morris*, 1949; *Khedroo*, 1970; *Wessberg* et al., 1979; and others) and **internal clamp fixation** (*Pohl*, 1941; *Penn* and *Brown*, 1944; *Thoma*, 1945, 1958; *Thoma* et al., 1945). Here, pins or screws are screwed in through the skin on both sides of the fracture in the mandible or affixed to the bone with the help of clamps. Stabilization of the fracture ensues extraorally through fixation rods or plastic bridges which are anchored to the ends of the pins projecting through the skin.

Direct fixation (osteosynthesis) ensues by means of retention elements which grip the bone immediately at the fracture ends.

Interosseous wiring (*Wassmund*, 1927; *Link*, 1937; *Gordon*, 1943; *Wheelock*, 1950; *Burch*, 1951; *Reichenbach*, 1954, 1957, 1959, 1969; *Thoma*, 1958; *Schwenzer*, 1967; and others) has been known longest. The fracture ends here are adapted to one another by wire sutures which are pulled through previously drilled holes. Interosseous wiring does not provide sufficient stabilization of the fragments. Additional splints therefore are necessary for immobilization (*Thoma*, 1958; *Köhler*, 1951; *Reichenbach*, 1957, 1959, 1969; *Schwenzer*, 1967; *Lentrodt* and *Höltje*, 1975).

Intermedullary wire fixation (*Scangall*, 1944; *Brown* et al., 1949; *Fries*, 1966) is less common. Here, a *Kirschner* wire is drilled into the mandible in an axially transverse direction. Usually, additional splints are not required.

Bone plating, by means of plates which are anchored in the bone with screws, allows a more stable fixation than the above-mentioned osteosynthesis methods. Plate systems which did not compress the ends of the fracture

(*Thoma*, 1958; *Hoffer* and *Arlotta*, 1961; *Roberts*, 1964; *Dott*, 1967; *Heiss* and *Grasser*, 1968; *Schilli*, 1969; *Brons* and *Boering*, 1970; *Spiessl* et al., 1971, 1972) have since been replaced by compression plates (*Luhr*, 1972; *Spiessl* et al., 1972, 1975; *Niederdellmann* and *Schilli*, 1972, 1973). Compression of the fragments provides the most stable fixation of the fracture ends, even when function is instituted (functional stability). Splints are not required after such a functionally stable osteosynthesis.

The procedures just outlined have their own particular indications, and are sometimes in competition with each other. It requires great experience to decide which method is the most advantageous to apply in an individual case. In the following, we have tried to set up generally valid rules, insofar as this is at all possible. Advantages and disadvantages of the individual procedures must be weighed against each other to be understood clearly.

Spontaneous healing can be expected if the fragments are only slightly mobile and not displaced and if there are no functional disturbances. In such cases, the therapy consists exclusively of avoiding extreme stresses on the fracture (liquid and soft diet only). Spontaneous healing may fail to occur if the situation has been evaluated incorrectly (mobility too great) or if the fracture has become infected. An infection is possible particularly if communication exists from the fracture gap into the oral cavity via a gingival pocket or a tear in the gingiva (a tooth in the fracture line). In such cases, therefore, an immobilizing splint should be applied, even when there is only minor fragment mobility.

With dentition, **dental splints** allow a sufficient reduction and fixation of the fragments in most cases. Lentrodt and Höltje (1975), Becker et al. (1976) as well as Schüle (1976), prefer the conservative treatment when there is adequate dentition.

Fractures within the dental arch can, in some cases, be treated with a **monomaxillary fixation.** The prerequisites are, first of all, an appliance which is stable in itself, either with an arch bar or a splint—horizontal interdental wiring is not suitable—and second, dentition which is sufficient for the fixation on both sides of the fracture. If these preconditions are fulfilled, then this method is preferred, because of its simplicity and minor incapacitation to the patient.

Intermaxillary fixation is required for all mandibular fractures outside the dental arch and also for a number of fractures within the arch—particularly fractures of the molar regions and multiple fractures. Here, an additional splint must be applied in the maxilla. In such cases, intermaxillary fixation provides sufficient immobilization of the fragments; if these are more severely displaced, however, osteosynthesis is usually necessary. The disadvantage of intermaxillary fixation is obvious: the patient is considerably compromised in eating, speaking, and in cleaning the teeth, by total mandibular immobilization. The patient is usually unable to work during the period of intermaxillary fixation. In addition, simultaneous fracture of the condylar head or neck contraindicates long periods of immobilization; in this situation, functional therapy should be instituted as early as possible.

If the dentition is not sufficient for attaching splints, e.g., in primary and mixed dentition, in the partially edentulous arch, and in the edentulous jaw, then the patient's splints or prostheses must be attached by **circumferential wiring.** A splint or denture attached by four circumferential wires can sufficiently stabilize a mandibular fracture in the anterior region, and also, although more rarely, in the buccal region. Intermaxillary fixation is achieved in such cases by **zygomaticomaxillary wire suspension of the mandible** (*Krüger*, 1967), a combined nasomandibular and zygomaticomandibular wiring. The two distal ends of the four circumferential wires are led around the malar arches and the two anterior ones are pulled through holes drilled in the lateral margins of the piriform aperture. After the maxillary prosthesis has been put in place and the mandible has been positioned in centric occlusion, the ends of the wires are twisted tight. Zygomaticomaxillary wire suspension of the mandible is indicated for fractures which require intermaxillary fixation, but where the dentition is not sufficient for attaching conventional splints. An additional disadvantage arguing against this is the possibility of an infection at the site of the wires' penetration of the mucosa; this can, however, usually be avoided by careful cleaning of the mouth. Today, the

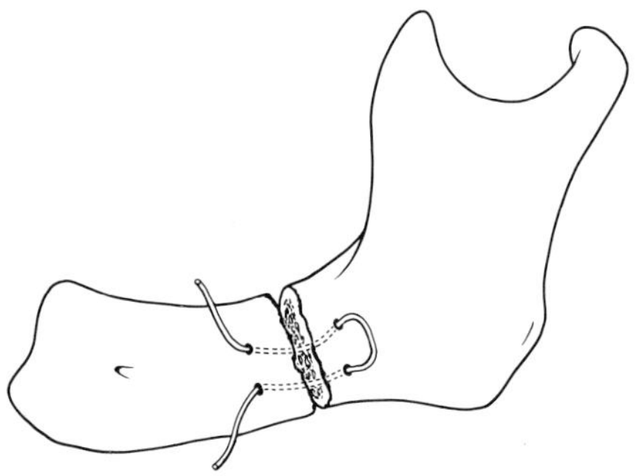
A

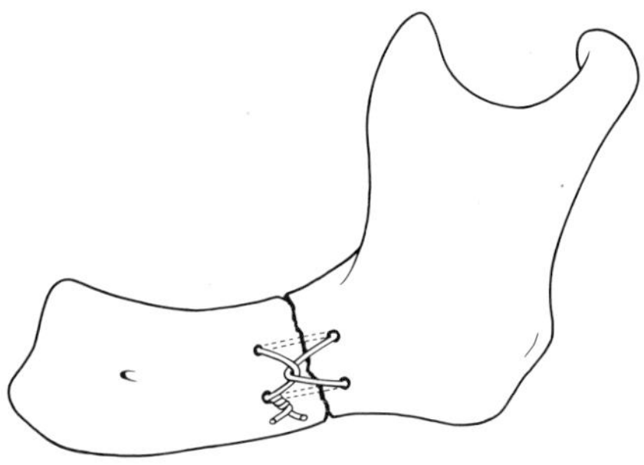
B

Figs. 8.1-25 A and B Neuner's interosseous wiring. This wire ligature is not functionally stable! Like other wire ligatures, it serves only to adapt displaced fragments. The stability must be provided by intermaxillary fixation. If indicated, monomaxillary fixation with an arch bar or a splint may suffice.

process has been largely replaced in adults by functionally stable osteosynthesis; for children, however, it is still the preferred procedure.

Skeletal pin fixation and **internal clamp fixation** are used predominantly for immobilization of the fragments in edentulous or sparsely dentulous parts of the mandible or in fractures outside the dental arch. Additional fixation through intraoral splints is advantageous. When intermaxillary fixation of the mandible is not used, great mechanical stress from muscular forces causes an osteoclastic reaction, with premature loosening of the screws. *Reichenbach* (1969) recommends, therefore, that the apparatus be removed after three weeks and replaced by Gunning splints. *Rowe* and *Killey* (1968) list the following as possible complications: damage to the inferior dental nerve, facial nerve and adjacent structures; loosening of the apparatus and development of cellulitis and necrosis of the bone at pin site, movement of the bone fragments, salivary fistula and traumatic injury to the apparatus.

Interosseous wiring serves the function of adaptating displaced bone fragments. It is not possible to connect the ends of the fractures to each other in a functionally stable manner through wire sutures alone. The crossed wire suture (Fig. 8. 1-25) which was described and designated as functionally stable by *Neuner* (1977), can, in conjunction with a monomaxillary arch bar, immobilize the ends of fractures within the dental arch enough that undisturbed callus healing can take place. A functionally stable fixation with primary healing, however, cannot be achieved with this method. The wire suture is not considered, therefore, as an independent therapeutic measure; its function always is only that of supporting intraoral splinting (*Thoma,* 1958; *Reichenbach,* 1957, 1959, 1969; *Schwenzer,* 1967).

Schwenzer (1967) considers displaced fractures in the dentulous jaw at the following locations to be indications for a wire suture:

- angle of the mandible,
- body of the mandible, especially outside the dental arch,
- ramus of the mandible,
- fractures at the base of the condylar process without dislocation of the condyle, if the surfaces of the fracture have completely lost contact with each other,
- open fractures.

In all cases, intermaxillary fixation with the help of intraoral splints also is undertaken. *Schwenzer* (1967) recommends that the splints be applied first, and the intermaxillary fixation undertaken, and only then that a decision be made with the help of radiographic examination about whether a wire suture is still necessary. The indication for interosseous wiring in dentulous and sparsely dentulous parts of the mandible in conjunction with *Gunning* splints, also recommended by *Schwenzer* in 1967, now can be regarded as dated because the performance of functionally stable osteosynthesis is better here. Interosseous wiring similarly may be necessary in children if a major displacement of the fragments is present. Here, the wire suture is usually applied in combination with zygomaticomaxillary wire suspension of the mandible (*Krüger*, 1964). Fixation at the mandibular inferior border will preclude damage to the tooth buds.

Compression osteosynthesis is the only method described which is functionally stable to the point that postoperative intermaxillary fixation is not necessary. The compression of the fragments is not a *conditio sine qua non* for primary healing of the fracture, but it does greatly increase the stability and thus indirectly guarantees a direct synthesis of the Haversian lamellar systems. Any movement in the fracture line, no matter how minor, facilitates the formation of callus and fibrous cartilage, and thus leads to secondary healing. Compression osteosynthesis is usually undertaken in the mandible with the help of dynamic compression plates (DCP) or Luhr plates which are anchored to the bone with screws (*Luhr*, 1972; *Spiessl* el al., 1972, 1975; *Niederdellmann* and *Schilli*, 1972, 1973).

Osteosynthesis via bone plating is not suited to all types of fractures. Comminuted fractures cannot generally be screwed to the point of absolute stability. In such cases, a reconstruction plate is better (Fig. 8.1-26); because of the greater surgical effort, however, this should, if possible, be implemented only in discontinuity defect fractures. Some diagonal fractures are not always suited to bone plating. Sagittal diagonal fractures, which occur very rarely, under certain circumstances can be screwed in a functionally stable manner with lag screws.

With comminuted fractures and diagonal fractures which cannot be stabely fixated, treatment should be performed with conventional splints and intermaxillary fixation, supported if necessary by interosseous wiring. In children, compression osteosynthesis should not be performed because of possible damage to the tooth buds. The advantage of immediate resumption of function would be less important here because the period of intermaxillary fixation would be significantly shorter in view of the more rapid healing in children.

The main advantage of functionally stable osteosynthesis is the elimination of intermaxillary fixation, which allows immediate postoperative masticatory function and cleaning of the teeth. The disadvantage is the necessity of operating twice—the plates and screws usually must be removed after about 3-12 months. An extraoral approach is necessary in many cases and the scar that arises must also be taken into account by the patient. Injuries to the marginal mandibular branch of the facial nerve usually can be avoided by precise surgical technique. In many cases, especially in fractures in the region of the chin, the intraoral approach is preferred in order to avoid an external scar; this may occasionally result in postoperative dehiscences of the mucosa and exposure of the plate. Fracture infections such as osteomyelitis, soft tissue abcesses and fistula formation are rare. They are more likely to appear if absolute functional stability is not achieved. These complications are, therefore, dependent principally on the precision of the surgical technique. *Reuter* and *Scharf* (1976) found more disturbances of sensation after functionally stable osteosynthesis than after conservative therapy. They attributed this, however, to the greater displacement in cases which were treated surgically, and not to iatrogenic injury.

The following are the indications for compression osteosynthesis:

a) Fractures in the edentulous or partially dentulous mandible.

Here, bone plating is the preferred method. No other method allows such reliable stabilization to be achieved. The best alternative would be the zygomaticomaxillary wire suspension of the mandible (*Krüger*, 1964). This allows fixation sufficient for secondary healing to be attained. This procedure is, however, more unpleasant for the patient than compression osteosynthesis. For this reason, it should be implemented only if the two operations and the external scar associated with bone plating are unacceptable to the patient.

b) Fractures in the dentulous mandible in asso-

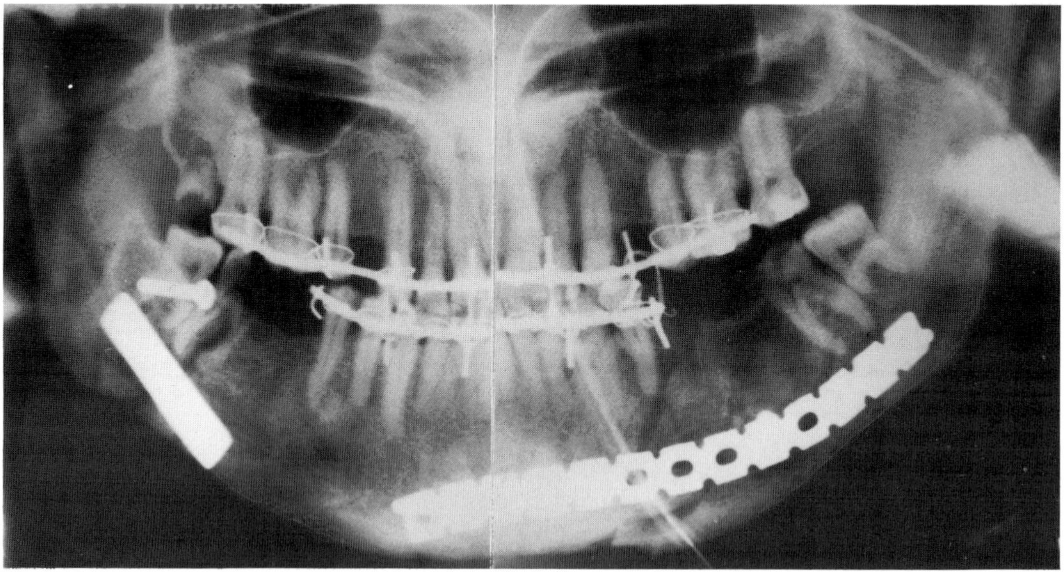

Fig. 8.1-26 Stabilization of a comminuted fracture in the left side of the mandible with a reconstruction plate. Another fracture in the region of the right angle of the mandible was treated with a normal Dynamic Compression Plate (DCP) with 4 screws and a lag screw.

ciation with fractures of the condyle or the condylar neck, which require functional therapy.

Compression osteosynthesis here offers the advantage of allowing the functional therapy of the condylar fracture to begin immediately after the operation (*Luhr*, 1972; *Becker* et al., 1975; *Spiessl*, 1975; *Schilli*, 1975, 1977; *Schmidt-Hoberg* and *Luhr*, 1976)

c) Displaced fractures of the angle, body, or ramus of the mandible, which require open reduction.

As interosseous wiring makes intermaxillary fixation necessary, bone plating is an alternative easy to choose; if there is already an open reduction, then it can be functionally stable at the same time. The removal of the plate, which is necessary later, is not usually significant in such cases.

d) Fractures in patients with epilepsy, hyperemesis, and respiratory diseases where intermaxillary fixation may be contraindicated.

e) Mandibular fractures that do not involve the TMJ

can be treated both with conservative methods as well as by compression osteosynthesis. The decision here can in many cases be left to the patient, depending on whether he prefers two operations or intermaxillary fixation. Experience has shown that many patients prefer the bone plating. If, however, a maxillary fracture or a fracture of the condylar process which requires intermaxillary fixation is present simultaneously, there would be little point in undertaking compression osteosynthesis.

f) Discontinuity defect fractures, especially after gunshot wounds,

can be bridged by a so-called reconstruction plate and then immobilized in a functionally stable manner (Fig. 8.1-26). Reconstruction plates are available in various lengths. They are also used to stabilize bone grafts. With comminuted fractures, individual pieces of bone can be attached to the plate with additional screws. Not infrequently, there is incomplete bony bridging of the defect. In such cases, a bone graft should be inserted; this can be attached with screws to the reconstruction plate which bridges the defect.

In keeping with an old rule of fracture treatment, a **tooth in the fracture line** always should be removed, even if it is still vital, because the connection of the fracture to the oral cavity via the periodontal space fosters infection through the gingival pocket (*Reichenbach*, 1954). Since the institution of that rule, the prerequisites for complication-free retention of vital teeth at the fracture line have become more favorable through improvement of the splints and, more importantly, through the possibility of functionally stable osteosynthesis. *Schönberger* (1956) found a 6% rate of postoperative fracture infection in 30 cases where the tooth at the fracture line was retained. The infection rate in 173 patients in whom a tooth at the fracture was prophylactically removed was 18%. *Götte* (1959), too, found more complications after prophylactic extraction of the tooth at the fracture site (20% of 60 cases) than when it was left in place (16.8% of 178 cases). The poorer results after prophylactic extraction are probably caused primarily by the fact that the teeth at the fracture line were left in place only in the most favorable instances while extraction was performed in unfavorable ones, e.g., in open, already infected fractures, extensive tears in the periodontal tissue and destruction of the alveolus. *Müller*, (1964) observed significantly more infection in the molar region of the mandible after leaving the teeth in place at the fracture site than in single-rooted teeth. He insists, therefore, on extracting molars which are situated at the fracture line but will allow anterior teeth and premolars to remain in place.

On the basis of these results, an unconditional requirement for extracting vital teeth at the fracture line can no longer be regarded as valid. *Ryberg* (1960) reported that after conservative treatment with splints within the first five days, over 50% of teeth situated at the fracture line could be preserved if they were radiologically complication-free.

The opinion of many authors (*Archer*, 1966; *Schwenzer*, 1967; *Rowe* and *Killey*, 1968; *Nasteff*, 1971; *G. O. Kruger*, 1972; *Trauner*, 1973; *E. Krüger*, 1974; and others) holds that teeth situated at the fracture site can be left in place if certain prerequisites are met. First among these is early treatment with a stable splint or by functionally stable osteosynthesis. Antibiotic cover is recommended, but this has significantly less value than the immobilization of the fracture ends. Further, the condition of the periodontium and of the tooth is important. Ragged gingival margins, broken alveolar walls, and fractures of the dental roots are hardly good preconditions for preserving a tooth in a fracture line. Similarly, when there is marginal periodontitis, complication-free healing cannot be expected. An individual decision must be made in every case whether a tooth in the fracture can be left in place. It is wise to remember the dictum: "If in doubt, have it out" (*Rowe* and *Killey*, 1968).

Devitalized teeth in a fracture line always should be removed, whether a periapical infection is already present or not (*Schönberger*, 1969). Impacted third molars always should be removed in the course of treatment if pericoronal inflammation is present. A completely unerupted third molar may be left in the fracture line if it is not open to the oral cavity and if the reduction of the fragments is not impeded thereby (*Schwenzer*, 1967; *Krüger*, 1974).

In the partially edentulous arch, which requires prosthetic treatment in any case, it is better to proceed according to the old rule and remove a tooth in the fracture site even if it is vital and the periodontium is tolerably well preserved.

The reduction of the fragments is easier, the earlier the treatment is undertaken.

Immediate reduction can be performed manually with fresh fractures. Usually a local anesthetic is required, and sometimes a general. The mandibular fragments are adjusted in centric occlusion and immobilized in this position by a splint. The adjustment of centric occlusion is required in the dentulous jaw even with surgical treatment through functionally stable osteosynthesis. In this case, several intermaxillary ligatures described by *Ernst* (1927, 1932) or *Kazanjian* (1933) are applied; these can be removed again after the operation.

Progressive reduction, with fractures which are difficult to reduce, can be undertaken with the help of elastic bands attached to the mandibular and maxillary splints (*Darnall*, 1923; *Wassmund*, 1927; *Moorehead*, 1934; *Winter*, 1934;

Ivy and *Curtis*, 1938; *Reichenbach*, 1954). The reduction should be completed within a few hours, and no later than 24 to 48 hours. If this is not successful, manual reduction or open reduction under local or general anesthesia is required.

After fixation of the fragments with splints, radiographic inspection is necessary. If this reveals that the reduction is imperfect, further measures, involving an open reduction with wire sutures or functionally stable osteosynthesis, are necessary.

References

Adams, W. M. (1956)
Internal wire fixation of facial fractures. Amer. J. Surg. 92: 12

Anderson, R. (1936)
Ambulatory method of treating fractures of the shaft of femur. Surg. Gynec. Obstet. 62: 865

Archer, W. H. (1966)
Die Chirurgie des Mundes und der Zähne. (Oral surgery.) vol. 2 3rd ed. Stuttgart – Wien – Zürich, Medica

Archer, W. H. (1966)
Oral surgery. 4th ed. Philadelphia – London, Saunders

Becker, R., D. Broxtermann, E. Esser, H. Meiners, and P. Topp (1976)
Indikationsstellung für verschiedene Osteosyntheseverfahren auf der Grundlage klinischer und experimenteller Untersuchungen. (Indications for various osteosynthesis methods on the basis of clinical and experimental studies.) Fortschr. Kiefer- u. Gesichtschir. 21: 296

Becker, R., E. Machtens, and J. Lenz (1975)
Möglichkeiten und Grenzen der Kompressionsosteosynthese. (Possibilities and limits of compression osteosynthesis.) Fortschr. Kiefer- u. Gesichtschir. 19: 87

Black, G. V.: quoted by Gilmer, T. L. (1881)

Brons, R., and G. Boering (1970)
Fractures of the mandibular body treated by stable internal fixation: A preliminary report. J. oral Surg. 28: 407

Brown, J. B., M. P. Fryer, and F. McDowell (1949)
Internal wire-pin immobilisation of jaw fractures. Plast. reconstr. Surg. 4: 30

Burch, R. J. (1951)
Treatment of displaced fractures of the edentulous mandibular angle. Oral Surg. 4: 1101

Converse, J. M. (1974)
External skeletal fixation of fractured mandibles. J. oral Surg. 1: 210

Converse, J. M., and F. W. Waknitz (1942)
External skeletal fixation of the mandibular angle. J. Bone Jt. Surg. 24: 154

Darnall, W. L. (1923)
Use of modified Baker anchorage in naval dental service. U.S. nav. med. Bull. 19: 42

Dechaume, M., M. Grellet, P. Franchebois, and M. Bonneau (1957)
Les fractures de l'apophyse coronoide de la mandibule. (Fractures of the coronoid process of the mandible.) Rev. Stomat. (Paris) 58: 677

Dingman, R. O., and P. Natvig (1964)
Surgery of facial fractures. Philadelphia – London, Saunders

Dott, W. A. (1967)
The problem of the fractured edentulous mandible. Oral Surgery Transactions 2nd Congress of the International Association of Oral Surgeons, p. 322, Copenhagen, Munksgaard.

Ernst, F. (1927)
Die zahnärztliche Behandlung der Unterkieferbrüche. (Treatment of mandibular fractures.) In Kirschner, M., and O. Nordmann: Die Chirurgie. (Surgery.) Vol. 4, 1, p. 842. Berlin – Wien, Urban & Schwarzenberg

Ernst, F. (1932)
Die Schienenverbände bei Ober- und Unterkieferbrüchen. (Splinting in maxillary and mandibular fractures.) In Bruhn, C., A. Kantorowicz, and C. Partsch: Handbuch der Zahnheilkunde. (Handbook of Dentistry.) Vol. 1, 4th ed., p. 115. München, Bergmann.

Fries, R. (1966)
Markdrahtung bei Unterkieferfrakturen. (Intramedullary wiring in fractures of the mandible.) Fortschr. Kiefer- u. Gesichtschir. 11: 225

Gilmer, T. L. (1881)
Fractures of the inferior maxilla. Illinois State dent. Soc. Trans. 67-104, Disc. 104-106

Gordon, S. D. (1937)
Immediate treatment of facial fractures. Canad. med. Ass. J. 37: 440

Gordon, S. D. (1943)
Wire suturing in the treatment of facial fractures. Canad. med. Ass. J. 48: 406

Götte, H. (1959)
Die Belassung von Zähnen im Bruchspalt in Abhängigkeit von der Art des Kieferbruchverbandes. (Leaving teeth in the fracture line, according to the type of splint.) Fortschr. Kiefer- u. Gesichtschir. 5: 333

Grimm, G. (1969)
Klinische Untersuchung mit Befunderhebung bei Gesichtsschädelverletzungen. (Clinical examination and diagnosis in facial skull injuries.) München, Barth.

Hagan, E. H., and D. F. Huelke (1961)
An analysis of 319 case reports of mandibular fractures. J. oral Surg. 19: 93

Hayward, J. R. (1962)
Treatment methods for jaw fractures. J. oral Surg. 20: 273

Heiss, J., and H. Grasser (1968)
Stabile Osteosynthese mit Platten. (Stable osteosynthesis with plates.) Dtsch. zahnärztl. Z. 23: 1085

Hoffer, O., and P. Arlotta (1961)
Behandlung von Unterkieferbrüchen mit Metallplättchen. (Treatment of mandibular fractures with metal plates.) Dtsch. zahnärztl. Z. 16: 807

Ivy, R. H., and L. Curtis (1938)
Fractures of the jaws. Philadelphia, Lea & Febiger

Kazanjian, V. H. (1933)
Treatment of automobile injuries of the face and jaws. J. Amer. dent. Ass. 20: 757

Kazanjian, V. H., and J. M. Converse (1974)
The surgical treatment of facial injuries. Baltimore, Williams & Wilkins. 2nd Ed. 1959, 3rd Ed. 1974

Khedroo, L. G. (1970)
External pin fixation for treatment of mandibular fractures: a reappraisal. J. oral Surg 28: 101

Köhler, J. A. (1951)
Diagnostik und Therapie der Kieferfrakturen. (Diagnosis and treatment of jaw fractures.) Heidelberg, Hüthig

Kruger, G. O. (1964)
Textbook of oral surgery. 2nd ed. St. Louis Mosby

Kruger, G. O. (1972)
Lehrbuch der Mund- und Kieferchirurgie. (Textbook of oral surgery.) Stuttgart – Wien – Zürich – Amsterdam, Medica

Krüger, E. (1964)
Indikation und Technik der operativen Kieferbruchbehandlung. (Indications and techniques for surgical treatment of jaw fractures.) Dtsch. zahnärztl. Z. 19: 1057

Krüger, E. (1974)
Lehrbuch der chirurgischen Zahn-, Mund- und Kieferheilkunde. (Textbook of oral surgery.) Vol. 2, Berlin, Buch- und Zeitschriften-Verlag "Die Quintessenz", 1st ed. 1974, 4th ed. 1981

Larsen, O. D., and A. Nielsen (1976)
Mandibular fractures. I. An analysis of their etiology and location in 286 patients. Scand. J. Plast. Reconstr. Surg. 10: 213

Lentrodt, J., and W.-J. Höltje (1975)
Indikation zur operativen bzw. konservativen Versorgung von Unterkieferfrakturen. (Indications for surgical and conservative care of mandibular fractures.) Fortschr. Kiefer- u. Gesichtschir. 19: 65

Lesney, T. A. (1953)
A method of immobilizing a common type of maxillary fracture. J. oral Surg. 11: 49

Link, K. H. (1937)
Zur Frage der Knochennaht bei Kieferbrüchen. (On the question of interosseous wiring in jaw fractures.) Zbl. Chir. 12: 988

Luhr, G. (1972)
Die Kompressionsosteosynthese bei Unterkieferfrakturen. (Compression osteosynthesis in mandibular fractures.) München, Hanser.

Moorehead, F. B. (1934)
A better method of treating fractures of the jaws. J. Amer. med. Ass. 102: 1655

Morris, J. H. (1949)
Biphase connector, external skeletal splint for reduction and fixation of mandibular fractures. Oral Surg. 2: 382

Müller, W. (1969)
Häufigkeit, Sitz und Ursachen der Gesichtsschädelfrakturen. (Frequency, site, and causes of facial skull fractures.) In Reichenbach, E.: Traumatologie im Kiefer-Gesichts-Bereich. (Maxillofacial traumatology.) p. 47 München, Barth

Müller, W. (1964)
Zur Frage des Versuchs der Erhaltung der im Bruchspalt stehenden Zähne unter antibiotischem Schutz. (On the question of attempting to retain teeth in the fracture line with antibiotic cover.) Dtsch. Zahn-, Mund- u. Kieferheilk. 41: 360

Nasteff, D. (1971)
Operationslehre der Mund-Kiefer-Gesichts-Chirurgie. (Techniques of oral and maxillofacial surgery.) Berlin, VEB Volk und Gesundheit

Neuner, O. (1977)
Maxillofaciale Traumatologie. (Maxillofacial traumatology.) Berlin – New York, de Gruyter

Niederdellmann, H. and W. Schilli (1972)
Funktionsstabile Osteosynthese im Unterkiefer. (Functionally stable osteosynthesis in the mandible.) Dtsch. zahnärztl. Z. 27: 138

Niederdellmann, H., and W. Schilli (1973)
Zur Plattenosteosynthese bei Unterkieferfrakturen. (Plate osteosynthesis in fractures of the mandible.) Dtsch. zahnärztl. Z. 28: 638

Parker, D. B. (1942)
Synopsis of traumatic injuries of the face and jaws. St. Louis, Mosby

Penn, J., and L. Brown (1944)
Year book of dentistry. Chicago, Year Book Publishers

Pohl, L. (1941)
Extraoral splinting of the edentulous mandible. Lancet 2: 389

Reichenbach, E. (1954)
Leitfaden der Kieferbruchbehandlung. (Guidelines for treatment of jaw fractures.) 6th ed. Leipzig, Barth

Reichenbach, E. (1957)
Verletzungen der Kiefer- und Gesichtsknochen und der benachbarten Weichteile. (Injuries of the jaw and facial bones and the adjacent soft tissues.) In Häupl. K., W. Meyer, and K. Schuchardt: Die Zahn-, Mund- und Kieferheilkunde. (Dentistry.) Vol. III/1, p. 639 München – Berlin, Urban & Schwarzenberg

Reichenbach, E. (1959)
Kritik einiger Neuerungen auf dem Gebiete der Kieferbruchbehandlung. (Criticism of some recent developments in the treatment of jaw fractures.) Fortschr. Kiefer- u. Gesichtschir. 5: 317

Reichenbach, E. (1969)
Die operative Behandlung der Unterkieferfrakturen. (Surgical treatment of mandibular fractures.) In Reichenbach, E.: Traumatologie im Kiefer-Gesichts-Bereich. (Maxillofacial traumatology.) München, Barth

Reichenbach, E., and W. Müller (1964)
Die Frakturen des Processus muscularis der Mandibula. (Fractures of the coronoid process of the mandible.) Zbl. Chir. 89: 1731

Reichenbach, E., and W. Müller (1966)
Der Mechanismus der Frakturen des Processus muscularis der Mandibula. (The mechanism of fractures of the coronoid process of the mandible.) Fortschr. Kiefer- u. Gesichtschir. 11: 211

Reuter, E., and F. Scharf (1976)
Spätfolgen nach Unterkieferfrakturen unter Berücksichtigung von Frakturverlauf, Dislokation und Behandlungsmethode. (Late sequelae following mandibular fractures with emphasis on fracture course, displacement and method of treatment.) Fortschr. Kiefer- u. Gesichtschir. 21: 307

Roberts, W. R. (1964)
The case for mandibular plating. Brit. J. oral Surg. 1: 200

Rowe, N. L., and H. C. Killey (1968)
Fractures of the facial skeleton. 2nd. ed. Edinburgh – London, Livingstone

Ryberg, J. (1960)
Statistische Untersuchungen zu den Frakturen mit Zähnen im Bruchspalt unter besonderer Berücksichtigung der Art der Schienung und deren Zeitpunkt. (Statistical studies of fractures with teeth in the fracture line, with special attention to the type of splinting and its timing.) Med. Diss. (thesis) Freiburg

Scangall, S. (1944)
Internal Kirschner fixation of the body of the edentulous mandible. Aust. J. Dent. 16: 198

Schilli, W. (1969)
Behandlungsmöglichkeiten bei Frakturen. (Treatment possibilities in fractures.) Therapiewoche 41: 2006

Schilli, W. (1975)
Indikation und Technik der stabilen Osteosynthese im Unterkiefer. (Indication and technique for stable osteosynthesis in the mandible.) Fortschr. Kiefer- u. Gesichtschir. 19: 79

Schilli, W. (1977)
Compression osteosynthesis. J. oral Surg. 35: 802

Schmidt-Hoberg, W., and H. G. Luhr (1976)
Technik und Ergebnisse der funktionellen Frühbehandlung von Unterkieferkörperfrakturen. (Technique and results of early functional therapy of fractures of the body of the mandible.) Fortschr. Kiefer- u. Gesichtschir. 21: 317

Schönberger, A. (1956)
Behandlung der Zähne im Bruchspalt. (Treatment of teeth in the fracture line.) Fortschr. Kiefer- u. Gesichtschir. 2: 108

Schönberger, A. (1969)
Die örtlichen Komplikationen bei Kieferverletzungen und ihre Behandlung. (Local complications in jaw injuries, and their treatment.) In Reichenbach, E.: Traumatologie im Kiefer-Gesichts-Bereich. (Maxillofacial traumatology.) p. 391. München, Barth

Schröder, H.: Quoted by Wassmund, M. (1927)

Schuchardt, K., N. Schwenzer, B. Rottke, and J. Lentrodt (1966)
Ursachen, Häufigkeit und Lokalisation der Frakturen des Gesichtsschädels. (Causes, frequency and location of fractures of the facial skeleton.) Fortschr. Kiefer- u. Gesichtschir. 11: 1

Schüle, H. (1976)
Fortschritte und Schwerpunkte der Behandlung von Mund - Kiefer - Gesichts - Verletzungen. (Advances and emphases in the treatment of maxillofacial injuries.) Fortschr. Kiefer- u. Gesichtschir. 21: 272

Schwenzer, N. (1967)
Zur Osteosynthese bei Frakturen des Gesichtsskeletts. (Osteosynthesis in fractures of the facial skeleton.) Stuttgart, Thieme

Spiessl, B. (1975)
Funktionsstabile Osteosynthese bei Unterkieferfrakturen – Problematik und Technik. (Functionally stable osteosynthesis in fractures of the mandible. Problems and techniques.) Fortschr. Kiefer- u. Gesichtschir. 19: 68

Spiessl, B., G. Schargus, and K. Schroll (1971)
Die stabile Osteosynthese bei Frakturen des unbezahnten Unterkiefers. (Stable osteosynthesis in fractures of the edentulous mandible.) Schweiz. Mschr. Zahnheilk. 81: 39

Spiessl, B., and K. Schroll (1972)
Gesichtsschädel. (The facial skeleton.) In Nigst, H.: Spezielle Frakturen- und Luxationslehre. (Textbook of fractures and dislocations.) Vol. I/1 Stuttgart, Thieme

Thoma, K. H. (1943)
A new method of intermaxillary fixation for jaw fractures in patients wearing artifical dentures. Oral Surg. 29: 433

Thoma, K. H. (1945)
Three fractures at the angle of the jaw: One treated by internal wiring, two by internal clamp fixation. Oral Surg. 31: 206

Thoma, K. H. (1958)
Oral surgery. St. Louis, Mosby

Thoma, K. H., M. Wenig, and S. I. Kaplan (1945)
Further uses of the peripheral bone clamp. Oral Surg. 31: 607

Trauner, R. (1973)
Kiefer- und Gesichtschirurgie. (Maxillofacial surgery.) 2nd ed., Vol. 2 München – Berlin, Urban & Schwarzenberg

Waldron, C. W., V. H. Kazanjian, and D. B. Parker (1943)
Skeletal fixation in the treatment of fractures of the mandible. J. oral Surg. 1: 59

Wassmund, M. (1927)
Frakturen und Luxationen des Gesichtsschädels. (Fractures and dislocations of the facial skeleton.) Leipzig, Meusser

Weiskopf, J. (1957)
Die Ätiologie der Frakturen des Processus muscularis mandibulae. (The etiology of fractures of the coronoid process of the mandible.) Dtsch. Stomat. 7: 17

Weiskopf, J. (1969)
Die Frakturen des Unterkiefers und ihre orthopädische Behandlung. (Fractures of the mandible and their orthopedic treatment.) In Reichenbach, E.: Traumatologie im Kiefer-Gesichts-Bereich. (Maxillofacial traumatology.) München, Barth

Wessberg, G. A., S. A. Shendel, and B. N. Epker (1979)
Monophase extraskeletal fixation. J. oral Surg. 37: 892

Wheelock, R. W. (1950)
Open reduction of fractured mandible. J. oral Surg. 8: 247

Winter, L. (1934)
Fractures of the mandible; a study of 200 cases. Dent. Cosmos 76: 316

Winter, L. (1943)
Mandibular fractures. Amer. J. Surg. 61: 367

2. Conservative Therapy

Eberhard Krüger

In the conservative treatment of mandibular fractures, fixation is undertaken indirectly through splints that are usually attached to the teeth or the alveolar process. Occasionally, especially in the poorly dentate jaw, extraoral appliances such as head-chin caps or rubber chin slings are used as supportive measures.

Since surgical methods have been perfected, especially that of compression osteosynthesis, conservative measures are used primarily only when good dentition remains. As in the past, such treatment retains its usefulness (*Dingman* and *Natvig*, 1964; *Rowe* and *Killey*, 1968; *Reichenbach*, 1969; *Weiskopf*, 1969; *Kazanjian* and *Converse*, 1959, 1974; *Lentrodt* and *Höltje*, 1975; *Becker* et al., 1976; *Krüger*, 1974; *Neumann-Lezius* and *Utz*, 1976; *Pfeifer* et al., 1975, 1976; *Virolainen* and *Aitasalo*, 1976, *Neuner*, 1977) despite the ever increasing tendency to handle such fractures by functionally stable osteosynthesis (bone plating, lag screws; *Spiessl* and *Schroll*, 1972, 1975; *Niederdellmann* and *Schilli*, 1972, 1973; *Schilli*, 1977).

Among fixation measures in the framework of conservative treatment are the monomaxillary splint in the mandible, and intermaxillary fixation with the aid of bimaxillary splints. In the edentulous or poorly dentate jaw, it is better to use a surgical technique. Combined intraoral and extraoral splints are used rarely. In non-displaced fractures of the mandible, where there is only slight mobility of the ends of the fracture, neither conservative nor surgical fixation measures need be applied.

2.1 Supervised Spontaneous Healing

We know from the course of bone fracture healing that spontaneous bony healing takes place in non-displaced fractures if the fracture ends are immobile or only slightly mobile against each other. This holds true for all infractions and fissures, as well as for a large proportion of greenstick fractures; it also occurs occasionally with complete fractures, most frequently here in fractures in the angle of the mandible (*Reichenbach*, 1957) and very rarely in fractures of the body and the ramus of the mandible. *Ganzer* (1943) strongly emphasized the possibility of spontaneous healing in his monograph "War Injuries of the Face and the Facial Skull": "It is quite surprising and accorded far too little consideration, how much nature is capable of achieving when it is simply left alone." With the help of clinical examples, he documents that healing and regeneration processes that go far toward re-establishing the original form are possible, even with gunshot fractures of the mandible, without fixation.

The **indication** for omitting fixation is a closed, only slightly displaced fracture with only slight fragment mobility and no existing occlusal disturbance. This is valid both for the dentulous and edentulous jaw (Fig. 8.2-1 and 8.2-2). With fractures inside the dental arch, there is usually a connection to the oral cavity through the periodontal pocket of the tooth in the fracture line. Still, there are even cases here in which the injury to the gingival margin is so minimal that immobilization can be omitted if the other prerequisites are present (Fig. 8.2-3).

Therapy consists exclusively of avoiding intense stress on the fracture. During the first two weeks, the patient should ingest only fluid nutrients and broths, slowly switching to normal fare after this period. The patient must be supervised on an out-patient basis until bony consolidation has appeared; this usually occurs after four to six weeks. The occlusion and the mobility of the fragments should be checked in weekly or biweekly follow-up examinations. The doctor also should be on guard against possible infections. If greater fragment mobility, occlusal disturbances or inflammatory reactions appear during the observation period, splint fixation should be undertaken immediately.

Fractures of the coronoid process require no therapy (*Dingman* and *Natvig*, 1964; *Rowe* and

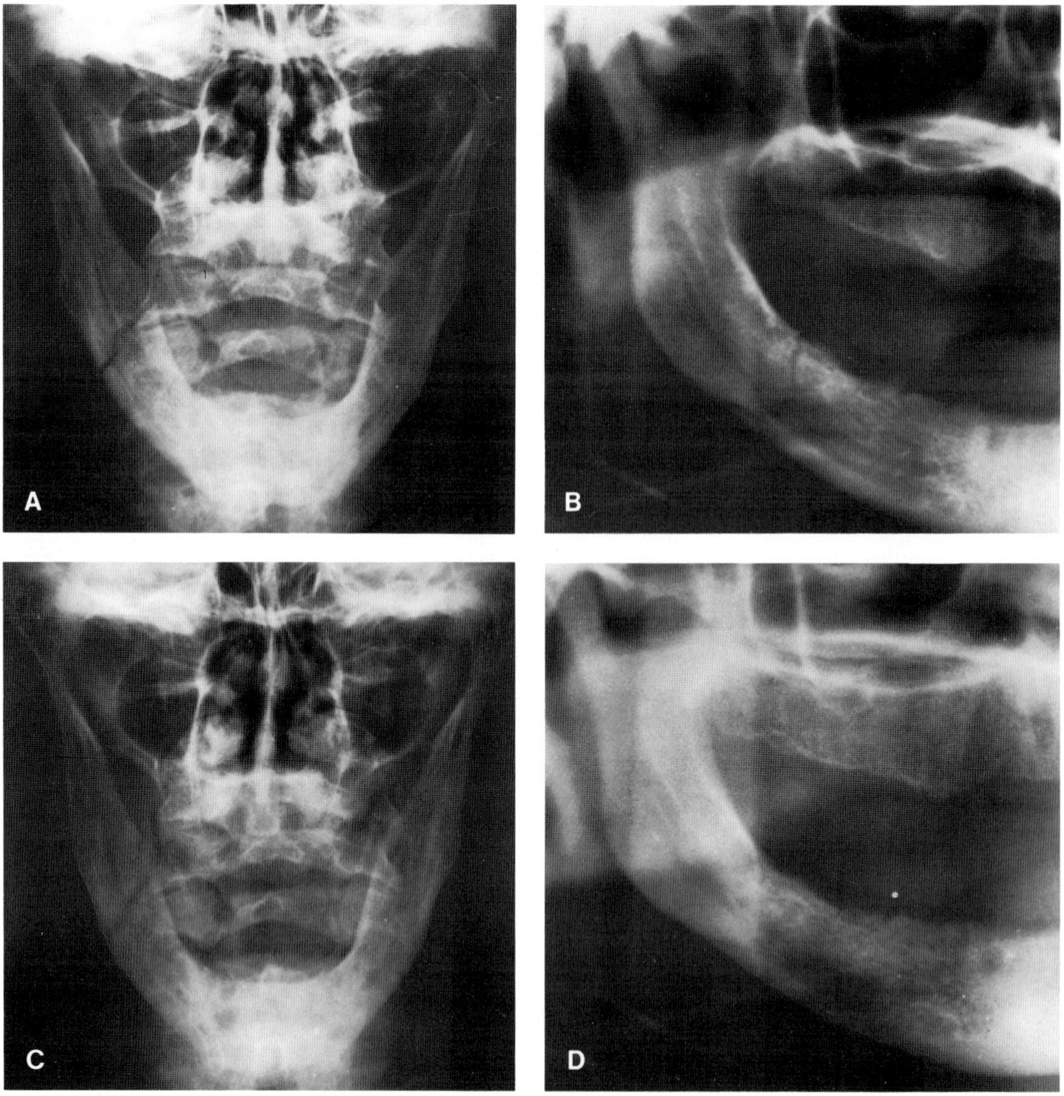

Figs. 8.2-1 A to D Controlled spontaneous healing of an undisplaced fracture of the right side of the mandible in an edentulous woman.

Figs. 8.2-1 A and B Radiographs of the fresh fracture. No attempt was made at immobilization. The patient was told to wear her dentures day and night and to take only liquid nutrients at first.

Figs. 8.2-1 C and D Radiographs after 8 months.

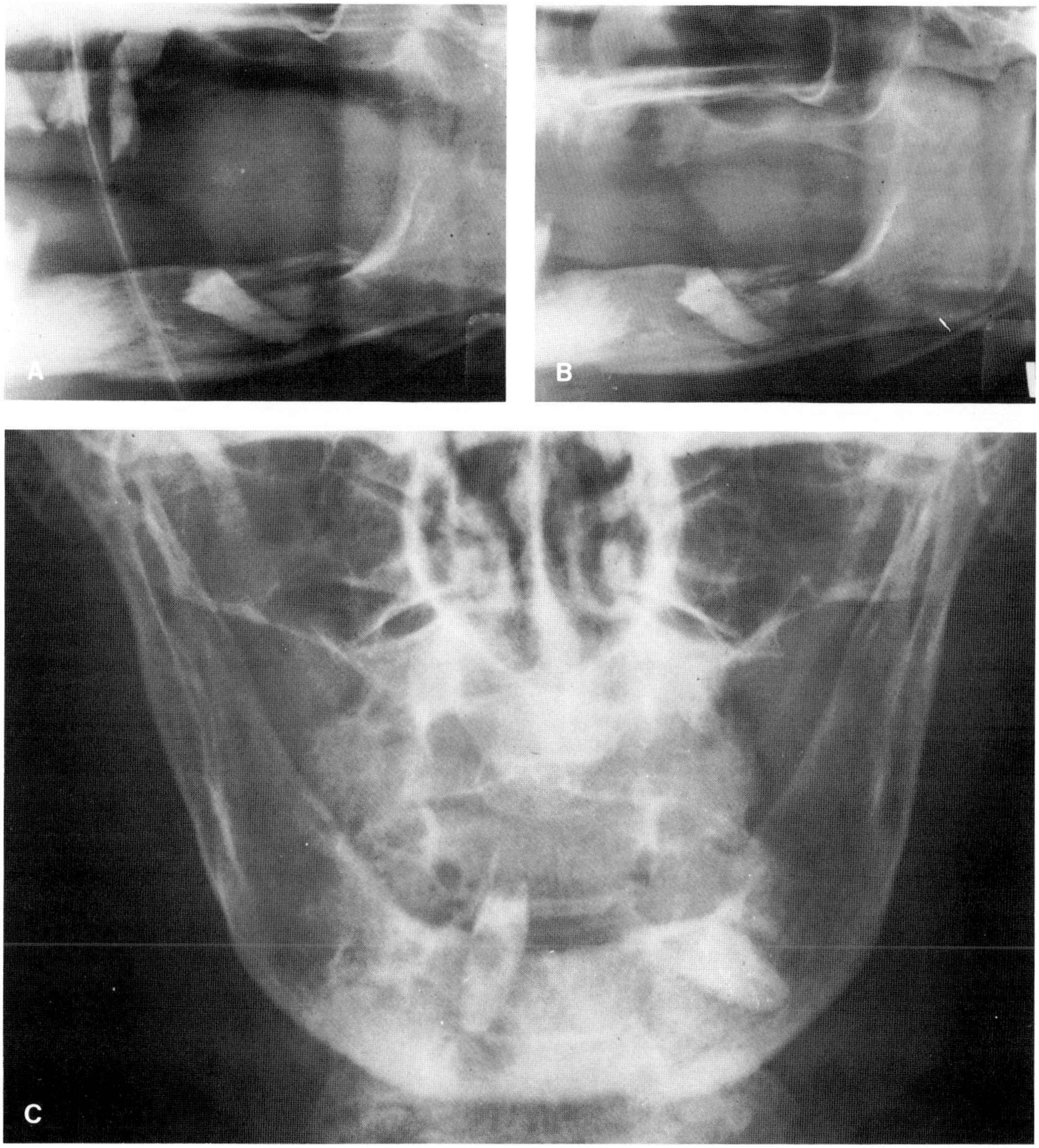

Figs. 8.2-2 A to C Controlled spontaneous healing of a slightly displaced oblique fracture of the left side of the mandible in the region of an impacted premolar.

Fig. 8.2-2 A Radiograph of the fresh fracture. The impacted premolar lies in the fracture line. There was no injury to the covering mucosa. The obliquely running fracture line provides broad adjacent surfaces for the fragments; therefore it was decided to dispense with immobilization. The course of bone healing was permitted to run without interference.

Figs. 8.2-2 B and C Radiographs prepared two months later. The fracture site was rigidly consolidated. The impacted premolar was removed surgically before new dentures were inserted.

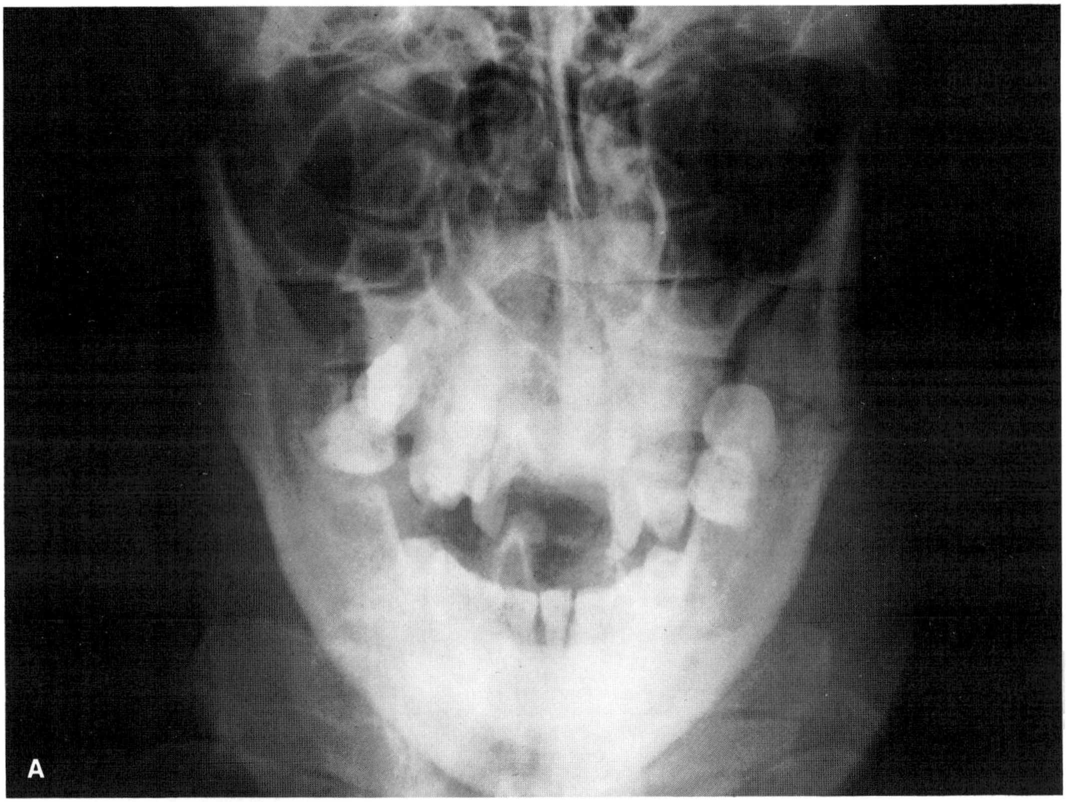

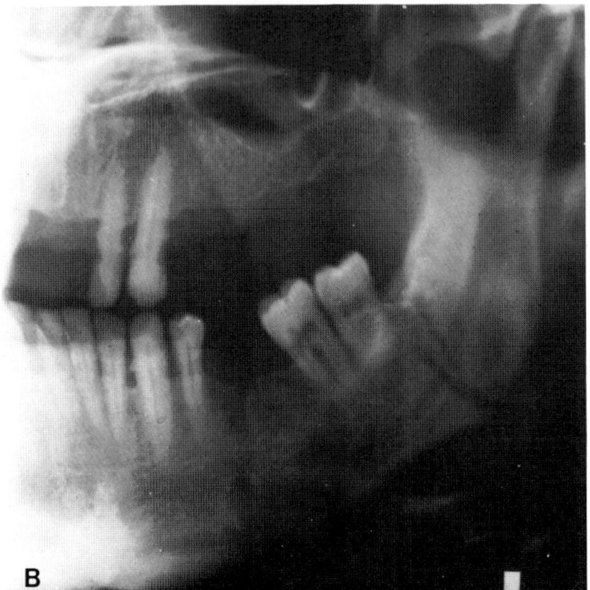

Figs. 8.2-3 A and B Non-displaced fracture in the region of the angle of the mandible in a partially edentulous dentition. There was no disturbance of occlusion. No immobilization was attempted. The patient continued to wear his partial denture and took only a soft diet at first. Bone healing was undisturbed.

Killey, 1968; *Weiskopf*, 1969). Often without any special measures, a fibrous fixation of the fracture ends ensues, through which, furthermore, the temporalis muscle can have an effect on the mandible. In other cases, the small fragment is pulled upward by muscle traction. The non-functioning of the temporalis muscle which results from this has proven to be of little importance. Any simultaneous mandibular or malar bone fractures must, however, be treated (*Weiskopf*, 1969; *Spiessl* and *Schroll*, 1972).

2.2 Monomaxillary Fixation

With fractures within the dental arch, the fragments can be stabilized, in cases with a favorable position, by a monomaxillary appliance fastened to the teeth. In the course of this, the mandible remains mobile as a whole so that masticatory function is maintained. Assuming that the splint does largely eliminate interfragmentary mobility, the immediate functional stress leads to static bony healing which is significantly faster (*Schrudde*, 1960; *Weiskopf*, 1969). Furthermore, retaining masticatory function constitutes a significant advantage over intermaxillary fixation for the patient.

The **indication** for monomaxillary fixation exists where there is sufficient dentition with a non- or slightly displaced and easily reduceable fracture in the chin region of the mandible (*Wassmund*, 1927; *Weiskopf*, 1969; *Kazanjian* and *Converse*, 1974; *Neuner*, 1977). *Dingman* and *Natvig* (1964) believe that monomaxillary fixation should be used only in exceptional cases, and prefer to treat most fractures within the dental arch with intermaxillary fixation. *Reichenbach* (1957) and *Krüger* (1974) limit the procedure to fractures in the anterior region while *Spiessl* and *Schroll* (1972) also include the premolar region.

The **technique** is determined by the requirement of sufficient stability in the splint and immediate manual reduction of the fragments. The reduction must be undertaken when the splint is applied. Fractures which cannot be easily reduced by hand require a bimaxillary appliance with intermaxillary rubber bands. *Thoma* (1958) recommends horizontal wiring according to *Risdon* (1929) for monomaxillary fixation. The use of this sort of horizontal fixation is inadvisable, because it is not stable enough to prevent interfragmentary movement without additional intermaxillary fixation. Similarly, none of the arch bars of the Jelenko, Winter, Erich, or Niro types possesses sufficient stability, and thus they should not be considered for monomaxillary fixation. The devices named have the further disadvantage of being injurious to the periodontal margin. The ligatures have a tendency, when being tightened, to turn in a gingival direction and to pull the arch bar to the gingiva. Intermaxillary fixation counteracts this tendency and thus these devices could be used for intermaxilary fixation, even though they are not suited for a monomaxillary one.

Before any splinting, the teeth must be repeatedly rinsed with a fluoride preparation to protect against demineralization processes and caries. This is particularly important when cold-curing acrylic is used to stabilize the arch bar (*Krüger* and *Chrissafis*, 1971).

The technique is determined primarily by the type of splint used. **The direct methods** which are considered for monomaxillary fixation are:

1. The wire-acrylic arch bar (*Schuchardt*, 1956, 1966)
2. The banded dental arch wire appliance (*Angle*, 1890; *Schröder*, 1971)

Usually a local anesthetic is administered for reduction of the fracture and applying the splint; if the displacement of the fragments is only minor, this may be omitted.

The wire-acrylic arch bar (*Schuchardt*, 1956, 1966; *Metz*, 1966) is made from a half-round soft stainless steel arch wire with cross-wires soldered to it*. The fixation ensues through individual ligatures for each tooth and application of cold-curing acrylic. The arch wire is adapted to the dental arch and the occlusal ends of the cross-wires are curved over the occlusal surface of the teeth. Thus, the bar is supported occlusally and cannot slip in a gingival direction when the ligature wires are tightened. This offers a decisive advantage over the Jelenko, Winter, Erich, and Niro type arch bars.

Ligature wires (soft, stainless steel 0.35 mm

* Manufacturer: Renfert, D-7700 Singen/Hohentwiel, Germany

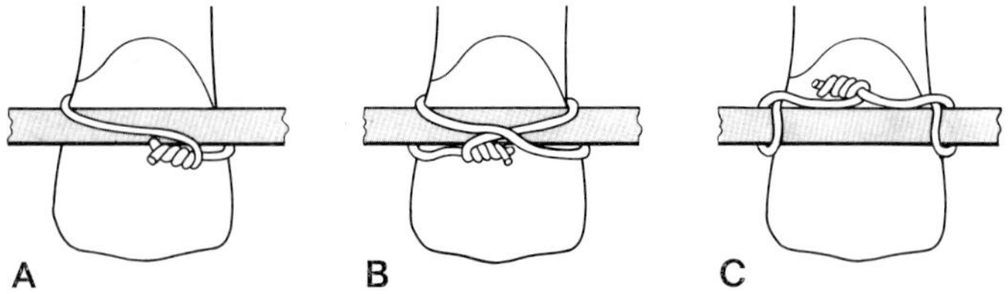

Figs. 8.2-4 A to C Various ligatures for the fixation of an arch bar.
Fig. 8.2-4 A Simple ligature.
Fig. 8.2-4 B Cross ligature.
Fig. 8.2-4 C Double ligature.

wires) are placed around the individual teeth. We use a ligature forceps designed by Korkhaus (Fig. 8.2-5 A) for this; alternatively, a needle-holder with a catch or a Pean hemostat could be used. The individual wires are cut to appropriate lenghts. One wire end is gripped by the ligature forceps and pulled in a lingual direction from the vestibule through the interdental space and subsequently led back through the neighboring interdental space from the lingual to the vestibular side. The ends of the wire then can be twisted together over the arch bar. It is best if all the ligature wires are first applied without the arch bar. The distal ends of the individual ligature wires are bent downward and the mesial ends are bent upward (Fig. 8.2-5 B). Only then is the arch wire positioned and fixed in place by twisting the pairs of wire ends. The distal end of a ligature wire is then situated gingivally the bar and the mesial end coronally (Fig. 8.2-5 C).
Another procedure is also possible: the arch bar can be fixed initially on each side with one ligature wire over the first premolar; every other ligature wire can then be applied individually and immediately twisted over the bar. This method of application requires more time.
Care must be taken when twisting the wires, that this is done only in one direction, e.g. clockwise, to avoid confusion when it is necessary to give the wires a few more turns for the final fixation. Twisting in one direction and then in the other increases the danger of breakage.
The simple ligature (Fig. 8.2-4 A) described above is usually sufficient, in the completely dentulous jaw, for complication-free fixation of the arch bar. With conically shaped teeth which have no points of contact with neighboring teeth, these ligature wires occasionally will slip off. In such cases, it is better to apply cross-ligatures (Fig. 8.2-4 B) or double ligatures (Fig. 8.2-4 C); in contrast to the simple ligatures, these have no orthodontic effects.
After all the ligature wires have been loosely twisted together, the ends of the fracture are reduced approximately by hand. The occlusion cannot be adjusted yet because the occlusal wires usually prevent it. The ligature wires are now tightened firmly. The twisted ends are shortened with a wire cutter to a length of 4 to 5 mm and adapted to the arch bar with a forceps (Fig. 8.2-5 C). Before the cold-curing acrylic is applied, the teeth are thoroughly rinsed with amine fluoride solution. The arch bar and the teeth should be dried and then the fluoride preparation applied. After about 2 minutes of effective time and further drying, another coating of amine fluoride is applied. This process should be repeated several times. The teeth and the arch bar should be treated once a week with amine fluoride during the entire duration of therapy. This is the only way demineralization of the enamel can be avoided while the appliance is in position (*Krüger* and *Chrissafis*, 1971).
Finally, the cold-curing acrylic is applied; this embeds the ends of the ligature wires and should also occupy the interdental spaces. Thus, undercuts present in the dental arch are used for retention of the arch bar. The acrylic coat must not be too voluminous; it should just embed the ends of the ligature wires and adjoin the vestibular coronal surfaces of the teeth to the width of the arch bar. The gingiva must always be left uncovered. No acrylic should be applied on either side of the fracture to the width of about two to three teeth, so that the arch wire can

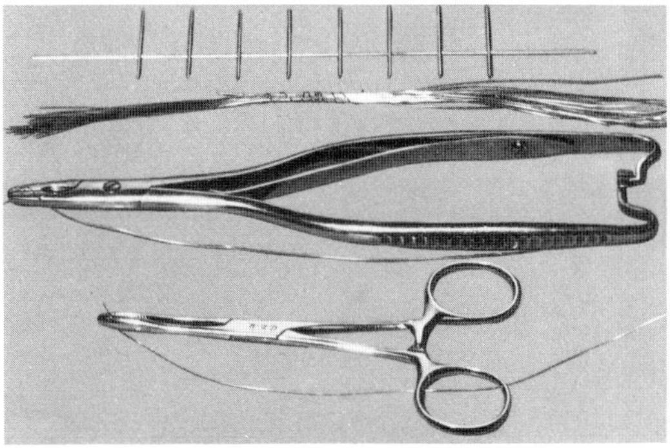

Figs. 8.2-5 A to E Placement of a wire-acrylic arch bar in the mandible.

Fig. 8.2-5 A Instruments: Top – arch wire and ligature wires; center – Korkhaus ligature forceps with ligature wires; bottom – Pean hemostat with ligature wire.

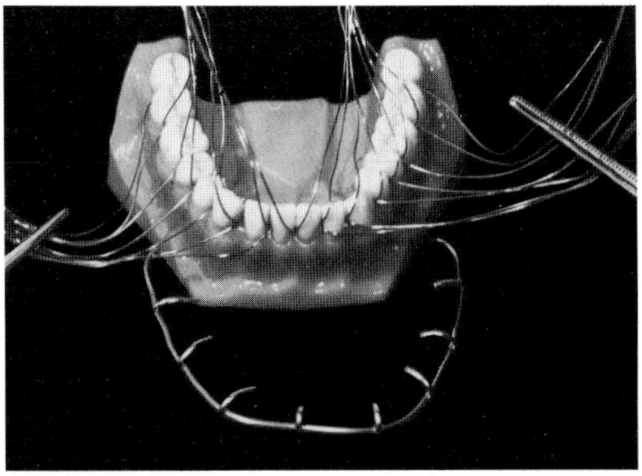

Fig. 8.2-5 B The ligature wires have been placed; the distal ends of the wires are bent down and the mesial ends are bent up and twisted with hemostats. The arch wire is at the front.

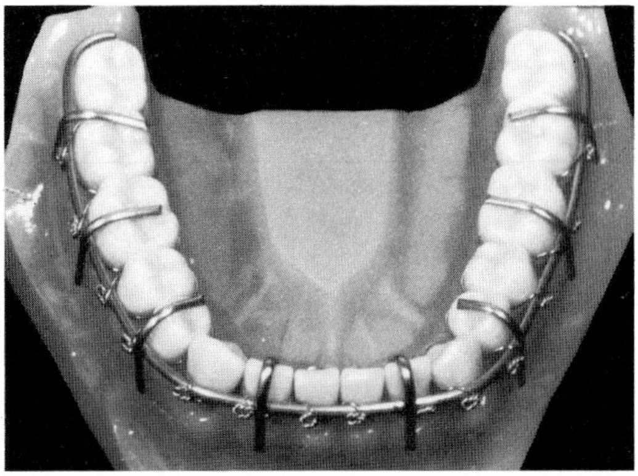

Fig. 8.2-5 C The arch bar bound with the ligature wires. The occlusal rests of the cross wires prevent sliding of the arch bar to the gingival margin when the ligatures are tightened.

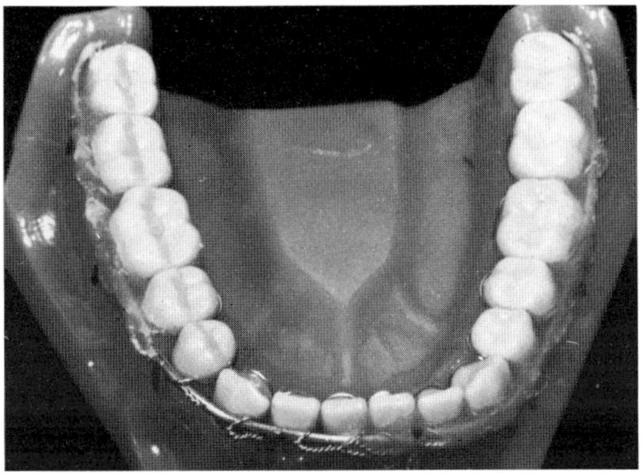

Fig. 8.2-5 D The arch bar is coated with cold-curing acrylic. The fracture site at 43 was spared to simplify reduction. The occlusal rests of the cross wires were removed.

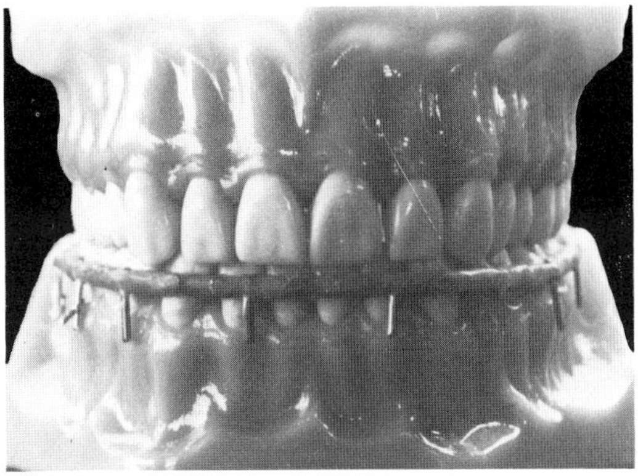

Fig. 8.2-5 E Following reduction of the fracture ends by adjustment of centric occlusion, the fracture site section of the arch bar also was coated with cold-curing acrylic. The gingival hooks of the arch bar may be used for fixation of the mandible in occlusion if corresponding wires are placed in the maxilla; such ligatures are not required for monomaxillary fixation.

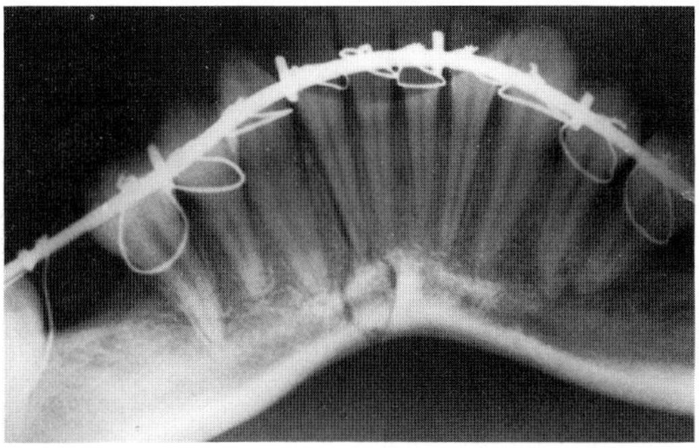

Fig. 8.2-6 A Monomaxillary fixation of a mandibular fracture at 43 with a wire-acrylic arch bar.

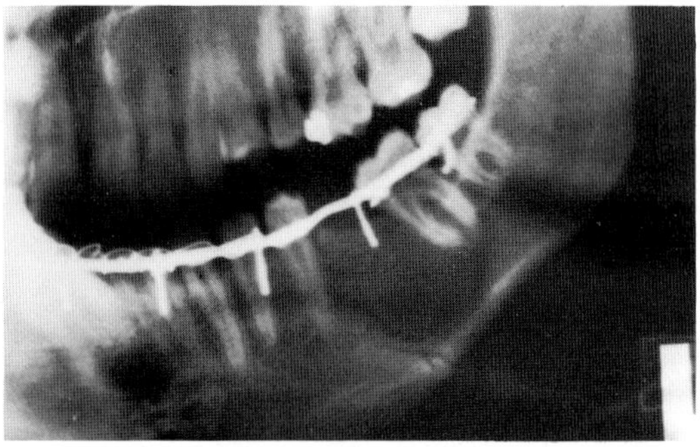

Fig. 8.2-6 B Monomaxillary fixation of a mandibular fracture at 35 with a wire-acrylic arch bar.

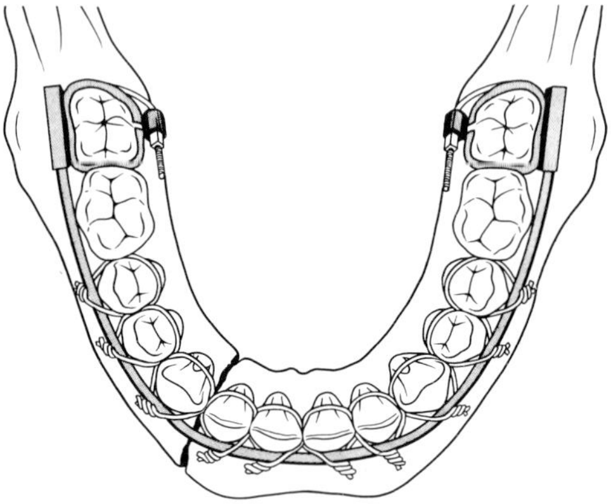

Fig. 8.2-7 Angle's banded arch wire appliance.

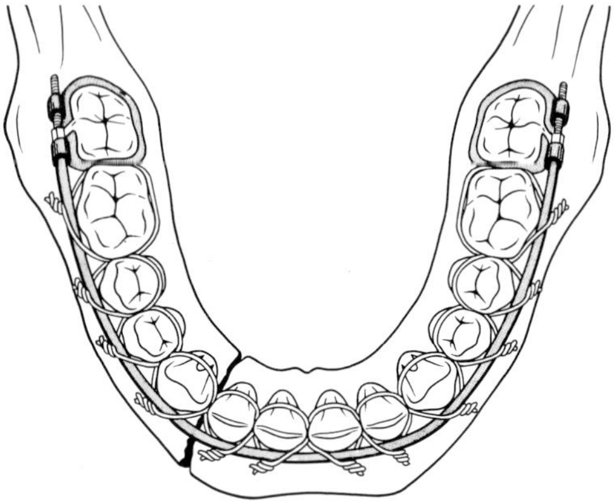

Fig. 8.2-8 Schröder's banded dental arch wire appliance.

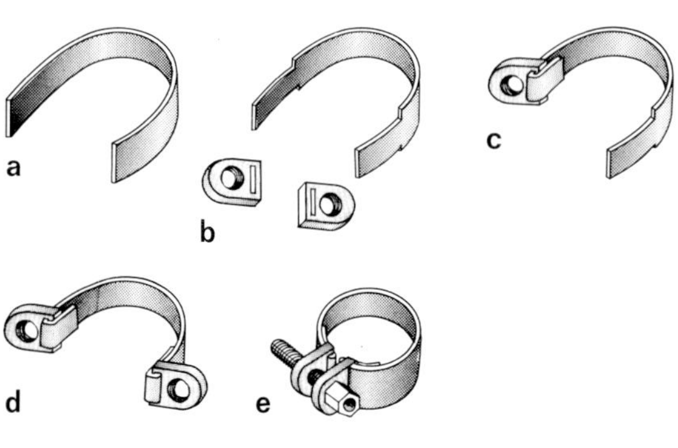

Fig. 8.2-9 Schlampp's modification of the Schröder band.
a) Band strip, 10 mm longer than the tooth circumference.
b) Band ends cut lash-like; ring with a screw-thread and holding ring without a thread.
c) The ring with a screw-thread is put on; the lash is bent inward.
d) Both rings are in place.
e) Completed screw band with bolt, in the head of which a channel has been engraved to take up the arch bar.

remain somewhat flexible for finer adjustment of the occlusion. When the plastic hardens, the splint retains enough stability so that the occlusal ends of the cross-wires can be cut off (Fig. 8.2-5 D). The gingival ends are not needed in the monomaxillary fixation, but can support intermaxillary rubber bands or wires.

After this, the occlusion can be adjusted to centric. An assistant presses the mandible firmly against the maxilla while the surgeon performs the final tightening of the ligatures adjacent to the fracture and then covers this part too with cold-curing acrylic (Fig. 8.2-5 D and Figs. 8.2-6 A and B).

To remove the splint after treatment is completed, the plastic coat is broken off piece by piece with forceps until the ends of the wires are exposed. These are then gripped by a ligature forceps, twisted open, cut through, and removed. Then the arch bar can be lifted off easily.

The **banded dental arch wire appliance** (*Angle*, 1890; *Schroeder*, 1911) developed from Angle's orthodontic apparatus. A previously prepared band, which is held with the help of a nut and bolt and which includes a channel to receive an arch bar, is applied to the last molar on each side. The two bands on the ends of the rows of teeth are connected with each other by an arch bar inserted into the channel. *Angle*'s band has the screw apparatus on the lingual and the channel on the buccal side (Fig. 8.2-7); the *Schröder* band has both the srew apparatus and the channel on the buccal side (Fig. 8.2-8). Before the bands are applied, molars which are in contact with their neighbors must be separated. The point of contact is encircled by a tight loop of wire; after 30 to 60 minutes, the interdental space is expanded enough for the band to be applied. The bands are contoured in such a fashion that they do not interfere with occlusion.

In 1944, *Schlampp* modified and dismantled the *Schröder* band in such a manner that it could be simply manufactured from a single band strip; thus, an extensive inventory of various size bands was no longer necesary. Other things needed in addition to the strip are a ring with a screw-thread, a holding ring without a thread, and a bolt with a thread on one end and a channel opening on the other. The width of the steel band used is 5 mm and the thickness of the band generally can be selected so that the teeth do not need to be separated. After the circumference of the tooth has been measured, a band 10 mm longer is cut. The ends are cut in a lappet fashion over a length of 7 mm, so that the eyelet-equipped rings can be pushed on. Care must be exercised here that the final position of the unthreaded holding ring is a mesial one and that of the ring with the thread is distal. The rings are mounted by bending back the ends of the lappets to the inside. The bolt can then be screwed in, whereby the crown band closes itself (Fig. 8.2-9).

Before screwing the band tight, the arch bar is fitted and inserted into the channels on both sides. The bands are then aligned in such a manner that the bar closely adjoins the dental arch. The arch bar is then stabilized by tightening the screw firmly and subsequently attaching it to the teeth with ligature wires. If the arch wire shows a tendency to slip gingivally when the ligatures in the anterior region are tightened, it is either fixed by an additional anterior band or a cross ligature is applied over the masticatory surfaces of each of the first premolars or the canines. These ligatures can be removed again in most cases after final fixation of the arch bar.

The stability of the device can be increased even more if the twisted ends of the ligatures wires are coated, following the suggestion of *Schuchardt* (1956), with cold-curing acrylic; the acrylic should also occupy the interdental spaces, without, however, touching the gingival margin (see above). By using the undercuts of the dental arch, the splint acquires additional rigidity. The cross-ligatures applied over the occlusal surfaces to avoid gingival slipping can be removed afterward.

After one of the devices described has been applied, the stability must be checked manually. An effort is made to shift the fragments in relation to each other. If there is still mobility, then the appliance is not stable enough and intermaxillary fixation is necessary. The same is true if occlusion and articulation are not trouble-free. The patient must be able to bring the teeth together in centric occlusion and perform masticatory movements without visible shifting of the fragments.

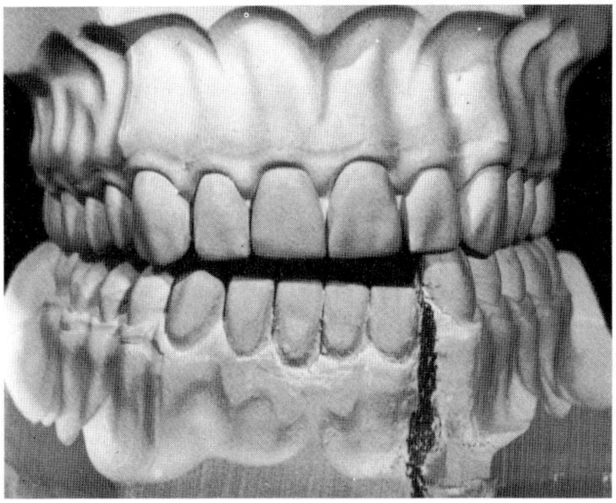

Figs. 8.2-10 A to E Suersen model operation for reduction of fragments in displaced fractures of the mandible.

Fig. 8.2-10 A Occlusal disturbance in a displaced fracture of the mandible between 32 and 33.

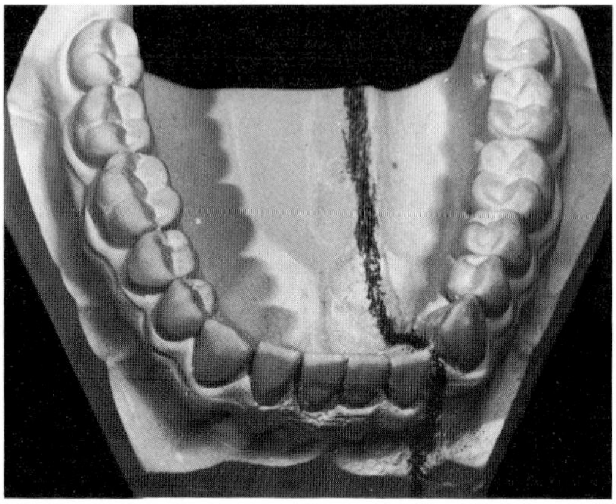

Fig. 8.2-10 B The fracture site has been drawn on the model.

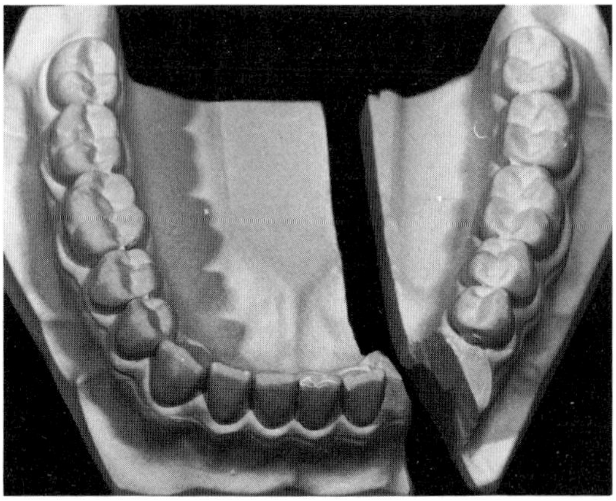

Fig. 8.2-10 C The mandibular model is sawn through at the fracture site. Tooth 3 3, in the fracture line, has been eliminated from the model.

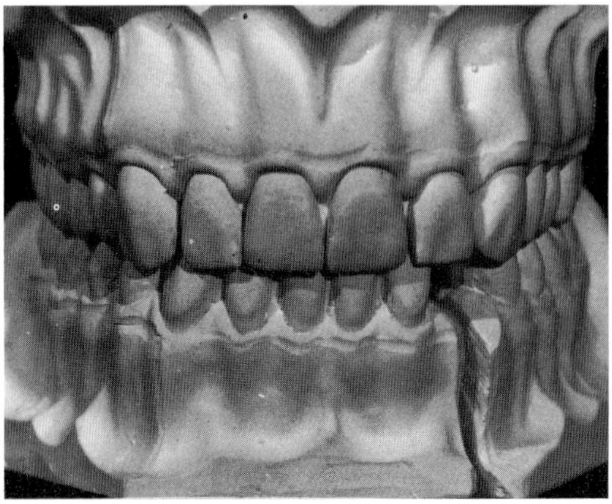

Fig. 8.2-10 D The model parts in proper occlusion.

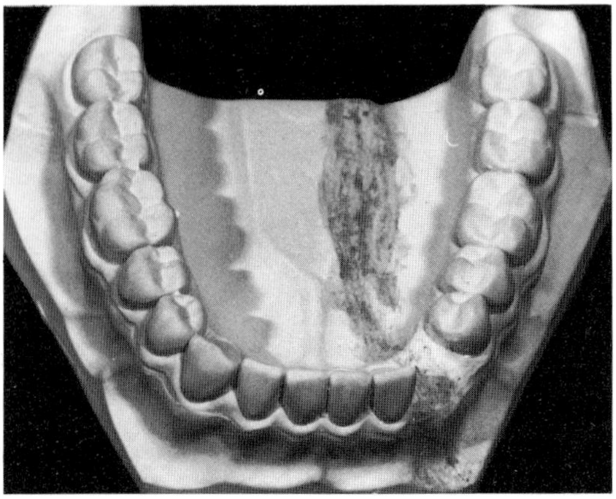

Fig. 8.2-10 E The joined model parts in proper position now may be used for the production of a splint.

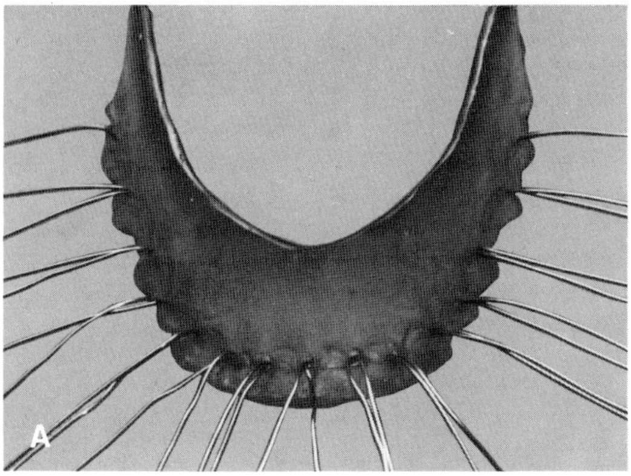

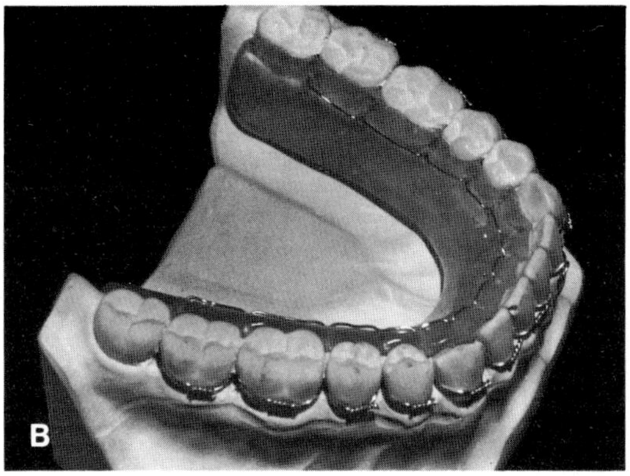

Figs. 8.2-11 A and B Mandibular lingual splint.

Fig. 8.2-11 A Acrylic plate with holes in the regions of the interdental spaces and wires drawn through. Befor insertion of the splint, the wire ends are drawn through the interdental spaces.

Fig. 8.2-11 B Mandibular lingual splint fastened on the model. The ends of the ligature wires have been twisted together over the buccal surfaces of the teeth.

In the case of an overbite of the upper over the lower anterior teeth, the arch bar must be situated deeply enough so that the occlusion is not disturbed. This is not always possible with a deep bite. In such cases, a lingual splint (see below) sometimes is the only possible solution.

Indirect methods, with the use of devices which are made in the dental laboratory from an impression, also can be used for monomaxillary fixation.

The following methods are considered:

1. Cast acrylic splints
   a) Lingual splint (*Hofer*, 1939)
   b) Sectional splint (*Kersting*, 1904; *Stout*, 1943; *Wirth*, 1955, 1956; *Neuner*, 1957, 1977)
2. Metal splints
   a) Cap splint (*Suersen*, 1871; *Meyer*, 1943, 1952; *Bolle*, 1952; *Rowe* and *Killey*, 1968)
   b) Open cap cplint (*Schröder*, 1911); cast metal splint (*Hering*, 1965; *Weiskopf*, 1969).

When the fragments are displaced, they are reduced as well as possible before the impression is taken. A local anesthetic may be necessary. Usually, the reduction is not so precisely correct that the splint made from the model can be put on without occlusal disturbance. The model thus obtained must, therefore, be corrected in most cases by an operation on the model in the laboratory. An impression from the undamaged maxilla also is necessary for this purpose. The maxillary model then serves as a standard for re-establishing the occlusion. If the maxillary and mandibular models do not fit together exactly, the mandibular model must be sectioned at the fracture site. Both parts should then be brought separately into occlusion with the maxillary model and subsequently connected to each other by casting with plaster. The model thus corrected provides the working basis for producing the splint (*Suersen*, 1871, Fig. 8.2-10).

The mandibular lingual splint (*Hofer*, 1939) is the simplest kind of cast acrylic splint. It adjoins the alveolar process and the dental arch on the lingual side, but leaves the occlusal surfaces free. Fixation ensues with ligature wires on the teeth. With a deep bite, the lingual splint may be the only one permitted by the occlusion. After it is properly positioned, the splint is provided with holes, drilled at each interdental space, through which the ligature wires are pulled.

A local anesthetic may be necessary for putting the splint in place. Before the splint is inserted, the ends of the ligature wires, which were left long, are pulled out from the lingual through the corresponding interdental spaces. By twisting the pairs of wire ends, the splint is firmly drawn on to the dental arch (Fig. 8.2-11). If the model operation was performed exactly, the mandibular fragments should fit into the splint as in a made to-order corset. After all of the ligature wires have been tightened, the occlusion and masticatory function must be sufficiently stabilized and free of problems. In order that the ligature wires do not become loose prematurely, it is recommended that the twisted ends, which are cut off short, be coated with cold-curing acrylic.

Sectional splints consist of lingual and buccal portions which grip the alveolar process and the dental arch on both sides and which are connected to each other in a hinge-like fashion. The buccal splint parts can be folded open; after the splint is positioned, it is closed. Using this principle, undercuts can be used to afford a more secure seat. The splints of *Kersting* (1904) and *Stout* (1943) have a lingual plate and two buccal splint parts which are flexibly connected in each case with the palatal portion, distal to the last tooth. In the middle, both the buccal portions are held together by a screw apparatus or a wire looped around an undercut button (Figs. 8.2-12 and 8.2-13). *Wirth*'s splint (1955, 1956) consists of two lingual and two buccal portions which are held together by continuous interdental wires (Fig. 8.2-14). The *Neuner* splint (1957, 1977) differs from the others in that the buccal bar adjoins only the dental arch and not the alveolar process. As with *Kersting*'s splint, is is locked with a screw. Missing teeth are replaced (Fig. 8.2-15). When the splint is in place, the mandibular fragments are reduced and held in occlusion by an assistant while the surgeon performs the locking. In many cases, a local anesthetic is necessary.

All cast acrylic splints have the disadvantage of allowing food particles and detritus to collect, which can give rise to gingivitis. The *Neuner* splint has an advantage over the others in leaving the gingiva uncovered, at least in the vestibule; it is thus accessible to cleaning efforts. The sectional splints of *Kersting*, *Wirth*, and *Neuner* can be taken off for the purpose of cleaning, but this should not be done, however, if at all avoidable, until two to three weeks have elapsed so that the ends of the fracture are not moved unnecessarily. Contamination of the splint can be avoided through tube feeding. This is usually only possible, however, with in-hospital treatment, and also largely reduces the advantage of omitting the intermaxillary fixation. The preference for the monomaxillary fixation stems, after all, from the fact that the mandible is kept functionally active and the patient can masticate almost normally (as long as he avoids hard foods).

After the final fixation of the splint, the stability should be checked manually in the region of the fracture and masticatory function should be inspected. If the ends of the fracture move visibly during this examination, intermaxillary fixation is necessary.

The **cap splint** (*Suersen*, 1871; *Meyer*, 1943; *Bolle*, 1952, 1954; *Rowe* and *Killey*, 1968) is a cast metal splint which holds each individual tooth with a cap (Fig. 8.2-16). After testing for fit, the splint is secured by cementing it onto the teeth. The advantages which are emphasized here are the great stability and the gentle treatment of the gingival margin (*Meyer*, 1952). The decisive disadvantage, however, is the covering of the occlusal surfaces and the difficulties this raises in occlusal inspection. This cannot be undertaken until after the splint is removed, i.e., after the fragments have consolidated. In such cases, it is not infrequent that correction of occlusion is necessary through grinding or prosthetic measures.

In practice, the models are mounted on an articulator. When there is displacement of the fragments, the model of the mandible must be sectioned. The model parts are then mounted separately (*Suersen*, 1871). If the cap splint is now modelled and mounted with a slight increase in vertical dimension, the disturbance of occlusion which actually results cannot be very significant.

The reduction of the fragments when the splint is put in place is somewhat problematical. In order to reduce the secretion of saliva, a preparatory subcutaneous injection of 0.5 mg atropine is recommended. It is best to press the mandibu-

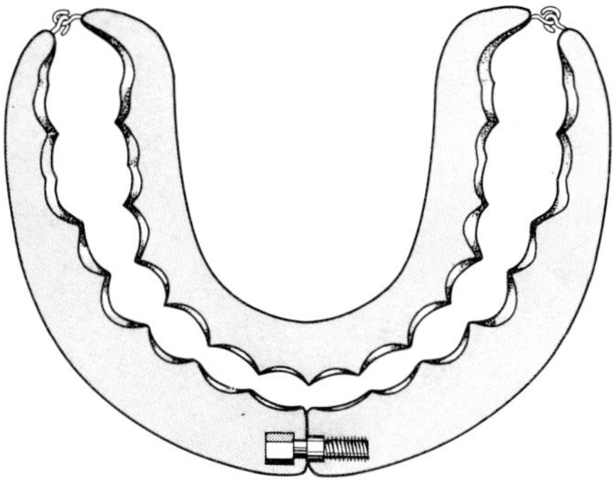

Fig. 8.2-12 Kersting sectional splint. The buccal segments, divided in the center, are connected with the lingual segment by hinges. Following placement of the splint, the buccal segments are held together with a screw connection.

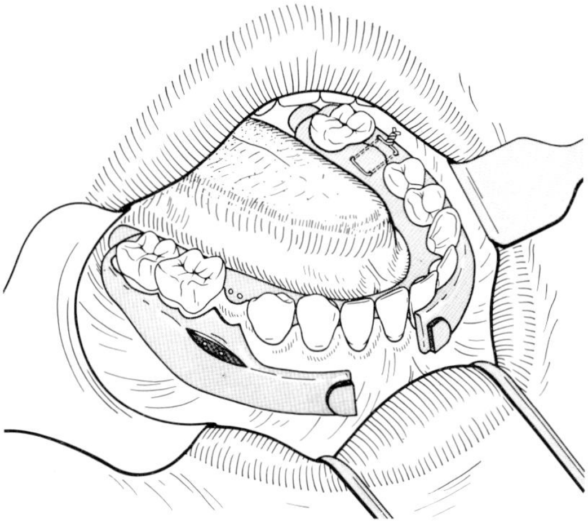

Fig. 8.2-13 Stout sectional splint. The buccal segments are connected to the lingual segment with hinges. In the center the buccal segments are held together with a ligature looped around undercut buttons. In the region of the missing teeth, additional bucco-lingual ligatures are placed; these are drawn through bur holes.

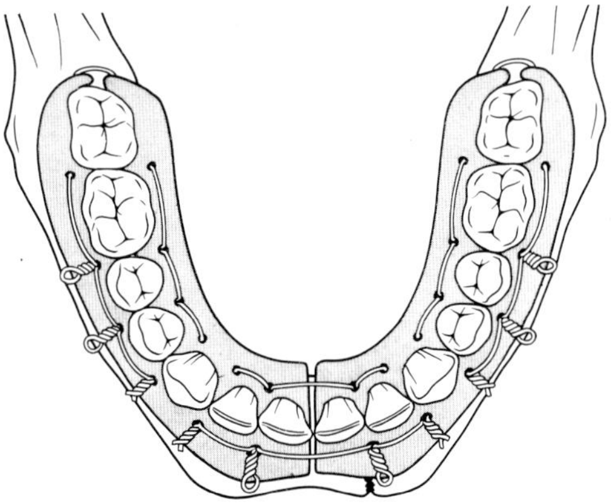

Fig. 8.2-14 Wirth sectional splint. Lingual and buccal segments are separate and are held together by interdental wires.

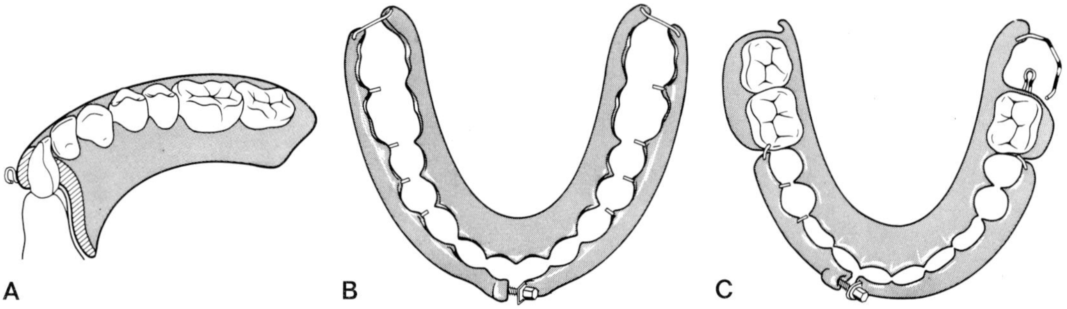

A B C

Figs. 8.2-15 A to C Neuner sectional splint. The vestibular gingiva remains exposed. The buccal parts are held together with a screw. Missing teeth are replaced.

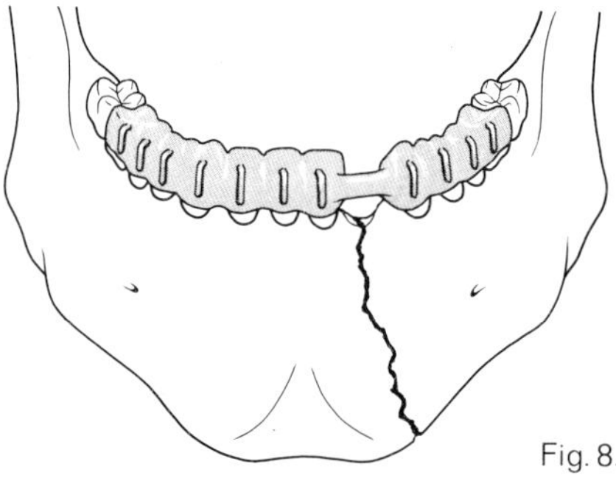

Fig. 8.2-16 Metal cap splint.

Figs. 8.2-17 A to C Rowe and Killey's metal cap splint.

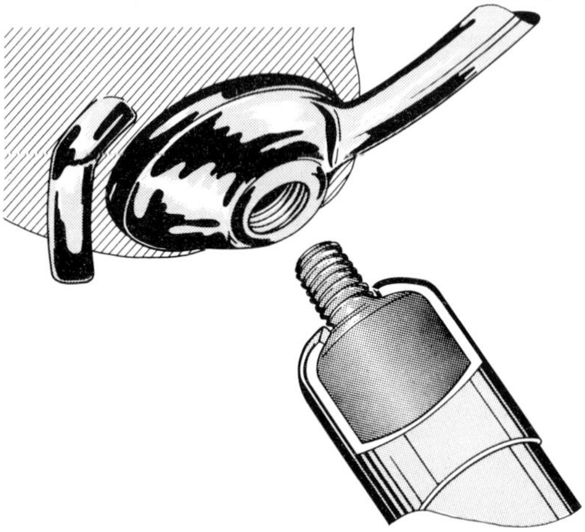

Fig. 8.2-17 A Locking plate with screws.

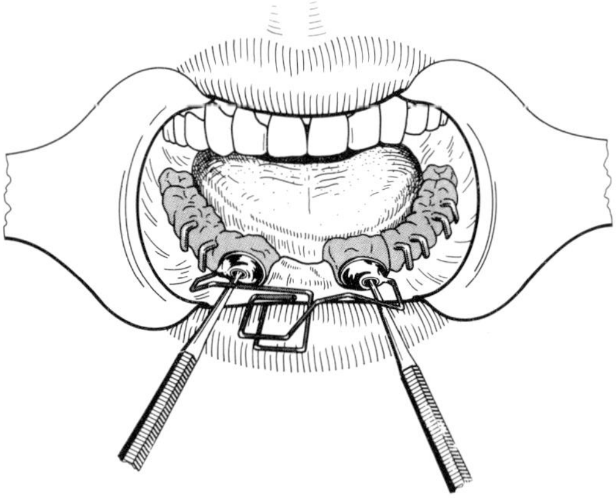

Fig. 8.2-17 B Cap splint components with locking plates to which localizing wires have been soldered. Following placement of the splint parts and reduction of the fragments, the localizing wires are connected with plaster and the locking plates are removed after the screws are loosened. The now correctly related locking plates are attached to each other with a connecting bar in the laboratory and the localizing wires are removed.

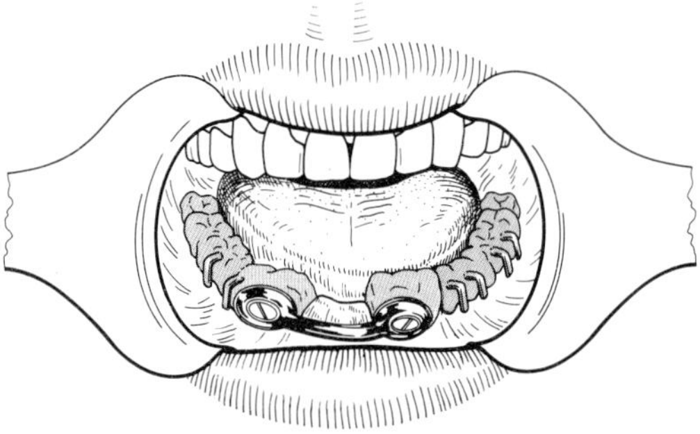

Fig. 8.2-17 C When the locking plates have been screwed in place, the splint components form a single unit with the connecting bar.

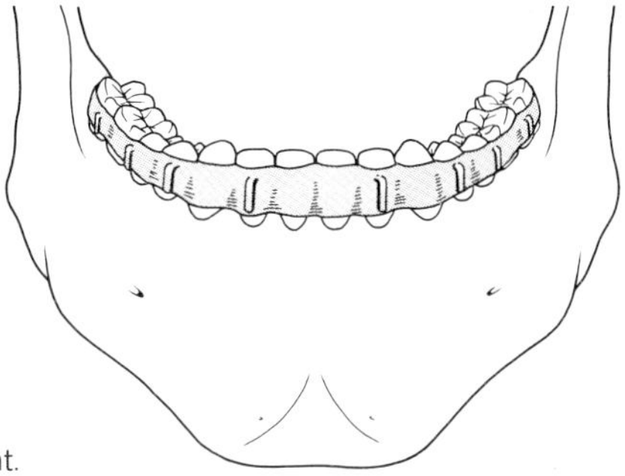

Fig. 8.2-18 Schröder open cap splint.

lar part firmly against the maxilla while the cement or cold-curing acrylic hardens. The cap splint is thereby held as a whole in centric occlusion, while the mandibular fragments are firmly pressed into the splint.

Rowe and *Killey* (1968) undertake the reduction of the fragments in a different manner. The cap splint is separated from the very beginning, and each fragment receives its own splint part. The parts are then connected with each other by a connecting bar with the help of locking plates.* (Fig. 8.2-17 A). A locking plate is fastened to each portion of the splint with a screw. The base for the locking plates must be worked into the wax model for the splint. A thread is cut into the cast splint and localizing wires are soldered to the locking plates with a high fusing silver solder.

Initially, both parts of the cap splint are adjusted and attached with cement. *Bradmun* (1960) recommends thinly mixed cold-curing acrylic for the fixation. In the maxilla, several ligatures are applied (e.g., as described by *Ernst*, 1927, 1932) for temporary intermaxillary fixation. The fragments then are reduced and intermaxillary fixation is established. The tie wires are fastened to the maxillary ligatures on one end and to the small hooks worked into the parts of the splint on the other. Then the locking plates are screwed tight. The localizing wires are led out of the mouth and bent without touching each other to form small squares (Fig. 8.2-17 B). The localizing wires then are connected with each other outside the mouth with plaster. After the screws are loosened, the locking plates, which are now positioned in correct relation to each other, are removed as a block, invested in the laboratory, and firmly connected by a soldered connecting bar. The localizing wires are then removed. The connecting bar is firmly inserted in the mouth through renewed screw fixation of the locking plates, whereby the two splint parts fuse into one unit (Fig. 8.2-17 C). Afterward, the intermaxillary fixation and the ligature wires in the maxilla are removed. A detailed description of this cap splint can be found in *Rowe* and *Killey* (1968).

* Manufacturer: F. H. Baxter, Ltd, Bradford, Yorks, England

The open cap splint (*Schröder*, 1911) leaves the occlusal surfaces exposed (Fig. 8.2-18). Thus, the major disadvantage of the cap splint, the impossibility of occlusal inspection, is eliminated. A disadvantage is the diminished rigidity from the cement or cold-curing acrylic fixation.

At present, **cast metal splints** (*Hering*, 1965, *Weiskopf*, 1969), which are considerably neater than the original open cap splint discussed by *Schröder*, generally are used. The cast metal splint encloses the dental arch with both a continuous lingual and a continuous buccal clasp. If the occlusion permits, the lingual and buccal splint parts are connected with each other via the molar and the premolar interdental spaces. If this is not possible without occlusal disturb-

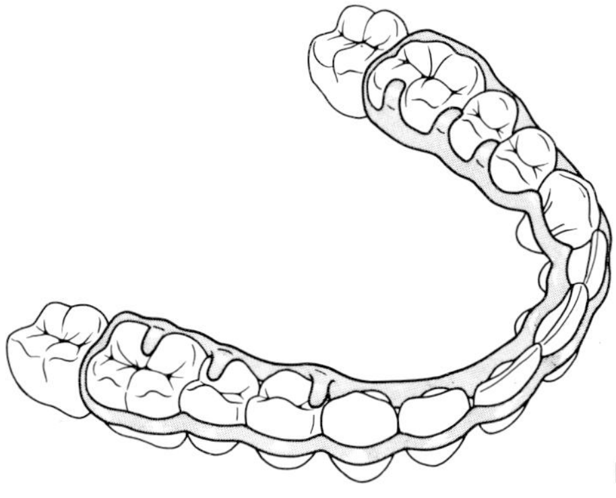

Fig. 8.2-19 Cast metal splint.

ance, small occlusal rests are mounted (Fig. 8. 2-19). Through precise measurement of the master model, it is possible to use undercut sites for retention.

Wire ligatures provide the fixation. These are wrapped around each individual tooth and twisted over the vestibular part of the splint as over an arch bar. In accordance with a suggestion of *Hering* (1965), the ligature wires also can be applied around the contact points of the teeth in the manner of separation ligatures and twisted together in the vestibule over the splint. The splint hold's the teeth together so that no separation occurs. The ligature wires are pulled through the interdental spaces before the splint is put in place. If ordinary interdental wires are used, the distal ends are bent back under and the mesial ends pulled through the corresponding recesses of the splint. If separation ligatures are used, each ligature wire is pulled through only one interdental space; the lingual ends are led out of the mouth upward and the vestibular ends are allowed to hang down.

After the ligature wires have been applied, the splint is put in place with an approximate reduction on the fragments. The ligature wires are twisted together over the buccal part of the splint, but still are not pulled tight. Centric occlusion is adjusted as an assistant presses the mandible firmly against the maxilla while the surgeon tightens the ligature wires. The cut ends are adapted to the buccal part of the splint and should be coated with cold-curing acrylic.

The follow-up treatment consists of keeping the oral cavity clean through careful brushing of the teeth and the splint after every meal. An inspection should be performed by the surgeon once or twice weekly, and the interdental spaces should be cleaned each time with a spray. A weekly rinse with a fluoride preparation is necessary.

After six weeks, the splint usually can be removed. Beforehand, the arch bar should be separated at the fracture site; an inspection should then be made to ascertain whether the ends of the fracture are sufficiently firm. If this is not the case, the arch bar parts are connected again. For this, a wire of the same thickness as the arch bar is laid over the site of the separation and fixed with at least two interdental wires on each side of the fracture. The cut ends of the ligature wires are coated with cold-curing acrylic (see also p. 265 and Figs. 8.2-36 B and C).

Cast acrylic splints and metal splints are removed and replaced if the ends of the fracture are not yet firm enough. After the final removal of the splint, the occlusion should be checked again and adjusted according to gnathological principles.

2.3 Intermaxillary Fixation

Intermaxillary fixation is necessary for all fractures in which no spontaneous healing is to be expected, where there is major displacement,

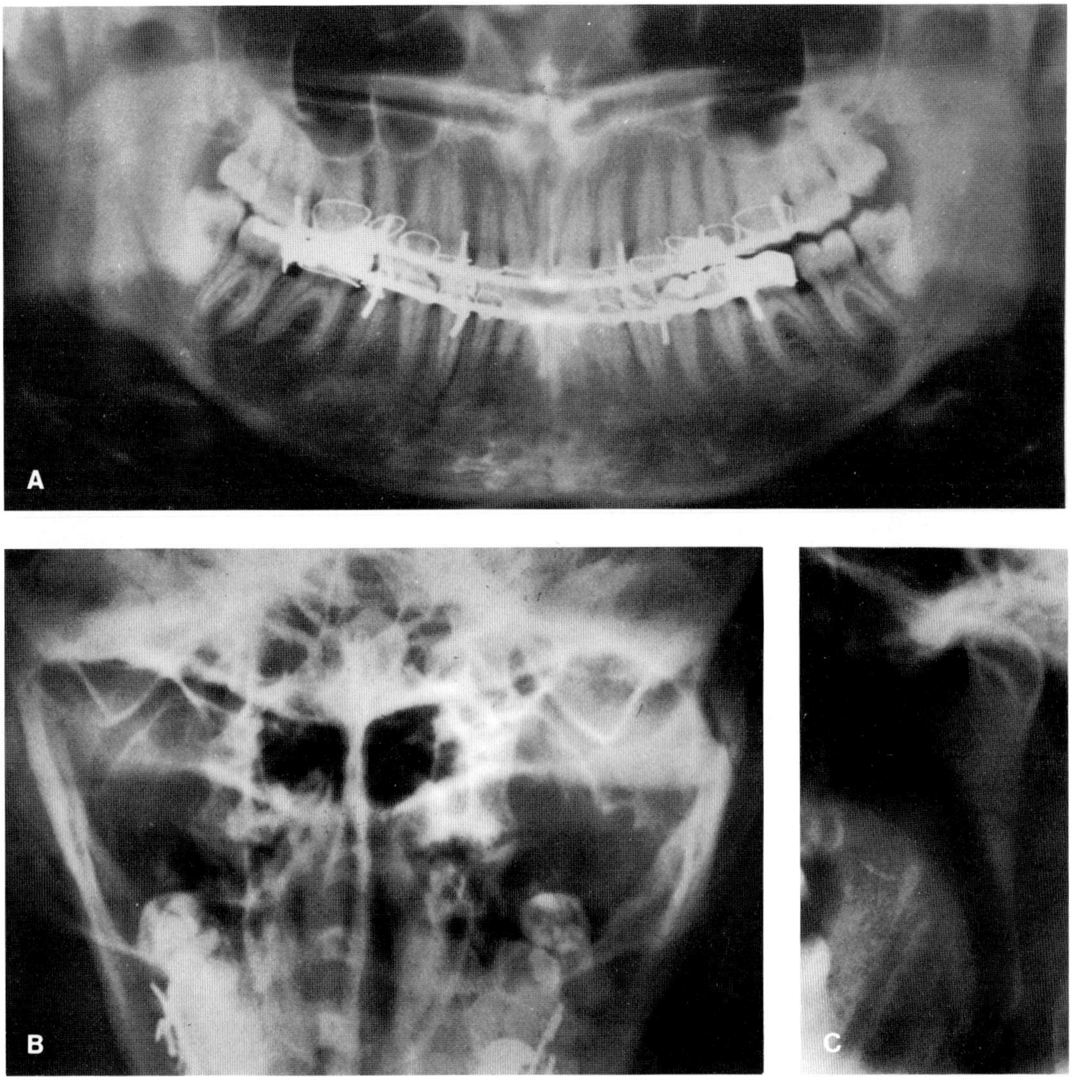

Figs. 8.2-20 A to C Indications for intermaxillary fixation in a fracture of the condylar neck with only slight displacement. Intermaxillary fixation is necessary in order that the good position of the fragments is not worsened by movements of the mandible. In this instance, the only slightly displaced fracture of the mandible cannot be treated by monomaxillary fixation.

Fig. 8.2-20 A Mandibular fracture at 43. Treatment was with wire-acrylic arch bar and intermaxillary fixation.

Figs. 8.2-20 B and C Additional slightly displaced fracture of the neck of the left condyle.

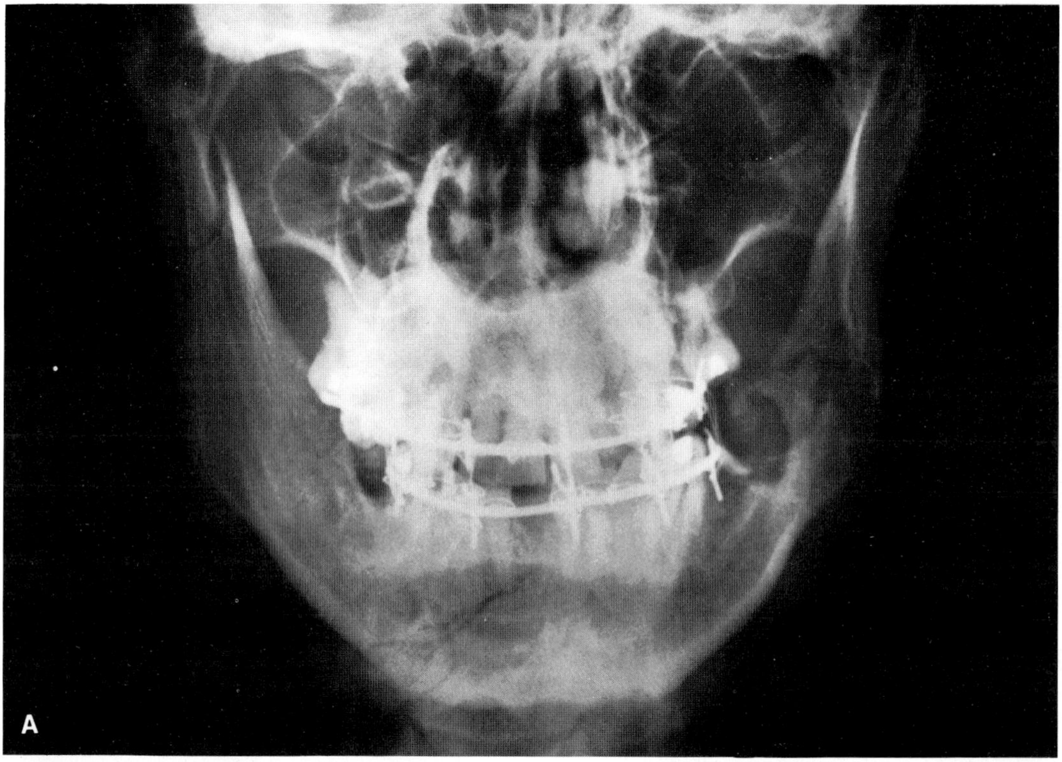

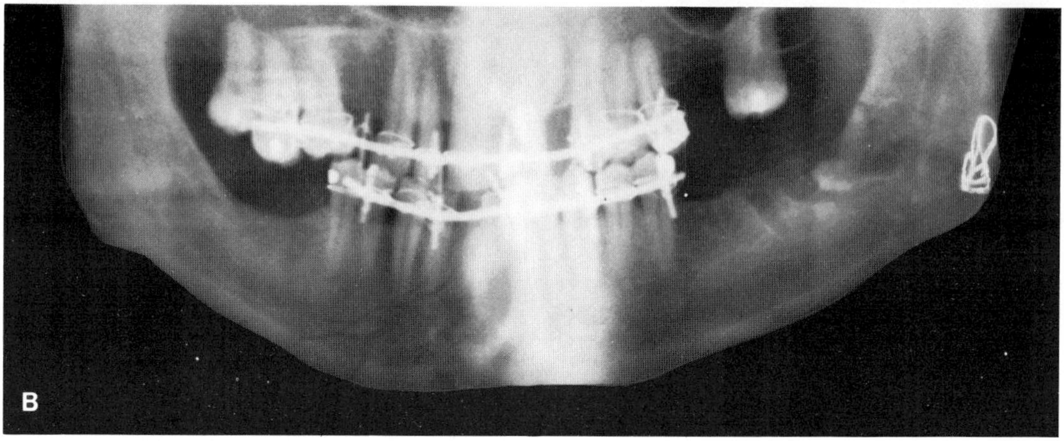

Figs. 8.2-21 A and B Indication for intermaxillary fixation in a non-displaced basal fracture of the right condylar process. In this case, the displaced fracture of the left angle of the mandible was not to be treated by functionally stable osteosynthesis.

Fig. 8.2-21 A A transversal fracture of the right side of the mandible without displacement, displaced fracture in the left angle of the mandible and basal fracture of the right condylar process. Intermaxillary fixation with wire-acrylic arch bar in the maxilla and the mandible.

Fig. 8.2-21 B Appearance following interosseous wiring. Because intermaxillary fixation is necessary for treatment of the joint fracture, there is no indication here for the more difficult compression plate osteosynthesis.

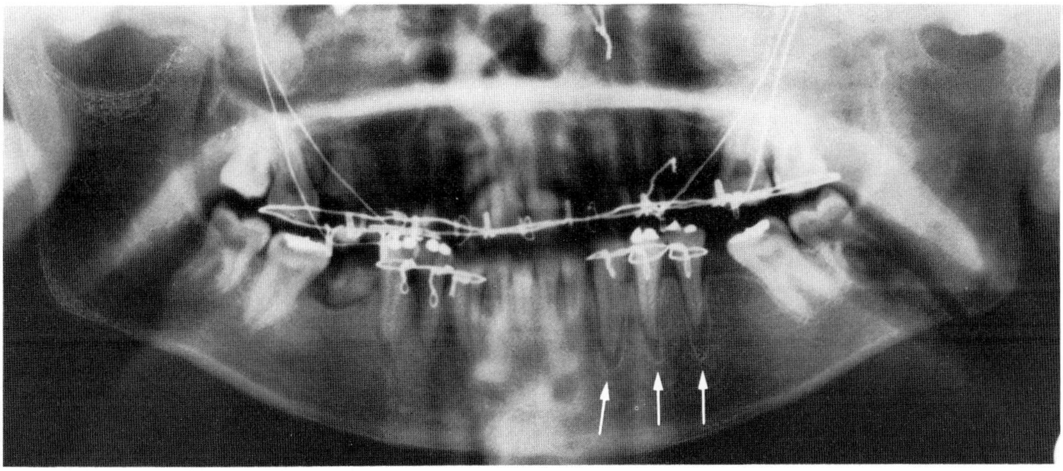

Fig. 8.2-22 Occlusal drift of teeth 33, 34, 35 with mobility after intermaxillary fixation with an insufficient number of ligatures.

where sufficient stability cannot be anticipated with monomaxillary fixation, and where surgical treatment through a functionally stable osteosynthesis is not undertaken. In the general section, we have already referred to the fact that a number of mandibular fractures, particularly those in which the TMJ is not involved, can be treated both conservatively through intermaxillary fixation as well as surgically through functionally stable osteosynthesis. These two methods thus compete in a number of cases. The decision can be left to the patient in this event. With fractures of the mandible in association with fractures of the condylar neck or condyle, which require an early functional treatment, intermaxillary fixation should not be used any more; here functionally stable osteosynthesis is to be preferred. The situation is different with fractures of the condylar neck which are not or only slightly displaced. Such fractures should be immobilized through intermaxillary fixation, because bony healing in the anatomically correct position can ensue here—in contrast to the greatly displaced fractures. If condylar fractures of this sort are combined with mandibular fractures, intermaxillary fixation also is the method of choice for the mandibular fracture (Figs. 8.2-20 and 8.2-21).

Intermaxillary fixation via tooth-supported appliances can be carried out only when sufficient natural teeth remain so that the ligatures may be fastened to them. If an insufficient number of teeth exist, they may loosen and, at worst, the teeth may be extracted with their bound ligatures. If that condition must be considered, it is better to undertake rigid internal fixation with compression plates, or to turn to a zygomatico-maxillary wire suspension of the mandible (see chapter 8.4). Even when there are sufficient remaining teeth, the danger of loosening or extraction must be considered if an insufficient number of these teeth are wired (Fig. 8.2-22). For that reason, one should adopt the rule that wire slings be placed about all of the remaining teeth.

Technique: The intermaxillary fixation can be undertaken rigidly through taut rubber bands (*Wassmund*, 1927; *Reichenbach*, 1954) or tie wires (*Schuchardt* and *Metz*, 1966) or elastically with a few rubber bands (*Kallenberger*, 1956). Usually the immobilization is made rigid for three weeks and elastic for a further three. In some cases, monomaxillary fixation can be instituted after a while. *Juniper* and *Awty* (1973) maintain that three to four weeks of intermaxillary immobilization is sufficient in 82% of the cases; they recommend that the rigidity of the fragments be checked after three weeks of immobilization

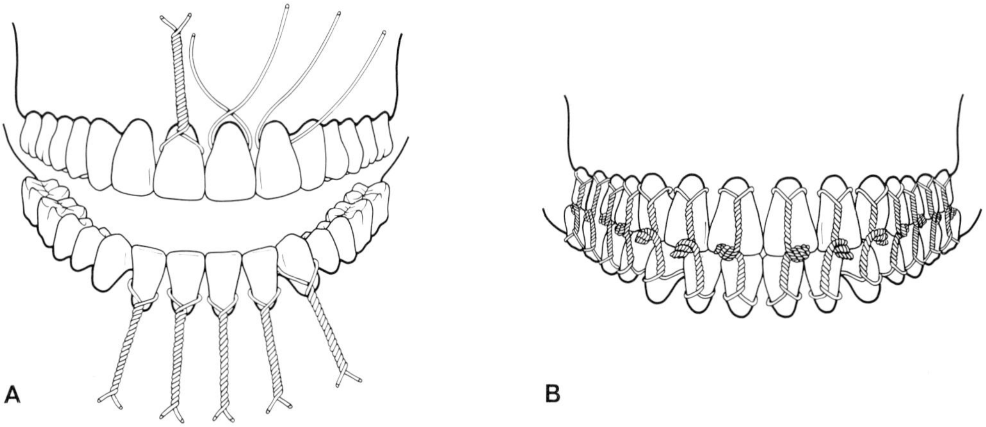

A

B

Figs. 8.2-23 A and B Gilmer's direct interdental wiring.

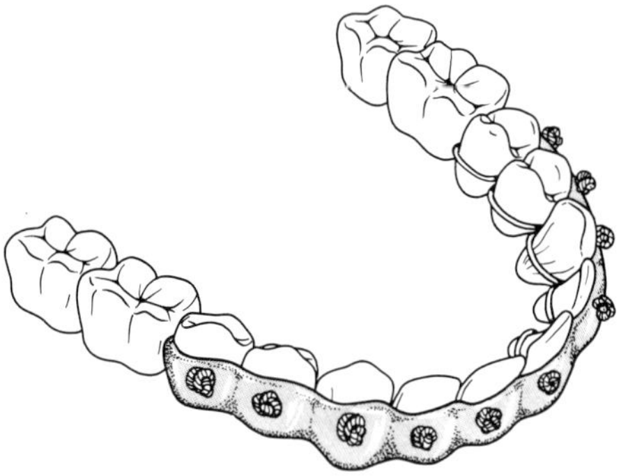

Fig. 8.2-24 Hering's interdental wiring with acrylic vestibular arch. The ligature ends are coated with cold-curing acrylic in the vestibular region. The ends of the ligatures are twisted to rosette shapes.

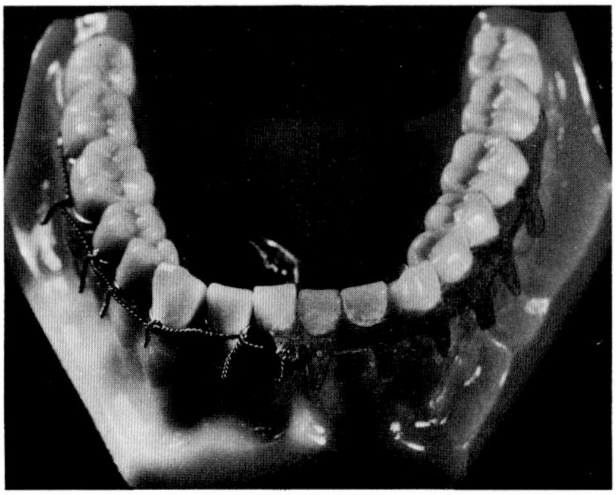

Fig. 8.2-25 Krüger's interdental wiring with acrylic vestibular arch. On the right side, the ligatures drawn to a cable arch wire are seen; on the left, acrylic has been placed.

and that the splint removed if there is consolidation.

Direct methods which are considered for the intermaxillary fixation are:

1. Interdental wiring
   a) Direct interdental wiring (*Gilmer*, 1887)
   b) Continuous or multiple loop wiring (*Stout*, 1943; *Obwegeser*, 1952)
   c) Interdental eyelet wiring (*Eby*, 1920; *Ivy*, 1922)
   d) Cable arch wire (*Risdon*, 1929)
   e) *Ernst*'s wire, (1927, 1932)
   f) *Kazanjian* button (1933)
2. Arch bar wiring
   a) Prefabricated arch bar, Jelenko, Winter, Erich, and Niro types (*Thoma*, 1958; *Kazanjian* and *Converse*, 1959, 1974; *Dingman* and *Natvig*, 1964; *Archer*, 1966; *Rowe* and *Killey*, 1968)
   b) Wire-acrylic arch bar (*Schuchardt*, 1956, 1966)
   c) Banded dental arch wire appliance (*Angle*, 1890; *Schröder*, 1917).

Interdental wiring is relatively easy to perform. Wire ligatures are applied in the maxilla and mandible, these are connected either directly by twisting the upper and lower wires ends together or with intermaxillary tie wires. The immediate reduction of the fragments is undertaken before the intermaxillary fixation after all the wire ligatures are applied and, if necessary, after the tooth in the fracture line has been extracted. Similarly, progressive reduction with rigid rubber bands is possible. The final fixation in centric occlusion should, however, ensue with tie wires. This method is not suited to an elastic intermaxillary fixation of mandibular fractures within the dental arch because the stability is insufficient in a horizontal direction. This is a considerable disadvantage in the conservative treatment of mandibular fractures within the dental arch. The method is very well suited to provisional emergency splinting and for fixation of the fragments before a functionally stable osteosynthesis. A local anesthetic is usually required for application of the ligatures. Any necessary tooth extractions should be performed after the ligatures have been placed but before the intermaxillary fixation.

Direct interdental wiring (*Gilmer*, 1887) is the simplest form of intermaxillary fixation. Single wire ligatures (0.25 mm soft steel wire) are applied around the teeth of the maxilla and mandible, and the ends are twisted over each tooth. If long-term intermaxillary fixation is necessary, as many teeth as possible should be provided with wire ligatures so that the muscular forces are distributed uniformly. For an emergency appliance, a few ligatures are enough. After the application of all the wires in the maxilla and mandible, manual reduction with adjustment of centric occlusion is undertaken. The wires of the maxillary teeth are then twisted together with the wires of the mandibular teeth (Fig. 8.2-23). If the occlusion cannot be adjusted manually, the twisted ends of the wires can be shortened to a length of 5 mm and bent back toward the gingiva; thus, they can serve to fasten intermaxillary elastic bands. An application of cold-curing acrylic will prevent the wire ends from bending up after the elastic bands have been applied. The elastic bands are replaced by tie wires after the reduction is complete.

According to a recommendation by *Hering* (1960), the entire vestibular dental arch can be strengthened with cold-curing acrylic. After the wire ligatures are applied, the twisted ends are shortened to a length of 2 cm. Acrylic then is applied to the vestibular surfaces of the dental crowns and the twisted ends of the ligature wires; it should also penetrate the interdental spaces. While the resin is still plastic, it is modelled into a buccal splint. The ends of the ligature wires are twisted into rosettes. They provide a means to fasten the tie wires or the rubber bands, and also can be coated with plastic afterward (Fig. 8.2-24).

The splint becomes even more stable if the twisted ends of the ligature wires of the second molar are twisted together with those of the first molar for two turns and then bent back at a right angle toward the gingiva. The same is done with the twisted ends of the first molar's ligature wires and those of the second premolar. This gives rise to a sort of cable arch wire, which then can be coated with cold-curing acrylic (*Krüger*, 1974, Fig. 8.2-25).

Continuous, or multiple loop wiring (*Stout*, 1943) is undertaken with a 0.5 mm soft steel wire. The buccal end is adapted to the dental arch

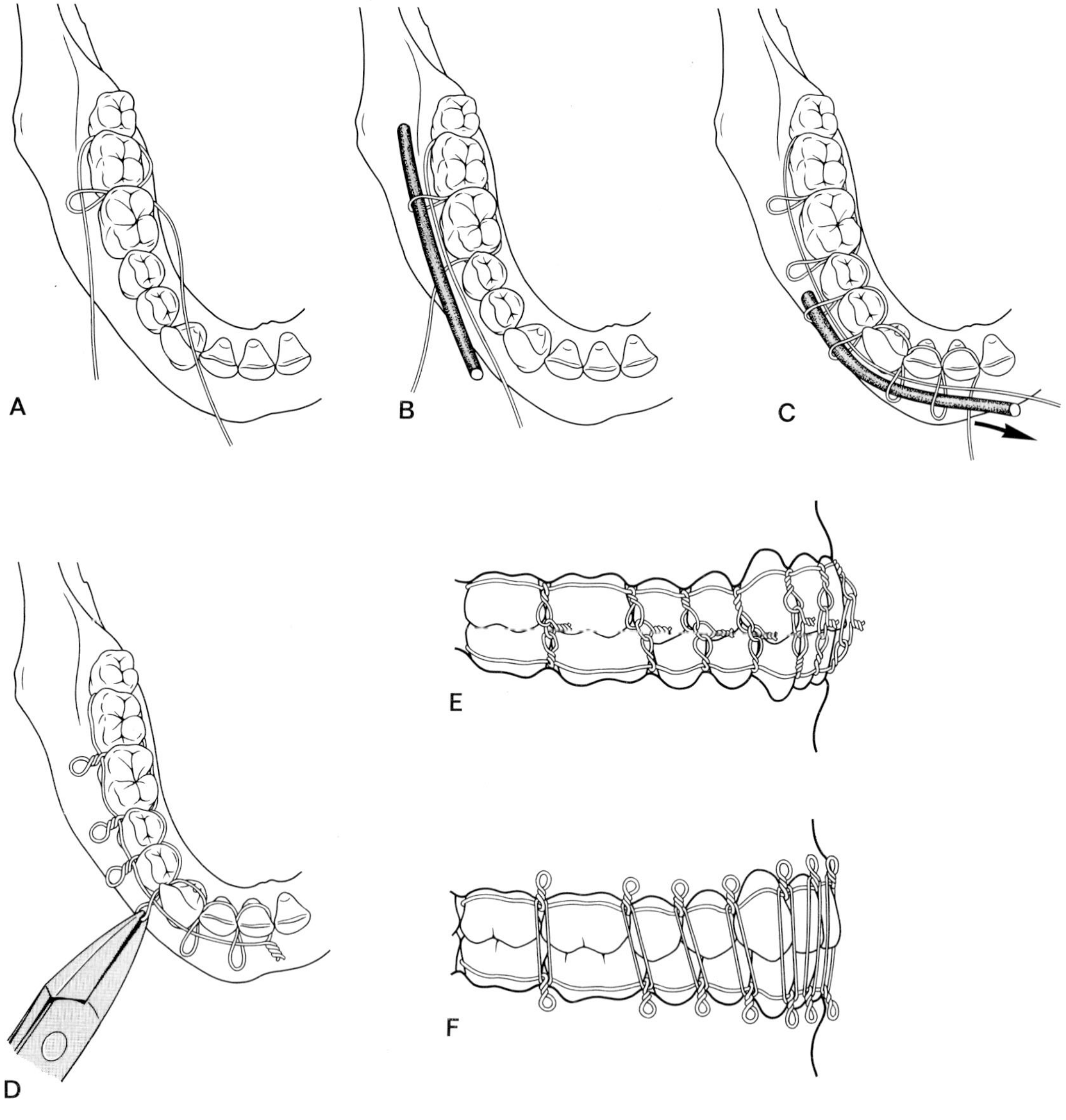

Figs. 8.2-26 A to F Stout's continuous, or multiple loop wiring.

Figs. 8.2-26 A and B The interdental loops are placed over a buccally adapted rod and around the buccal wire end.

Fig. 8.2-26 C When the loops have been completed on one side, the rod is withdrawn.

Fig. 8.2-26 D The loops are tightened with a ligature pliers.

Fig. 8.2-26 E Intermaxillary fixation with tie wires.

Fig. 8.2-26 F Intermaxillary fixation with elastic rings. The loops are bent gingivally for this purpose.

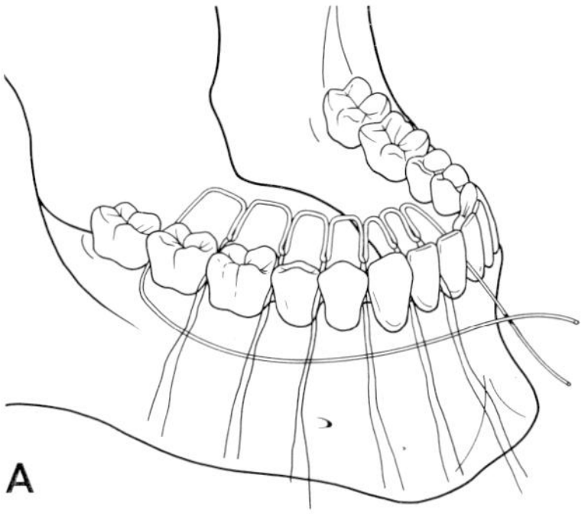

A

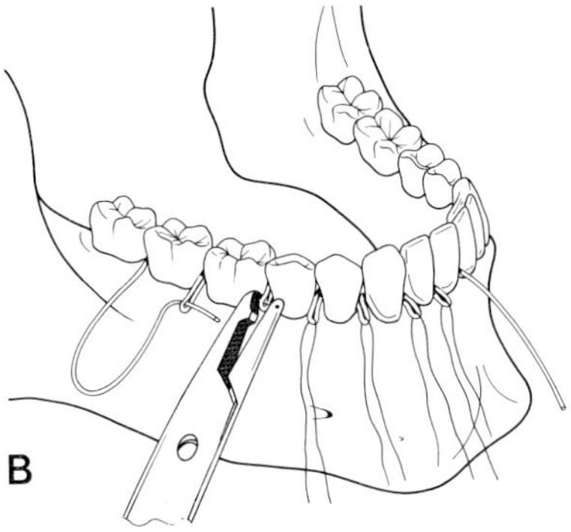

B

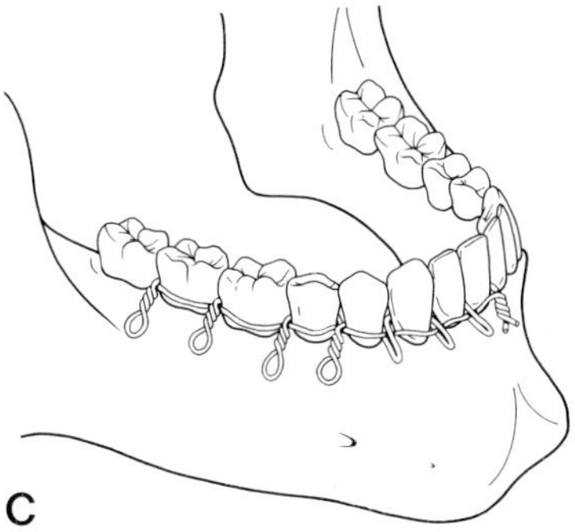

C

Figs. 8.2-27 A to C Obwegeser's placement technique for continuous loop wires.

Fig. 8.2-27 A Pulling the pre-shaped loops through the interdental spaces with silk ligatures.

Fig. 8.2-27 B Pulling the buccal end of the wire through the loops.

Fig. 8.2-27 C Tightening the loops.

and should only be long enough to reach the other side, proceeding somewhat beyond the midline. The lingual end, which must be significantly longer, is then brought through the adjacent mesial interdental space in a buccal direction, formed into a loop around the short buccal wire and led back through the same interdental space in a lingual direction (Fig. 8.2-26 A). The end of a pliable round rod, approximately 3 to 4 mm thick, which previously has been adapted to the dental arch, then is inserted into the loop. The lingual wire is pulled tight and led in a buccal direction through the next interdental space (Fig. 8.2-26 B), brought around the rod and once again led through the same interdental space. In this manner, all the teeth of a quadrant are encircled by the lingual end of the wire. The continuous loop formation is interrupted when there is a gap in the dental arch. The buccal and the lingual ends of the wire are twisted together until the gap has been bridged, after which the loop formation is continued in the same way as before. At the midline, the lingual end is only led through to the labial side and not back again. It is loosely twisted with the buccal end. Then the round rod is pulled out with a rotating motion (Fig. 8.2-26 C). The individual uniform loops are now tightened with a ligature forceps by a few twists above the buccal wire, which causes this to be pressed into the interdental space and the lingual wire to be firmly adapted to the tooth cervix (Fig. 8.2-26 D). After tightening, a smaller loop should remain behind; this should be bent back in an occlusal direction to provide a means for receiving the tie wires which are to be applied after the fracture ends are reduced (Fig. 8. 2-26 E). If a progressive reduction is anticipated, the loops are bent back toward the gingiva to hold elastic bands (Fig. 8.2-26 F).

Obwegeser (1952) modified the technique of applying this splint. He used soft stainless steel wire of 0.6 mm thickness. The wire is preformed, so that the interdental loops can be pulled simultaneously through the interdental spaces with the help of silk ligatures (Fig. 8.2-27 A). Round loops are formed from the two strands of the interdental wire which have been pressed together with a special forceps. One end of this tool is fitted with a hole and the other with a spike which penetrates it. With it, the distal end

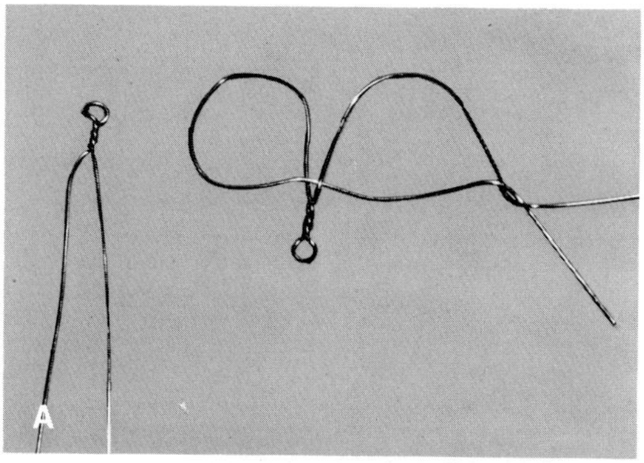

Fig. 8.2-28 A to C Interdental eyelet wiring.

Fig. 8.2-28 A Left – wire with eyelet; right – eyelet wire.

Fig. 8.2-28 B Complete eyelet ligature et 4 7, 4 6; twisted eyelet ligature 4 5, 4 4; wire for an eyelet ligature placed at 4 2, 4 1.

Fig. 8.2-28 C Intermaxillary fixation by means of tie wires.

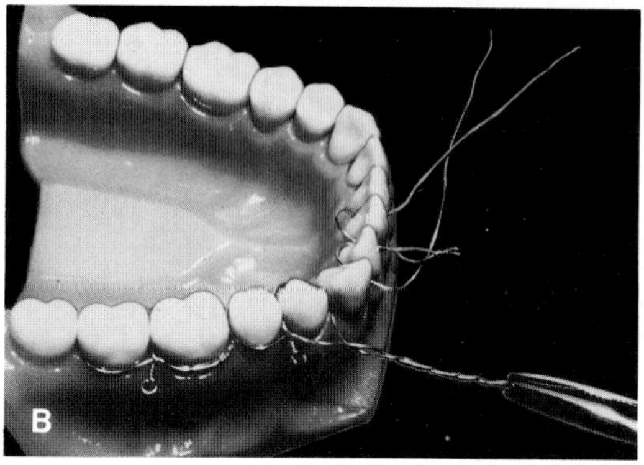

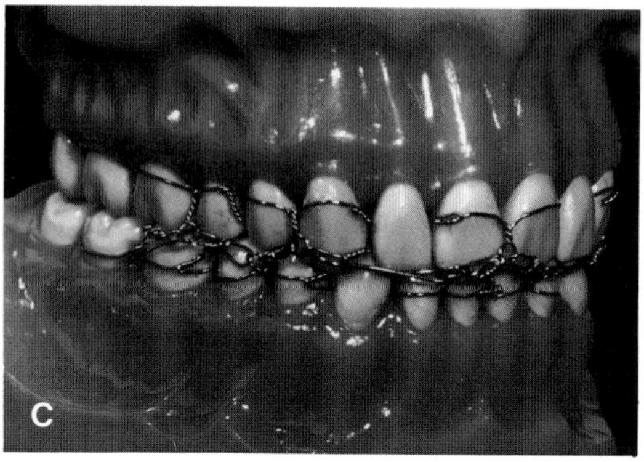

of the wire is led forward along the arch (Fig. 8. 2-27 B) and twisted with the mesial end of the wire. The loops are tightened with the special forceps on top of the buccal wire, whereby this is pressed into the interdental space and the lingual part of the ligature is tightly adapted to the neck of the tooth, just as in the original *Stout* method (Fig. 8. 2-27 F).

Interdental eyelet wiring (*Eby*, 1920; *Ivy*, 1922) is undertaken with 0.35 mm soft steel wire. For one eyelet wire which encircles two adjacent teeth, a 15 cm wire is needed. An eyelet is formed in the middle by twisting the ends around a dental bur (Fig. 8. 2-28 A). To treat a fracture in a complete dentition, 14 eyelet wires are necessary. An arrangement with 11 wires is also recommended by *Rowe* and *Killey* (1968):

- in the maxilla, one eyelet wire between the central incisors and one each between the canines and the first premolars and between the second premolars and the first molars, and
- in the mandible, one eyelet wire between the central and lateral incisors, between the two premolars and between the first and second molars.

The two ends of an eyelet wire are pulled from the buccal side through the interdental space of the two teeth to which the eyelet wire is to be applied. The eyelet then is situated on the buccal side of the interdental space. One wire end is then brought through the neighboring distal interdental space and the other is brought through the neighboring mesial one in a buccal direction. The distal end is pulled through the eyelet and twisted with the mesial end at the level of the mesial interdental space; the eyelet is pulled into the interdental space in the course of this procedure (Fig. 8. 2-28 B). The tie wires should be applied in a V-pattern with a cross-

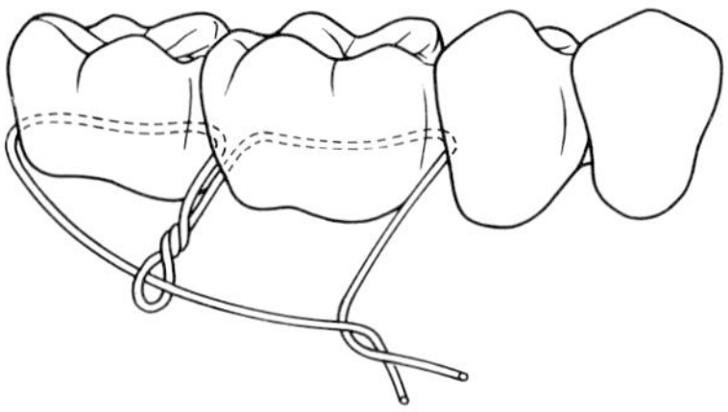

Fig. 8.2-29 A The buccal wire runs through the eyelet. When the ligature is tightened, the eyelet is drawn into the interdental space.

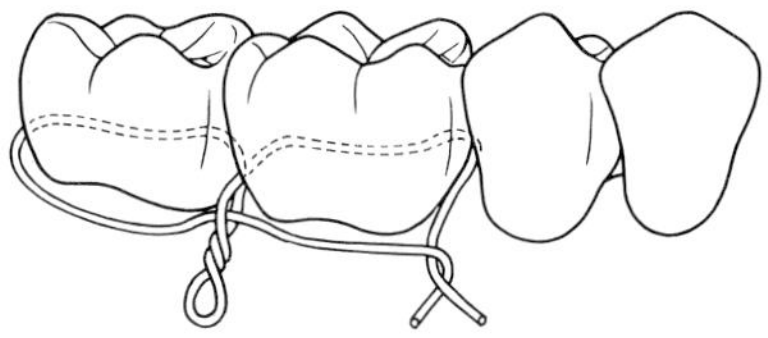

Fig. 8.2-29 B The buccal wire lies between the interdental wires. The eyelet cannot be drawn into the interdental space when the ligature is tightened.

Fig. 8.2-30 William's modification of eyelet wiring: the buccal wire is drawn through an additional loop.

bracing effect; this prevents anterior and lateral movement even when the wires are slightly loosened (Fig. 8.2-28 C).

The tie wires are drawn through the eyelets, which is not always easy if they are situated deep in the interdental space. Then they must be gripped with a pointed forceps and pulled out somewhat, so that the ends of the tie wires, which are best bent back into a small hook, can be drawn through. If elastic bands are to be applied, it is better to proceed as with continuous or multiple loop wiring, and pull the distal buccal wire end through the interdental wires instead of through the eyelet (Fig. 8.2-29).

Williams (1968) recommended a further modification: in the prior preparation of the wires, an eyelet is formed initially in the customary manner. Then one end of the wire is passed back through the eyelet, forming a second loop, and is finally secured by a further twist with the other end (Fig. 8.2-30). In an overclosed bite, it may be necessary to mount the eyelet on the palatal side of the maxilla in the anterior region.

Ernst's wires (1927, 1932) and the *Kazanjian* buttons (1933) each are applied around two adjacent teeth. The arrangement is the same as with the eyelet wiring. The application technique previously has been described in the section on emergency appliances (see pp. 112 f. and Figs. 4-16 to 4-18).

For the **cable arch wire** (*Risdon*, 1929), a 0.7 – 1 mm soft steel wire is needed. A ligature is applied with this wire around the last tooth of the arch on each side. The ends must be long enough that they extend beyond the midline adjacent to the row of teeth after being twisted together. The twisted ends of the two wires are then twisted together at the midline. Individual ligatures of 0.35 mm soft stainless steel wire are applied around the remaining teeth and twisted together over the cable arch (Fig. 8.2-30). The bent-back and cut wire ends can receive the tie wires or elastic bands or can be twisted directly with the corresponding wire ends of the opposite half of the jaw.

Arch bar wiring has the advantage over interdental wiring of greater stability in the horizontal direction. The arch bar therefore is better suited to elastic intermaxillary fixation than interdental wiring. Moreover, a transition from an intermaxil-

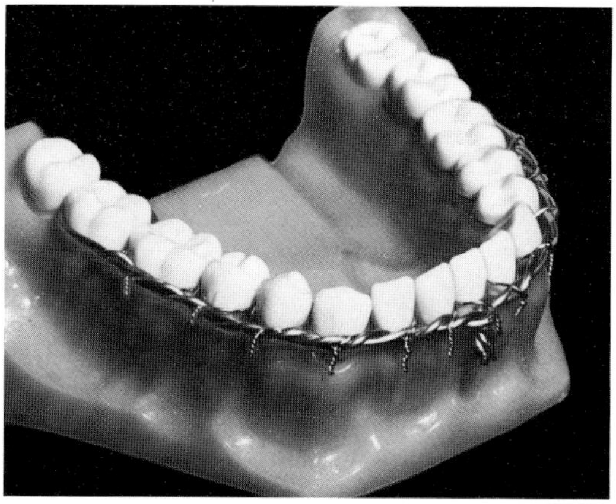

Fig. 8.2-31 Cable arch wire.

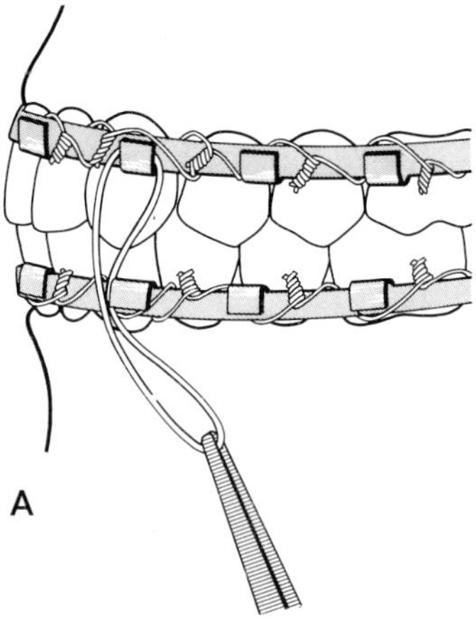

A

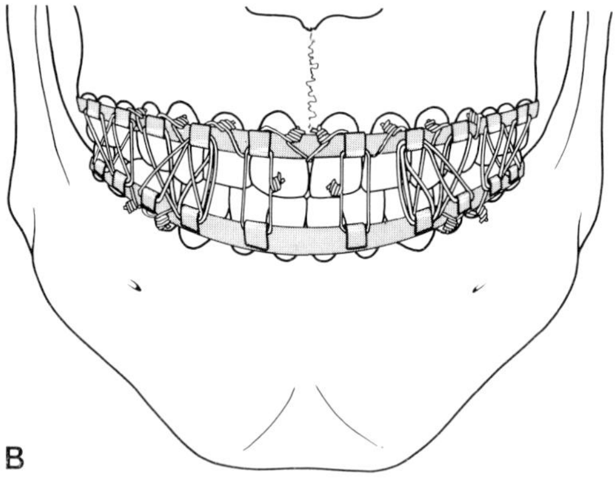

B

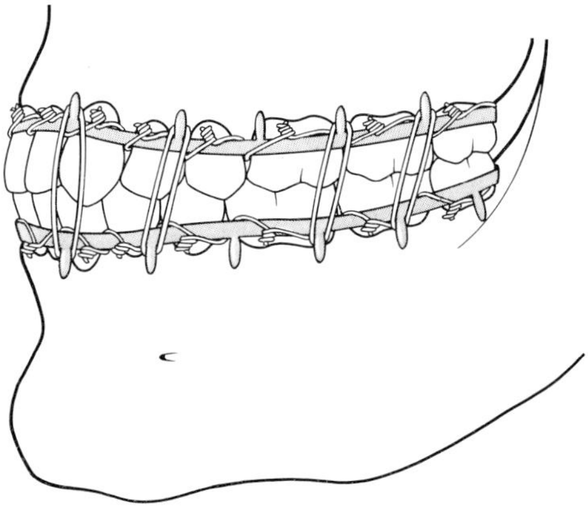

C

Fig. 8.2-32 A Erich arch bars in the maxilla and the mandible. An elastic band is placed for intermaxillary fixation.

Fig. 8.2-32 B Erich arch bars with intermaxillary tie wire fixation.

Fig. 8.2-32 C Winter arch bars with intermaxillary tie wire fixation.

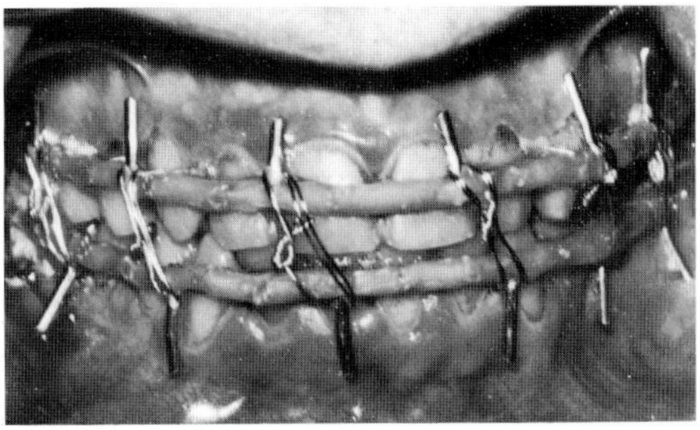

Fig. 8.2-33 Schuchardt's wire-acrylic arch bar with intermaxillary fixation with tie wires.

lary fixation to a monomaxillary one is possible during the treatment period.
The reduction of the fragments can be undertaken before the ligatures are pulled tight. One customary method is to insert a divided arch bar which allows the fragments to be adjusted separately by immediate reduction or elastic bands.
The prefabricated arch bar of malleable metal is available in various types (Jelenko, Winter, Erich, Niro) from dental supply houses. The arch bar, which is provided with small hook attachments, can be contoured easily by hand. The hooks serve to receive the elastic bands or the tie wires, and must therefore be pointed toward the gingiva when the arch bar is applied. The bar should extend up to and encircle the last tooth on each side distally. It is cut to size in the proper length, bent back on the ends, and fixed to the teeth with ligature wires made from 0.35 mm soft stainless steel (Fig. 8.2-32). As with *Schuchardt*'s wire-acrylic arch bar (1956, 1966), all ligatures may be applied at one time to the teeth of one side of the jaw. Only then is the arch bar, which previously has been cut to size and contoured, inserted and secured. On the other hand, the bar can also be fixated with two ligatures, with each subsequent ligature applied to the already positioned bar.
When the ligatures are firmly tightened, as a rule the arch bar slips in a gingival direction until it finally rests on the gingiva. This is a decisive disadvantage in comparison with *Schuchardt*'s wire-acrylic arch bar, which prevents gingival slipping by an occlusal support during tightening. In the maxilla, the arch bar is tied on firmly right away; this is done in the mandible only if the fracture is situated outside the dental arch or if the ends of the fragments are not displaced. When there is displacement with shoulder formation within the dental arch, the ligature wires are first tightened only loosely. The fracture then is manually reduced, for which a local anesthetic is usually necessary. After reduction and adjustment of centric occlusion, the ligatures are tightened firmly in the mandible as well, and the intermaxillary tie wires or elastic bands are applied (Fig. 8.2-32 A to C). The intermaxillary fixation causes the splints to be pulled away somewhat from the gingiva again, which relieves the marginal periodontium. Despite this, periodontal damage may still occur during the prolonged period of fixation.
For better stabilization of this dressing, cold-curing acrylic can be applied after the intermaxillary fixation, as with *Schuchardt*'s wire-acrylic arch bar. The bars are thus additionally supported in the interdental spaces, and the ends of the ligature wires coated with acrylic cannot become loose.
The wire-acrylic arch bar (*Schuchardt* et al. 1956, 1961, 1966) already has been described as one of the splints for monomaxillary fixation. For intermaxillary fixation, an arch bar is applied in both the maxilla and the mandible (Figs. 8.2-33 to 8.2-35). Care must be taken here that the lower arch bar is situated deeply enough when there is an overbite of the upper anterior teeth, so that the occlusion is not disturbed. After the teeth have been rinsed with an amine fluoride solution and a cold-curing acrylic has been applied, the occlusal layers are cut off and their

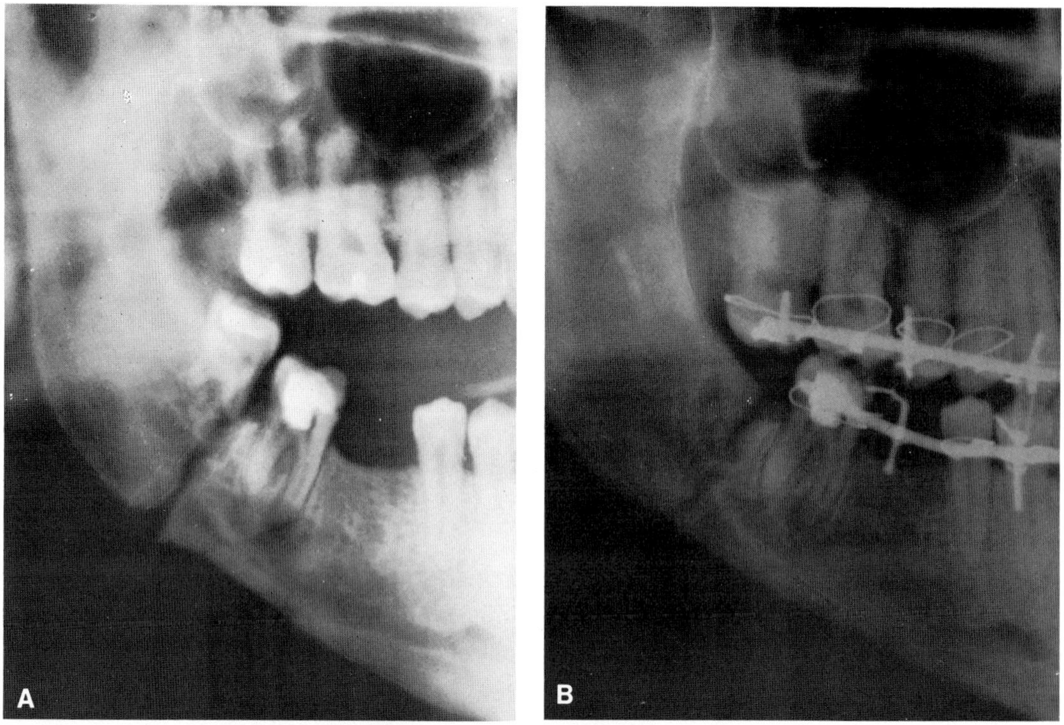

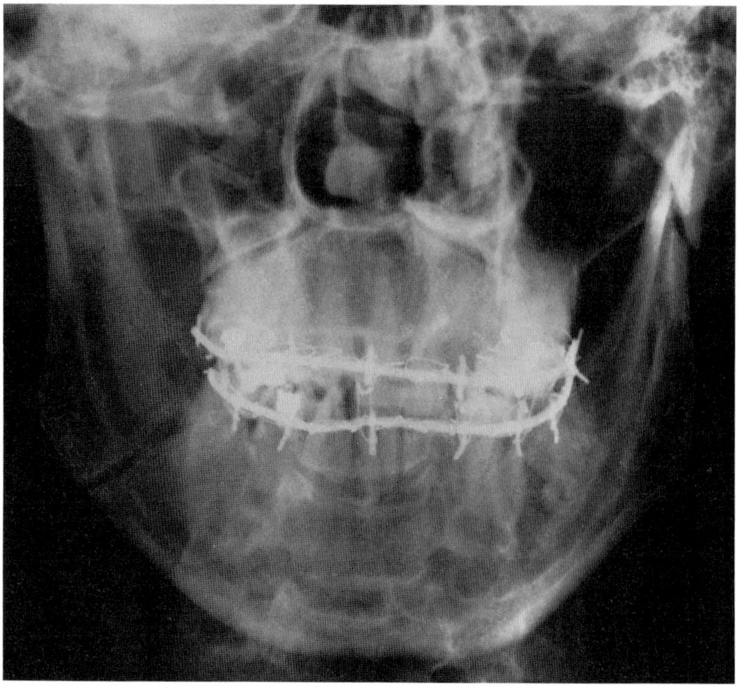

Fig. 8.2-34 A Fracture in the posterior tooth region of the right side of the mandible; 48 in the fracture line.

Fig. 8.2-34 B Condition following extraction of the third molar, placement of wire-acrylic arch bars and tie wire intermaxillary fixation. The small fragment is not included in the appliances. As there is no displacement, surgical measures for fixation are not required.

Fig. 8.2-35 Radiograph after treatment of a fracture of the right angle of the mandible and a left sided fracture of the condylar neck with wire-acrylic arch bars and intermaxillary fixation. All fragments are in proper position; surgical procedures are not necessary.

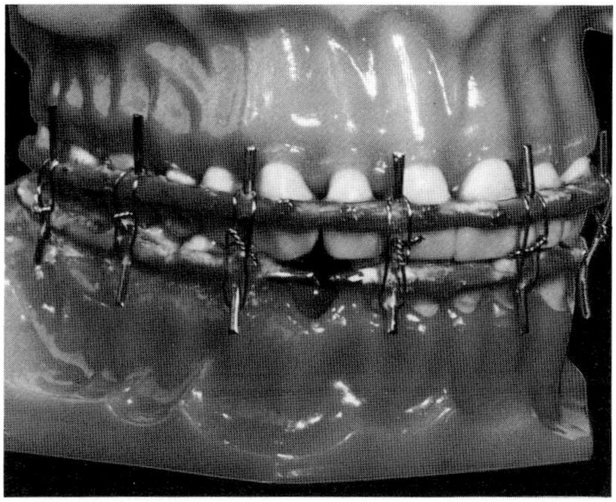

Figs. 8.2-36 A to C Principle of split wire-acrylic arch bar to simplify reduction of the fragments.

Fig. 8.2-36 A The arch bar is divided at the fracture site. Both fragments are fixed in centric occlusion by intermaxillary tie wires.

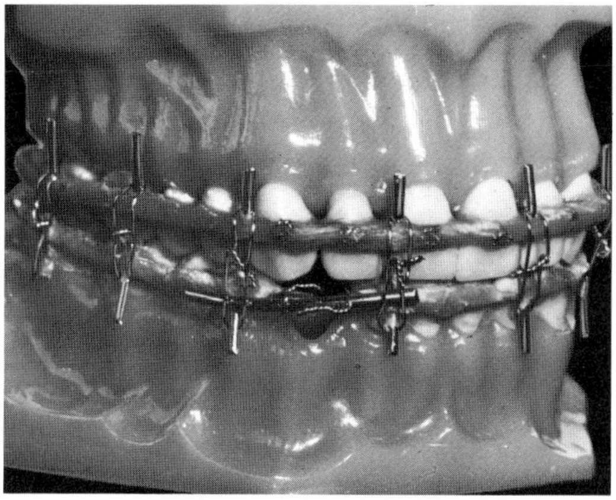

Fig. 8.2-36 B The separation site is bridged with a piece of arch bar wire held in place by two wire ligatures.

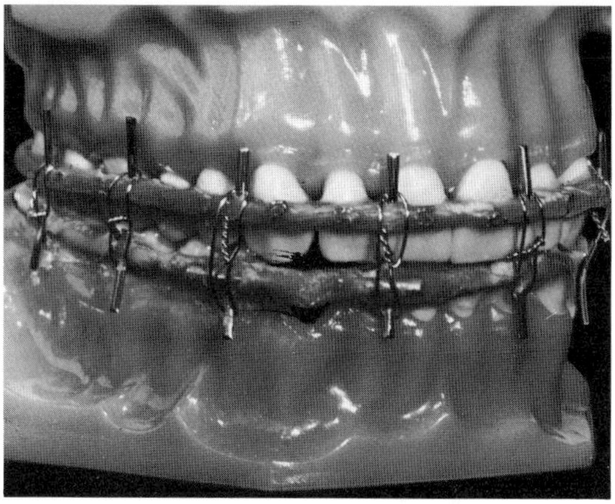

Fig. 8.2-36 C The bridging wire is coated with acrylic. Thus, the mandibular arch bar has become a stable unit again.

cut surfaces smoothed with a grinding stone.
There are various possibilities for reduction of fragments fractured within the dental arch:
For one, a space can be left in the acrylic coating at the fracture site and the ligatures adjacent to it, and the occlusion can be adjusted manually or with taut elastic bands. The ligatures near the fracture are subsequently tightened. The arch bar in this area then is also coated with acrylic.
Another possibility consists of separating the mandibular splint at the fracture site and adjusting each fragment separately through manual manipulation or with elastic bands; subsequently, a rigid fixation is performed with tie wires. Once this is accomplished, the arch bar parts are connected to each other again. A piece of arch bar wire which is fixated with ligatures on each side of the fracture and with a plastic coat provides the bridging (Figs. 8.2-36 to 8.2-38).
The gingival hooks of the arch bar provide a means of receiving the tie wires or elastic bands. The wire-acrylic arch bar is stable enough for the elastic fixation to ensue with a few elastic bands, which permit a movement of the

Figs. 8.2-37 A to C Reduction of a mandibular fracture with a split wire-acrylic arch bar.

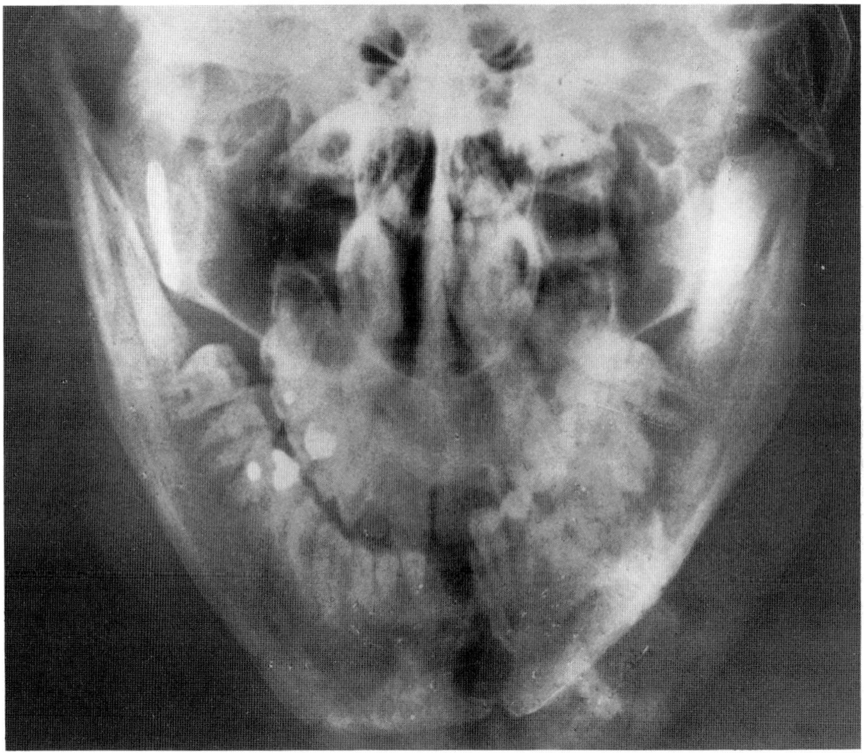

Fig. 8.2-37 A Mandibular fracture at 32, fracture of the left condylar neck and the right coronoid process.

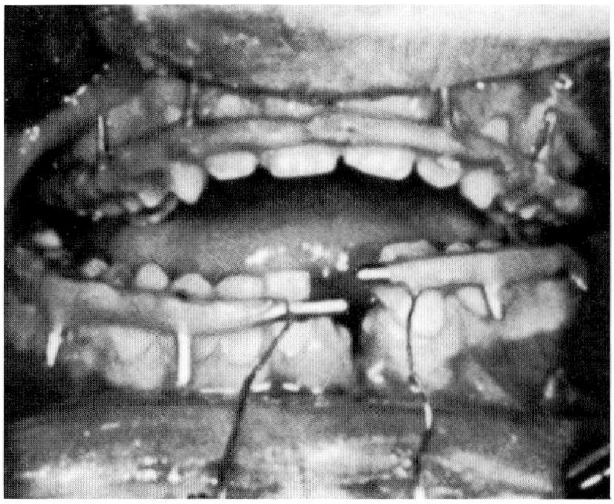

Fig. 8.2-37 B Wire-acrylic arch bar in the maxilla, split wire-acrylic arch bar in the mandible.

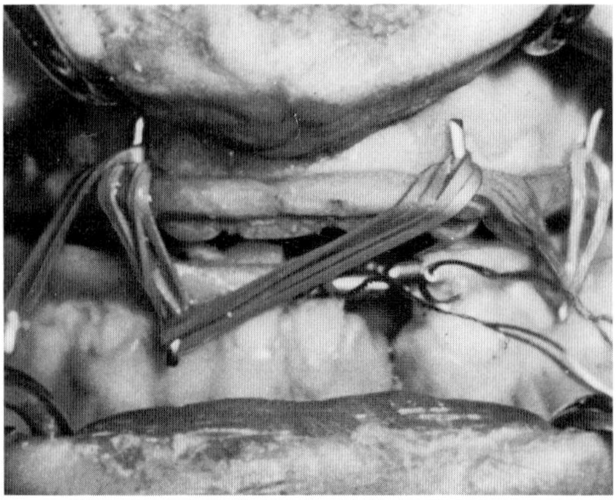

Fig. 8.2-37 C Reduction with elastic bands.

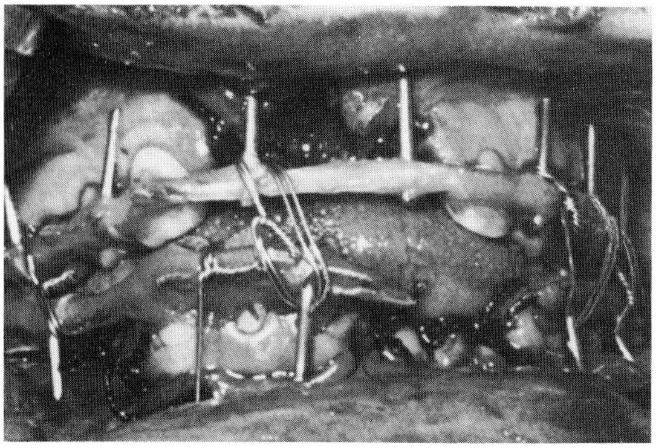

Fig. 8.2-38 A The fragments of a mandibular fracture were reduced separately; the arch bar components for the mandibular fragments are attached to the arch bar of the maxilla by intermaxillary tie wires. A circumferential wire in the region of the right canine provides additional fixation for the arch bar whose interdental wires have little retention on the conically shaped anterior teeth.

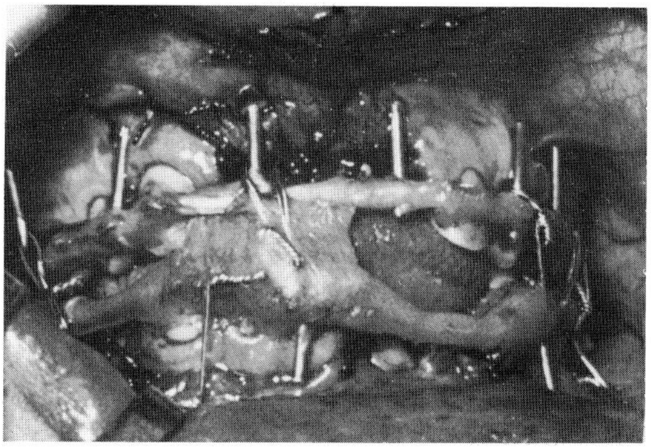

Fig. 8.2-38 B Connection of both arch bar components by wire and acrylic.

mandible and an opening of the arches. After two to three weeks, an elastic fixation usually replaces the rigid fixation with tie wires or taut elastic bands.

The splint can present problems with an over-closed bite. These can be overcome by applying a small bar on each side only in the molar and premolar region, or by the lingual application of the bar in the anterior region (Fig. 8.2-39).

The wire-acrylic arch bar can be enlarged and completed in the mouth through the application of acrylic. Thus, saddles can be applied in edentulous sections of the jaw, if necessary. The use of cold-curing acrylic allows the arch bar to be transformed into an individually fitted jaw fracture splint with simple means and without having recourse to a dental laboratory; this splint is superior to most of the other direct splints with regard to stability and firmness of seat, and is equivalent to the best indirect splints.

The banded dental arch wire appliance (*Angle*, 1890; *Schroeder*, 1917) is used primarily for monomaxillary fixation (see pp. 244 f.). If the twisted ends of the ligature wires are bent back gingivally and stiffened with an acrylic coat, intermaxillary tie wires or elastic bands also can be applied. Similarly, an arch bar with soldered cross wires like those on *Schuchardt*'s wire acrylic arch bar can be used.

Indirect splints are used only rarely for intermaxillary fixation. The strong point of these appliances, which are produced in the laboratory from an impression, lies in monomaxillary fixation.

The mandibular lingual splint (*Hofer*, 1939) also can be used for intermaxillary fixation, in conjunction with interdental wiring, an arch bar, or an acrylic splint in the maxilla. In this case, the ends of the ligature wires used to immobilize the lingual splint are bent back in a gingival direction and strengthened with acrylic. They can provide a means of holding the tie wires or elastic bands. In the case of an over-closed bite, the lingual splint is much to be preferred because it does not interfere with the occlusion. In the maxilla, eyelet wires which are mounted in the anterior region on the palatal side are best in such cases.

Sectional splints and **cap splints** can be used for intermaxillary fixation if hooks also are mounted on the buccal part for the tie wires or elastic bands.

Following completion of the splinting and reduction procedures, and intermaxillary fixation of the mandible in centric occlusion, it is necessary that a **radiograph** be taken. If this film indicates that displacement of the fragments per-

Figs. 8.2-39 A to D Arrangement of the wire-acrylic arch bar in an over-closed bite.

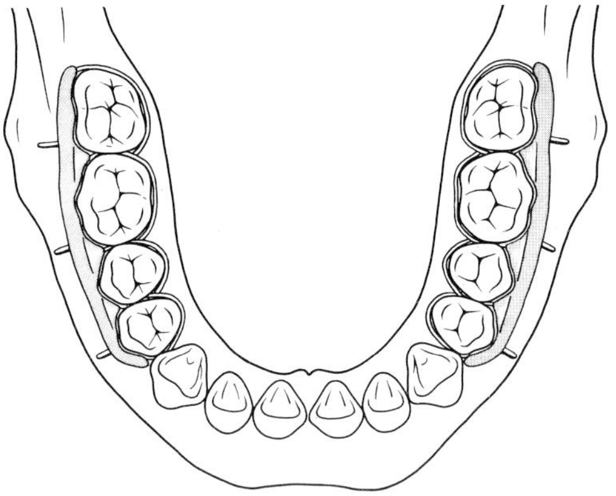

Fig. 8.2-39 A Two split arch bars in the posterior tooth regions of the mandible.

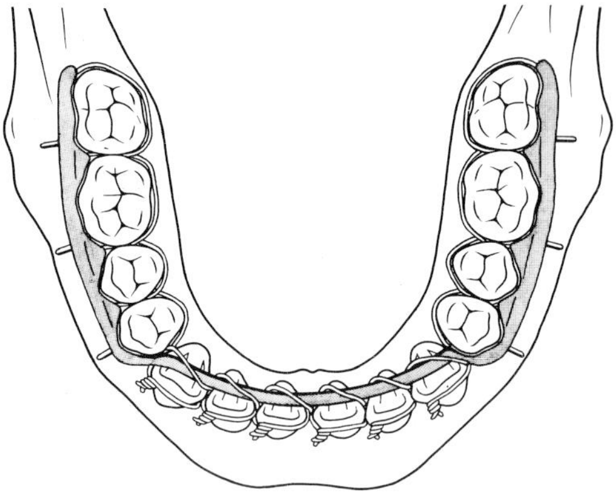

Fig. 8.2-39 B Arch bar in lingual position anteriorly and buccal position posteriorly.

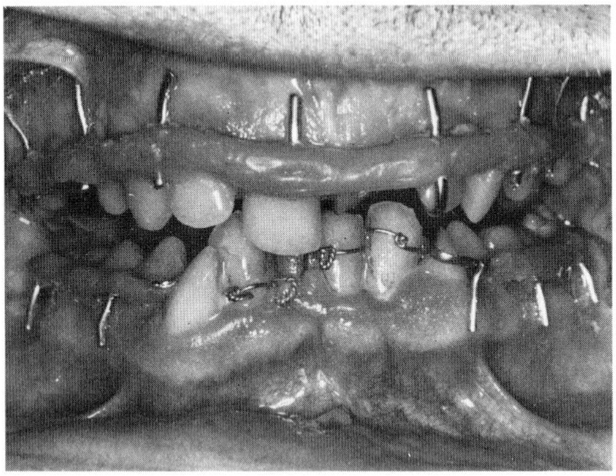

Fig. 8.2-39 C Wire acrylic arch bar *in situ* in over-closed bite.

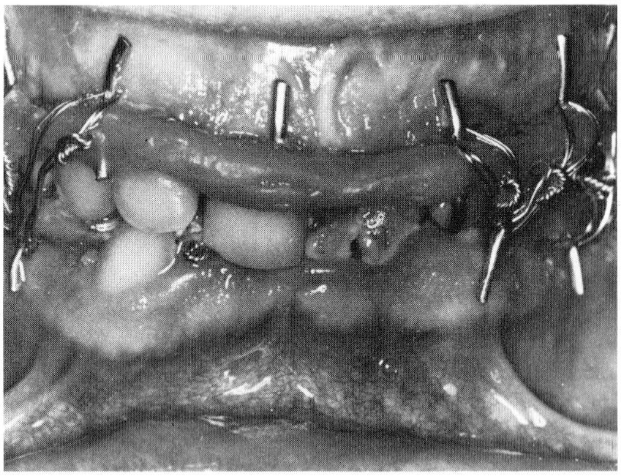

Fig. 8.2-39 D Appearance following intermaxillary fixation.

sists, surgical measures are required as a rule. In such instances, one either proceeds to interosseous wiring to supplement intermaxillary fixation or a rigid internal fixation with a compression plate or lag screw osteosynthesis is carried out (Fig. 8. 2-40).

The follow-up treatment, as with monomaxillary fixation, consists primarily of careful cleaning of the oral cavity and the teeth. During rigid intermaxillary fixation, patients may receive only fluid nourishment. While this is in effect, only the buccal surfaces of the teeth are accessible to cleaning with a toothbrush and rinsing with a fluoride preparation. It is therefore particularly important to clean the interdental spaces and the splints carefully with a spray at least once a day. After two to three weeks, the rigid fixation is replaced by elastic fixation. Patients may then remove the elastic bands to eat, and normal cleaning of the teeth with the toothbrush can be resumed. The elastic bands are subsequently put back. The elastic fixation is instituted for an additional period of about three weeks after the two-to three-week rigid immobilization. After this time has elapsed, the splint usually can be removed. In the case of fractures within the

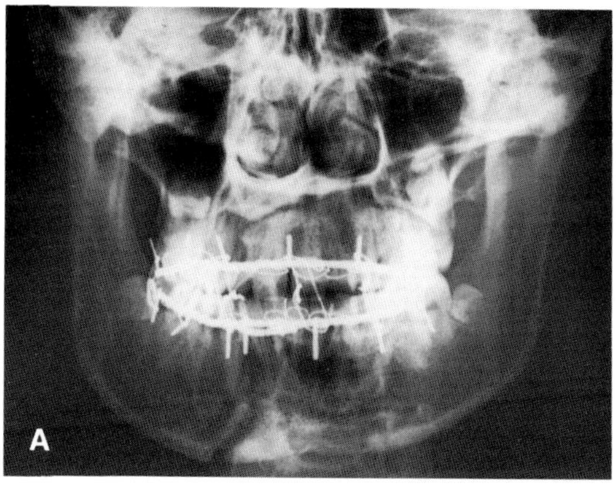

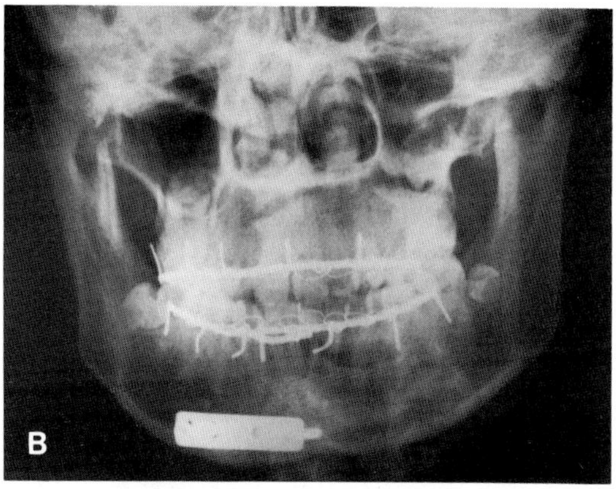

Figs. 8.2-40 A to D Incomplete reduction of a fracture of the mandible after intermaxillary fixation: indication for surgical treatment.

Fig. 8.2-40 A Fracture gaping at the border of the mandible after intermaxillary fixation of the mandible in centric occlusion.

Fig. 8.2-40 B Appearance after rigid internal fixation by means of a compression plate.

Fig. 8.2-40 C The gaping fracture between 43 and 42 is clearly visible.

Fig. 8.2-40 D Complete reduction following compression plate osteosynthesis.

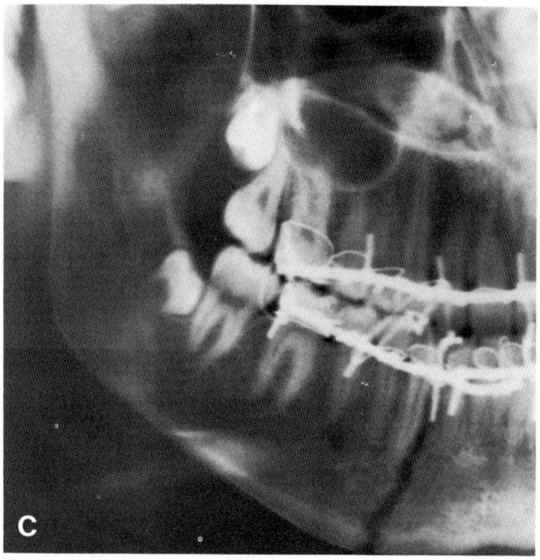

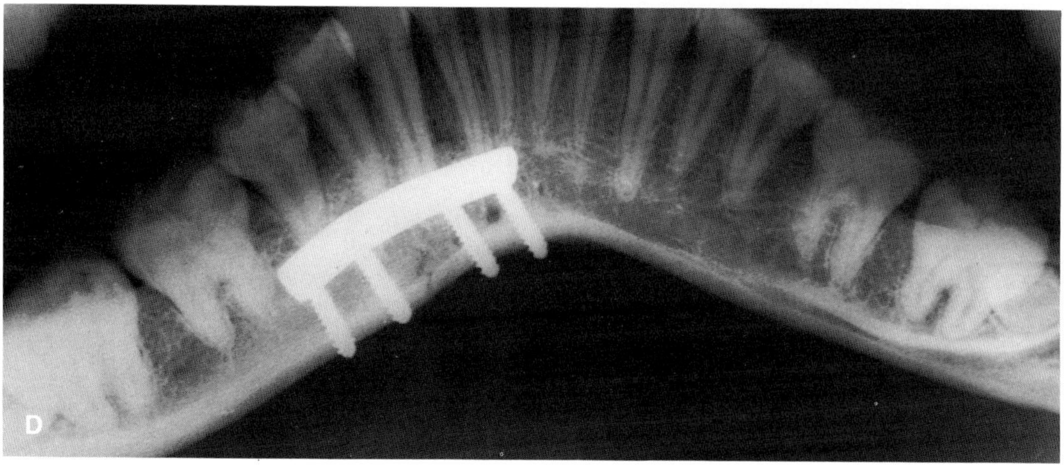

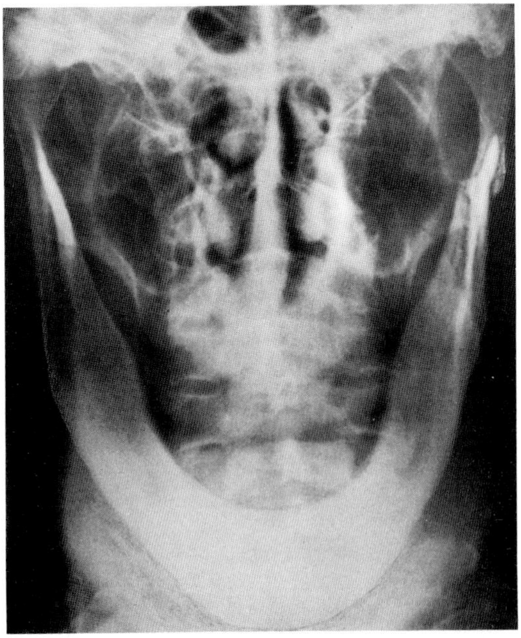

Fig. 8.2-41 A Fracture of the base of the left condylar process with only minor displacement in an edentulous patient.

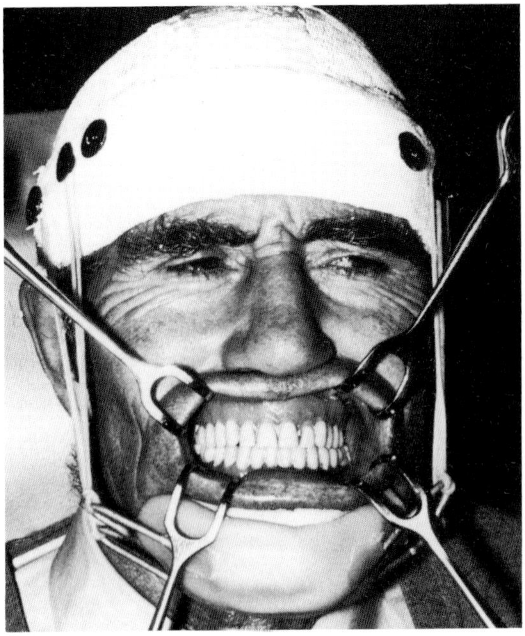

Fig. 8.2-41 B Treatment with plaster head gear and chin cap. Buttons are mounted on the head gear to receive elastic bands. The patient wears his dentures.

dental arch, the arch bar is first separated at the fracture site. If the fracture site does not prove to be firm enough yet, the parts of the splint are connected with each other again (see p. 265) and the elastic bands are reapplied. If necessary, the mandibular splint alone can be left in position, as monomaxillary fixation.

2.4 Conservative Treatment of Fractures in the Edentulous and Insufficiently Dentulous Mandible

If there are not enough teeth present for the attachment of the splint in the treatment of a displaced mandibular fracture, a surgical measure, especially functionally stable osteosynthesis, is usually undertaken today. Non-displaced fractures with fracture ends which are not very mobile require no fixation (see Supervised spontaneous healing, pp. 237 ff.).

Beyond this, there are some fractures with only minor displacement and mobility which can be supported sufficiently with simple extraoral dressings. In such cases, the patient's dentures are used for intraoral support. If these are missing, occlusal dentures (bite blocks) made from impressions, or base plates as devised by *Gunning* (1886-1887), can be used in partially dentulous or edentulous jaws. The patient must be able to close the mouth with the prostheses or the prepared plates in the correct occlusion. The mandible is then supported at the chin with a chin cap which is attached to a headgear appliance with elastic bands. A chin cap can be made from acrylic, and metal bars or hooks can provide a way to receive elastic bands. If a plaster headgear appliance is used, several buttons can be molded on in the temple region (Fig. 8.2-41).

Extraoral and intraoral appliances should be worn by the patient at all times during the first three weeks. The bite blocks or plates are removed from the mouth only for cleaning after eating, and the chin cap taken off only for eating. After two to three weeks, the extraoral appliance does not have to be worn all the time, and after four weeks, usually it can be left off completely.

2.5 Results and Complications

The results of the conservative treatment of mandibular fractures which have been reported in the literature must be characterized throughout as favorable. Complications and poor healing results are relatively rare.

Complications from the Splint

Muska (1971) reported on the complications of intermaxillary immobilization. There is a danger of **aspiration** of blood or vomitus if the intermaxillary tie wires or elastic bands cannot be removed quickly enough. *Muska* (1971) describes a case in which massive hemorrhaging from a tongue injury a week after the accident cost the patient his life. The intermaxillary fixation proved to be an obstacle in the removal of blood from the oral cavity and in applying a pressure dressing. Heart failure ensued before the intermaxillary tie wires could be removed. The autopsy revealed that a major branch of the lingual artery had been severed in the tongue wound.

In 1976, *Freitag* and *Höhnle* documented **dental dislocations** as a side effect of intraoral splints in 173 retrospectively investigated conservatively treated cases of mandibular fractures. There were dislocations of individual teeth in 18.5% and dislocations of several adjacent teeth in 8.7% (serial dislocations, see Fig. 8.2-22). In order to avoid orthodontic effects of this sort, care must be taken that the arch bar fits the dental arch everywhere and that the muscular forces are transmitted equally to all teeth. Ligatures which cause occlusal alteration in the teeth are to be avoided.

All splints, when they are worn for a long time, can cause **demineralization** of the **tooth enamel** as the manifestation of carious processes (Figs. 8.2-42 A and B). This is particularly true for *Schuchardt's* wire acrylic arch bar. Experimental investigations by *Krüger* and *Chrissafis* (1971) revealed that the cause of this alteration is not the cold-curing acrylic's acidic effect. If constitutional factors are disregarded, the cause appears to be retention of contamination in a narrow gap between splint and tooth surface which is inaccessible to a mechanical cleaning. Our efforts therefore must be directed toward keeping the space between the splint and the surfaces of the teeth as small as possible by limiting the use of the plastic. Furthermore, care must be taken that contamination of the inaccessible areas be held to a minimum through careful and regular brushing of the teeth—this holds for all splints. By means of intensive preparatory treatment of the dental crowns with a fluoride preparation, the acid solubility of the enamel can be reduced to such a degree that the caries-inducing splints can be worn, in a majority of cases, without damage to the tooth enamel. Additional rinsings once each week are particularly recommended. These anti-caries measures allowed *Krüger* and *Chrissafis* (1971) to reduce the demineralization processes of the tooth enamel to a minimum with *Schuchardt*'s wire acrylic arch bar. In a retrospective investigation, 89% of the patients showed no enamel alteration after wearing the wire acrylic arch bar for at least six weeks (Fig. 8.2-42 C); in the remaining 11%, minor enamel demineralization was ascertainable on not more than four teeth.

Disturbances of Fracture Healing

Infections of the fracture site are the most frequent complication after conservative treatment of mandibular fractures. *Köhler* (1951) found fracture infections in 20% of the cases, of which half had soft tissue abscesses. *Reither* (1956) found a 10.5% fracture infection rate in 458 cases. *Andrä* and *Sonnenberg* (1966) observed fracture osteomyelitis in 13.9% of mandibular fractures when no antibiotic was administered. Institution of antibiotic therapy reduced the complication rate to 9.9%. In 1961, *Paschke* and *Berz* reported a fracture infection rate of over 7.8% among 385 conservatively treated mandibular fractures. These values are exceptionally high, and cannot be regarded as a

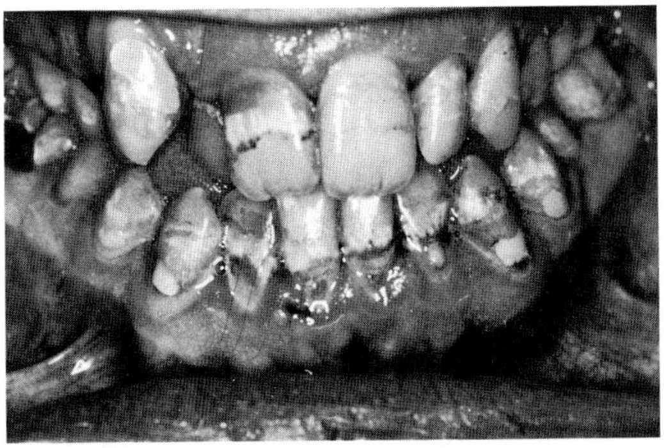

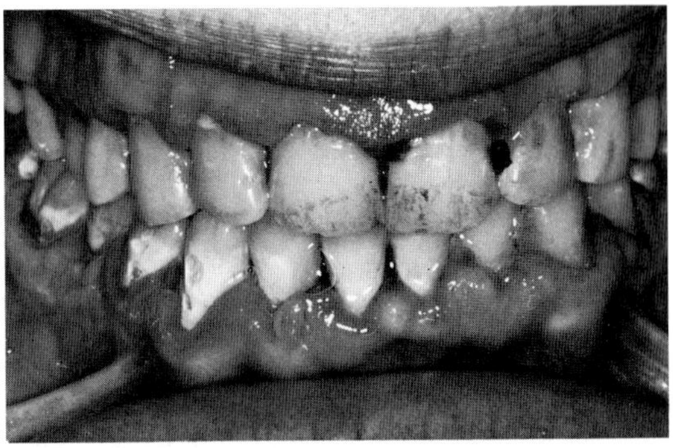

Figs. 8.2-42 A and B Decalcification zone at the enamel, and cervical caries following 6-week intermaxillary fixation with wire-acrylic arch bars.

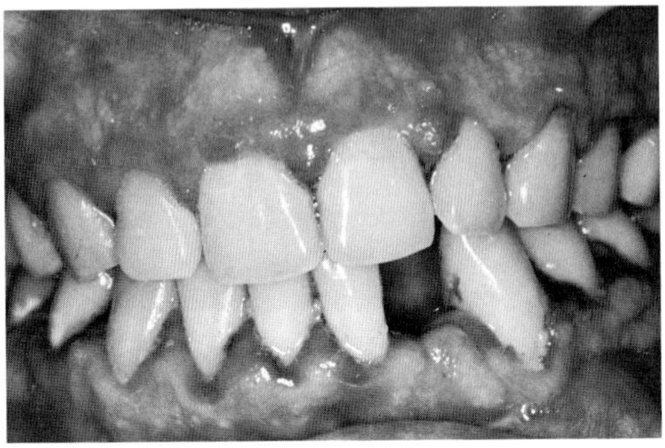

Fig. 8.2-42 C Undamaged enamel following 6-week intermaxillary fixation with wire acrylic arch bars and previous application of amine fluoride solution.

standard today. *Schuchardt* et al. (1960) found a significantly more favorable incidence, 5.2 % of 1174 cases, as did *Trauner* (1973) with 2.7 % of 522, *Claudi* and *Spiessl* (1975) with 3.4 % of 67, and *Höltje*, *Luhr*, and *Holtfreter* (1975) with 3.7 % of 1,614 cases. In a retrospective investigation of 104 cases treated in the Department of Oral and Maxillofacial Surgery in Bonn, we found a fracture infection rate of 1,9 %. It is worthy of note that the fracture infection rate after functionally stable osteosynthesis, 3.2 to 4.5%, is not significantly greater than that of conservative treatment (*Höltje*, *Luhr*, and *Holtfreter*, 1975; *Claudi* and *Spiessl*, 1975).

The time of the treatment plays a decisive role in the development of a fracture infection. *Heidsieck* analyzed 111 cases with displaced mandibular fractures in 1954 (non-displaced fractures were not considered). Of these, 65 % healed without complications; here treatment ensued after an average of 9.4 days. In the remaining 35 % with fracture infections, treatment began after an average of 14.5 days. The fracture treatment therefore should usually be undertaken within the first week.

The extent to which **teeth at the fracture site** are factors in the formation of a fracture infection cannot be clearly established. In 1956, *Schönberger* found inflammatory complications in 18 % of 173 cases after extracting the tooth at the fracture site, and in 6 % of 30 cases in which teeth were left in place at the fracture. In this latter group, the teeth were all vital, with tolerably intact periodontium, while there was significantly greater damage to the tooth socket and a high rate of tooth mortification in the first group. With *Götte* (1959), the rate of complication after extraction was 20 % (60 cases) and 16.8 % (178 cases) when the tooth was left in place. *Neal* et al. (1978) found infections in 23% (69 cases) after extraction and in 13% (113 cases) after leaving the tooth in place. These quoted results should not give rise to the conclusion that the teeth at the fracture site should always be left in place. *Müller* (1964) ascertained that the incidence of fracture osteomyelitis was significantly greater when molars are left in place in the fracture line than after being extracted in the course of the fracture treatment. With monoradicular teeth, there were no perceptible differences.

Schönberger (1969) recommends the following procedure to reduce the incidence of fracture osteomyelitis with teeth at the fracture site:

1. Devitalized teeth and root stumps should be removed, with the exception of monoradicular teeth with a complication-free root canal filling and a normal apical appearance in the radiograph.
2. Vital teeth in the anterior and premolar regions may be left in place if the tooth socket is in tolerably good condition. Molars should usually be removed.

A further cause of fracture infection is **insufficient immobilization** of the fragments in fractures within the dental arch, with exposure to the oral cavity. Early treatment, therefore, with a complication-free stabilization of the fragments is an important prerequisite for avoiding fracture infections. Supportive antibiotic therapy is certainly advantageous, but does not have the same value as early treatment of the fracture.

In rare cases, an **actinomycotic infection** can appear. Case histories have been published by *Spreter von Kreudenstein* (1936), *Zitka* (1951), *Portwich* and *Schlegel* (1960), *Schuchardt* (1964), *Rowe* and *Killey* (1968), and *Trauner* (1973). The actinomycetes penetrate into the tissue over the fracture gap, which is open to the oral cavity.

Disturbances of sensitivity not infrequently occur after fractures of the mandible. The inferior alveolar nerve is rent or even severed when the fracture takes place. The damage is minor if the fragments are slightly or not at all displaced and increases with increasing displacement. *Reuther, Hausamen* and *Esswein* (1976) found primary disturbances of sensitivity in 465 of 1086 mandibular fractures (42.8%). In this series, it was possible to examine 244 of the affected patients later. Of these, 93 had permanent alterations of sensitivity, while the condition had cleared up in the others. Extrapolated to the total patient group, 16.3 % had permanent nerve injuries. These injuries were classified as follows: 4.9% anesthesias, 7.9% hypesthesias, 2.3% paresthesias, and 1.2 % hyperesthesias. *Müller* (1967) to the contrary found only 30 (1.3 %) instances of permanent damage to the mandibular nerves in a series of 2258 mandibular fracture patients.

No distinction was made in these statistics between patients treated conservatively and those treated surgically. *Reuter* and *Scharf* (1976) made the distinction and found hypesthesia in 4 % of conservatively managed patients; following wire osteosynthesis they recorded hypesthesia in 16% and anesthesia in 3% and after rigid internal fixation by means of compression plate or lag screw osteosynthesis they noted hypesthesia in 13% of their subjects. The low rate of disturbed sensitivity noted following conservative treatment is explained by the associated minor displacement; more severely displaced fractures were treated surgically.

In our own mandibular fracture patients we have found four subjects, in a series of 64 (6.25 %) available for follow-up examination, who had disturbances of sensitivity of the mental nerve after conservative treatment; three of these had hyesthesia and one anesthesia.

Occlusal disturbances persist if the reduction was not precisely performed. In 1943, *Wassmund* observed a 12.6 % occlusal disturbance rate in 323 retrospectively investigated cases. *Köle* (1956) and *Trauner* (1973) found an 0.8 % rate with 530 cases, and *Neumann-Lezius* and *Utz* found an 0.9 % rate with 1.352 cases (including maxillary fractures). *Reuter* and *Scharf* (1976) assessed the occlusal situation not only on the basis of clinical criteria, but also through the application of Kerr occlusal indicator wax in the dorsal contact position. The occlusion was characterized as good if there was a great deal of contact surface perceptible in the Kerr wax. In 64 cases, the incidence of occlusal disturbances was 22%. The incidence was only 16% after wire osteosynthesis and intermaxillary fixation, and only 6% after functionally stable osteosynthesis. In our own experience, we found occlusal disturbances in 7.7% of 104 cases of conservatively treated mandibular fractures.

Pseudarthroses are relatively rare: two were observed among 1.500 cases (0.1%) by *Wassmund* (1943), eight in 556 cases (1.4%) by *Hermann* et al. (1960), five in 385 cases (1.3%) by *Paschke* and *Berz* (1961), one in 67 cases (1.5%) by *Claudi* and *Spiessl* (1975), four in 530 cases (0.8%) by *Köle* (1956) and *Trauner* (1973), and 14 among 577 cases (2.5%) by *Mathog* and *Boies* (1976). In 104 of our own cases which we investigated retrospectively, we found one pseudarthrosis (0.96%).

The causes of pseudarthrosis formation are insufficient immobilization of the fragments, infection of the fracture, and in older patients, delayed callus formation.

References

Andrä, A., and I. Sonnenberg (1966)
Die Bruchspaltostitis als Komplikation bei Unterkieferbrüchen in Beziehung zum primär vitalen Zahn am oder im Bruchspalt. (Fracture site osteitis as a complication in mandibular fractures in relation to the vital tooth in or adjacent the fracture site.) Dtsch. Stomat. 16: 336

Angle, E. H. (1890 a)
A new method for the treatment of fracture of the maxilla. Int. dent. J. 11: 330

Angle, E. H. (1890 b)
The Angle system of treating fractures of the maxillary bones. Brit. J. dent. Sci. 33: 484

Archer, H. W. (1966 a)
Oral Surgery. 4th ed., Philadelphia, W. B. Saunders

Archer, H. W. (1966 b)
Chirurgie des Mundes und der Zähne. (Oral Surgery.) 3rd. ed., vol. 2. Stuttgart – Wien – Zürich, Medica

Becker, R., D. Broxtermann, E. Esser, H. Meiners, and P. Topp (1976)
Indikationsstellung für verschiedene Osteosyntheseverfahren auf der Grundlage klinischer und experimenteller Untersuchungen. (Indications for various osteosynthesis techniques on the basis of clinical and experimental investigations.) Fortschr. Kiefer- u. Gesichtschir. 21: 296

Bolle, R. (1952)
Über gegossene Kappenschienen zur Behandlung von Kieferbrüchen. (Cast cap splints for the treatment of jaw fractures.) Dtsch. zahnärztl. Z. 7: 815

Bolle, R. (1954)
Über die Behandlung der Kieferbrüche im zahnärztlichen Institut der Universität Göttingen in den Jahren 1949-1953. (Treatment of jaw fractures in the Dental College of the University of Göttingen in the period 1949-1953.) Dtsch. Zahnärztebl. 8: 759

Bradnum, P. (1960)
An improved method of fixation of silver cap splints. Brit. dent. J. 108: 302

Claudi, B., and B. Spiessl (1975)
Ergebnisse bei konservativer und operativer Behandlung von Unterkieferfrakturen (ohne Kollumfrakturen). (Results with conservative and surgical treatment of mandibular fractures; except fractures of the TMJ.) Fortschr. Kiefer- u. Gesichtschir. 19: 73

Dingman, R. O. and P. Natvig (1964)
Surgery of facial fractures. Philadelphia – London, W. B. Saunders

Eby, J. D. (1920)
Principles of orthodontia in the treatment of maxillofacial injuries. Int. J. Orthodont. 6: 273

Ernst, F. (1927)
Die zahnärztliche Behandlung der Unterkieferbrüche. (Dental treatment of mandibular fractures.) In Kirschner, M. and O. Nordmann: Die Chirurgie. (Surgery.) Vol. 4,1 Berlin – Wien, Urban & Schwarzenberg, p. 842

Ernst, F. (1932)
Die Schienenverbände bei Unter- und Oberkieferbrüchen. (Splints in mandibular and maxillary fractures.) In Bruhn, C., A. Kantorowicz, and C. Partsch, eds.: Handbuch der Zahnheilkunde. (Handbook of dentistry.) 4th. ed., Munich, I. F. Bergmann, vol. 1, p. 115

Freitag, V., and T. Höhnle (1976)
Zahnreihenluxation als Nebenwirkung von intraoralen Schienenverbänden. (Dental dislocations as side effects of intraoral splints.) Dtsch. zahnärztl. Z. 31: 640

Ganzer, H. (1943)
Die Kriegsverletzungen des Gesichts und Gesichtsschädels. (War injuries of the face and facial skeleton.) Leipzig, J. A. Barth

Gilmer, T. L. (1887)
A case of fracture of the lower jaw with remarks on treatment. Arch. Dent. 4: 388

Götte, H. (1959)
Die Belassung von Zähnen im Bruchspalt in Abhängigkeit von der Art des Kieferbruchverbandes. (Leaving teeth within the fracture line in dependence on the type of splinting.) Fortschr. Kiefer- u. Gesichtschir. 5: 333

Gunning, T. B. (1866/67)
The treatment of fracture of the lower jaw by interdental splints. N.Y. med. J. 3: 433; and 4: 11 and 274

Heidsieck, C. (1954)
Über die Behandlungsergebnisse bei Unterkieferfrakturen. (Results of treatment of mandibular fractures.) Dtsch. Stomatol. 4: 271

Hering, H.-J. (1960)
Eine einfache Methode der Kieferbruchschienung mit Hilfe von schnellhärtendem Kunststoff. (A simple technique for splinting jaw fractures with cold-curing arylic.) Dtsch. Zahnärztebl. 14: 742

Hering, H.-J. (1965)
Eine einfache Methode zur Befestigung von gegossenen Kieferbruchschienen. (A simple method for attaching cast metal splints.) Zahnärztl. Welt 66: 652

Herrmann, M., H. H. Grasser, and I. Beisiegel (1960)
Die Kieferbrüche an der Zahn-, Mund- und Kieferklinik in Mainz von 1949-1959. (Jaw fractures in the Mainz Dental College from 1949 to 1959.) Dtsch. zahnärztl. Z. 15: 657

Hofer, O. (1939)
Neuere Erkenntnisse in der Zahn-, Mund- und Kieferchirurgie. Über Frakturen der Kiefer. (Recent developments in oral surgery. Fractures of the jaws.) Zbl. ges. Zahn-Mund-Kieferheilk. 4: 327

Höltje, W.-J., H.-G. Luhr, and M. Holtfreter (1975)
Untersuchungen über infektionsbedingte Komplikationen nach konservativer oder operativer Versorgung von Unterkieferfrakturen. (Studies of infection-elicited complications after conservative or surgical care of fractures of the mandible.) Fortschr. Kiefer- u. Gesichtschir. 19: 122

Ivy, R. H. (1922)
Observations of fractures of the mandible. J. Amer. med. Ass. 79: 295

Juniper, R. P., and M. D. Awty (1973)
The immobilization period for fractures of the mandibular body. Oral Surg. 36: 157

Kalienberger, K. (1956)
Die Brüche des Unterkiefers. (Fractures of the mandible.) Fortschr. Kiefer- u. Gesichtschir. 2: 1

Kazanjian, V. H. (1933)
Treatment of automobile injuries of the face and jaws. J. Amer. dent. Ass. 20: 57

Kazanjian, V. H., and J. M. Converse (1959)
Surgical treatment of facial injuries. 2nd ed., Baltimore, Williams and Wilkins Co. (3rd ed. 1974)

Kersting, G. (1904)
Behandlung von Unterkieferfrakturen. (Treatment of mandibular fractures.) Dtsch. med. Wschr. 30: 390

Köhler, J. A. (1951)
Diagnostik und Therapie der Kieferfrakturen. (Diagnosis and treatment of jaw fractures.) Heidelberg, A. Hüthig

Köle, H. (1956)
Ergebnisse von Kieferbruchkontrollen im Zeitraum 1948-1959. (Results of jaw fracture follow-ups in the period 1948-1959.) Fortschr. Kiefer- u. Gesichtschir. 2: 115

Krüger, E. (1974)
Lehrbuch der chirurgischen Zahn-, Mund- und Kieferheilkunde. (Textbook of oral and maxillofacial surgery.) Berlin, Buch- und Zeitschriften-Verlag "Die Quintessenz", vol. 2 (4th ed. 1981)

Krüger, E. and S. Chrissefis (1971)
Kariesprophylaxe durch lokale Anwendung von Aminfluoriden bei der Versorgung von Kieferbruchpatienten mit der Drahtkunststoffschiene nach Schuchardt. (Caries prevention by local application of amine fluoride in the care of jaw fracture patients with Schuchardt's wire-acrylic arch bar.) Dtsch. zahnärztl. Z. 26: 1227

Lentrodt, J., and W.-J. Höltje (1975)
Indikationen zur operativen bzw. konservativen Versorgung von Unterkieferfrakturen. (Indications for surgical and conservative care of mandibular fractures.) Fortschr. Kiefer- u. Gesichtschir. 19: 65

Löhers, H.
Quoted by Röse, C. (1893): Über Kieferbrüche und Kieferbruchverbände. (About jaw fractures and splints.) Jena

Mathog, R. H., and L. R. Boles, Jr. (1976)
Nonunion of the mandible. Laryngoscope (St. Louis) 86: 908

Metz, H.-J. (1966)
Indikation und Technik der Drahtbogen-Kunststoffschiene nach Schuchardt. (Indication and technique of the wire-acrylic arch bar of Schuchardt.) Fortschr. Kiefer- u. Gesichtschir. 11: 124

Meyer, W. (1943)
Elementarbegriffe der Kieferbruchbehandlung. (Fundamental concepts of treatment of jaw fractures.) Dtsch. zahnärztl. Wschr. 46: 395

Meyer, W. (1952)
Die Orthopädie und das marginale Parodontium. (Orthopedics and the marginal periodontium.) Dtsch. zahnärztl. Z. 7: 225

Müller, W. (1964)
Zur Frage des Versuchs der Erhaltung der im Bruchspalt stehenden Zähne unter antibiotischem Schutz. (Maintenance of teeth in the fracture line under antibiotic cover.) Dtsch. Zahn- Mund- Kieferheilk. 41: 360

Müller, W. (1967)
Häufigkeit und Art der Spätfolgen bei 2733 Frakturen des Gesichtsschädels. (Frequency and sort of late sequelae in 2733 fractures of the facial skull.) Fortschr. Kiefer- u. Gesichtschir. 12: 220

Muska, K. (1971)
Einige Bemerkungen zu Komplikationen bei der intermaxillären Verschnürung. (Some comments about complications in intermaxillary fixation.) Dtsch. zahnärztl. Z. 26: 822

Neal, D. C., F. Wayne, and B. Alpert (1978)
Morbidity associated with teeth in the line of mandibular fractures. J. oral Surg. 36: 859

Neumann-Lezius, G., and W. Utz (1976)
Ergebnisse konservativer und operativer Kieferbruchbehandlung. (Results of conservative and surgical treatment of jaw fractures.) Dtsch. zahnärztl. Z. 31: 103

Neuner, O. (1957)
Vereinfachte Schienungstechnik zur Behandlung von Unterkieferfrakturen. (Simplified splinting technique for the treatment of mandibular fractures.) Dtsch. zahnärztl. Z. 12: 726

Neuner, O. (1977)
Maxillofaciale Traumatologie. (Maxillofacial traumatology.) Berlin – New York, de Gruyter

Niederdellmann, H., and W. Schilli (1972)
Funktionsstabile Osteosynthese im Unterkiefer. (Functionally stable osteosynthesis in the mandible.) Dtsch. zahnärztl. Z. 27: 138

Niederdellmann, H., and W. Schilli (1973)
Zur Plattenosteosynthese bei Unterkieferfrakturen. (Plate osteosynthesis in fractures of the mandible.) Dtsch. zahnärzt. Z. 28: 638

Obwegeser, H. (1952)
Über eine einfache Methode der freihändigen Drahtschienung von Kieferbrüchen. (A simple method for free-hand wire splinting of jaw fractures.) Öst. Z. Stomat. 49: 652

Paschke, H. and A. Berz (1961)
Die Frakturen der Kiefer-Gesichtsknochen und die statistische Auswertung derselben am Krankengut der Universitätsklinik für Zahn-, Mund- und Kieferkranke in Erlangen aus den Jahren 1950-1960. (Fractures of the maxillofacial bones and their statistical evaluation in the patients of the University Dental College in Erlangen in the years 1950-1960.) Dtsch. Zahnärztebl. 18: 681

Pfeifer, G., W. Busch, and B. Rottke (1975)
Verlauf und Auswirkung des Therapiewandels bei Frakturen des Gesichtsschädels. (Course and effect of changes in therapy in fractures of the facial skeleton.) Fortschr. Kiefer- u. Gesichtschir. 19: 62

Pfeifer, G., H.-G. Luhr and W. Höltje (1976)
Grenzen und Möglichkeiten der konservativen und operativen Kieferbruchbehandlung. (Limits and possibilities of conservative and surgical treatment of jaw fractures.) Dtsch. zahnärztl. Z. 31: 101

Portwich, G., and D. Schlegel (1960)
Die cervico-faciale Aktinomykose. (Cervicofacial actinomycosis.) Med. Mschr. 14: 726

Reichenbach, E. (1954)
Leitfaden der Kieferbruchbehandlung. (Guidelines for treatment of jaw fractures.) 6th ed., Leipzig, J. A. Barth

Reichenbach, E. (1957)
Verletzungen der Kiefer- und Gesichtsknochen und der benachbarten Weichteile. (Injuries of the maxillofacial bones and the adjacent soft tissues.) In Häupl, K., W. Meyer, and K. Schuchardt: Die Zahn-, Mund- und Kieferheilkunde. (Dentistry.) Munich, Urban & Schwarzenberg, Vol. III/1, p. 639

Reichenbach, E. (1969)
Die operative Behandlung der Unterkieferfrakturen. (Surgical treatment of mandibular fractures.) In: Reichenbach, E.: Traumatologie in Kiefer-Gesichts-Bereich. (Traumatology of the maxillofacial region.) Leipzig – Munich, J. A. Barth

Reither, W. (1956)
Der Erfolg der Kieferbruchbehandlung an der Klinik für Zahn-, Mund- und Kieferkrankheiten der Universität München in den Jahren 1945-1953. (Success of treatment of jaw fractures at the University of Munich Dental College in the years 1945-1953.) Dtsch. zahnärztl. Z. 11: 1300

Reuter, E., and F. Scharf (1976)
Spätfolgen nach Unterkieferfrakturen unter Berücksichtigung von Frakturverlauf, Dislokation und Behandlungsmethode. (Late sequelae of fractures of the mandible, with special attention to course of the fracture, displacement, and method of treatment.) Fortschr. Kiefer- u. Gesichtschir. 21: 307

Reuther, J., J-E. Hausamen, and W. Esswein (1976)
Neurologische Störungen nach Frakturen im Kiefer- und Gesichtsbereich. (Neurologic disorders after maxillofacial fractures.) Fortschr. Kiefer- u. Gesichtschir. 21: 290

Risdon, F. (1929)
The treatment of fractures of the jaws. Canad. med. Ass. J. 20: 260

Rowe, N. L., and H. C. Killey (1968)
Fractures of the facial skeleton. 2nd. ed., Edinburgh – London, Livingstone

Schilli, W. (1977)
Compression osteosynthesis. J. oral Surg. 35: 802

Schlampp, H. (1944)
Die Kieferbrüche und ihre Behandlung mit der Profilschiene. (Jaw fractures and their treatment with profile splints.) Berlin, Berlinische Verlagsanstalt

Schönberger, H. (1956)
Behandlung der Zähne im Bruchspalt. (Treatment of teeth in the fracture line.) Fortschr. Kiefer- u. Gesichtschir. 2: 108

Schönberger, A. (1969)
Die örtlichen Komplikationen bei Kieferverletzungen und ihre Behandlung. (Local complications in jaw injuries, and their treatment.) In Reichenbach, E.: Traumatologie im Kiefer-Gesichts-Bereich (Traumatology of the maxillofacial region.) Leipzig – Munich, J. A. Barth, p. 391

Schröder, H. (1911)
Handbuch der zahnärztlich-chirurgischen Verbände und Prothesen. (Handbook of oral surgical dressings and prostheses.) Vol. 1. Frakturen und Luxationen der Kiefer. (Fractures and dislocations of the jaws.) Berlin, H. Meusser

Schröder, H. (1917)
Anatomischer Charakter, Prognose und zahnärztliche Behandlung der Unterkieferschussbrüche. (Anatomical character, prognosis, and dental treatment of mandibular gunshot injuries.) In Klapp, R., and H. Schröder: "Die Unterkieferschussbrüche." (Mandibular gunshot fractures.) Berlin, H. Meusser

Schrudde, J. (1960)
Die Knochenbildung unter funktionellen Gesichtspunkten. (Bone formation with respect to function.) Dtsch. Zahn- Mund- Kieferheilk. 32: 97

Schuchardt, K. (1956)
Ein Vorschlag zur Verbesserung der Drahtschienenverbände. (A proposal for improving arch bar splinting) Dtsch. Zahn- Mund-Kieferheilk. 24: 39

Schuchardt, K. (1964)
Mikrobiologische und klinische Beobachtungen und Erfahrungen bei der zervikofazialen Aktinomykose. Klinischer Teil. (Clinical observations and results in cervicofacial actinomycosis.) Fortschr. Kiefer- u. Gesichtschir. 9: 259

Schuchardt, K., L. M. Brichetti and N. Schwenzer (1960)
Frakturen des Gesichtsskelettes. (Fractures of the facial skeleton.) Stoma (Heidelb.) 13: 159

Schuchardt, K., M. Kapovits and B. Spiessl (1961)
Technik und Anwendung des Drahtbogenkunststoffverbandes. (Technique and application of the wire-acrylic arch bar.) Dtsch. zahnärztl. Z. 16: 1241

Schuchardt, K., and H. J. Metz (1966)
Injuries of the facial skeleton. In Gibson, T.: Modern trends in plastic surgery. Vol. 2. London, Butterworths.

Spiessl, B. (1975)
Funktionsstabile Osteosynthese bei Unterkieferfrakturen.–Problematik und Technik. (Functionally stable osteosynthesis in fractures of the mandible.–Problems and technique.) Fortschr. Kiefer- u. Gesichtschir. 19: 68

Spiessl, B., and K. Schroll (1972)
Gesichtsschädel. (Facial skull.) In Nigst, H.: Spezielle Frakturen- und Luxationslehre. (Special treatment of fractures and dislocations.) Vol. I/1. Stuttgart, Thieme

Spreter von Kreudenstein, T. (1936)
Beiträge zur Therapie der Kieferaktinomykose. (Treatment of actinomycosis of the jaw.) Dtsch. Zahn- Mund- Kieferheilk. 3: 678

Stout, R. A. (1943)
Intramaxillary wiring and intermaxillary elastic traction and fixation. In: Manual of standard practice of plastic and maxillo-facial surgery. Military Surgical Manuals I. Philadelphia – London, W. B. Saunders Co., p. 272

Süersen, W. (1871)
Über Verletzungen resp. Frakturen des Ober- und Unterkiefers. (Injuries and fractures of the maxilla and the mandible.) Dtsch. Vjschr. Zahnheilk. 11: 261

Thoma, K. H. (1958)
Oral Surgery. St. Louis, The C. V. Mosby Co.

Trauner, R. (1973)
Kiefer- und Gesichtschirurgie. (Maxillofacial Surgery) Vol. 2. Munich – Berlin – Vienna, Urban & Schwarzenberg

Virolainen, E., and K. Altasalo (1976)
Surgical and conservative treatment of mandibular fractures. A follow-up study. J. oral Surg. 5: 265

Wassmund, M. (1927)
Frakturen und Luxationen des Gesichtsschädels. (Fractures and dislocations of the facial skeleton.) Leipzig, H. Meusser

Wassmund, M. (1943)
Die freihändige Versorgung der Brüche des Unterkiefers, einschliesslich der Schußbrüche. (Free-hand care of mandibular fractures including gunshot fractures.) Berlin, Berlinische Verlagsanstalt

Weiskopf, J. (1969)
Die Frakturen des Unterkiefers und ihre orthopädische Behandlung. (Fractures of the mandible and their orthopedic treatment). In Reichenbach, E.: Traumatologie im Kiefer-Gesichts-Bereich. (Maxillofacial traumatology.) Leipzig – Munich, J. A. Barth, p. 217

Williams, D.
Quoted by Rowe, N. L. and H. C. Killey (1968)

Wirth, F. (1955)
Eine kombinierte Kunststoff-Draht-Kieferbruchschiene. (A combined acrylic-arch bar splint for fractures of the jaw.) Zahnärztl. Rdsch. 64: 425

Wirth, F. (1956)
Die Kombination der Draht- und Prothesenschiene bei der Kieferbruchbehandlung. (The combination of arch bar and prosthesis splint in treatment of jaw fractures.) Fortschr. Kiefer- u. Gesichtschir. 2: 97

Zitka, E. (1951)
Klinische und therapeutische Erfahrungen bei cervikofacialer Aktinomykose. (Clinical and therapeutic experience in cervicofacial actinomycosis.) Öst. Z. Stomat. 48: 11

3. Interosseous Wiring

Norbert Schwenzer

3.1 Biomechanical Principles of Interosseous Wiring

Interosseous wiring is the surgical union of two or more bone fragments with the aid of wire ligatures. Drilling holes in the bone is required for the purpose.

The technique, in use since the beginning of the 19th century, was not adopted widely because of associated complications, e.g., injury to teeth, osteomyelitis, fracture line abscesses, fistula formation, disturbances in occlusion, and pseudoarthrosis. Analyses of the source of failures (*Link*, 1937; *Dietrich*, 1951; *Andrusch*, 1959) pointed to poor asepsis and the use of wires not resistant to corrosion; copper or Randolph wires were found unsuitable. Above all, however, failures were ascribed to the insufficient stabilization effect of the wire ligature. For a long period, therefore, purely conservative methods were given preference in the treatment of fractures of the jaw. Only the increased frequency of facial skull fractures and the resulting need for a more rational fracture therapy led to reconsideration of interosseous wiring and to the development of an absolutely safe and widely applicable technique.

Before that development could be completed, however, a series of fundamental studies of the mechanical and biological reactions of the wire ligature was required.

The wire material used at the time was an "austenitic," soft, monofilament chromium-nickel-steel material (V_4AS) of the following composition:

0.7 % C, 1.0 % Si, 2.0 % Mn, 16.5-18.5 % Cr, 10.5-13.5 % Ni, 2.0-2.5 % Mo.

The physico-mechanical properties were:

Tensile strength	50-70 kp/mm^2
Limit of elasticity	21 kp/mm^2
Ductile strength	45 % min.
Modulus of elasticity	20-300 kp/mm^2
Specific gravity	7.9 g/cm^2

The method of production of the wire was drawing.

Diameters of 0.35, 0.4, and 0.5 mm were used for the wire ligatures.

The greatest strain to which a 100 mm strip of wire could be put before a break occurred was 6.4 kp (0.35 mm diameter), 8.4 kp (0.4 mm) or 16.2 kp (0.5 mm; *Schwenzer*, 1966, 1967).

The question of shape of the wire ligature for maximal stability was investigated as well, in that five different shapes of the ligature (Fig. 8.3-1) were tested on a model for tensile force and deflection. These studies indicated that greatest stability was achieved when two parallel wires were used, each with two bur holes. The stability of this design increased with increasing vertical distance between the drilled holes. The effective strain, e.g., during biting, is only one-fourth of the experimental value.

The ligature design in which only a single hole is utilized, the second wire being drawn through the same hole as the first and proceeding around the margin of the mandible in a figure of eight ligature, was the second most stable. The mechanically poorest form was the simple figure of eight ligature. The weakest points in all of the forms tested was at the site of the drilled hole and at the point at which the wires twisted together. Under the influence of tension or bending forces, the wires became untwisted or tore into the bone.

These observations made on a model were substantiated in animal experiments on fractured rabbit mandibles (Fig. 8.3-2). These studies demonstrated that it is possible to hold the fragments in constant position without additional fixation, and sometimes even to develop bony consolidation (*Schwenzer* and *Dieckmann*, 1971). In man, however, this is not possible.

Taking into consideration the various muscular forces, the complex movements of the mandible, and the great forces developed during mastication, man absolutely requires additional fixation of the fractured mandible with splints. Interosseous wiring alone is not able to provide functional stability, even when the diameter of the wire is increased. The ligature affords only

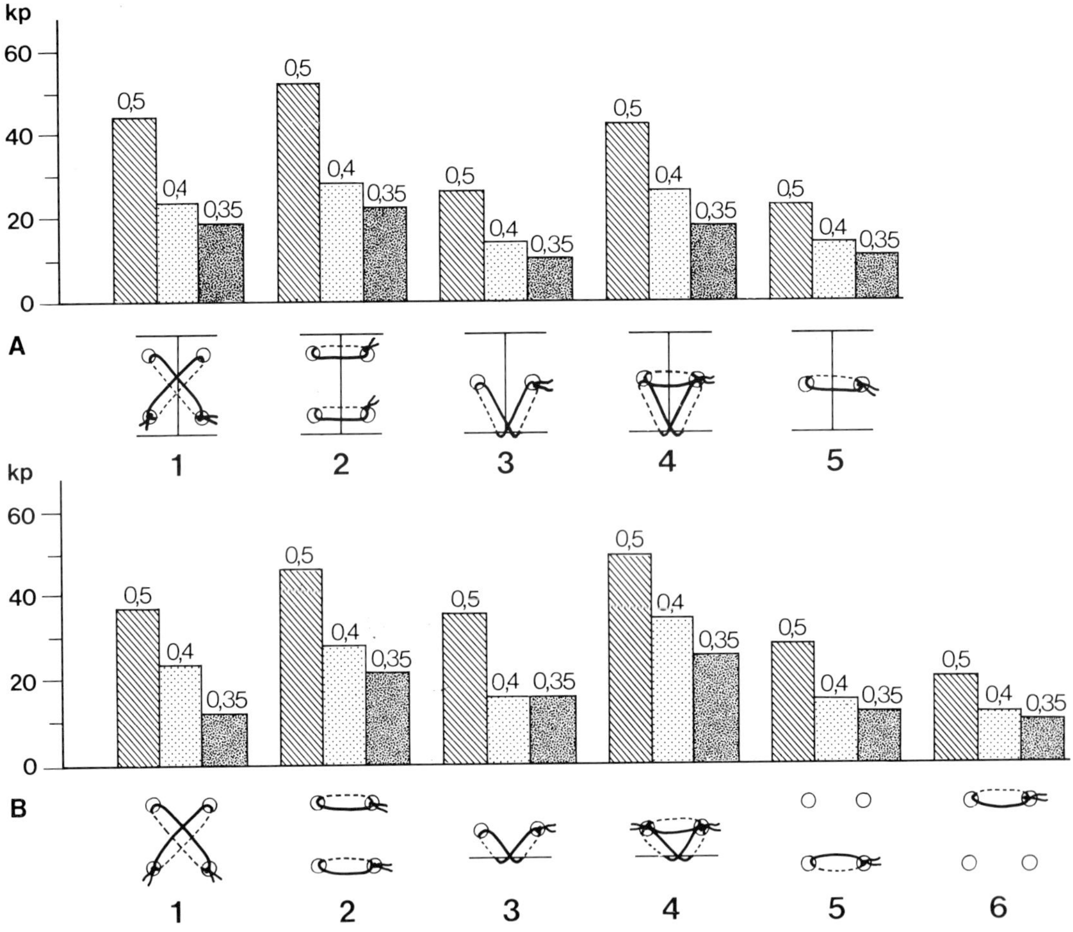

Fig. 8.3-1 Experimental responses of various shapes of wire ligatures to force (A) and bending (B); wire diameters 0.5, 0.4 and 0.35 mm. The weakest point of the wire ligature in each instance is at the bur holes and at the twisted joints. Ligature No. 2 was the most stable. If only two bur holes are placed, ligature No. 4 is the most stable.

resting stability. The wire ligature fixes the fragments in exact anatomical relationship following reduction of the fracture and thus provides the prerequisite for sound healing of the fracture. Earlier mobilization of the immobilized jaw frequently is made possible. Primary healing of the bone, as is sought via plate osteosynthesis, is unattainable. Instead, as a rule, indirect healing of the bone occurs.

The use of heavier wire does not lead to better stability, as has been confirmed by animal experiments (*Dieckmann*, 1970). The usual wire diameter used in the human mandible, 0.4 mm, has been found to be entirely adequate. Heavier wires (more than 0.5 mm diameter) are less flexible and adapt less well to the contours of the bone. During twisting of the wires, uneven strains may develop at the portal of the drilled hole, and bone tears may develop in thin bone lamellae. Furthermore, the question of removal

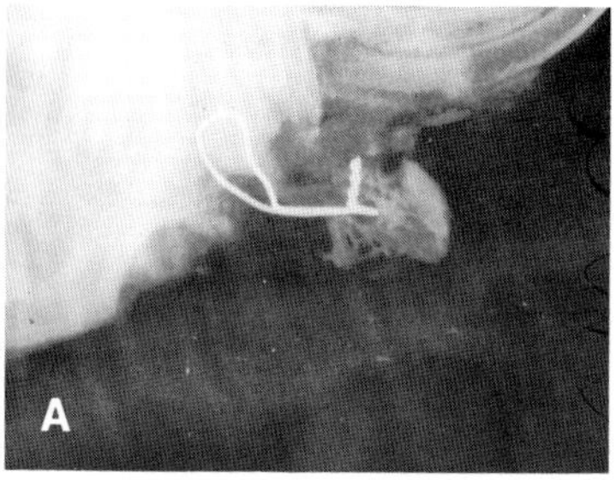

Fig. 8.3-2 A Pseudoarthrosis and sequestrum formation four weeks following immobilization of a fractured rabbit mandible with a wire ligature in the shape of a figure of eight; design that proved to be the least suitable.

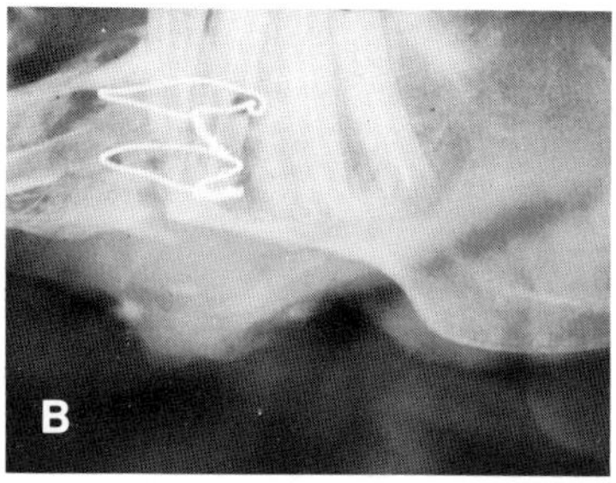

Fig. 8.3-2 B The fragments in the fractured rabbit mandible could be held in normal position with a parallel wire ligature.

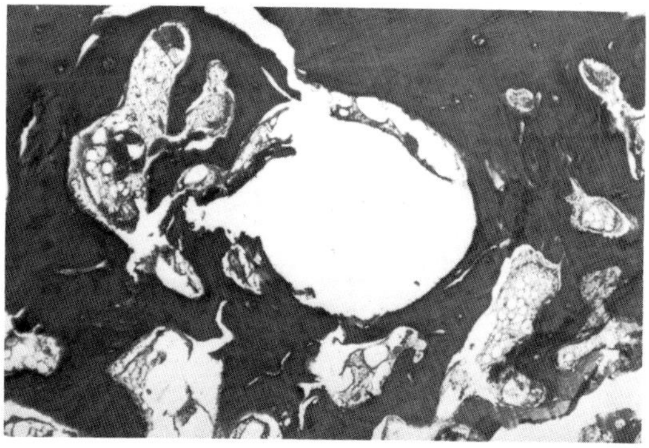

Fig. 8.3-3 Bur hole in the rabbit mandible (H & E stain, 130 X) placed with a low-speed sharp bur. The bone shows no evidence of injury.

of the osteosynthesis wires becomes more important as the equilibrium between metal and bone shifts in favor of the former.

In this connection, therefore, one must examine the extent to which injury to the bone and soft tissue may arise from the material used for the osteosynthesis. Studies by *Schwenzer* and *Renner* (1972), *Grasser* (1972) and *Steinhilber* (1976) have shown that appropriate use of the wire does not lead to corrosion and associated toxic effects. Microscopic examination and electron beam microanalyses of wire surfaces and cuts on used wires have provided no evidence of structural changes. Nor have there been any disturbances of wire structure itself. However, when wire is manipulated improperly, e.g., when it is crushed with forceps, even high quality steel is subject to corrosion damage. This damage can be avoided with proper care. The stainless steels react completely passively in tissue and in tissue cultures and have no cytotoxic effects. The V_4AS wire introduced in 1954 (480 mV) fulfills all the requirements made of a material to be used for osteosynthesis (*Hicks*, 1964).

No disadvantageous effects on fracture healing were found in animal experiments with wire ligatures. Rather, in fact, in the region of the prepared holes, normal bone deposition was present when these holes were prepared with low-speed, sharp burs (Fig. 8.3-3). The studies of used wires showed, with respect to corrosion changes, that no changes affecting success appeared as a rule. Minor microscopically demonstrable surface changes following long-term placement of the wire, found after wire had been in place in one subject for 66 months, did not lead to weakening of the material. Greater corrosion, therefore, with its undesirable effects, is not likely even when the

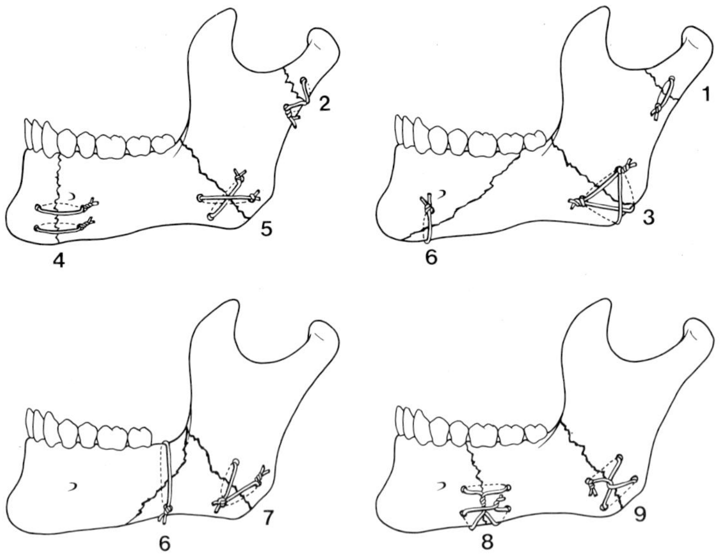

Fig. 8.3-4 Various wire ligature shapes.
(1) simple ligature
(2) figure-of-eight ligature
(3) combined simple and figure-of-eight ligature (Schwenzer, 1967)
(4) double ligature
(5) crossed ligature
(6) circumferential wiring
(7) triangular wiring
(8) Brons (1970) wiring
(9) Neuner's (1977) wire ligature.

wires are in place for long periods. The wires therefore need not be removed; this has been confirmed by clinical observations as well. For the use of wire ligatures, therefore, one can draw the following conclusions from experimental results:
Interosseous wiring is an excellent type of osteosynthesis useful in a variety of applications. It can lead to success when the following caveats are observed:

1. The wire ligature is not functionally stable. Additional means of immobilization of the fractured mandible, with splints, is indispensable.
2. Only monofilament V_4AS steel wire may be used.
3. The holes drilled into the bone must not be too close to the fracture line.
4. Low-speed drills must be used and the bone must be kept moist by spraying with Ringer solution to avoid heat damage.
5. The diameter of the drilled hole should be only slightly greater than that of the wire being used.
6. Increasing the diameter of the wire does not improve stability. As a rule, a diameter of 0.4 mm suffices for interosseous wiring of the mandible.

This discussion of interosseous wires and their application, as they are related to mandibular fractures, can be extrapolated as well to interosseous wires used in the treatment of fractures of the midface. Here, contrary to the bending forces that predominate in the mandible, however, the principal forces that arise are tension forces (*Schwenzer,* 1975), which provide much better conditions. In consequence, as a rule, supplemental fixation devices are superfluous.

3.2 Shapes of Interosseous Wire Ligatures

The diversity of interosseous wire ligatures is underlined by the fact that a whole series of ligature types has clinical application. As noted in the previous section, there are mechanically stable, as well as less stable forms of interosseous wires. In addition to the anatomical peculiarities, e.g., tooth roots, mandibular canal, the selection of a particular type of ligature depends as well on the type of fracture and the course of the fracture line. The following suture shapes may be used (Fig. 8.3-4):

1. Simple ligature
The most frequent form of ligature, especially when it is necessary to secure small fragments or when there is only a small surgically prepared approach. It is appropriate for fixation of the coronoid and the condyloid process and for intraoral wire ligatures. This type of ligature has a low resistance to bending.

2. Figure-of-eight ligature
Not suitable for tension forces, because the crossed loop can slip into the fracture line. Less desirable than the previous form from the point of view of bending resistance as well. Is easily applied, however, because the wire is introduced into both holes from the outside.

3. Simple ligature combined with figure-of-eight ligature
Most stable form in respect to tension and bending forces when there are only two holes. This form permits fixation in the vertical via the shoulder that passes around the edge of the mandible. It is appropriate for almost all transverse and oblique fractures of the body of the mandible, and may be used in fractures of the condylar neck as well. We prefer this ligature shape.

4. Double ligature
It is the most stable ligature mechanically against tension and bending forces. Its stability increases with increasing distance between the prepared holes. In the edentulous mandible, the upper pair of drilled holes may be placed above the mandibular canal. In the dentulous mandible, this usually is not possible because of the danger of root injury. The applicability of this form of suture, therefore, is limited.

5. Crossed ligature
Crossed ligatures are mechanically less desirable than parallel ligatures. If it is possible to place two holes in each fragment, this design provides no advantages. Almost the same effect may be attained with the ligature described under (3), above.

6. Transcircumferential wiring
This form of wiring, described by *Thoma* (1958), is well adapted to oblique fractures. It is a combination of wire ligature and cerclage and can be placed from intra- or extraorally.

7. Modifications
In addition to these basic varieties, further modifications are known. These include the triangular ligature (7), the wire arrangement described in 1970 by *Brons* (8), and the crossed wire ligature described by *Neuner* (1977) with a single loop (9). These wire ligatures require the placement of three or four bur holes. They too, however, are not functionally stable so that the range of indications for their use is not fundamentally greater than that of ligatures with two parallel wires. According to various reports, they are said to permit very early functional therapy because of their better stability conditions.

From case to case—and that is one of the great advantages of interosseous wiring—one must modify techniques, e.g., to stabilize several fragments, as may be necessary in crushing fractures. In addition, combinations with circumferential wiring are required occasionally, this supplemental step serving in adaptation of fragments as well as immobilization of denture splints.

3.3 Indications for Interosseous Wiring

Interosseous wiring has demonstrated its usefulness in a whole series of fracture types, in that it reliably adapts displaced fragments after reduction and until bony consolidation, thus contributing to the restoration of form and function. It is used as a supportive measure only in connection with dental splints in the following forms of mandibular fractures associated with displacement of fragments:

1. Fractures in edentulous or largely edentulous mandibles (Fig. 8.3-5)
2. Fractures of the horizontal ramus distal to the most posterior tooth (retrodental fractures)
3. Fractures of the angle of the jaw (Figs. 8.3-6 and 8.3-7)

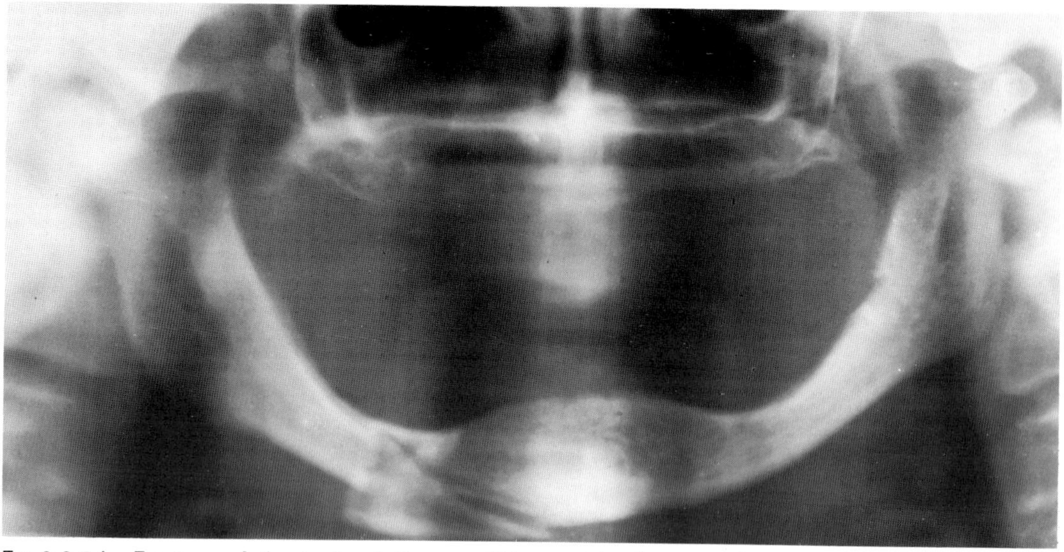

Fig. 8.3-5 A Fracture of the body of the mandible at right; fracture of the condylar process at left. Edentulous jaws.

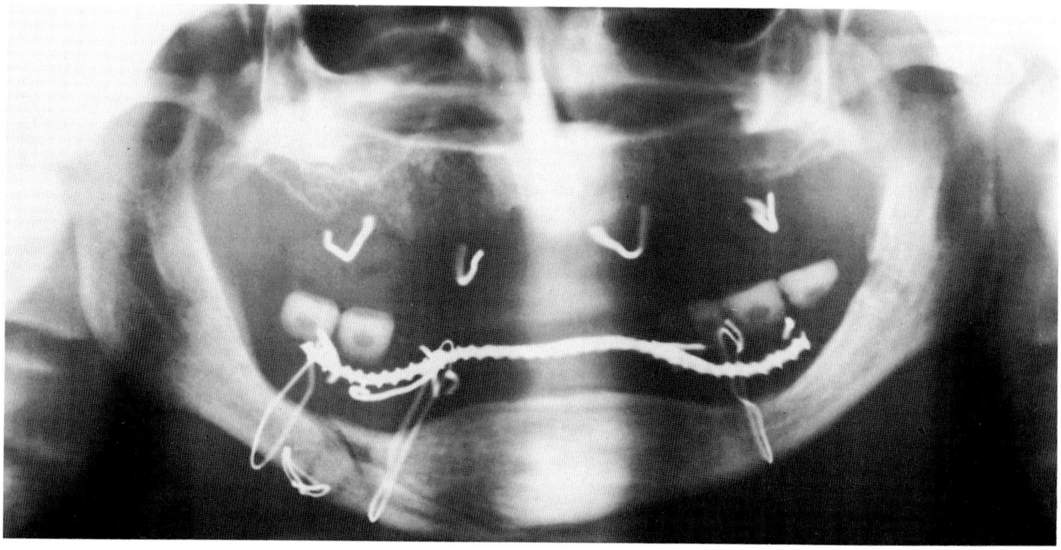

Fig. 8.3-5 B Wire ligature and splinting of the mandible by fixation of the mandibular denture with three circumferential wires.

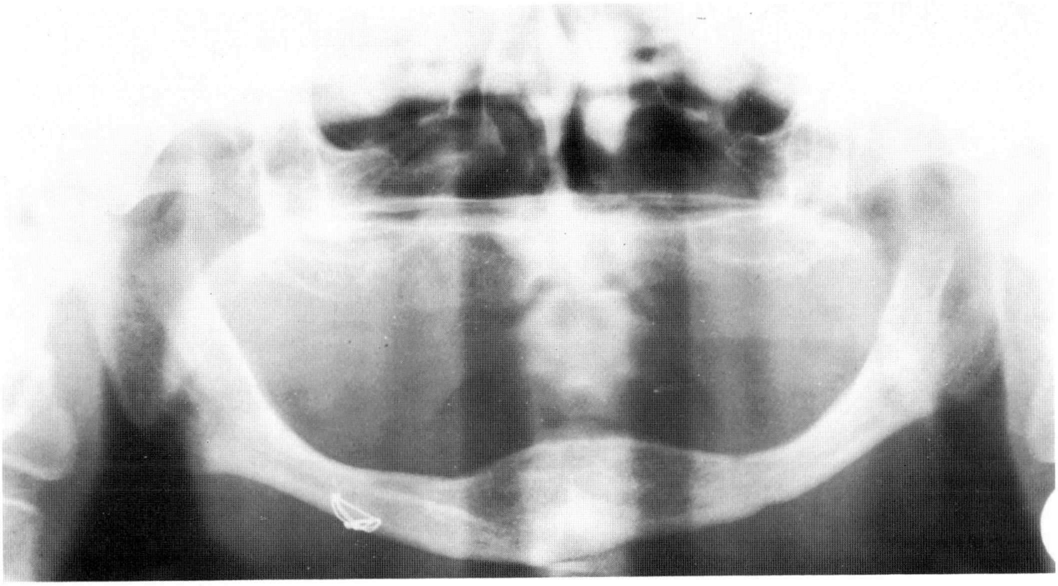

Fig. 8.3-5 C Appearance two years later. Wire ligatures healed without irritation.

4. Fractures open to the oral cavity or to the environment
5. Bilateral fractures of the body of the mandible (Fig. 8.3-8)
6. Severely displaced diagonal or horizontal fractures of the ascending ramus
7. Deep fractures of the condylar process lacking fragment contact at the base
8. Severely displaced fractures of childrens' mandibles in the primary and mixed dentition stages (Fig. 8.3-9)

In principle, interosseous wiring is required in all instances in which fragment reduction is not possible by conservative measures and functionally stable osteosynthesis is not planned. Interosseous wires serve to maintain the position after reduction. Interosseous wiring may be indicated immediately in a series of types of fractures, as in open fractures with exposed fragments, and especially when several single fragments are present, as in fractures associated with gunshot wounds and in the edentulous mandible. Indications may appear secondarily as well, however, as when reduction of fractures within the dentulous dental arch by conservative techniques leads to difficulties.

Especially in comminuted fractures in which several small fragments must be reduced and immobilized precisely in their original positions, placement of interosseous wires is the method of choice. It is superior to all other techniques of osteosynthesis requiring extensive exposure of the bone and implantation of larger pieces of metal.

Interosseous wiring is also indicated for use in combined fractures of the maxilla and the mandible in which intermaxillary immobilization is necessary anyway.

For fixation of fragments in the child's mandible, in which the tooth buds should not be injured

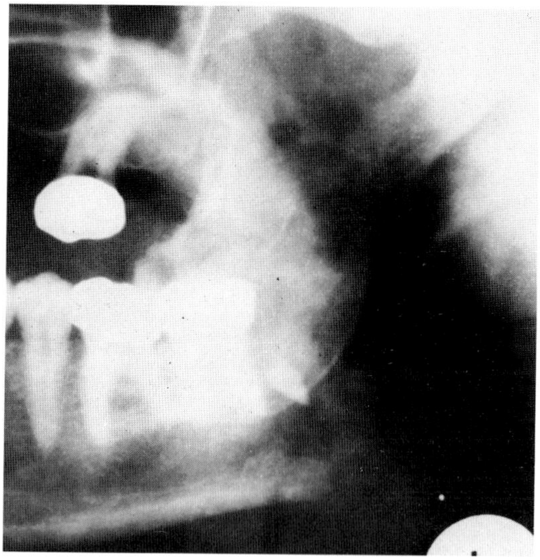

Fig. 8.3-6 A Iatrogenic mandibular fracture associated with an attempt to extract the left mandibular third molar.

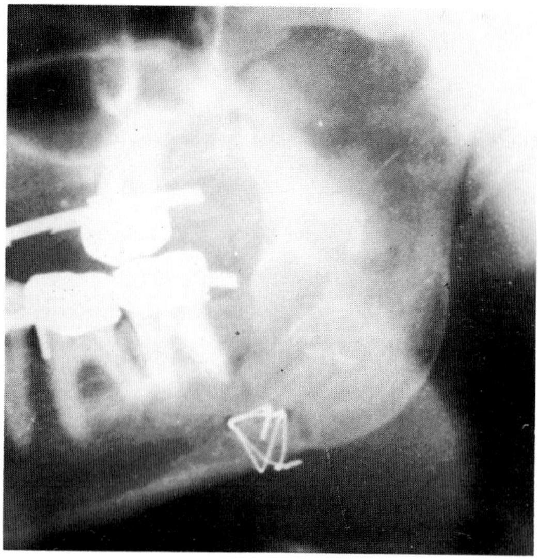

Fig. 8.3-6 B Appearance following removal of the root, placement of arch bars, and interosseous wiring.

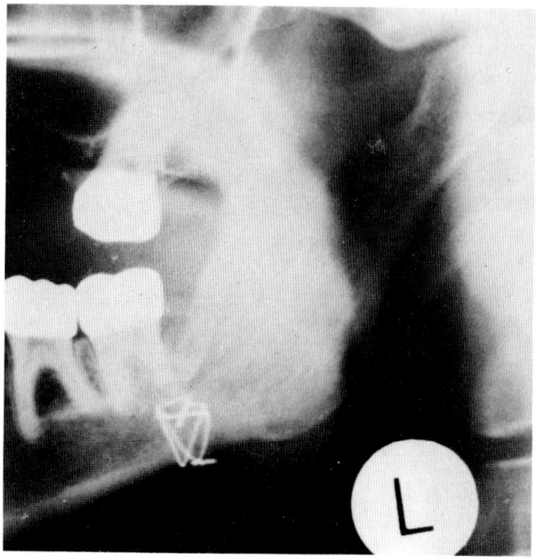

Fig. 8.3-6 C Appearance one year later.

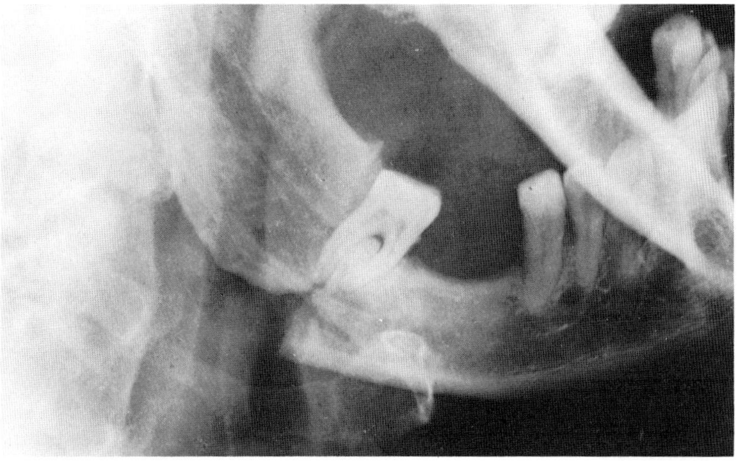

Fig. 8.3-7 A Typical fracture of the angle of the mandible with elevation of the ascending ramus. The third molar is in the fracture line.

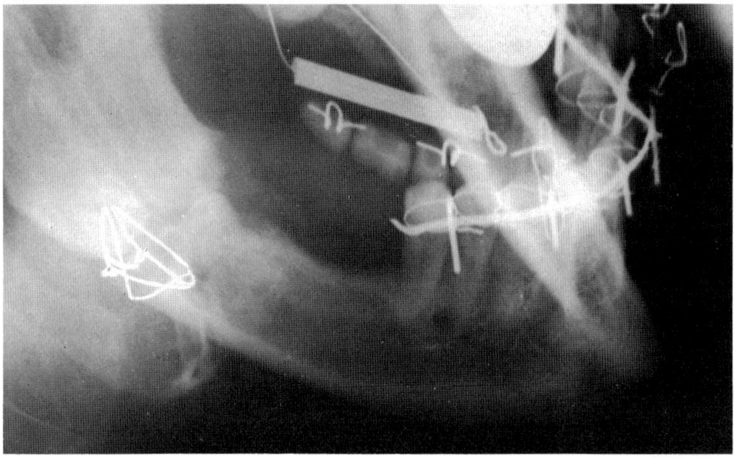

Fig. 8.3-7 B Appearance following intermaxillary fixation with the aid of a maxillary denture fastened by means of circumzygomatic wiring and a mandibular arch bar and open reduction with interosseous wiring.

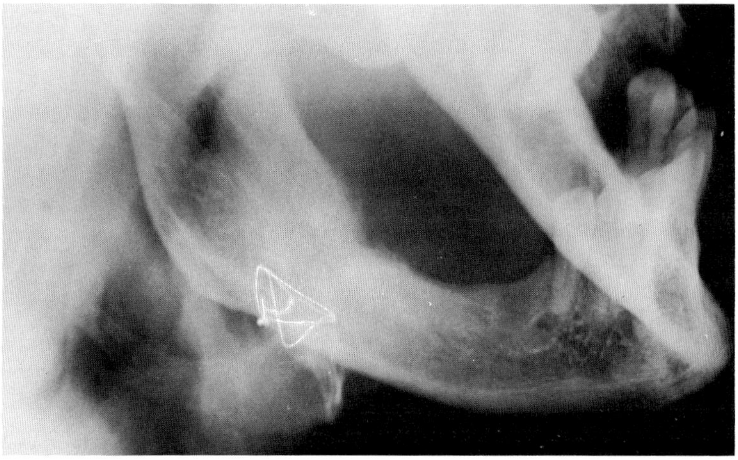

Fig. 8.3-7 C Appearance one year later.

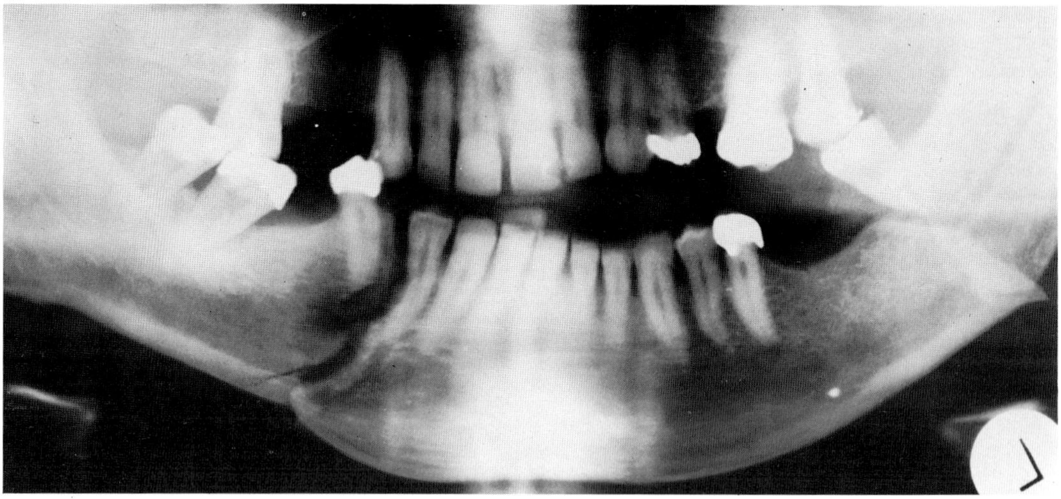

Fig. 8.3-8 A Bilateral fracture of the mandible treated with two wire ligatures and intermaxillary fixation via tooth-borne arch bars. Teeth in the fracture lines were extracted.

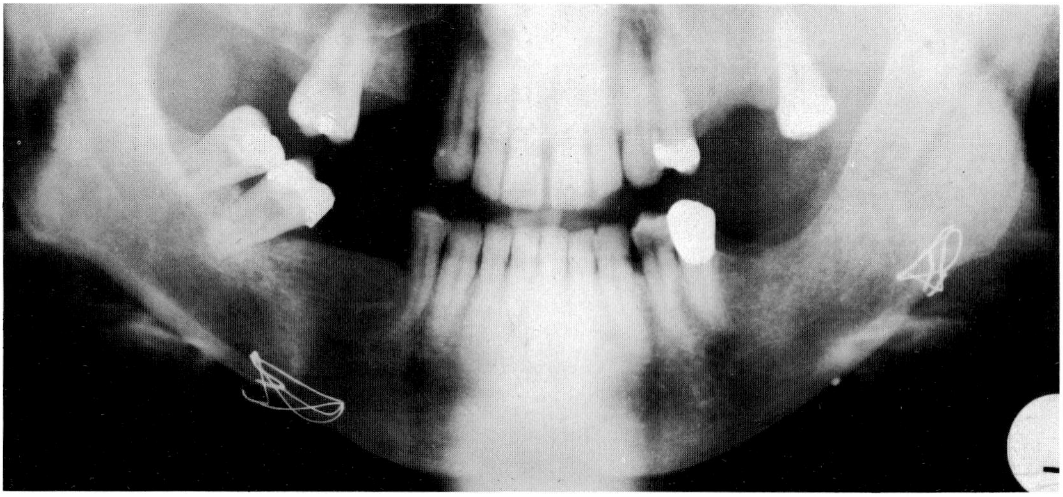

Fig. 8.3-8 B Appearance one year later. There is bony consolidation; the fragments are in normal position.

under any circumstances, interosseous wiring provides the only possible method of osteosynthesis (Fig. 8.3-9). By placing the holes for the wire in the region of the inferior border of the mandible or in the external cortical layer, such injury can be avoided in every instance (*Schwenzer*, 1969).

For fixation of bone transplants following comminuted fractures associated with loss of bone, interosseous wires have demonstrated their usefulness, just as they have in pseudoarthroses.

The method also is applicable for osteosynthesis in the region of the temporomandibular joint; opinions about specific techniques, e.g., whether a completely dislocated condylar process should be removed at all costs and then be replanted in dislocation fractures, vary. Most German authors are rather guarded in their approaches to fractures of the temporomandibular joint and prefer purely conservative measures (*Kristen* and *Singer*, 1976; *Günther* et al., 1966; *Schwenzer*, 1977; *Becker* and *Austermann*, 1981).

3.4 Technique of Interosseous Wiring

Instrumentation

As a rule, the wire ligature can be placed in the mandible with a steel wire of 0.4 mm diameter. Depending on the size of the fragments, thinner wires (0.35 or 0.2 mm) may be used. The latter size is especially useful as a threading wire.
The required instrumentarium consists of two bone-holding forceps, one or two sharp bone hooks, a low-speed handpiece and rose or *Lindemann* burs, pointed and flat forceps, a wire cutter and a *Pean*'s forceps, or a needle holder with a ratchet to twist the wire ends (Fig. 8-3-10). Either a bent blunt hemostat or a *Spiessl* forceps (Fig. 8.3-10 A) may be used to guide the wire.

Splints

With teeth present, the planned splint should be placed before open reduction. Any of the directly placed splints are appropriate (see Chapter 6). Note that the arch bar must be separated in the region of the fracture, lest the open reduction be made more complicated.
If anterior teeth are present to make intermaxillary fixation possible, placement of denture saddles is not necessary for fractures of the retrodental region, as a rule.
In fractures of the edentulous jaw, *Gunning* splints which are placed immediately following wiring must be available. These are placed with circumferential wires in the mandible and with circumzygomatic or permaxillary wires in the maxilla as supplemental immobilization.
The time for the subsequent intermaxillary fixation is given variously in the literature. Ten days (*Neuner*, 1977) is the shortest interval; 4 to 6 weeks (*Freihofer* and *Sailer*, 1975) the longest. It depends largely on the type of fracture. On the average, we have used intermaxillary fixation for 3 to 4 weeks.

Removal of the Tooth within the Fracture Line

The required extraction of a tooth in the line of the fracture usually is undertaken before open reduction. The socket must be covered by means of a mucoperiosteal flap subsequently. With severe displacement, this is not always possible, so that definitive intraoral wound closure sometimes must be done following open reduction and osteosynthesis.

Tooth extraction in the fracture line is indicated when:

1. The tooth represents interference to reduction of the fracture.
2. The fracture line continues to the fundus of the socket so that a root tip and half a root extend into the fracture line (Fig. 8.3-8 A).
3. Apical osteitis or advanced marginal periodontitis exists.
4. Root fractures are present.
5. An unerupted or semi-erupted tooth, e.g., third molar, lies in the fracture line (Fig. 8.3-7 A).

The indications for extraction should be more limited with an old fracture than a new one, because of possible infection. The remarks of *Ryberg* (1960) should be considered in this connection; her studies indicate that the earlier the fracture is immobilized, the better the chances for maintenance of a tooth lying in the fracture line.
In principle, **extraoral**, **intraoral**, as well as **combined** intra- and extraoral techniques are possible (*Kazanjian*, 1933; *Schröder*, 1966; *Paul* and *Acevedo*, 1968; *Reichenbach*, 1969; *Schwenzer* and *Steinhilber*, 1974; and *Archer*, 1975). The type of procedure selected depends on the location of the fracture, the manner in which it occurred, and the extent of accompanying soft tissue damage. As a rule, nasal intubation anesthesia is preferred because it permits undisturbed adjustment of the occlusion. Nevertheless, reduction is possible with conduction or local anesthesia. In all instances in which there is exposure to the oral cavity, whether through a mucosal injury or the existence of a tooth in the fracture line, antibiotic cover for 5 to 6 days is suggested.

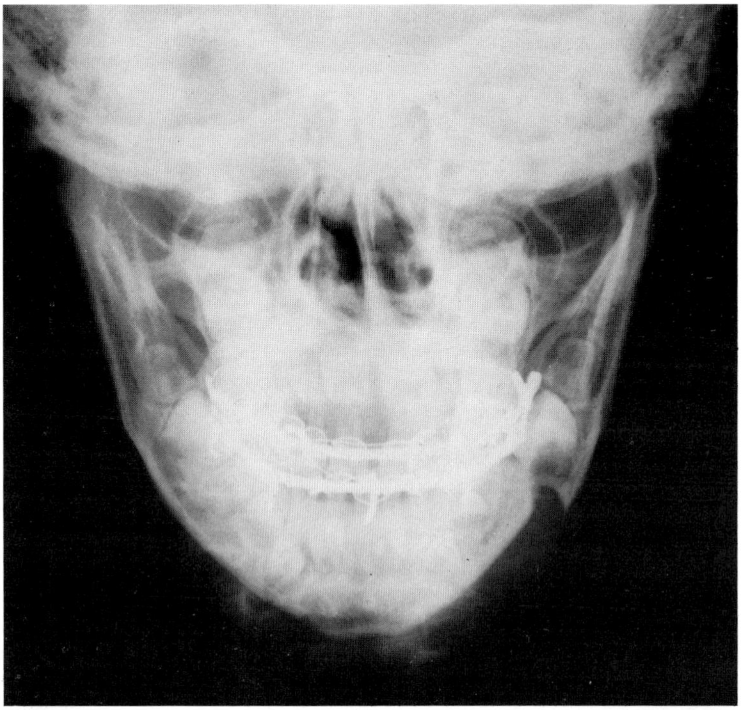

Fig 8.3-9 A Mandibular fracture in a 6-year-old girl. The tooth bud in the fracture line impedes reduction of the fracture.

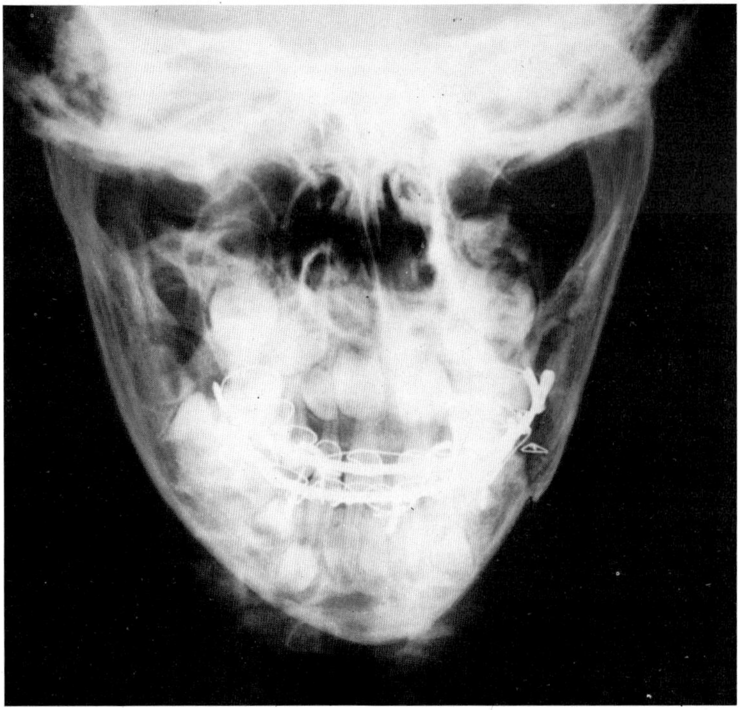

Fig. 8.3-9 B Appearance following extraction of the bud of the first molar and intraoral interosseous wire placement.

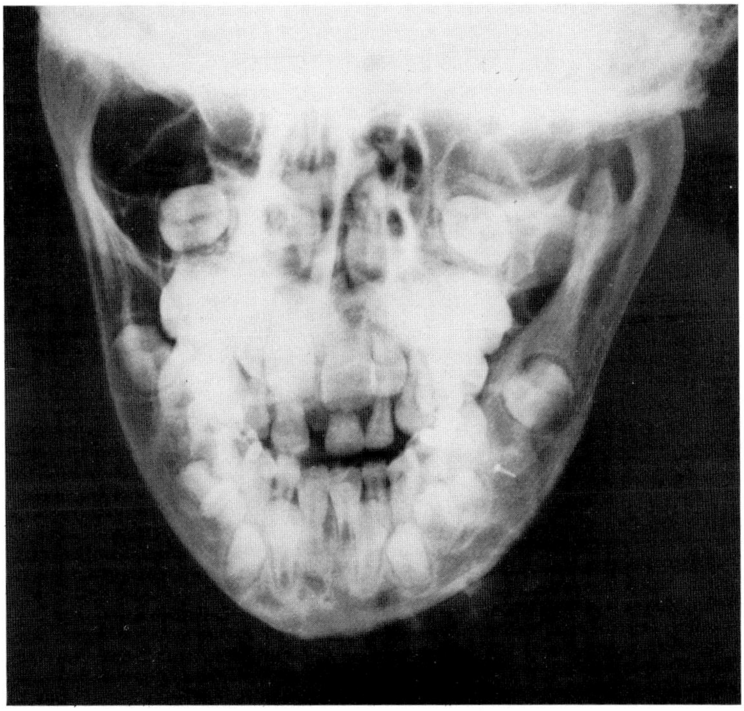

Fig. 8.3-9 C Appearance two years later.

3.4.1 Extraoral Approach

The extraoral approach has the advantage of providing a better view; it is suitable for all fractures of the body or the angle of the mandible and the condylar process. It serves as well in all perforating soft tissue-bone injuries. The patient is positioned in such a manner that the mandible-neck site to be operated is in an observable position; the head is deflected. In fractures of the chin, the head is bent backwards in a straigth position. The fracture site is exposed via an incision approximately 5 cm long, at least two fingerbreadths below the inferior border of the mandible with the natural folds of the skin taken into consideration. If the line of the incision lies in a neck fold, the later scar will be barely visible. Especially with fractures of the angle of the mandible and in the molar region, the incision should not be placed too high because the course of the mandibular branch of the facial nerve must be heeded. The arch-shaped line between the mastoid and the greater horn of the hyoid bone, as previously described by *Spiessl* and *Schroll* (1972), serves as an orientation line here as well. The skin and the platysma are elevated from the fascia of the neck to the margin of the mandible. The facial artery and vein must be ligated when the fracture is in the region of the angle of the mandible. The mandibular branch of the facial nerve crosses both of these vessels at the level of the inferior border of the mandible and remains above the site of the incision in the soft tissue (see also Chapter 8, Section 5.1.1.1 and Fig. 8.5.1-2). In fractures within the masseter-pterygoid sling, the insertion of the muscle must be separated, at least in part, from the bone. This is true as well for deep fractures of the condylar process. The periosteum is incised along the mandibular border and the fracture site is exposed. The periosteum is reflected

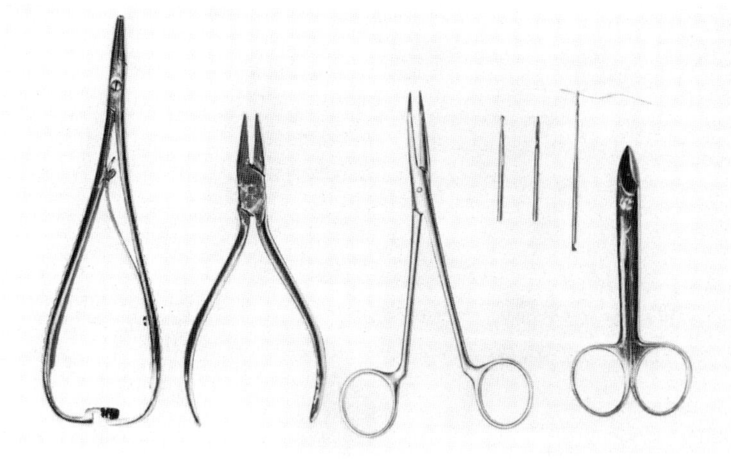

Fig. 8.3-10 A Instrumentation for placement of interosseous wires. From left to right: ligature forceps to twist the wires, flat forceps, Spiessl forceps, burs, wire cutter.

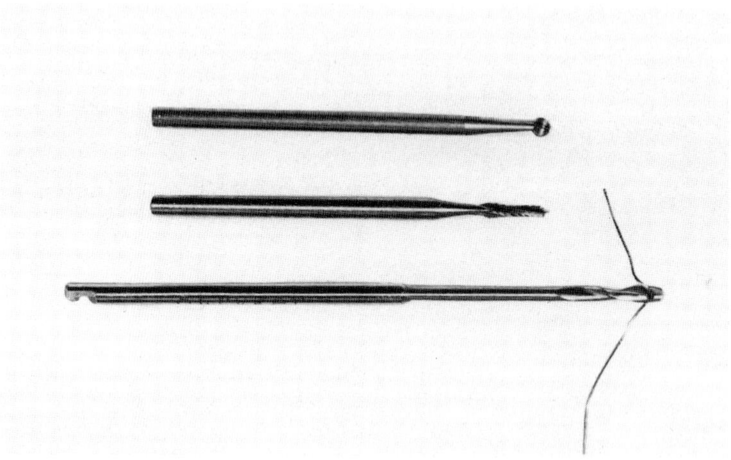

Fig. 8.3-10 B Various burs for use in placing the bur hole; (top): rose bur, Lindemann bur; (bottom): bur with hole to permit wire to be drawn through.

chiefly on the outer surface. Following removal of the hematoma from the fracture line, the bone fragments are reduced with the aid of bone forceps and bone hooks.

When reduction has been completed, bur holes are placed 6 to 8 mm from the fracture line; these should lie below the mandibular canal. Continuous spraying with Ringer solution protects the bone from overheating and simultaneously rinses the bone debris from the bur hole. Placement of a metal spatula serves to protect the soft tissue from damage by a slipping bur. In the dentulous mandible, we prefer placement of two bur holes only, and a combined horizontal and figure-of-eight wire ligature running around the inferior border of the mandible (Fig. 8.3-11). When the wire has been drawn through the prepared holes, the ends are twisted together on the external surface of the mandible and cut to a 5 mm stub. The twisted ends are placed along the mandible or countersunk into a bur hole. Two parallel wires can be placed in the edentulous mandible; here the upper pair of holes must be placed above the mandibular canal.

Following placement of suction drainage, the

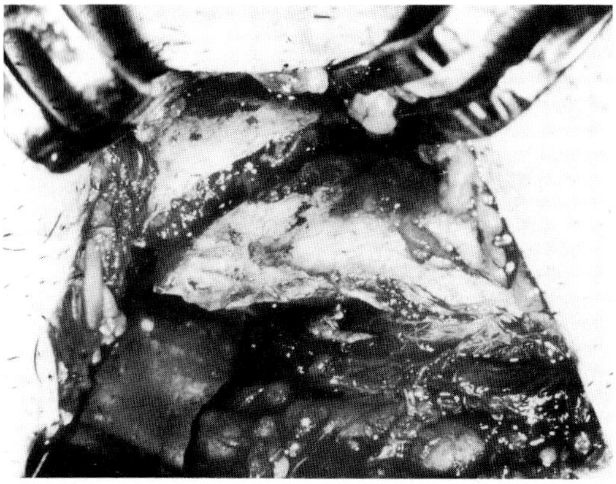

Fig. 8.3-11 A Fracture in the angle of the mandible exposed from extraoral approach. The ascending ramus is displaced laterally.

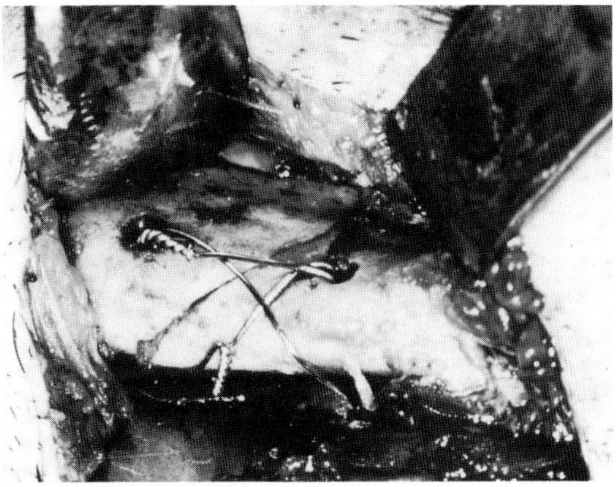

Fig. 8.3-11 B The fragments have been reduced; the interosseous wires have been placed (horizontal loop combined with figure-of-eight ligature).

wound is closed in layers. In this process, care must be taken that the insertions of the masseter and pterygoid muscles be fixed carefully in place. The skin suture must be atraumatic. It is desirable to check occlusion immediately after placement of the wire ligatures and to assure intermaxillary fixation at that time. Separated splints must be connected immediately.

For fractures of the region of the temporomandibular joint, a preauricular incision on the tragal canthus may serve to provide access. In this way, one reaches the back side of the ascending ramus. This difficult access route is particularly appropriate for high fractures of the condylar neck, while the submandibular access is better for fractures of the condylar base (*Thoma*, 1958; *Krüger*, 1974; Fig. 8.3-12).

3.4.2 Intraoral Approach

The intraoral approach is considered for fractures of the ascending ramus, especially for fractures of the coronoid process and of the angle of the mandible. Reduction and immobilization of a fracture of the condylar process can proceed via an intraoral approach too, although with greater technical difficulties. Access is via an incision on the leading edge of the ascending ramus that continues to the vestibule in the molar region, in a manner similar to that used in surgery for prognathism. In the body of the mandible, a curved or a trapezoid incision may be used. In addition, the possibility for placement of additional extraoral puncture incisions for placement of the bur holes exists, as in rigid internal fixation by means of compression plates and lag screws (see Chapter 8.5 and 8.6).

Furthermore, an interosseous wire may be placed directly in association with the surgical removal of an impacted tooth or one that lies in the fracture line, the existing incision being used (Fig. 8.3-13). That may become particularly necessary in the extraction of third molars in the fracture line if displacement occurs during the extraction. In the edentulous mandible, the mandibular ridge incision is suggested (*Dingman* and *Natvig*, 1964).

The bur hole in the dorsal fragment is placed from the socket in the direction of the buccal external cortical layer. The second hole is directed from the external cortical layer toward the socket, so that the inner layers of the bone are not included (Fig. 8.3-14 A). *Rowe* and *Killey* (1968) guide the wire transalveolarly from the lingual to the buccal corticalis (Fig. 8.3-14 B). If no teeth are present, orientation is by way of the oblique line.

Placement of an interosseous wire extending throughout the entire corpus requires either exposure of the bone on the lingual side as

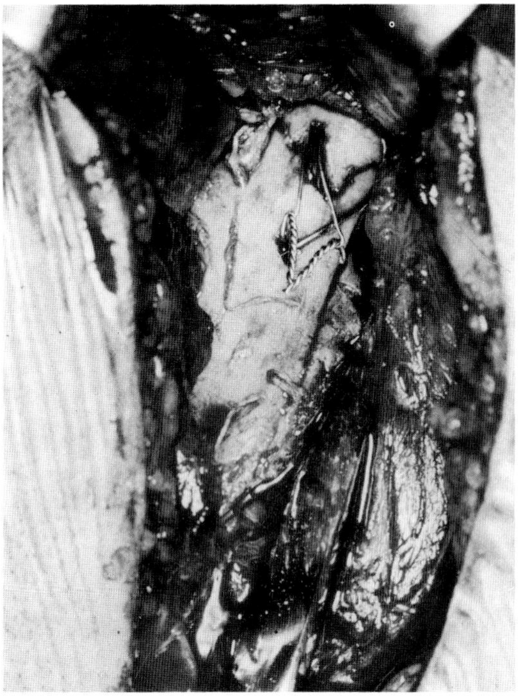

Fig. 8.3-12 Interosseous wire in a fracture of the base of the condylar process, placed from a submandibular incision (horizontal loop combined with figure-of-eight ligature).

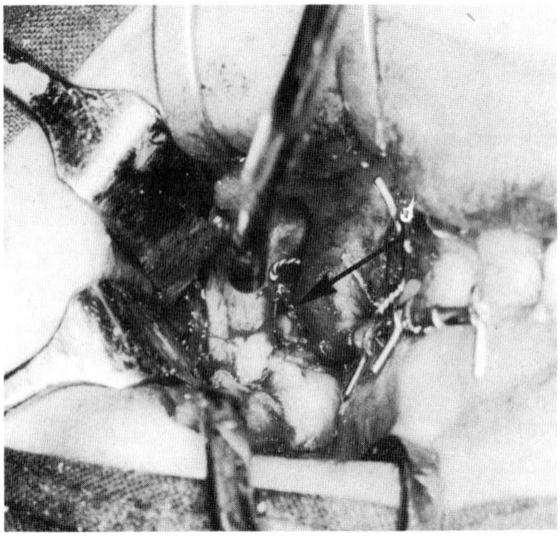

Fig. 8.3-13 Intraoral interosseous wire following third molar extraction. The wire (arrow) has been led only through the external cortical layers.

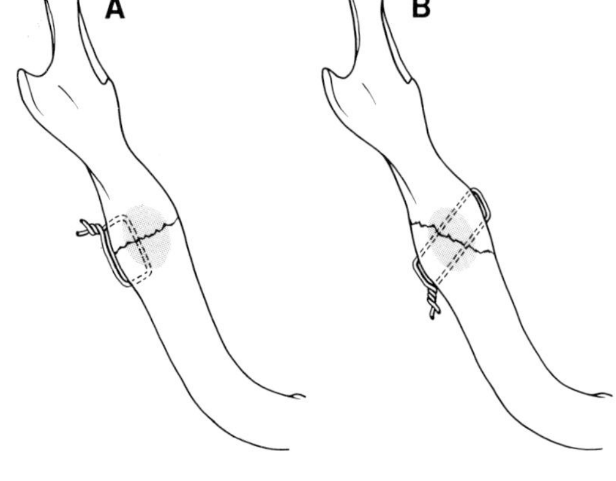

Figs. 8.3-14 A and B Course of the wire in intraoral placement of an interosseous wire.

Fig. 8.3-14 A Ligature through the buccal cortical layer.

Fig. 8.3-14 B Ligature through the lingual and buccal cortical layers (*Rowe* and *Killey*, 1968).

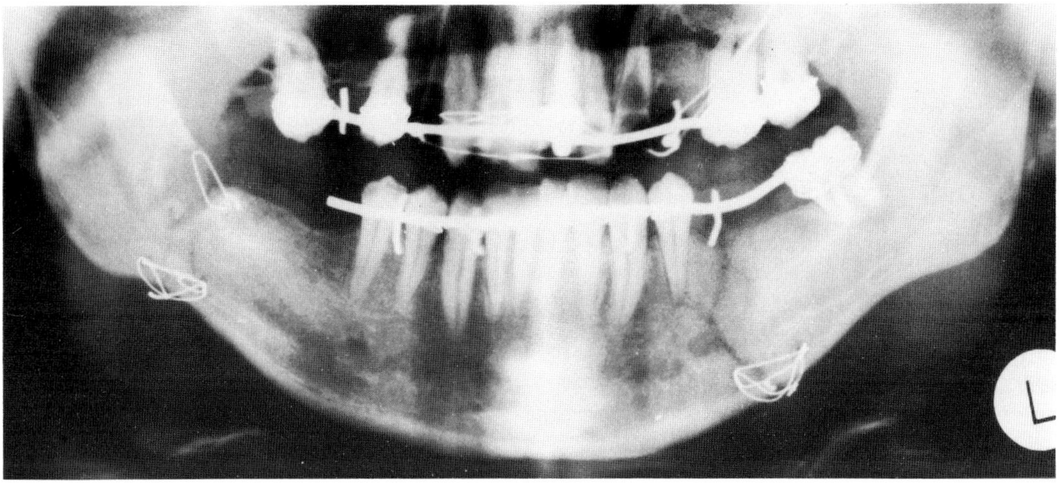

Fig. 8.3-15 A Bilateral fracture of the mandible and midface fracture. The fracture at the right angle of the mandible was immobilized with intra- and extraoral interosseous wires.

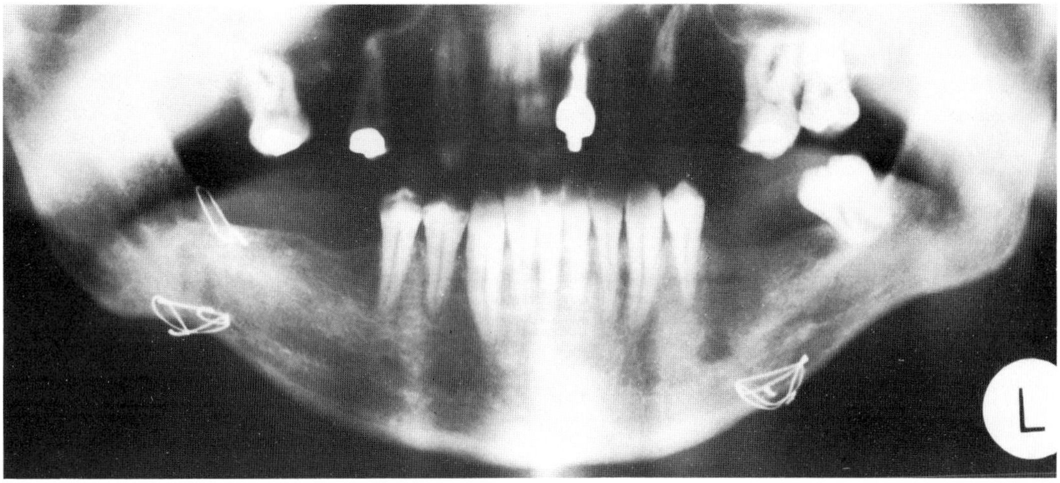

Fig. 8.3-15 B Appearance 7 months later.

well (*Hooley* and *Friedman*, 1967) or extreme displacement of the fragments if one proceeds only from the buccal side. In this case, however, there is the possibility of strain—if not tearing—of the mandibular vessels and the nerve. With extensive laceration of the oral mucosa, one must decide in each instance how the bur holes are to be placed.

The view is better in the chin region because it is possible to separate the soft tissue well and to expose the inferior border of the mandible so that it may be clearly seen.

When the oral mucosa is not torn and when no tooth extraction is necessary, we prefer the extraoral approach because it affords better stabilization of the fracture.

Placement of a *Redon* drain to carry off secretions is desirable. The needle described by

Schwenzer is used to lead the drain from the oral vestibule to the fissure of the mouth after the oral mucosa has been pierced. We in the Tübingen Department of Maxillofacial Surgery have used this technique for a long time for orthopedic surgery (*Schmelzle* and *Rolffs*, 1974).

A combined intra-extraoral approach is especially useful in fractures with soft tissue injuries which have led to exposure of the bone. This approach also may become necessary when it is not possible to achieve satisfactory reduction or immobilization via intraoral means (Fig. 8.3-15).

The removal of interosseous wires placed intraorally, especially in the region of the third molar, is necessary in a large number of instances because the relatively thin oral mucosal covering does not afford sufficient soft tissue support, especially when there is atrophy of the bone in the region of the former socket. The danger of perforation of the wire is always present.

Interosseous wires along the inferior border of the mandible, to the contrary, only rarely lead to irritation because here the soft tissue layer is sufficiently thick. The removal of the wires along the border of the mandible and in the ascending ramus may be done from an intraoral approach if the procedure is necessary.

3.5 Results

Interosseous wiring surely is one of the more frequently used methods of osteosynthesis in the facial skeleton. Review of the more recent literature indicates that this method is one of the more reliable methods, too. Nonetheless, some complications have been described. Thus, *Freihofer* and *Sailer* (1975) report a 7% complication rate in 178 interosseous wires placed via the intraoral approach in the mandible. The complications range from occlusal disturbances and delayed healing (in 5 patients each) to pseudoarthrosis and osteomyelitis in one patient each. Investigations of *Schmieg* and *Niemzcyk* (1975) in Tübingen revealed that among 33 fractures of the angle of the mandible treated by intraoral placement of interosseous wires, two patients developed fracture line abscesses and the wires became exposed in two others. No disturbance of bone healing occured. In a comparison with 74 conservatively treated fractures of the angle of the mandible, there were four fracture line abscesses. In a survey of 36 comminuted fractures of the mandible by *Dieckmann* and *Niederdellmann* (1975) of the same Department, there were no fracture line abscesses after interosseous wiring.

The experience of *Schegg, von Allmen* and *Neuner* (1975) with 450 interosseous wires provided 12 instances of infections of longer duration. Pseudoarthroses occurred in two mandibles in old men. Similar results are reported by *Renner* (1969), who checked 42 wire sites in the mandible: 23 at the angle, 17 in the body, and 2 in the alveolar process. Only in one instance was their a disturbance of healing, associated with a fracture of the angle. The patient suffered from post-traumatic osteoporosis (*Sudeck's* atrophy).

Brons (1970) described 73 interosseous wires in the mandible. In this series, bony apposition occurred within 4 to 20 weeks along the fracture line, depending on the fracture site. The type of wire ligature that he used (0.6 mm) permitted him to achieve consolidation of the fracture without additional immobilization in some instances. In this procedure, especially possible in edentulous mandibles, the upper pair of holes was placed above the mandibular canal.

A retrospective survey published by *Höltje, Luhr* and *Holtfreter* (1975) included 170 cases in which wire ligatures had been placed. There were 2 infiltrates, 5 abscesses, 4 instances of osteomyelitis, and one late infiltrate. In 220 compression osteosyntheses, there were only 2 abscesses and 3 delayed infiltrations, i.e., the complication rate was lower.

Any critical evaluation of results will indicate that interosseous wiring is a reliable and useful type of osteosynthesis in fractures of the mandible. It has a wide range of indications for use because it may be used with almost all types of fractures. Although various tendencies exist to obviate intermaxillary fixation, one should recognize clearly that no functional stability is thus attained—as has been demonstrated experimentally. In view, therefore, of the avoidance of needless complications that could give the technique a bad name, one should accept the disadvantage of additional immobilization. Of course one must vary the duration of immobilization from patient to patient. The advantage of the technique, that the removal of the osteosynthesis wire is not necessary as a rule, should also be weighed in the evaluation of the technique.

3.6 Errors and Dangers in Interosseous Wiring of the Mandible

Various errors may endanger the success of interosseous wiring. These mistakes, which apply in part to other techniques for osteosynthesis, rest in part on clumsy surgical technique and, in part, on lack of attention to principles of immobilization. They may be summarized as follows:

1. Insufficient Immobilization
   Supplemental immobilization of the mandible by intermaxillary fixation is the most important requirement for undisturbed healing. As a rule, it is not enough to immobilize the fragments with an interosseous wire itself. Supplemental intra- and intermaxillary immobilization are required.
2. Improper Manipulation of the Wire
   Even stainless steel wire can be weakened and damaged along its surface by multiple bending and squeezing with forceps, making it less resistant to forces of corrosion. Care therefore must be taken that the wire does not come into contact with base metal instruments. In addition, those wire components that are to remain in the bone should not be grasped. The places at which the instrument grasps the wires as they are being twisted must be cut off.
3. Leaving a Tooth in the Fracture Line
   Leaving a tooth in the fracture line can lead to an infection of the site. That infection, in the best case, appears after bony healing is complete; in the worst case, it arises during the phase of healing. The indications for extraction (see p. 287) therefore must be followed carefully. In the case of an infection, the relationship of teeth adjacent the fracture line should be checked again.
4. Bone Damage
   Injury to the bone may arise from overheating resulting from excessively rapid drilling and insufficient spraying with physiological saline solution. Necrosis is especially possible in small bone fragments; this may lead to sequestration.
5. Root Injury
   If the bur holes are placed too high in the dentulous jaw, the danger of injury to the roots arises. If the nerve-vessel entry at the apical foramen is injured in the process, the danger of gangrene—and associated loss of the tooth and infections of the fracture line—arises. The possibility of root damage exists in the intraoral approach as well if the external cortical layer is pierced too far away from the fracture line or insufficiently deep.
6. Injury to the Inferior Alveolar Nerve
   Care should be taken when the bur holes are placed that these are near the inferior border of the mandible or the alveolar process. Perforation of the mandibular canal offers the danger of a nerve lesion and the associated temporary or permanent anesthesia. In the dentulous jaw, a ligature shape should be chosen in which only two bur holes are placed near the inferior border of the mandible.
7. Injury to the Facial Nerve
   Injury to the facial nerve may be either the result of drawing a hook along the nerve or cutting through it while exposing the line of fracture. The latter is possible if the approach is made too close to the inferior border of the mandible so that the mandibular branch of the facial nerve is injured. The danger of separation exists as well when ligation of the facial artery is undertaken too closely to the mandibular border. Lesions of several or all facial nerve branches can arise especially during the exposure of condylar neck fractures via a preauricular incision. If the nerve has been damaged by a bone hook, as a rule, it recovers.

References

Andrusch, L. (1959)
Die Indikation und Anwendung der Knochendrahtnaht und Drahtumschlingung bei Frakturen im Kiefer-Gesichtsbereich (Indications for and application of interosseous and circumferential wiring in the maxillofacial region). Med. Diss., Rostock

Archer, H. W. (1975)
Oral and Maxillofacial Surgery, vol. 2. Philadelphia – Toronto – London, W. B. Saunders

Becker, R., and K.-H. Austermann (1981)
Frakturen des Gesichtsschädels. (Fractures of the facial skull.) In Schwenzer, N., and G. Grimm: Zahn-Mund-Kiefer-Heilkunde. Spezielle Chirurgie. (Dentistry. Oral and maxillofacial Surgery.), Vol. 2, Stuttgart, Thieme

Brons, R. (1970)
Stabiele interne fixatie bij Corpus mandibulae frakturen (Stable internal fixation in fractures of the mandibule). Med. Diss., University of Groningen

Dieckmann, J. (1970)
Experimentelle und klinische Untersuchungen zum Stabilitätsproblem bei der Drahtnaht am Gesichtsskelett. (Experimental and clinical studies of the stability problem associated with interosseous wiring on the facial skeleton). Med. Diss. Würzburg

Dieckmann, J., and H. Niederdellmann (1975)
Operative Versorgung von Mehrfachfrakturen im Unterkiefer durch Drahtosteosynthese. (Surgical treatment of multiple fractures of the mandible by interosseous wiring). Fortschr. Kiefer- u. Gesichtschir. 19: 97

Dietrich, K. (1951)
Indikation bei der Verwendung der Drahtnaht in der Kieferbruchhandlung (Indications for interosseous wiring in treatment of jaw fractures). Dtsch. zahnärztl. Z. 6: 414.

Dingman, R. O., and P. Natvig (1964)
Surgery of Facial Fractures. Philadelphia – London, W. B. Saunders

Freihofer, H. P., and H. Sailer (1975)
Erfahrungen mit der enoralen Drahtosteosynthese bei Unterkieferfrakturen. (Experience with intraoral wire osteosynthesis in mandibular fractures). Fortschr. Kiefer- u. Gesichtschir. 19: 104

Grasser, H. (1972)
Metallose–Gefahr durch Osteosynthese-Materialien. (Danger from materials used in osteosynthesis). Dtsch. zahnärztl. Z. 27: 413

Günther, H., N. Schwenzer, and H. J. Metz (1966)
Fraktur, Luxation und Kontusion des Kiefergelenkes. (Fracture, dislocation and contusion of the temporomandibular joint). Fortschr. Kiefer- u. Gesichtschir. 11: 173

Hicks, J. H. (1964)
Corrosion in surgical implants. Chem. and Ind. 28: 1240

Höltje, W. J., H. G. Luhr and M. Holtfreter (1975)
Untersuchungen über infektionsbedingte Komplikationen nach konservativer oder operativer Versorgung von Unterkieferfrakturen. (Studies of complications caused by infections following conservative or surgical treatment of mandibular fractures). Fortschr. Kiefer- u. Gesichtschir. 19: 122

Hooley, J. R., and G. L. Freedman (1967)
"Degloving" in treatment of fracture of the mandibular symphysis. J. oral Surg. 25: 236

Kazanjian, V. H. (1933)
Treatment of automobile injuries of the face and jaws. J. amer. dent. Ass. 20: 757

Kristen, K., and R. Singer (1976)
Therapie and Prognose der Luxationsfrakturen des Kiefergelenkes beim Jugendlichen. (Treatment and prognosis of fractures of the temporomandibular joint in children). Fortschr. Kiefer- u. Gesichtschir. 21: 314

Krüger, E. (1974)
Lehrbuch der chirurgischen Zahn-, Mund- und Kieferheilkunde (Textbook of oral surgery). vol. 2, 1st ed. Berlin, Buch- und Zeitschriften-Verlag "Die Quintessenz" (4th ed. 1981)

Link, K. H. (1937)
Zur Frage der Knochennaht bei Kieferbrüchen. (The question of interosseous wiring in jaw fractures). Zbl. Chir. 17: 988

Neuner, O. (1977)
Maxillo-faciale Traumatologie (Maxillofacial traumatology). Berlin – New York, Walter de Gruyter

Paul, J. K., and A. Acevedo (1968)
Intraoral open reduction. J. oral Surg. 25: 516

Reichenbach, E. (1969)
Traumatologie im Kiefer-Gesichtsbereich (Traumatology of the maxillofacial region). Leipzig – München, J. A. Barth

Renner, H. (1969)
Zum Problem der Metallschädigung bei der Osteosynthese des Gesichtsskelettes mit Stahldraht (Metal damage in osteosynthesis of the facial skeleton with steel wire). Med. Diss. Würzburg

Rowe, N. L., and H. C. Killey (1968)
Fractures of the facial skeleton. Edinburgh – London, Livingstone

Ryberg, N. L. (1960)
Statistische Untersuchungen zu den Frakturen mit Zähnen im Bruchspalt unter besonderer Berücksichtigung der Art der Schienung und deren Zeitpunkt (Statistical study of fractures having teeth in the fracture line, with special attention to the type of splinting and its timing). Med. Diss. Freiburg

Schegg, H. K., G. v. Almen, and O. Neuner (1975)
Erfahrungen mit der Drahtosteosynthese nach Neuner bei der funktionellen Kieferbruchhandlung (Experiences with the Neuner interosseous wiring in functional treatment of jaw fractures). Fortschr. Kiefer- u. Gesichtschir. 19: 101

Schmelze, R., and J. Rolffs (1974)
Die intraorale Redon-Drainage bei Osteotomie im aufsteigenden Unterkieferast (Intraoral Redon drainage in osteotomy of the ascending ramus of the mandible). Fortschr. Kiefer- u. Gesichtschir. 18: 148

Schmieg, E., and H.-M. Niemczyk (1975)
Intraorale Drahtosteosynthese bei Kieferwinkelfrakturen (Intraoral wire osteosynthesis in fractures of the angle of the mandible. Fortschr. Kiefer- u. Gesichtschir. 19: 107

Schröder, F. (1966)
Apparate zur Reposition und Fixation der Kieferfrakturen (Devices for reduction and fixation of jaw fractures). Fortschr. Kiefer- u. Gesichtschir. 11: 117

Schwenzer, N. (1966)
Das mechanische und biologische Verhalten der Drahtnaht bei der Osteosynthese (The mechanical and biological response of interosseous wires in osteosynthesis). Dtsch. zahnärztl. Z. 21: 266

Schwenzer, N. (1967)
Zur Osteosynthese bei Frakturen des Gesichtsskelets (Osteosynthesis in fractures of the facial skeleton). Stuttgart, G. Thieme

Schwenzer, N. (1969)
Operative Frakturbehandlung bei Kindern (Surgical treatment of fractures in children). Dtsch. zahnärztl. Z. 24: 316

Schwenzer, N. (1975)
Zur Frage der Metallschädigung und Stabilität bei der Drahtosteosynthese am Mittelgesicht (The question of damage to metal and stability in interosseous wiring of the midface). Fortschr. Kiefer- u. Gesichtschir. 19: 145

Schwenzer, N. (1977)
Grundlagen der Kieferbruchbehandlung. (Fundamentals of treatment of jaw fractures.), Cologne, Deutscher Ärzteverlag

Schwenzer, N., and J. Dieckmann (1971)
Tierexperimentelle Untersuchungen zum Stabilitätsproblem bei der Drahtnaht am Gesichtsskelett (Animal experimental investigation of the stability problem in interosseous wiring of the facial skeleton. Stoma 24: 153

Schwenzer, N., and H. Renner (1972)
Experimentelle Untersuchungen zum Problem der Metallschädigung bei der Drahtosteosynthese am Gesichtsskelett (Experimental investigations of the question of metal damage in interosseous wiring of the facial skeleton). Dtsch. Zahn-, Mund- u. Kieferheilk. 58: 145

Schwenzer, N., and W. Steinhilber (1974)
Traumatologie des Gesichtsschädels (Traumatology of the facial skull). Munich, E. Banaschewski

Spiessl, B., and K. Schroll (1972)
Gesichtsschädel (Facial skull). In Nigst, H.: Spezielle Frakturen- und Luxationslehre (Textbook of fractures and dislocations). vol. 1/1. Stuttgart, G. Thieme

Steinhilber, W. (1976)
Die operative Behandlung von Mittelgesichtsfrakturen. Metallurgische, tierexperimentelle und klinische Untersuchungen (Surgical treatment of midface fractures. Metallurgical, animal experimental and clinical studies). Berlin, Buch und Zeitschriften-Verlag "Die Quintessenz"

Thoma, K. H. (1958)
Oral Surgery. St. Louis, C. V. Mosby Co.

4. Circumferential Wiring and Zygomatico-Maxillary Wire Suspension of the Mandible

Eberhard Krüger

Tooth-borne splints customary in conservative therapy cannot be applied in the nearly or completely edentulous jaw. In such instances it is possible to fix the patient's dentures, or occlusal splints, or base plates as devised by *Gunning* (1866/1867) surgically to make immobilization of the mandible possible. However, these surgical measures do not serve osteosynthesis, but rather only the fixation of the splints.

4.1 Circumferential Wiring

Circumferential wiring of the mandible is the simplest method of immobilizing a splint. The mandible is simply circumscribed with several wires, the ends of which are twisted together over the existing denture or a base plate. The technique was used first by *Baudens* (1840), who applied silk circumferential ligatures in oblique fractures of the mandible and fixed the ends of the ligatures about a molar.
Robert (1852) placed a silver wire circumferential ligature. After *Gilmer* (1881), *G. V. Black* was the first American to use the technique himself; Gilmer personally recommended circumferential wiring over a splint attached to the teeth. The method was used particularly for immobilization of mandibular dentures in fractures of the edentulous and nearly edentulous mandible (*Gordon*, 1937; *Ivy* and *Curtis*, 1938; *Parker*, 1942; *Björn*, 1952; *Götte*, 1957; *Thoma*, 1958, *Krüger*, 1964, 1974; *Reichenbach*, 1969; and others). Today, however, it has been replaced largely by functionally stable osteosynthesis. Only in the treatment of mandibular fractures of children does the technique maintain a place (see Chapter 13).
Single circumferential wires can serve to provide supplementary fixation of an arch bar in edentulous sections of a jaw; in these regions a denture saddle made of cold curing acrylic is placed (Figs. 8.4.-1 to 8.4-3).
Four circumferential wires are best used to fix a lingual splint or a partial denture. These are placed on both sides in the canine and molar regions.
A monomaxillary fixation of this sort provides sufficient fixation only in fractures in the anterior region of the partially dentulous mandible or in the deciduous dentition. In most instances it will not be possible to avoid intermaxillary fixation. If the dentition of the maxilla is sufficient to support immobilization of a conventional splint, intermaxillary fixation may be undertaken in the usual manner (Fig. 8.4-4). In the alternative, if the dentition of the maxilla is insufficient, a

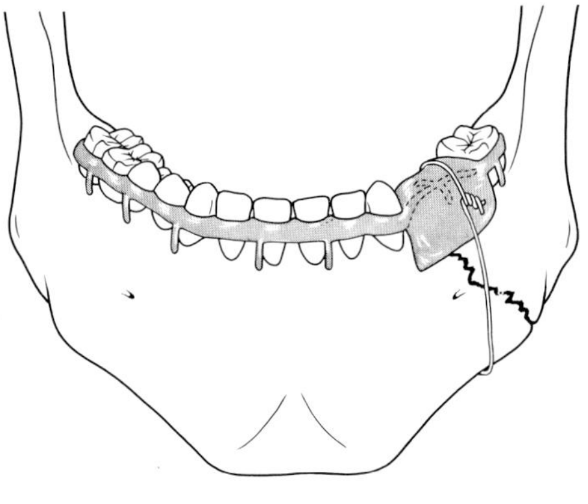

Figs. 8.4-1 Circumferential wiring as a supplemental measure for fixation of a wire-acrylic arch bar in an edentulous region filled with a denture saddle.

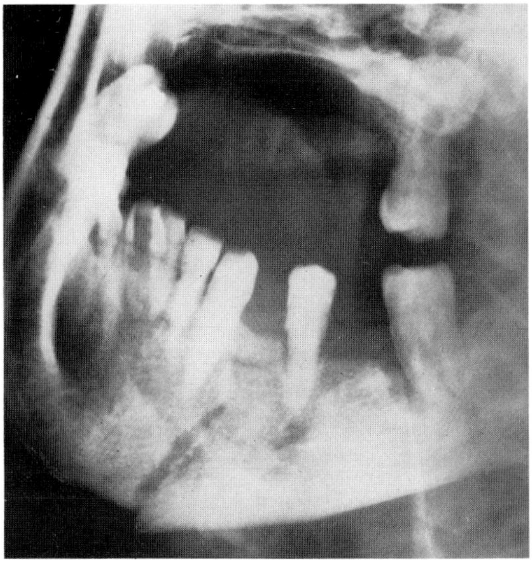

Fig. 8.4-2 A Posterior mandibular fracture. 3 3 is in the fracture line; 3 4 and 3 6 are missing; 3 5 and 3 7 have severe marginal periodontitis involvement.

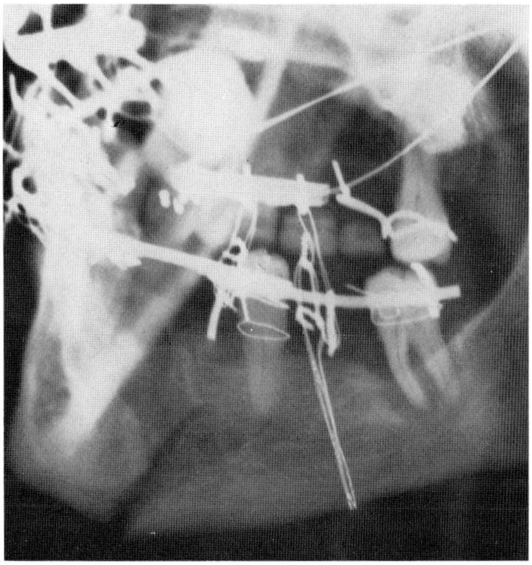

Fig. 8.4-2 B Appearance following intermaxillary fixation. There is a wire-acrylic arch bar in the mandible with denture saddles in the edentulous regions. A circumferential wire has been placed between 3 5 and 3 7 for improved fixation of the arch bar. A wire-acrylic arch bar with channels and a palatal plate has been placed in the largely edentulous maxilla and supplementally fixed by circumzygomatic wiring.

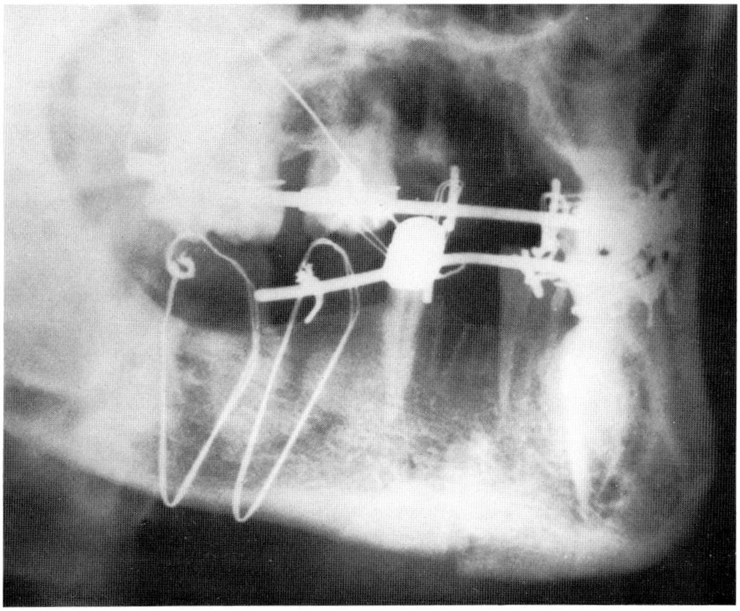

Fig. 8.4-3 The free end saddle of a wire-acrylic arch bar has been fixed in place with two circumferential wires.

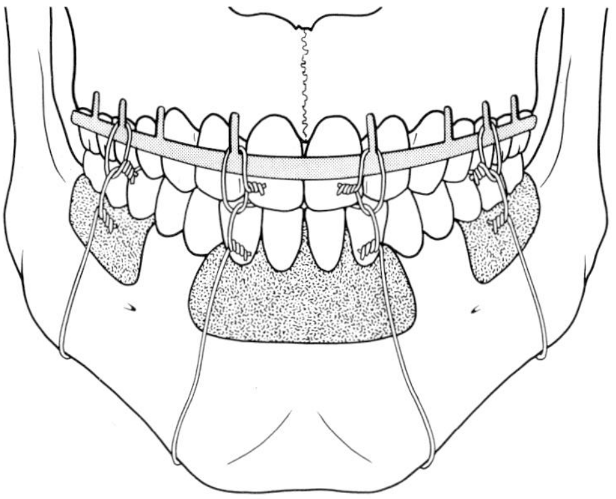

Fig. 8.4-4 Mandibular partial denture retained with 4 circumferential wires. For intermaxillary fixation a wire-acrylic arch bar has been placed in the completely dentulous maxilla.

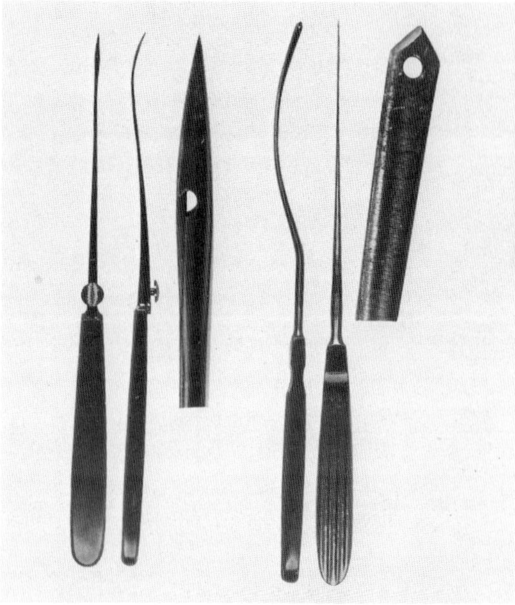

Fig. 8.4-5 Punches for placement of circumferential wires. The wire is drawn through the eyelet.

zygomatico-maxillary wire suspension is necessary (see below).

Technique: An awl (Fig. 8.4-5) pierces the tissue below the border of the mandible extraorally and is led along the lingual side of the bone while maintaining contact with the bone until it pierces the mucosa of the floor of the mouth. Now a wire is drawn through the eye of the awl, which is guided around the mandible and back into the oral cavity on the buccal side. After cutting through the wire at the eye, the awl can be drawn back empty. The ends of the wire are see-sawed snugly against the mandible and twisted together over a splint or a denture (Fig. 8.4-6).

A technique used in the past, in which the wire was guided about the mandible with a long cannula intended for use in lumbar puncture (*Thoma*, 1958; *Kazanjian* and *Converse*, 1959, 1974; *Reichenbach*, 1969) may be deemed outdated today.

Direct circumferential wiring without the use of a splint has been suggested for fixation of oblique fractures of the mandible (*Thoma*, 1958; *Kazanjian* and *Converse*, 1959, 1974). Surgical opening of the mucoperiosteum over the mandible is required for this purpose. Buccally and lingually, trapeze-shaped flaps are elevated. Following placement of two circumferential wires, the mucosa is sutured closed over them (Fig. 8.4-7). We do not use this technique because the stability attained is not sufficient to assure interfragmentary immobilization.

4.2 Zygomatico-Maxillary Wire Suspension of the Mandible

Zygomatico-maxillary wire suspension (*Krüger*, 1964, 1973) affords intermaxillary fixation of the fractured mandible when there is otherwise insufficient dentition: the mandibular denture or a base plate is bound in place with four circumferential wires. Intermaxillary fixation proceeds via two circumzygomatic wires and two wires inserted through the margin of the pyriform aperture (Fig. 8.4-8).

Rowe and *Killey* (1955, 1968) recommend two circumferential wires in the mandible for the fixation of *Gunning* splints in the edentulous

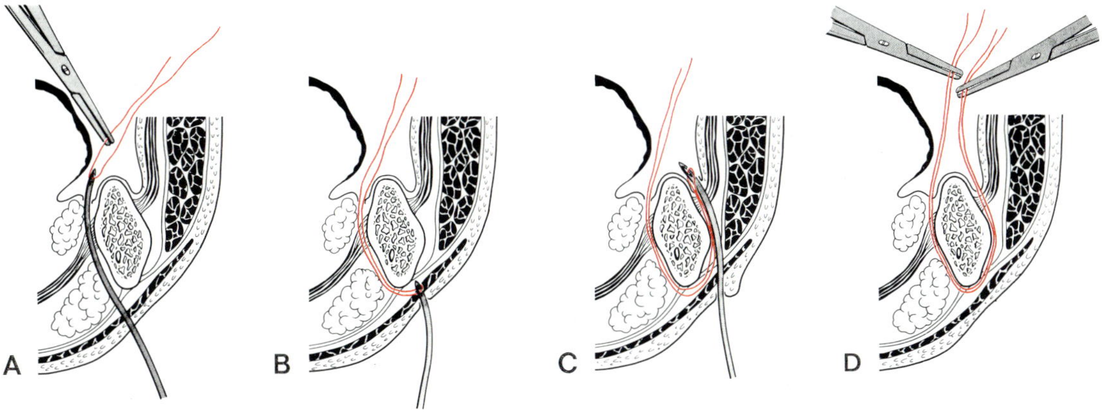

Figs. 8.4-6 A to D Technique of circumferential wiring.

Fig. 8.4-6 A The extraorally inserted punch passes through the floor of the mouth and picks up a wire lingual to the mandible.

Fig. 8.4-6 B The punch is passed around the mandible with the doubled wire.

Fig. 8.4-6 C The punch passes through the buccal mucosa.

Fig. 8.4-6 D The now completely placed circumferential wire may be tightened over a denture or a denture saddle.

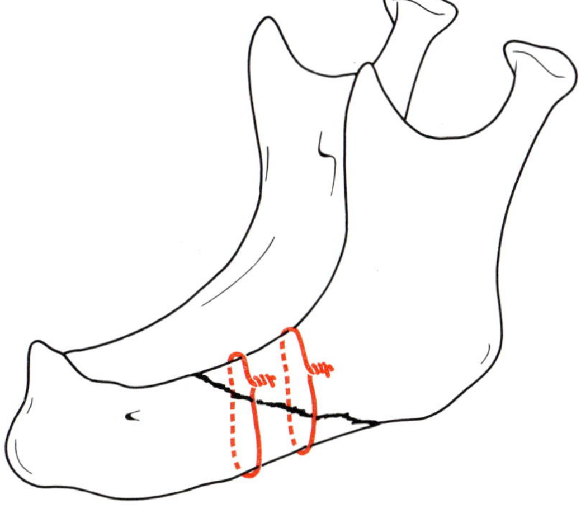

Fig. 8.4-7 Submucosal circumferential wire in oblique fractures of the mandible.

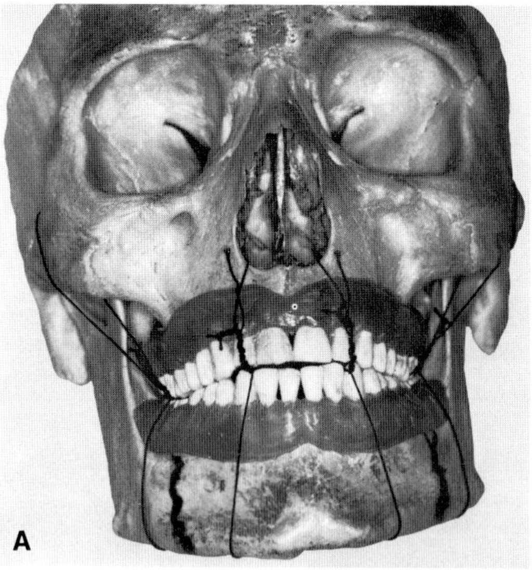

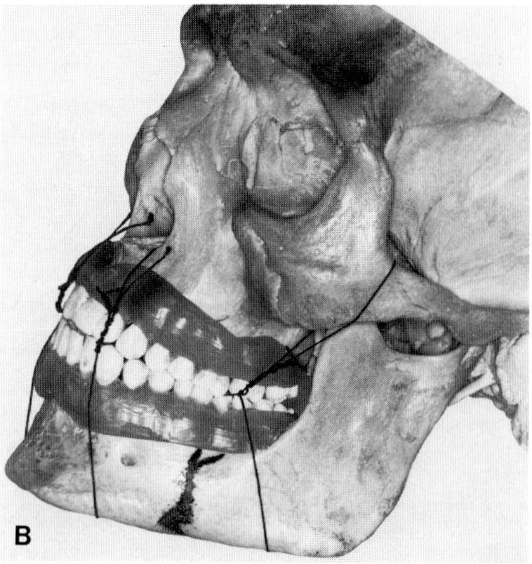

Figs. 8.4-8 A and B Principle of zygomatico-maxillary wire suspension of the mandible with circumzygomatic wiring and fixation on the bony margin of the piriform aperture for treatment of fractures of the mandible in patients with edentulous mandible and maxilla. The mandibular denture is bound up with 4 circumferential wires whose long ends are looped around the zygomatic arches or drawn through bur holes at the piriform aperture. After tightening of the suspension wires, the mandible and its denture are pulled tightly against the maxillary denture.

mandible, and two perialveolar wires for the same purpose in the maxilla. *Thoma* (1943, 1958) describes a form of nasomandibular wiring: the mandible is fixed to the pyriform aperture with two wires, with the upper denture locked between maxilla and mandible. *Hayward* (1962) immobilizes the maxillary denture by suspension at the malar ridges and the pyriform angle.

My own procedure (*Krüger*, 1964) guarantees greater stability through suspension at four points (Fig. 8.4-8). The method may be used when splints cannot be placed because of the absence of enough teeth and when intermaxillary fixation is indispensable. The zygomatico-maxillary wire suspension of the mandible replaces the bimaxillary splints otherwise attached to the teeth. The technique has been largely replaced today by rigid internal fixation. An indication for its use is present in adults, when the patient's suitability for surgery is limited through systemic disease or advanced age. In children, the method remains the technique of choice, now as in the past, when intermaxillary fixation is necessary (see Chapter 13).

Technique: The presence of maxillary and mandibular dentures is a prerequisite for the use of the procedure in the edentulous or partially edentulous jaw. If, in an accident, the dentures are broken, they must be repaired as a preliminary step. If dentures are not present, *Gunning*-type base plates or bite blocks are necessary. These must be made from impressions. When there is displacement of the fragments in the region of the body of the mandible, reduction of the sawed sections of the model can cause difficulties if occlusion between the mandible and the maxilla is not possible because of lack of sufficient teeth or complete absence of teeth. In such instances one can attempt to hold the mandibular fragments in the proper position while the impression is being taken. Local anesthesia is required for this purpose as a rule. If the mandibular model is characterized by the formation of a shoulder despite these efforts, it is separated with a saw cut; the frag-

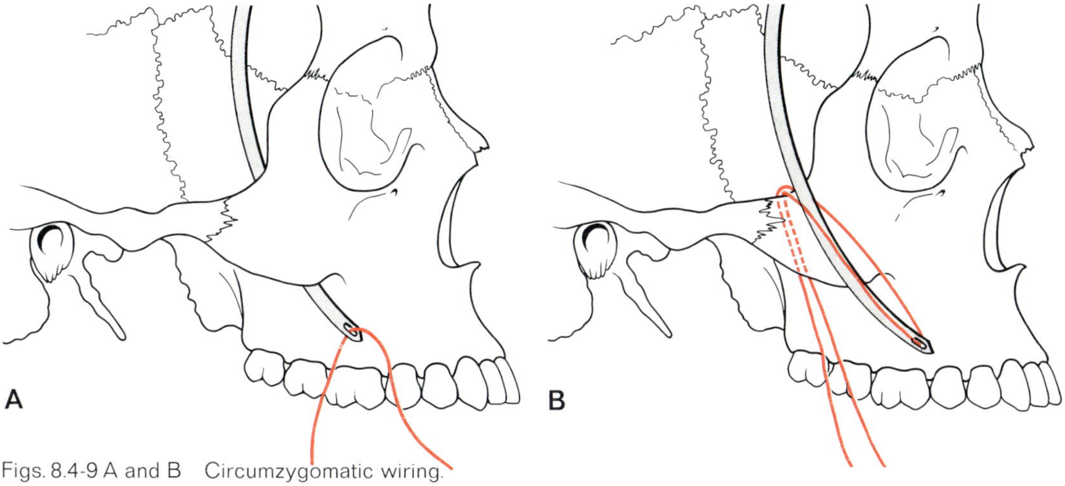

Figs. 8.4-9 A and B Circumzygomatic wiring.

Fig. 8.4-9 A The punch pierces above the zygomatic arch and is guided medial to the arch through the vestibule. The wire is taken up here.

Fig. 8.4-9 B The punch is guided around the zygomatic arch and returned to the vestibule lateral to the arch. Then the punch is drawn out empty.

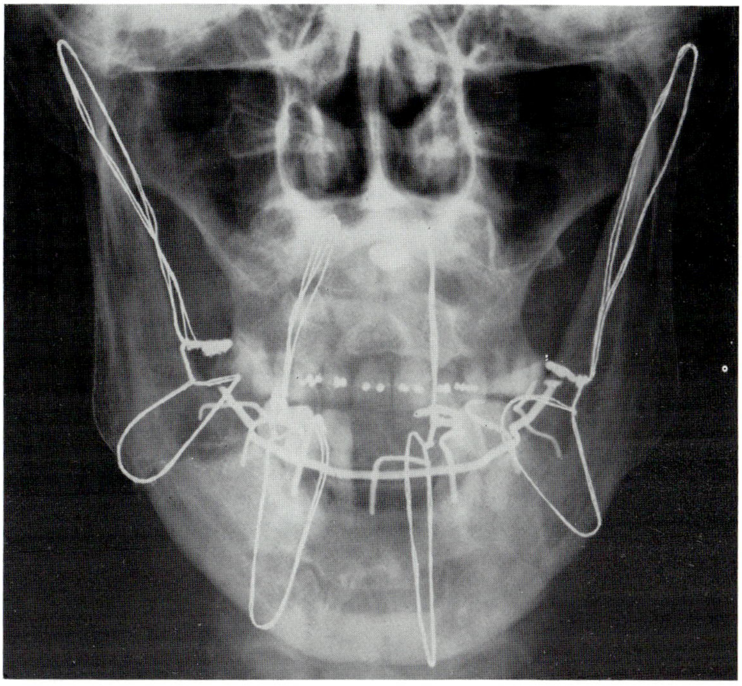

Fig. 8.4-10 Zygomatico-maxillary wire suspension of a bilaterally fractured mandible, using the complete maxillary denture and the partial mandibular denture. The fracture sites are in the posterior region at the right side and in the left canine region; both sites are included in the appliance so that sufficient stability is assured.

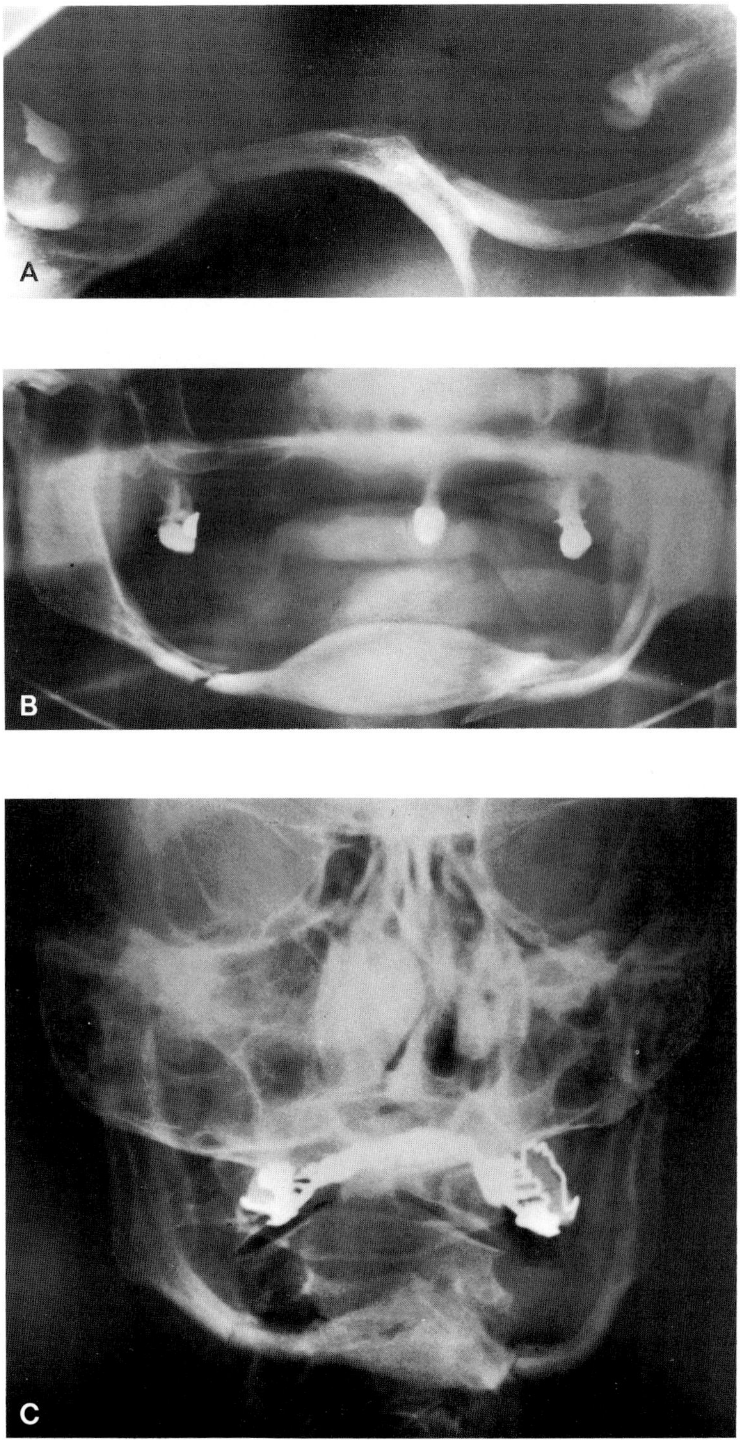

Figs. 8.4-11 A to C Bilateral fracture in the edentulous and severely atrophied mandible of a woman with coronary insufficiency. A long period of surgery is beyond consideration because of the patient's poor health. Furthermore, rigid internal fixation by means of compression plates is difficult in extremely atrophic mandibles, as here at least on the right side. For these reasons, in this instance zygomatico-maxillary wire suspension of the mandible is the treatment of choice for this patient.

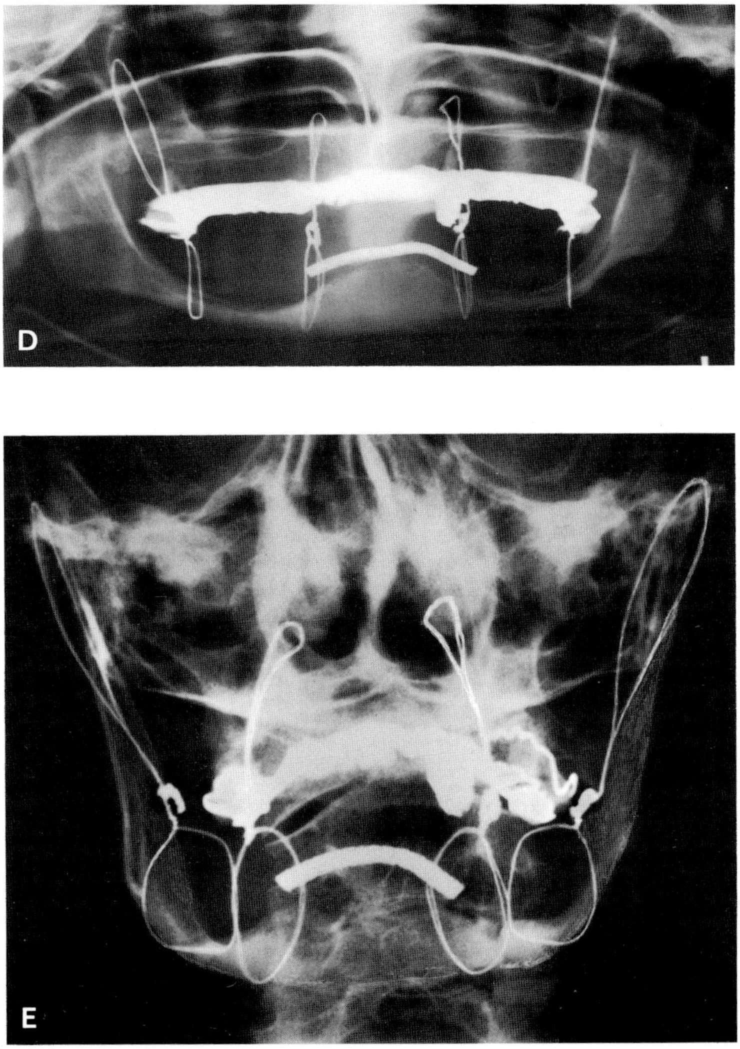

Figs. 8.4-11 D and E Radiographs following zygomatico-maxillary suspension of the mandible incorporating the patient's dentures. Following the relatively short surgery which the patient tolerated well, the fragments consolidated without any complications.

ments are reduced visually in a manner such that the shoulder is eliminated. Occasionally it may be necessary to correct the base plate during the operation. If necessary, it may be sectioned at the fracture site and the pieces then placed into the desired position with cold-curing acrylic. In this procedure, an assistant holds the base plate pieces firmly to the mandibular fragments while the latter are held in the correct position.

The operation is undertaken with the patient under general anesthesia. As a first step, the mandibular denture or the newly prepared base plate is attached with four circumferential wires. When the wires are twisted together, the fracture ends are reduced simultaneously; these must fit into a previously worn denture as though it were a corset. If an impression-formed base plate is used, it is desirable that its base be lined with gutta percha to avoid formation of pressure points. Then circumzygomatic wires are placed around both arches. A punch is used

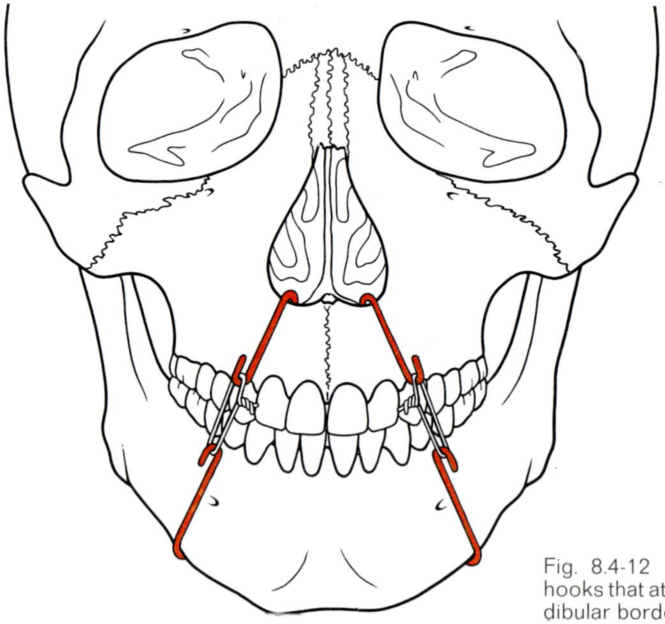

Fig. 8.4-12 Dal Pont's intermaxillary fixation with hooks that attach to the piriform aperture and the mandibular border.

to pierce the skin as far anteriorly as possible and is guided medially downward along the arch until it passes through the mucosa in the oral vestibule. One end of the wire is drawn through the eye of the awl and the needle is pulled back to be passed over the arch and returned to the vestibule lateral to the zygomatic arch, piercing the oral mucosa for the second time at the same site. When the wire has been clipped at the eye of the awl and drawn out, the awl is withdrawn (Fig. 8.4-9).

To place the anterior suspension wires, the piriform aperture must be exposed through an incision in the vestibule. The nasal mucosa is elevated bilaterally in the region of the pyriform angle and a hole is placed on each side, the nasal mucosa being retracted and protected. After placement of the wires, the mucosal incision is sutured and the wire ends perforate the mucosa through the incision site to appear in the oral cavity.

Then the maxillary denture or base plate is inserted, the mandible is brought into centric occlusion, and the suspension wires are twisted together with the circumferential wires of the mandible (Figs. 8.4-10 and 8.4-11). The twisted ends should be coated with cold-curing acrylate.

Follow-up treatment: Point-shaped wounds persist in the vestibule and on the floor of the mouth at the sites where the wires pierce the tissue. These sites cannot heal as long as the apparatus is worn. Lest purulent infections arise at these wounds, careful oral hygiene is required, with mouth rinses following each meal and frequent cauterization with gentian violet solution. If a submucosal or sublingual abscess forms nonetheless, it must be incised and drained; the wires need not be removed prematurely. The splint remains *in situ* four to six weeks. Loosening of the wires, especially at the piriform aperture, is possible during this time. At the end of the period, the suspension wires are removed through the mouth. The mandibular denture held in place with the circumferential wires is permitted to remain *in situ* for two to three additional weeks in cases of fracture of the body of the mandible. In the event of loosening of the denture, the circumferential wires are tightened. In fractures of the angle of the jaw and the ascending ramus, the circumferential wires are removed at the same time as the suspension wire.

Complications are rare following circumferential wiring and zygomatico-maxillary suspension of the mandible. Most likely to occur are infections at the wires. We found 8 instances of infection in a series of 38 patients; all of these were managed by incision and antibiotic therapy and premature removal of the wires was not necessary in any instance. Further complications were not observed (*Krüger* and *Rivas*, 1975).

4.3 Nasomandibular Hook Fixation

The technique described by *Dal Pont* (1967) achieves intermaxillary fixation through two pairs of metal hooks supported in the maxilla on the floor of the nose and in the mandible along its margin. The hooks are inserted by piercing through the mucosa in the oral vestibule. Following insertion of the maxillary and mandibular dentures, the upper and lower hooks are connected with each other by means of wires or elastic bands (Fig. 8.4-12). The indication for use of this method also has been largely limited by functionally stable osteosynthesis.

References

Baudens, L. B. (1840)
Fracture de la mâchoire inférieure (Fracture of the mandible.) Bull. Acad. Méd. (Paris) 5: 341

Björn, H. (1952)
Circumferential wiring. Dtsch. zahnärztl. Z. 7: 302

Black, G. V.
Quoted by Gilmer, T. L. (1881)

Dal Pont, G. (1967)
A new method of intermaxillary bone fixation. In: Husted, E. and E. Hjørting-Hansen, eds.: Oral Surgery. Trans. 2nd Congress of the International Assn. of Oral Surgeons. Copenhagen, Munksgaard, p. 325

Gilmer, T. L. (1881)
Fractures of the inferior maxilla. Illinois State dent. Soc. Trans., 67-104, discussion, 104-106

Götte, H. (1957)
Die Verwendung der perimandibulären Drahtumschlingung in der Kieferbruchbehandlung. (The use of circumferential wiring in treatment of jaw fractures.) Dtsch. zahnärztl. Z. 12: 1050

Gunning, T. B. (1886/1887)
The treatment of fracture of the lower jaw by interdental splints. N. Y. med. J. 3: 433 and 4: 11 and 279

Hayward, J. R. (1962)
Treatment methods for jaw fractures. J. oral Surg. 20: 273

Ivy, R. H., and L. Curtis (1938)
Fractures of the jaws. Philadelphia, Lea & Febiger

Kazanjian, V. H., and J. M. Converse (1959)
The surgical treatment of facial injuries. Baltimore, Williams and Wilkins, 2nd ed. (3rd ed. 1974)

Krüger, E. (1964)
Indikation und Technik der operativen Kieferbruchbehandlung. (Indications for and technique of surgical treatment of jaw fractures.) Dtsch. zahnärztl. Z. 19: 1057

Krüger, E. (1974)
Lehrbuch der chirurgischen Zahn-, Mund- und Kieferheilkunde. (Textbook of oral surgery.) Vol. 2, Berlin, Buch- und Zeitschriften-Verlag "Die Quintessenz" 1st ed. (4th ed. 1981)

Krüger, E., and L. A. Rivas (1975)
Operative Behandlung von Frakturen des Unterkiefers im Wachstumsalter. (Surgical treatment of fractures of the mandible during the growth period.) Fortschr. Kiefer- u. Gesichtschir. 19: 201

Parker, D. B. (1942)
Synopsis of traumatic injuries of the face and jaws. St. Louis, C. V. Mosby

Reichenbach, E. (1969)
Die operative Behandlung der Unterkieferfrakturen. (The surgical treatment of mandibular fractures.) In: Reichenbach, E: Traumatologie im Kiefer-Gesichts-Bereich. (Traumatology of the maxillofacial region.) Munich, J. A. Barth

Robert, G. A. (1852)
Nouveau procédé de traitement des fractures de la portion alvéolaire de la mâchoire inférieure. (A new procedure for treatment of fractures of the alveolar part of the mandible.) Bull. gén. Thér. (Paris) 42: 22

Rowe, N. L., and H. C. Killey (1968)
Fractures of the facial skeleton. 2nd ed. Edinburgh – London, Livingstone

Thoma, K. H. (1943)
A new method of intermaxillary fixation of jaw fractures in patients wearing artificial dentures. Oral Surg. 29: 433

Thoma, K. H. (1958)
Oral Surgery. St. Louis, The C. V. Mosby Co.

5. Rigid Internal Fixation by Means of Compression Plates

5.1 General Principles–Peculiarities of Mandibular Compression Plate-Osteosynthesis

Wilfried Schilli

The experiments of *Schenk* and *Willenegger* (1964), and *Rahn* (Chapter 5.2) have shown that primary healing of the bone can be expected only if there is absolutely rigid fixation of the fragments. Only when absolute immobility is not maintained in the vicinity of the fracture is there a danger of infection to the damaged region. This immobility takes on particular importance in the mandible because all fractures in the tooth-bearing section are contaminated with bacteria. The attached gingiva, which is firmly connected with the periosteum, tears at the slightest displacement of the break. Fractures passing through dental alveoli are in particular danger. Every small movement of the fragments against each other causes saliva, which is high in bacterial content, to be pumped into the fracture gap. Using splinting elements which clamp to the bone therefore involves an increased danger of infection in the line of fracture, as the foreign body in the damaged area facilitates the commencement of infection. It is thus understandable that efforts in jaw surgery to use *Lane*'s simple small bone plates, which had been used previously in surgery of the extremities, repeatedly ended in failure. However, often the only possible route to precise repositioning of the fragments is that of surgical exposure of the fracture and open reduction. It seems only logical, then, to immobilize them in this position with plates and screws.

Methods of this type for use in the maxillary and mandibular regions are reported by, among others, *Christiansen* (1945), *Thoma* et al. (1948), *Case* (1950), *Reichenbach* (1953), *Rank* et al. (1954), *Shira* (1954), *Pini* (1959), *Hoffer* and *Arlotta* (1951), and *Battersby* (1967). Because of the difficulty of achieving reliable stability and because of recurring infection of the fracture and subsequent osteomyelitis, all of these authors have limited the indication for this osteosynthesis procedure to special individual instances. As reliably rigid fixation was not possible with the available fine screws and plates, additional intraoral dental splinting and intermaxillary fixation was recommended by *Thoma* et al. (1948), *Reichenbach* (1953), and *Shira* (1954).

In order to overcome this disadvantage, several authors attempted to form the plates three-dimensionally (*Smith* and *Robinson*, 1954; *Levignac*, 1956; *Palfer-Sollier*, 1956). The plates, which mostly encircled the mandible, were exceptionally stable, but practically incapable of adaptation. The same was true for the L-splint developed by *Robinson* and *Yoon* in 1963; this was a plate with an angular profile, with a so-called inlay part recessed in a groove into the bone. This plate cannot be bent to fit the various possible anatomical situations of the bone. For this reason, we have recommended small cuts in the inlay part of the plate to make a certain amount of flexibility possible (*Schilli*, 1969).

All of these procedures have great disadvantages. If the plates were easily and precisely adaptable to the surface of the bone, it was only at the price of instability. The easily adaptable plates were dimensionally insufficient for the functional forces prevalent in the mandible. If the plates were stabilized by profiles or by some other three-dimensional reinforcement, then they could not be fitted individually to the surface of the bone. The mounting surface on the bone was small and thus the fixation often insufficient. Moreover, the exact reduction of the fragments was often lost when the fastening screws were tightened. The end result in these cases, then, was that the fragments adapted themselves to the position of the plate. Because the reduction of the fragments in the dentulous and partially dentulous jaw must be exact to the millimeter, these procedures were unsuitable for routine treatment. An additional complicating factor is the sufficient bone thickness which is a precondition for the use of stable plates and screws. In the mandible, bone thickness of this amount is generally found only in the vicinity of the inferior border.

Under the leadership of the Swiss Association for the Study of Internal Fixation (ASIF), a trend has established itself in extremity surgery toward functionally stable internal fixation for fractures. The main goal of this surgical treatment for broken bones is the restoration of full function as early as possible, which permits institution of an active and painless movement therapy for the muscles and joints. The precondition for this is a constant state of absolute immobility of the bone fragments during the healing process. This sort of rigid internal fixation, which precludes even microscopic movements of the bone fragments with absolute certainty, is the precondition for primary healing safe from infection. In order to achieve this sort of absolute stability, the fragments are pressed against each other by initial stress and ingeniously thought-out auxiliary devices. This interfragmentary compression increases friction and thus yields stability. Interfragmentary compression of this type can be produced statically or dynamically. With static compression, the fragments are pressed against each other through the pressure produced by an internal fixation implant. The classical examples of these are lag screws (see section 6) and compression plates (see section 5.2 and 5.3). In dynamic compression, the interfragmentary pressure is produced through functional forces.

Pauwels (1940) has shown that the most favorable site for internal fixation is the spot where the muscularly determined tensile forces are the greatest. This tension band principle allows stable fixation with relatively weak devices stressed with tension forces, as a tension band neutralizes the tensile forces which pull the fragments apart and transforms them into pressure forces. If a stable internal fixation plate must, for anatomical reasons, be mounted in the pressure zone region, an additional tension band must be applied in the region of traction to nullify the functionally produced traction and to maintain the interfragmentary pressure. This can, in general, have smaller dimensions than the actual compression plate. The traction side in the mandible lies in the lingual-cranial region in the area of the alveolar process (section 5.1.1). Fracture fixations are therefore functionally the most favorable in the region of the alveolar process. This is the reason why such favorable prognoses exist for tooth-borne splints. Internal fixation to the bone in this favorable traction region in the dentulous sections is only conditionally possible, if at all, because of the danger of injuring the teeth. *Michelet* et al. (1973) and *Souyris* et al. (1973) tried to solve the problem with small, easily bendable plates. These are fixed in the region of the alveolar process with short screws which grip only the outer cortex. *Champy* et al. (1976) have reported good results with this method.

In internal fixation in the region of the inferior border of the mandible, i. e., in a biomechanically unfavorable pressure area, a tension band must be applied in the vicinity of the alveolar process in order to maintain the interfragmentary pressure and thus the absolute rigidity. References to this have been made by *Snell* and *Dott* (1969), and *Brons* and *Boering* (1970) in particular, as well as *Spiessl* and *Schroll* (1972). This additional tension band can be achieved by interdental ligatures or a tension band arch bar if the fracture lies in the tooth bearing region, or by a small two- or three-finger plate in the region of the alveolar process.

With the use of individually adaptable stable plates in the region of the inferior border of the mandible, interfragmentary pressure is produced by the special configuration of the screw holes. In 1968, *Luhr* became the first to introduce this method into maxillofacial surgery. He used self-tapping screws with conically formed heads, screwed eccentrically into the conically formed plate holes, which pressed the fragments against each other. For producing the pressure, the ASIF system uses the cortex screws, which are widely used in surgery of the extremities and have pre-cut threads, and the dynamic compression hole of *Perren* et al. (1969; see p. 349 ff.).

5.1.1 Surgical Approach

5.1.1.1 Extraoral Approach

All internal fixation systems with plates which use special hole and screw configurations to

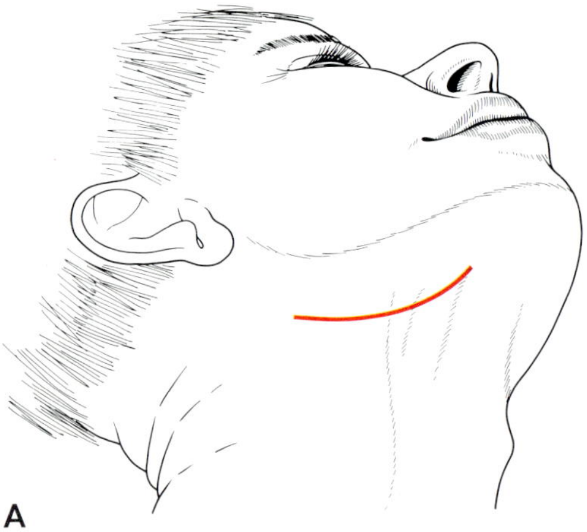

Fig. 8.5.1-1 A Line of incision for extraoral exposure of the inferior border of the mandible. The incision extends parallel to and about 2 cm below the border of the mandible. If at all possible, an existing fold in the skin should be used as the incision site.

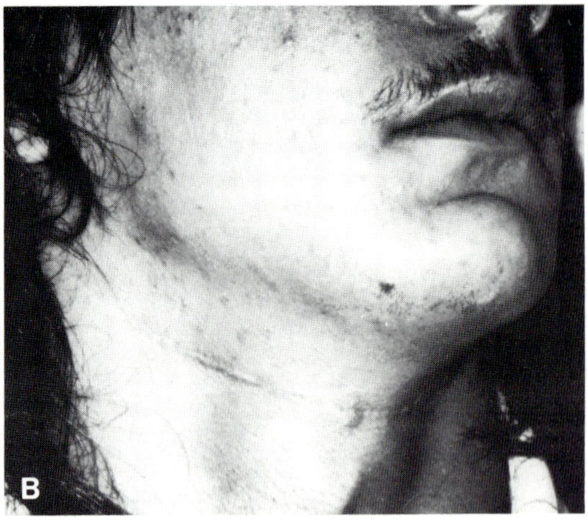

Fig. 8.5.1-1 B The scar from a submandibular incision after osteosynthesis via the extraoral approach.

produce the interfragmentary pressure are applied at the inferior border of the mandible. This region is displayed most distinctly through an extraoral approach. The site of the incision for the angle and the horizontal ramus of the mandible lies parallel to the inferior border of the mandible, in a fold of skin about 2 cm below it (Fig. 8.5.1-1). The skin and the subdermal fat underneath are separated by an incision perpendicular to the skin surface. The platysma is then exposed as a fine plate of muscle with a fiber direction transverse to the incision.

Particular attention must be paid to the marginal mandibular branch of the facial nerve. *Dingman* and *Grabb*'s anatomical studies (1962) revealed that the mandibular branch was always situated above the inferior border of the mandible in the anterior region; in the section between the facial artery and the angle of the mandible, it was found to be above this boundary in 81 % of the cases and below this boundary by up to 1 cm in 19 %. Between the angle of the mandible and the facial artery, only 21 % of the sample had a single branch of the mandibular ramus, 67 % had two, 9 % three and 3 % four. All branches crossed the facial vein on the superficial surface. The facial artery was crossed either superficially or deeply, or both.

In general, the marginal mandibular branch of the facial nerve is situated beneath the platysma. Rarely however, it is so near the inner layer that it might be injured when the muscle is separated. Therefore, the sharp separation of the platysma and possibly necessary ligation of vessels should be performed as far as possible in a caudal direction. For this reason, the cranial tissue fragments should not be pulled upward before the division of the platysma.

The mandibular branch of the facial nerve is most easily found by looking for the facial vein and following it to the inferior border of the mandible. If the nerve is found in this course, then it should be exposed (Fig. 8.5.1-2). The facial vein and artery are then tied off beneath the nerve. In further dissection, the nerve is pulled up out of the operative area together with the soft tissue portions of the cheek. An electrical nerve stimulator facilitates the location of the mandibular branch. With this disposable battery-powered device (Fig. 8.5.1-3) the nerve can be located precisely.

If the nerve is not found in the course of dis-

Figs. 8.5.1-2 A and B Appearance at surgery: exposure of the marginal mandibular branches of the facial nerve.

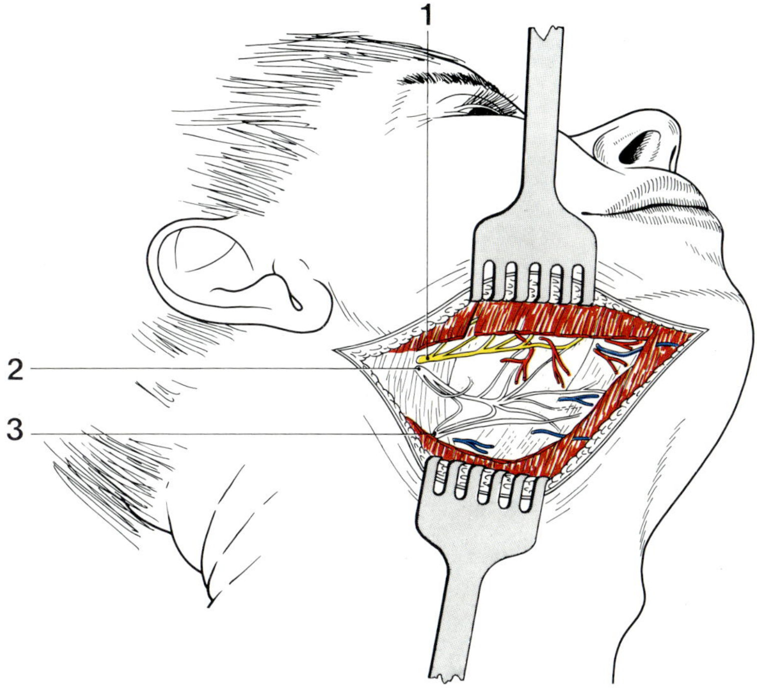

Fig. 8.5.1-2 A A view of the superficial cervical fascia under the separated platysma. Beneath is the mandibular ramus (1), which consists of two branches between the angle of the mandible and the facial vessels in 67 %, in 21 % there is one branch, 9 % have three branches, and 3 % four branches. In the inferior region are situated the cervical branches of the facial nerve (2) and the cranial branch of the cutaneus colli nerve (3).

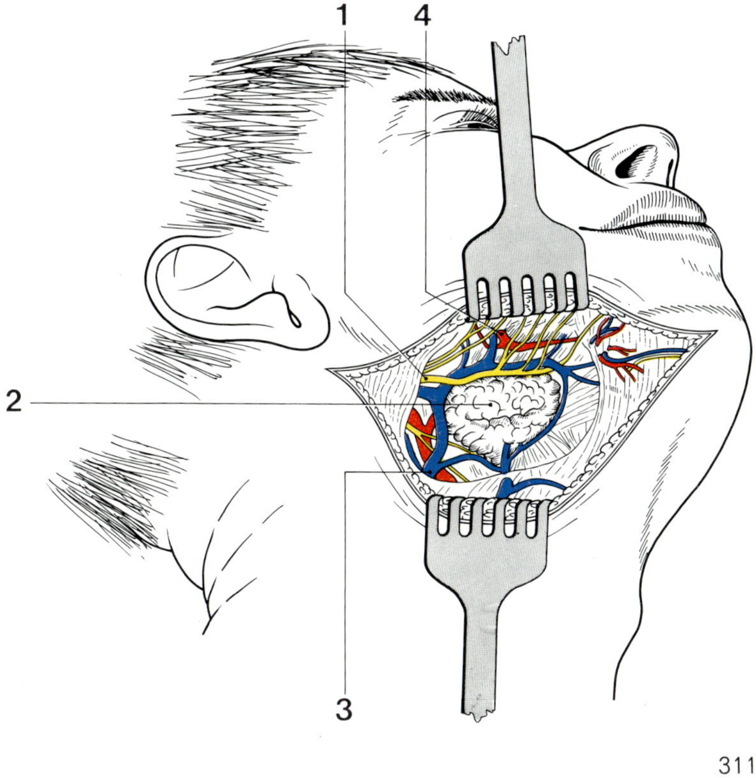

Fig. 8.5.1-2 B After the superficial cervical fascia has been separated, the mandibular ramus (1) and the facial vessels can be exposed. The submandibular gland (2) is situated deeper down. All branches of the mandibular ramus cross the facial vein (3) superficially, while the facial artery (4) may be crossed superficially, deeply, or both.

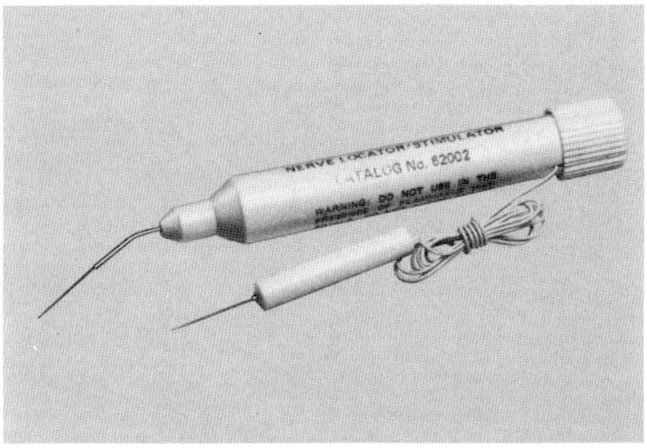

Fig. 8.5.1-3 Electric nerve probe. This disposable device is delivered in a sterile package. Inspection of light indicates whether it is ready for operation. The small needle electrode on the cable is inserted anywhere under the patient's skin. The intensity of the electrical nerve stimulation is variable; for rough orientation, it is set initially at maximum strength and the weakest setting is used for direct searching for the nerve.

section up to the height of the inferior border of the mandible, it is located higher and exposing it is superfluous.

The mandibular branch must not be confused with the cervical branches of the facial nerve, which innervate the platysma. Stimulation of the nerve branches situated in front of the facial vessels and below the inferior border of the mandible can likewise effect movements of the corner of the mouth, although these fibers have no connection with the lip muscles. These movements are probably induced by contractions of the platysma.

After the muscle layer is separated, the platysma is folded upward with the flap of skin. The angle of the jaw, enveloped by the masseter-pterygoid sling, can usually be readily identified. The bone is exposed through sharp separation and dissection of the periosteum.

For displaying the anterior sections of the mandible, especially of the chin, we use a curved incision. This, too, is situated about 2 cm below the palpable mandibular border. The subdermal layer of fat usually is relatively thick. There is no danger of injuring a nerve if the incision is not extended distally beyond the region of the canines (Fig. 8.5.1-4).

The periosteal sheath is shifted to the side only as far as is necessary for trouble-free exposure of the region of the fracture and application of the plate. After the operation is completed, the wound is closed at several levels. The wound cavity is drained with suction drainage. With small clean wounds, a very small dimensioned drainage, such as that used in hand surgery, is sufficient (Manovac, Fig. 8.5.1-5). The outer skin closure is performed with hair-fine interrupted sutures or with a running burried suture. It is to be expected that even with the greatest care in suturing technique, an unattractive, clearly perceptible scar will remain behind in about 13 to 15% (*Schilli* and *Härle*, 1976; *Prein et al.* 1976). This is a distinct disadvantage of this approach.

5.1.1.2 Intraoral Approach

Investigations of primary fracture healing and the resistance to infection of absolutely rigid fixed bone fragments permit osteosynthesis from an intraoral approach as well, as contamination with saliva does not represent any significant danger when there is absolute stability.

Experiences with reconstruction plates in tumor surgery have shown that even if the metal is exposed in the mouth, there is no certainty of infection. A great advantage of the intraoral approach is the possibility of inspecting the occlusion at all times. The result is an easier repositioning and inspection of the positioning during the placement of the device. For this reason, and because the danger of scar formation or nerve damage does not exist, more and more authors prefer the intraoral approach (*Souyris* et al., 1973).

The incision is situated within movable mucosa, about 2 mm to the side of the muco-labial fold. The incision line extends parallel to the alveolar process in the vestibule (Fig. 8.5.1-6). The

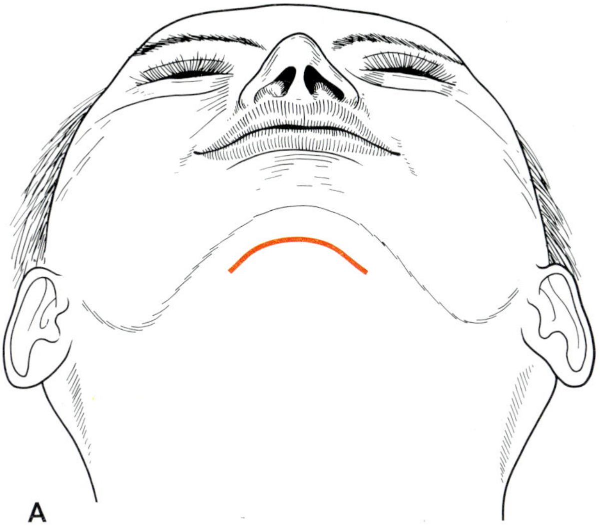

Fig. 8.5.1-4 A Curved incision line for the extraoral exposure of the chin region.

A

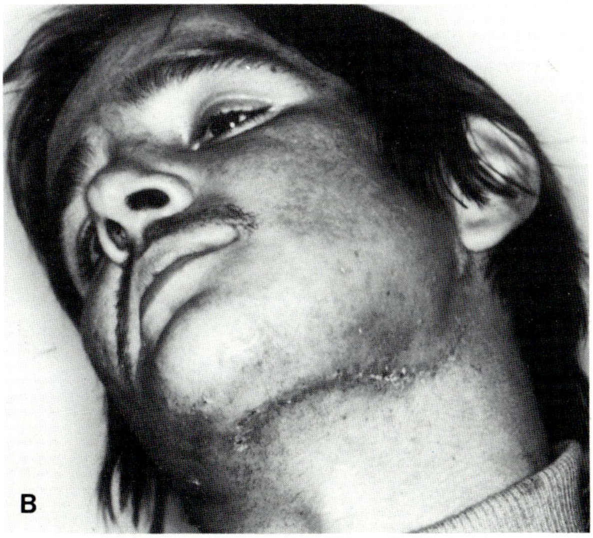

Fig. 8.5.1-4 B The scar after a curved submental and submandibular incision.

B

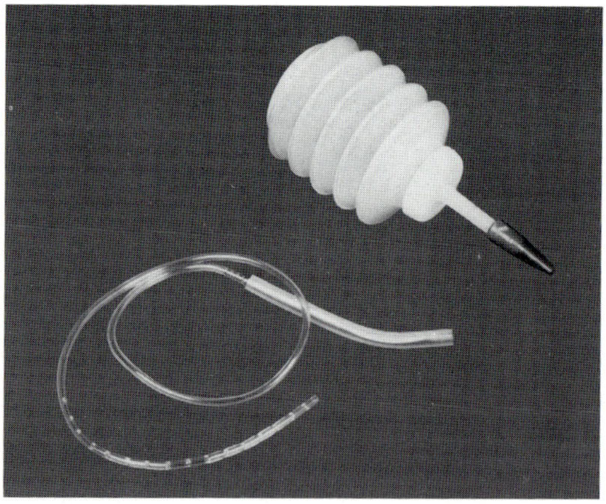

Fig. 8.5.1-5 Small suction drainage (Manovac). The perforated end of the hose is situated in the wound and the suction hose is led from the wound through the skin or the mucosa with the help of the needle. The drainage hose must be immobilized with a suture or adhesive plaster at the exit site on the skin or the mucosal membrane.

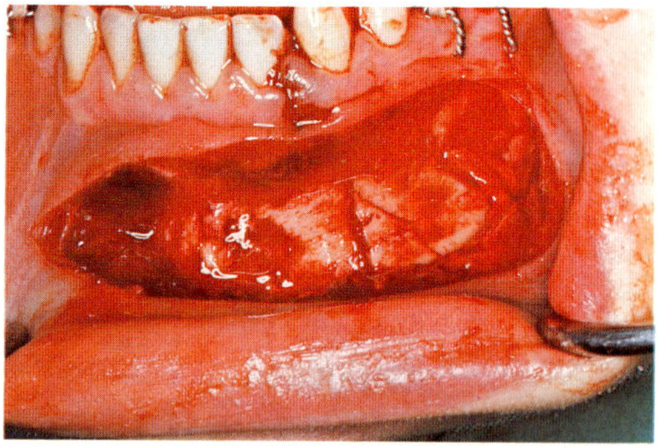

Fig. 8.5.1-6 Intraoral incision line for exposure of the inferior border of the mandible. The incision line is situated completely in the area of the movable mucosa and extends parallel to the muco-labial fold. After the mucosa is incised through, the soft tissue is separated down to the bone.

mucosa and the connective tissue underneath it are incised perpendicular to the surface of the mucosa to a depth of about 2 mm. Then the mental nerve must be separated through blunt dissection in the vicinity of the mental foramen. When the nerve is found, it is freed along its main branch with fine forceps and dissection scissors (Fig. 8.5.1-7 and 8.5.1-8). In the remaining area of the incision, the soft tissue is reflected from the bone to about the level of the root tips. Soft tissue and periosteum are shifted to the side with a periosteal elevator and thus the bony outer surface of the mandible is exposed. If there is sufficient mobilization of the branches of the mental nerve, the buccal region of the inferior border of the mandible also can be clearly exposed. For holding back the tissue, Homann hooks have proven particularly convenient (Fig. 8.5.1-9). When the Homann hooks are used, the mandible is simultaneously pressed against the maxilla. If the reduction is correct, the fragments are thus immobilized. This prepares the fracture for the osteosynthesis with plates or lag screws. Boring holes and cutting threads seems simple in the mental region, extending up the premolars. In order to avoid injury to the soft tissue, a protective casing should always be used. In the distal area, the inferior border can be exposed intraorally approximately to the angle of the mandible and, if necessary, drilling for a lag screw osteosynthesis in a sagittal direction can be undertaken. Any drill holes which are to extend vertically to the mandibular ramus must be drilled transbuccally through a small puncture incision. The ASIF has developed special instruments for this, which are also used for rigid internal fixation in orthopedic maxillofacial operations in the mandibular ramus. In essence, however, transbuccal work can be performed with any protective casing (Fig. 8.5.1-10).

After completion of internal fixation, the mucous membrane wound is closed with interrupted sutures or a continuous suture; here, too, suction drainage with a Manovac tube seems advantageous. The tube is led out intraorally from the mucosa in the vestibule. The tightness of the sutures can be checked easily during the suction. If the screwing takes place transbuccally, the tube can be led out through the puncture incision (Fig. 8.5.1-11). The drain usually is removed on the second or third day. In uncomplicated cases, drainage can ensue through a

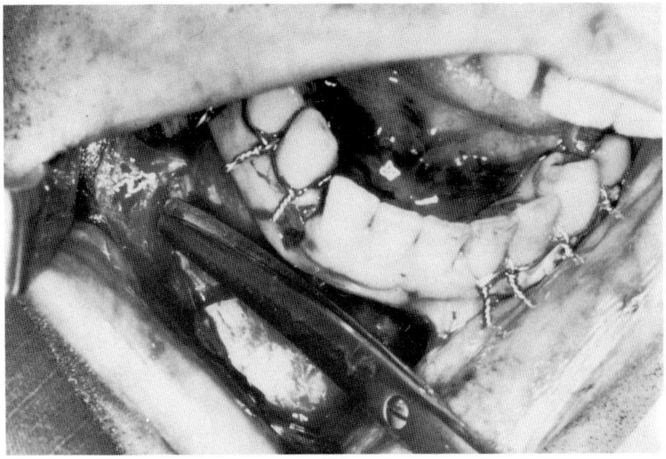

Fig. 8.5.1-7 When the periosteum is carefully reflected in a caudal direction, the mental foramen and the mental nerve become visible in the region of the root apices of the first premolars. The freed periosteum is grasped with forceps and the nerve is dissected free with a pair of curved dissection scissors.

Figs. 8.5.1-8 A and B The mental nerve after being dissected free. Good approach to the bone, even in the vicinity of the mental foramen.

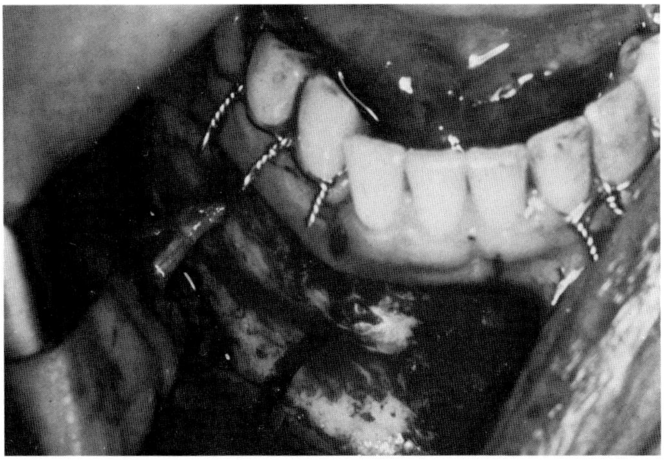

Fig. 8.5.1-8 A The fracture is situated in front of the mental foramen between 43 and 42.

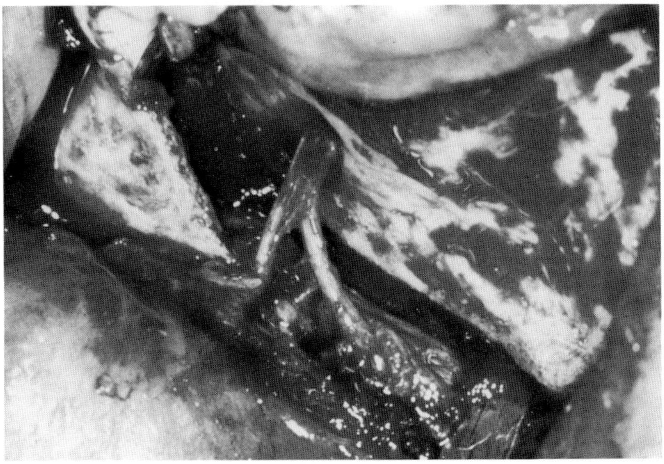

Fig. 8.5.1-8 B The fracture is situated behind the mental foramen between 46 and 45.

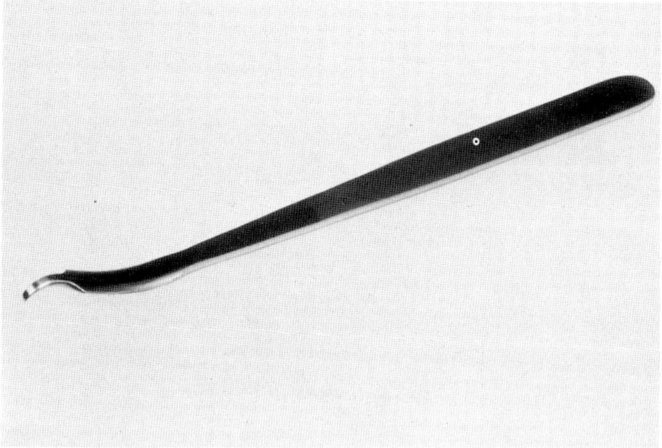

Fig. 8.5.1-9 Homann hook. The point of the hook is pushed around the inferior border of the mandible.

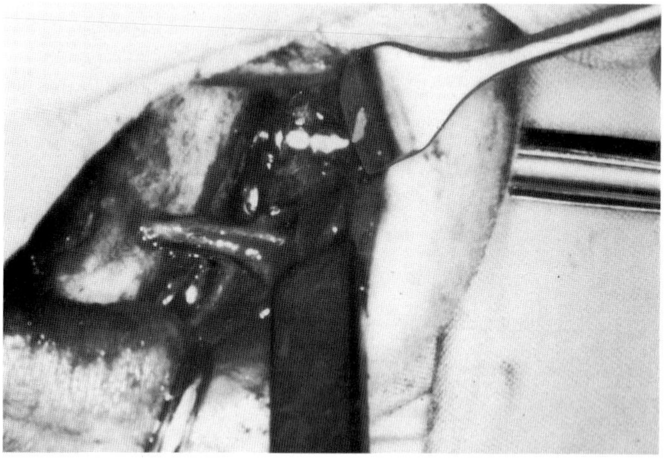

Fig. 8.5.1-10 Transbuccal drilling through a protective sleeve. A closed scissors is initially inserted through a small puncture incision in the outer skin into the oral cavity. A tap sleeve is slid through along this perforation as a protective casing; vertical drilling of and screwing into the bone can then be performed through the casing.

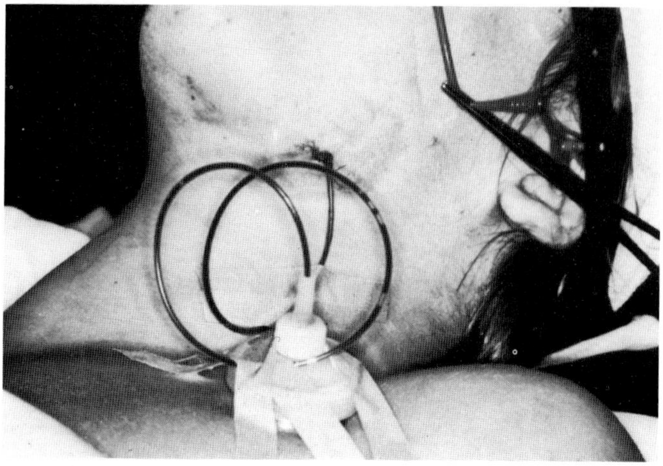

Fig. 8.5.1-11 Suction drainage through the Manovac. The hose was led out through the puncture incision after transbuccal drilling.

simple rubber drain instead of the suction drainage. This, too, is removed after two to three days.

5.1.2 Postoperative Treatment and Complications

An osteosynthesis only fulfills the requirement of functional stability if function can be resumed immediately after the operation without endangering the stabilization. The forces which prevail in the mandible for masticatory functions are extraordinarily great. In individual cases, values of over 100 kp have been measured. To avoid overburdening the internal fixation mechanically at these peak values, therefore, it is recommended that the patient be advised to use caution and restraint in his chewing.
In the tooth-bearing and partially dentulous jaw, the absolute first priority is the exact re-establishment of the occlusion. This is generally instituted through preoperative intermaxillary fixation by means of wire ligatures. They can be removed at the end of the operation. In osteosynthesis with an intraoral approach, it is advisable to maintain the intermaxillary fixation for a few days to protect the soft tissue wound and the intraoral sutures, and to nourish the patient during this period with fluid through a naso-gastric tube inserted while the patient is anesthetised. The wound's condition thus remains clean, and the intraoral sutures, which are endangered during postoperative swelling, remain tight.
In special circumstances—such as, for example, the necessity of further anesthesia or vomiting—requiring immediate release of the intermaxillary fixation, this is possible at any time. The interdental wire ligatures are removed at the same time.
The rigid internal fixation is not infection prone and thus prophylactic antibiotic treatment is superfluous. Such treatment is limited to patients in whom there is massive visible contamination of the wound area. If, in the course of the postoperative treatment, an infection of the wound area appears with swelling and pus formation, it is treated as any abscess. If increased redness and swelling appears shortly after internal fixation, a few sutures should be loosened in the vicinity of the greatest swelling and any pus which appears is aspirated. The wound cavity is drained. In the case of abscess formation, an incision is made in the area of the greatest swelling; drainage should be provided. The bacteria can be identified from the pus emitted or from the wound secretions and an antibiotic sensitivity test performed. Before these results are available, a broad-spectrum antibiotic should be prescribed in a sufficiently high dosage. This can be replaced, if necessary, by an appropriate antibiotic after the specific sensitivity is known.
The appearance of a wound infection, which can come between the 6th and 10th day, is never an indication for removal of the osteosynthesis materials. Even if a chronic inflammation persists, usually it can be kept under control with antibiotic treatment and local drainage sufficient to permit bone healing in other areas of the fracture. In any case, the precondition is an absolutely secure stable fixation of the bony fragments and reliable positioning of the osteosynthesis materials. A single loose screw can endanger the success of the treatment.
In order to provide additional stability for the wound, it is advisable to effect intermaxillary immobilization in osteosynthesis cases with infection. Only if there is still no resolution of the infection after three weeks and metal parts are distinguishable through the drainage cavity, should the foreign bodies be removed.
In the rare cases of osteomyelitis following fracture—which can only be diagnosed unequivocally at the end of the first month—a new compression osteosynthesis may need to be applied.

5.1.3 Removal of the Metal

Generally, mounted plates are removed from the region of the face. The covering soft tissue layer is too thin; thus, injuries can result even from inconsequential blows. The removal of the plates is omitted only when the patient is old and in poor health. The removal of the plates from the mandible can almost always be done intraorally and under local anesthesia. A general anesthetic is more advantageous only with plates in the molar region and at the angle of the mandible, because of the accompaning muscle relaxation. These plates, too, are exposed from the intraoral side, and the screws are screwed out through a small transbuccal puncture incision. Plates and screws which have been used once must not be used again because of the danger of corrosion.

References

Battersby, T. G. (1967)
Plating of mandibular fractures. Brit. J. oral Surg. 4: 194

Brons, R., and G. Boering (1970)
Fractures of the mandibular body treated by stable internal fixation: a preliminary report. J. oral Surg. 28: 407

Case, J. (1959)
Metacarpal plates and screws in edentulous fractured mandibles. Ref. Intern. Dent. Congr., London

Champy, M., J. P. Lodde, J. H. Jaeger, and A. Wilk (1976)
Ostéosynthèses mandibulaires selon la technique de Michelet. I. Bases biomécaniques. (Michelet's technique for plate osteosynthesis. I. Biomechanics.) Rev. Stomatol. Chir. Maxillofac. 77: 569

Christiansen, G. W. (1945)
Open operation and tantalum plate insertion for fracture of the mandible. Oral Surg. 3: 194

Dingman, R. O., and W. C. Grabb (1962)
Surgical anatomy of the mandibular ramus of the facial nerve based on the dissection of 100 facial halves. Plast. reconstr. Surg. 29: 266

Hoffer, O., and P. Arlotta (1961)
Behandlung von Unterkieferbrüchen mit Metallplättchen. (Treatment of mandibular fractures with small metal plates.) Dtsch. zahnärztl. Z. 16: 807

Levignac, J. (1956)
Sur le traitement chirurgical des fractures de la mandible. (Surgical treatment of fractures of the mandible.) Rev. franç. Odonto-stomat. 3: 209

Luhr, H. G. (1968)
Zur stabilen Osteosynthese bei Unterkieferfrakturen. (Stable osteosynthesis in mandibular fractures.) Dtsch. zahnärztl. Z. 23: 754

Michelet, F. X., J. Deymes, and B. Dessus (1963)
Osteosynthesis with miniaturized screwed plates in maxillo-facial surgery. J. max.-fac. Surg 1: 79

Palfer-Sollier, M. (1956)
L'ostéosynthèse par gouttières vissées en durallium dans les fractures mandibulaires (avec ou sans perte de substance). (Osteosynthesis with Durallium screw splints in mandibular fractures with or without loss of hard tissue.) Rev. franç. Odonto-Stomat. 3: 587

Pauwels, F. (1940)
Grundriß einer Biomechanik der Frakturheilung. (Outline of the biomechanics of fracture healing.) Verh. dtsch. Ges. Orthop. 34: 62

Perren, S. M., J. Russenberger, S. Steinemann, M. E. Müller, and M. Allgöwer (1969)
A dynamic compression plate. Acta orthop. scand. Suppl. 125: 29

Pini, C. E. (1959)
Le osteosintesi mediante plachette mettaliche nelle fratture della mandibola. (Metal plate osteosynthesis in fractures of the mandible.) Minerva stomat. 8: 105

Prein, J., A. Eschmann, and B. Spiessl (1976)
Ergebnisse der Nachuntersuchung bei 81 Patienten mit funktionsstabiler Unterkieferosteosynthese. (Follow-up examination results in 81 patients with functionally stable osteosynthesis of the mandible.) Fortschr. Kiefer- u. Gesichtschir. 21: 304

Rank, B. K., A. R. Wakerfield, and G. S. Gunter (1954)
Internal fixation of the mandibular fractures. Brit. J. plast. Surg. 7: 279

Reichenbach, E. (1953)
Zur Frage der operativen Knochenbruchbehandlung im Bereich des Gesichtsschädels. (Surgical bone fracture treatment in the region of the facial skull.) Dtsch. Zahn-, Mund- u. Kieferheilk. 17: 376

Robinson, M., and Ch. Yoon (1963)
The "L" splint for the fracture mandible: a new principle of plating. J. oral Surg. 21: 395

Schenk, R. K., and H. Willenegger (1964)
Histologie der primären Knochenheilung. (Histology of primary bone healing.) Langenbecks Arch. klin. Chir. 308: 440

Schilli, W. (1969)
Behandlungsmöglichkeiten bei Frakturen. (Treatment choices in fractures.) Therapiewoche 41: 2006

Schilli, W., and F. Härle (1976)
Die funktionsstabile Osteosynthese – ein Problem des operativen Zugangs. (Functionally stable osteosynthesis: a problem of surgical approach.) Fortschr. Kiefer- u. Gesichtschir. 21: 300

Shira, R. B. (1954)
Open reduction of mandibular fractures. J. oral Surg. 12: 95

Smith, A. E., and M. Robinson (1954)
Individually constructed stainless steel bone onley splint for immobilization of proximal fragment in fractures of the angle of the mandible. J. oral Surg. 12: 170

Snell, J. A., and W. A. Dott (1969)
Internal fixation of certain fractures of the mandible by bone plating. Plast. reconstr. Surg. 43: 281

Souyris, F., B. Caravel, and J. P. Reynaud (1973)
Ostéosynthèses mandibulaires par plaques vissées sans blocage: méthode originale et résultats après 5 ans. (Mandibular osteosynthesis with screw plates without intermaxillary fixation: An original technique and results after 5 years.) Rev. Stomatol. Chir. Maxillofac. 74: 253

Spiessl, B., and K. Schroll (1972)
Gesichtsschädel. (Facial skull.) In H. Nigst: Spezielle Frakturen- und Luxationslehre. (Textbook of fractures and luxations.) Vol. I/1 Stuttgart, G. Thieme

Thoma, K. H., D. J. Holand, W. H. Woodbury, J. G. Burrow, and E. L. Sleeper (1948)
Fractures cases treated by means of internal fixation. J. oral Surg. 1:90

5.2 Compression Plate Osteosynthesis through the Luhr System

Hans-Georg Luhr

5.2.1 Introduction

The treatment of mandibular fractures is not problematical as long as the fractures are in sufficiently dentulous mandibular segments and as long as adherence to certain principles is maintained during treatment (see section 2). However, if the teeth are absent as supporting elements for splints, neither reduction nor sufficient fixation of fragments is possible without surgery. The surgical treatment methods common in the past for fractures in the partly dentulous or edentulous segments of the mandible involved some substantial difficulties with respect to the fixation of fracture ends which was stable during function. An osteosynthesis that is stable during function appeared possible most readily with application of the principle of axial compression which was advocated long ago by the Belgian surgeon *Danis* (1949). It was clear that, for anatomic reasons, the traction devices used in surgery of the extremities by the Swiss Association for the Study of Internal Fixation (ASIF)* for the creation of axial pressure (*Müller* et al., 1963) could not be applied to the mandible. This realization led to the development of a self-tightening compression plate (*Luhr*, 1968; Fig. 8.5.2-1). Self-tightening compression plates also have been developed for surgery of the extremities (*Perren* et al., 1969; *Allgöwer*, 1969; *Mittelmeier*, 1968) and were modified and developed further, in part for the special needs of maxillofacial surgery (*Spiessl* et al., 1971; *Spiessl* and *Schroll*, 1972; *Niederdellmann* and *Schilli*, 1972; *Becker* and *Machtens*, 1973; *Schilli* et al., 1973; *Becker*, 1974; *Niederdellmann*, 1974, 1975; *Spiessl*, 1975; *Schilli*, 1975).

* Arbeitsgemeinschaft für Osteosynthesefragen (AO).

5.2.2 Principles of Construction and Material of the Compression Screw Plate (CSP)

With the goal of osteosynthesis that is stable during function, an osteosynthetic union was developed for treatment of mandibular fractures which does justice to the particular anatomic and functional conditions in the mandibular region in its construction, and to the properties of the materials used. By far the greatest stability can be achieved in the mandible by use of plates provided with screws. Bone plates and screws of stainless steel or chromium-cobalt alloys were used, among others, by *Thoma* (1948, 1952), *Bigelow* (1943), *Pini* (1959), and *Hoffer* and *Arlotta* (1961). *Robinson* and *Yoon* (1957, 1963) have described an L-shaped profile splint in which the short leg of the L is inserted in a milled bone groove. Further modifications of the simple bone plates without compression holes originated with *Smith* and *Robinson* (1954), *Beal* and *Levignac* (1955), *Palfer-Sollier* (1956), *Heiss* and *Grasser* (1968), *Schilli* (1969), and *Spiessl* (1969). The clinical experience, that despite rigid fixation and correct surgical technique, the commonly used plates with screws often led to delayed healing of fractures or no healing at all (*Brand*, 1937; *Eggers* et al., 1951) results from a frequently far from ideal adaptation of the fragments. If the insertion of the screw is slightly off center, the result can even be distraction of the fracture ends. Since at least some authors, such as *Thoma* (1952, 1958) and *Shira* (1954), emphasize the need for additional immobilizing procedures even for simple plates with screws, these methods have not become accepted. In contrast, the principle of axial compression for better adaptation and meshing of the fracture ends, combined with a distinct increase in the stability of the osteosynthesis, appeared to be a promising means of avoiding the disadvantages of the formerly used rigid plate and screw method. These considerations led to the development of a self-

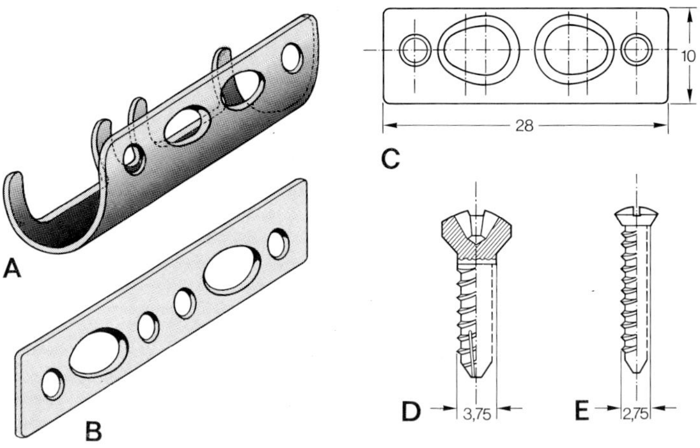

Fig. 8.5.2-1 Compression screw plate (CSP)

Fig. 8.5.2-1 A CSP with basal groove-shaped profile. The plate, whose groove surrounds the inferior border of the mandible, is extremely stable and permits axial compression of the fracture by means of eccentric holes (compression screw holes–CSH) and so-called compression screws with conical heads (CS).

Fig. 8.5.2-1 B Straight CSP (without basal groove). This type of plate is adapted easily in difficult anatomic conditions of the mandibular surface and is used primarily with the intraoral surgical technique.

Fig. 8.5.2-1 C Top view of the CSP with 2 eccentric compression screw holes (CSH) and 2 retention screw holes (RSH).

Fig. 8.5.2-1 D Compression screw (CS) with conical head.

Fig. 8.5.2-1 E Retention screw which, after axial compression of the fragments by the large screws, additionally protects the fragments from bending stress.

compressing plate. This compression screw plate (CSP), with eccentric holes in the plate and the use of screws with cone-shaped heads, realizes in a simplified way the principle of axial compression (*Luhr*, 1968). The compression screw plate (CSP) with a basal groove (Fig. 8.5.2-1 A) encompasses the inferior border of the mandible and thus guarantees additional stabilization of the fragments. The straight type of plate without a basal profile can more easily be adapted to the often irregular shape of the bone surface and is suited especially for treatment of fractures by means of an intraoral approach (Fig. 8.5.2-1 B).

Principle of Operation of the Compression Screw Plate

The two central holes in the plate close to the fracture line have an eccentric shape, with the smaller hole diameters—always located on the outside—corresponding to the diameter of the screw shaft (Fig. 8.5.2-1 C). The inner edges of the eccentric holes are bevelled at a slope of 45°, corresponding to the angle of the cone-shaped heads of the compession screws, so that the largest possible contact surface between screw head and plate, and thus a precise direction for the screw during the compression process, is guaranteed. Drilling in the bone is done within the small diameter of the eccentric holes in the plates (Fig. 8.5.2-2 A), and one compression screw is screwed into each hole (Fig. 8.5.2-2 B). During the final phase of screw insertion—after the outer and inner cortical layer is already completely perforated with screw threads—the conical heads of the compression screws are pulled into the largest diameter of the eccentric holes. In this process, the two screws move toward each other, carry the fracture ends along, and put them under pressure with one another (Fig. 8.5.2-2 C). The distance which each of the two individual compression screws can traverse during its gliding motion is 1.6 mm, which means that during the compression process, the maximum path of the screws as they advance toward each other is 3.2 mm. The pressure forces exerted on the fracture are in the range of 30 to 40 kp, as was shown in animal experiments. In clinical use, however, the magnitude of the force exerted cannot be measured in individual cases. But this has no practical significance, as the

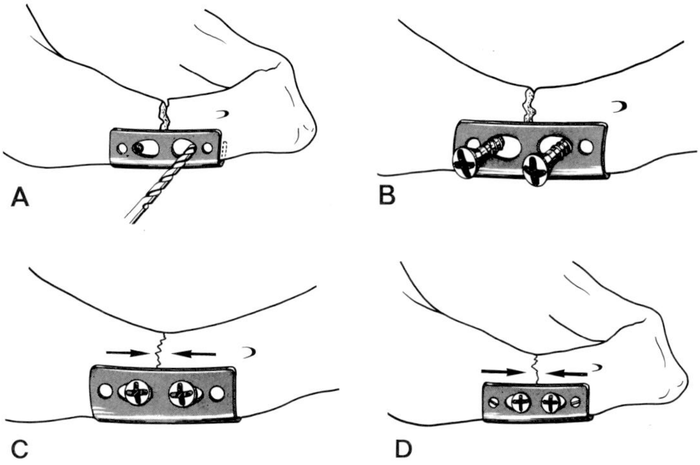

Fig. 8.5.2-2 A The region of the mandible under the small diameter of the eccentric plate holes is perforated by a surgical drill.

Fig. 8.5.2-2 B While the compression screws are inserted, the fracture gap is still open.

Fig. 8.5.2-2 C During the last phase of screw insertion, the conical screw heads slip into the great diameter of the holes; thus the fracture ends are pulled together and positioned by high pressure (arrows indicate the direction of the forces exerted).

Fig. 8.5.2-2 D After insertion of the smaller retention screws, the treated fracture is protected against bending forces.

effective pressures (force per unit area) at the contact surfaces of the superposed bony prominences represent, for each fracture, an individual entity that cannot be measured.

After the compression process of the actively functioning compression screws is concluded, the plate is stabilized by means of two additional retention screws (Fig. 8.5.2-2 D). These are centered and screwed into the bone through the outer small plate holes and secure the fragments against possible rotational stress. The active compression screws used are self-threading Duodriv screws, which have been used extensively and successfully in surgery of the extremities. In combination with the appropriate screwdriver, the cross slit guarantees flawless guidance of the screw and secure transmission of force. The screw holes are pre-drilled in the bone with a spiral drill of 3.0 mm diameter. The Duodriv screws, which are equipped with milled grooves, and which have sharp threads, cut the threads in the bone itself.

The retention screws have a considerably smaller diameter, but they are also self-threading; here, a surgically drill of 24 mm diameter is used for preliminary drilling.

We consider cutting of threads in advance in the bone as unnecessary because of the limited height of the threads. Positive results in more than 1000 cases have convinced us that self-threading screws guarantee absolutely firm anchoring of the screws in the bone if there is precise correspondence between advance drilling and the diameter of the screws. The use of self-threading screws offers the advantages of requiring fewer instruments and allowing a simpler surgical technique.

Properties of the Material for Vitallium® Plates

The austhenitic stainless steels used in bone surgery, for example, type AISI 316 according to U.S. specifications, are usually subject to corrosion. In stainless steel, homogeneous, electrolytically polished surfaces and avoidance of any damage to the protective passive layer during the operation are pre-requisites for reduction of frictional corrosion to a low level. These steels must remain entirely undamaged on their surface if they are to exhibit their maximum corrosion resistance (*Bechtol* et al., 1959). In electrolytes (tissues) containing halogen and oxygen, stainless

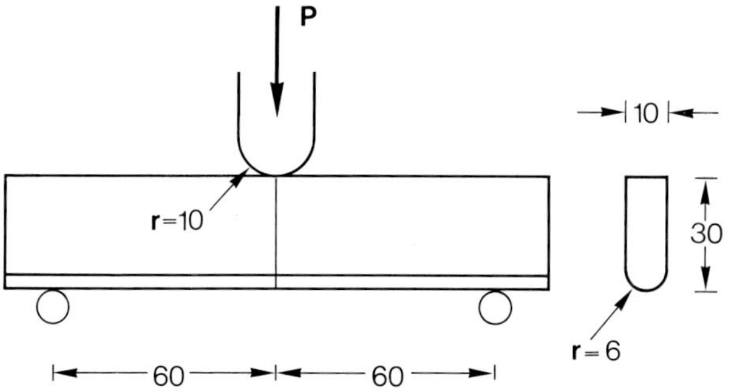

Fig. 8.5.2-3 For each osteosynthesis junction to be tested, one pair of test pieces is joined at the lower edges. Next, the model junction is placed on two bars, each 60 mm from the interface of the test pieces, and stressed with a single load (P). Under a greater load, the model is bent, and the gap at the lower edge between the two test pieces opens up. The gap width at the lower edge, when the load is increased in equal steps, is a measure of the stability of the osteosynthesis being tested. The following rule applies: the narrower the width of the gap, the more stable the osteosynthesis (see also Fig. 8.5.2-5).

steel is subject to pitting, which can become noticeable after several years and carries the danger of localized metallosis. Removal of the metal is then necessary after 2 to 5 years. This is true especially for self-tightening compression plates, in which, in accord with their method of action, considerable frictional forces are created between the screw heads and the edges of the plate holes during the compression phase. Therefore the use of stainless steel has been discontinued for compression plates. Other metals, e.g., titanium or tantalum, do have considerably better corrosion resistance than stainless steel, but their stability characteristics are inadequate, so that implants must have very thick dimensions in order to provide comparable stability. The materials just mentioned therefore seemed to us to be unsuitable for the self-tightening compression plate.
Vitallium®, the cobalt-chromium-molybdenum alloy, however, has the desired characteristics, including remarkable resistance to corrosion due to tension and friction (*Cohen*, 1962) as well as excellent stability properties. In bone surgery, Vitallium was used for the first time in 1936 by *Venable* and *Stuck* (1947) after preliminary study in animal experiments. When initial difficulties in the fabrication of Vitallium implants had been overcome, the alloy became firmly established in bone surgery on the basis of its superior corrosion resistance. Already up to 1956, more than 10 million surgical Vitallium implants had been used. Vitallium has the particular advantage that it can remain in the organism for an unlimited time (*Venable* and *Stuck*, 1947). Thus the need for removal of the implant is eliminated, so that a second operation can be avoided.

5.2.3 Fundamental Research

5.2.3.1 Physical and Technical Studies on the Stability of Internal Fixation

Since the stability, i.e., the resistance to the action of mechanical forces, is one of the main criteria for the suitability of a method of internal fixation, it was tested in experimental models for a number of diverse methods used in mandibular surgery. Test substances were prism-shaped pieces of PVC synthetic of 10 mm thickness, 30 mm height, and 75 mm length. Pairs of these pieces were joined by the method to be tested, in the manner of a clinically used type of internal fixation. The test model was then placed on edge on two supports and stressed with a single load at the center (Fig. 8.5.2-3). This load exposed the test model, similar to the clinical situation, to bending stress. A measure of the stability of the test model is the width of the gap between the two synthetic pieces being tested opposite to the plate or wire fixation. The more stable the fixation, the smaller is the width of the gap.

Methods of internal fixation tested (Fig. 8.5.2-4):

1. Two wire ligatures (0.5 mm) running horizontally in parallel

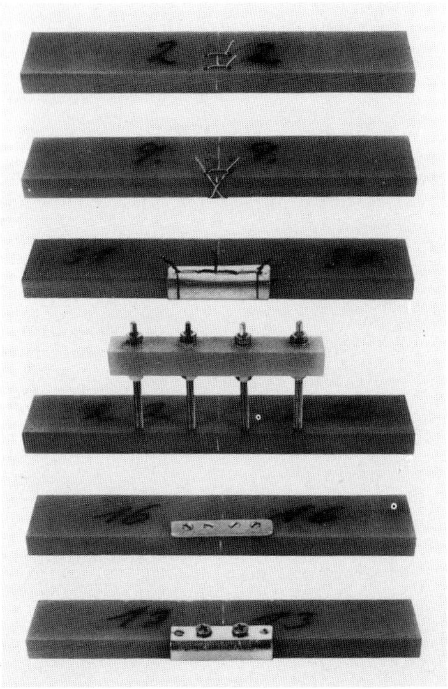

Fig. 8.5.2-4 Models of the osteosynthesis tested.
(1) Two parallel wire ligatures (wire thickness 0.5 mm).
(2) A horizontal wire ligature combined with a figure-of-eight ligature.
(3) Groove-shaped splint 38 mm in length, of 0.5 mm thick stainless steel, attached with three 0.5 mm thick wire ligatures (similar to the method advocated by *Hayward* 1962).
(4) "Pin fixation" as modified by *E. Becker* (1957, 1958). Four percutaneous osteosynthesis screws are connected by a 10 x 10 mm thick bar of cold-curing arylic (Paladur®).
(5) Normal 4-hole bone plate (Venable bone plate, 38 mm, Vitallium).
(6) Compression screw plate (CSP), 38 mm.

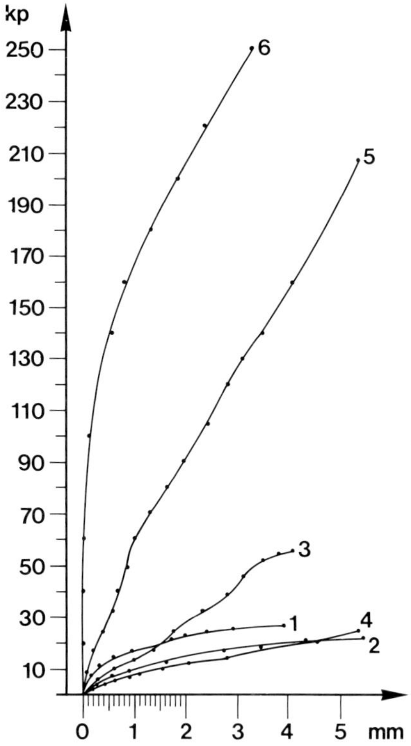

Fig. 8.5.2-5 Stability of different types of osteosyntheses under bending stress. The figure shows the gap width between pairs of test pieces as a function of the load. Even relatively small loads of 20 kp lead to loosening of osteosyntheses 1 to 4 (gap widths several millimeters). The usual screw plate system (5) is already considerably more stable, but it is excelled by far by the compression screw plate (6).

2. Wire ligature (0.5 mm) running horizontally, combined with a figure-of-eight ligature
3. Groove-shaped plate of 0.5 mm stainless steel, combined with wire ligatures
4. Pin fixation with "extracutaneous" synthetic bridge of *E. Becker* (1957)
5. Vitallium bone plate of *Venable* (1947, length 38 mm)
6. Compression screw plate (CSP) of *Luhr* (1968)

Results

Figure 8.5.2-5 shows the stability of the various methods of internal fixation. Wire ligatures No. 1 and No. 2 as well as ligature No. 3 (grooved splint, combined with wire ligatures) and fixation No. 4 (pin fixation) are not stable under stress. Even under low bending stress of 10 to 15 kp, gap widths up to 2 mm occur. Under clinical conditions, for this method of osteosynthesis one has to count on considerable motion in the

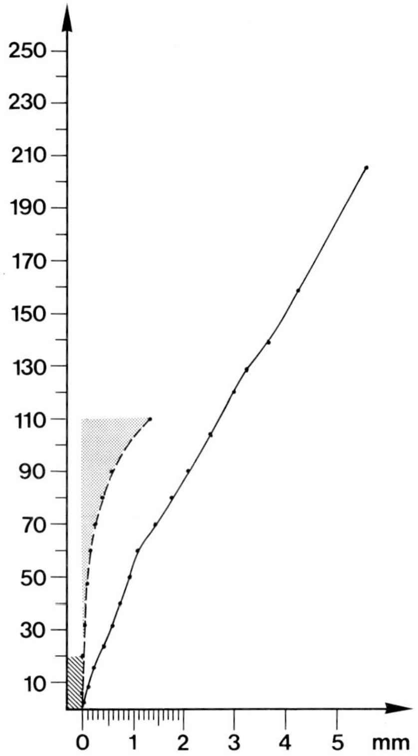

Fig. 8.5.2-6A The usual screw plate system shows permanent deformation—even though only to a limited extent—beginning at 20 kp, but increases steeply at higher values. Relatively stable junction, completely elastic only up to 20 kp (elasticity region shown shaded).

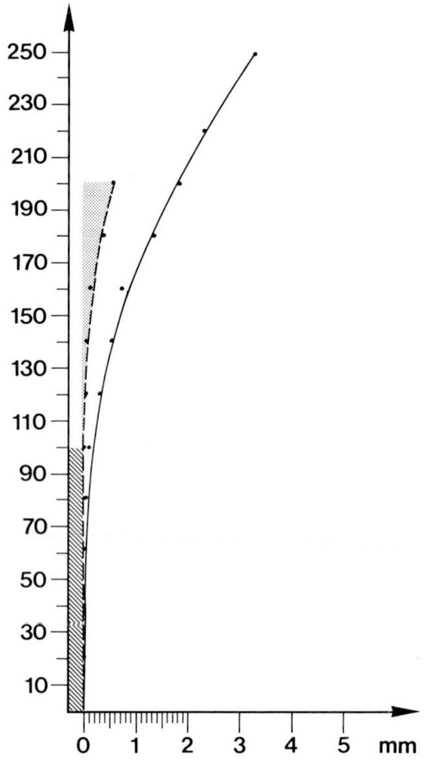

Fig. 8.5.2-6B Compression screw plate can be bent only minimally up to 100 kp; in this region there is no permanent deformation. Very stable junction, which is completely elastic up to 100 kp (elasticity region shown shaded).

fracture gap and displacement of the fracture ends even with limited stress on the fracture. The Vitallium bone plate—No. 5—provides much better stability.

However, if the so-called permanent deformation, i.e., the width of the gap, is measured which remains after the stress on the entire connector is removed, the simple rigid 4-hole bone plate is definitely inferior to the compression screw plate (No. 6). Figure 8.5.2-6A shows that such a permanent deformation already sets in at a load of 20 kp on the simple bone plate, and that it becomes considerable in the region up to 100 kp. In contrast, the CSP fixation (No. 6) possesses superior mechanical characteristics. Within a load limit of 100 kp, this compression plate is completely elastic and, at the same time, shows extremely high stability against bending, which is not even approximated by any of the other methods of internal fixation (Fig. 8.5.2-6B). In summary, the physical and technical studies in model experiments show the superior stability of the compression screw plate with concomitant complete elasticity up to a load limit of 100 kp. Thus, the CSP most closely satisfies the mechanical demands for rigid internal fixation under functional stress.

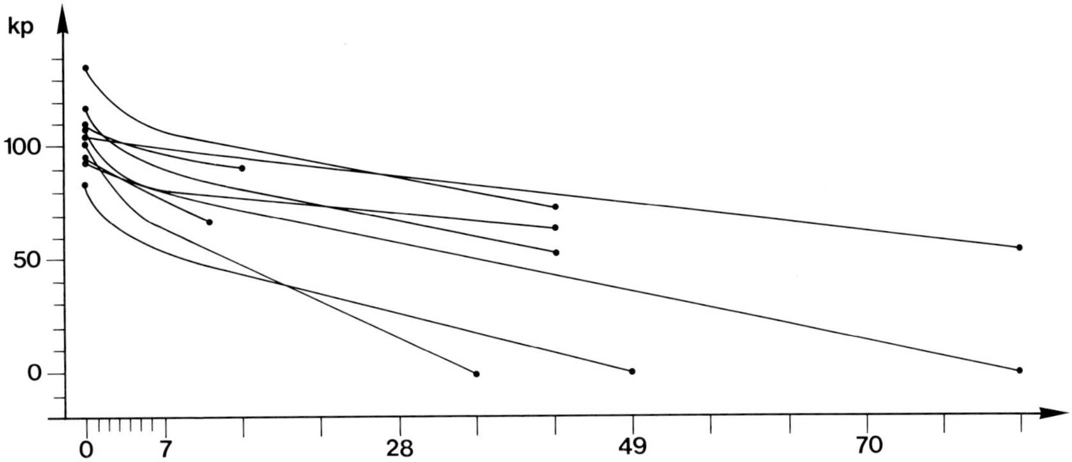

Fig. 8.5.2-7 Pressure curves after experimental osteotomies (from *Perren* et al., 1969). Curves are distinctly flatter than, but basically similar to, those in Fig. 8.5.2-8.

5.2.3.2 Measurement of Pressure Forces during Healing of Fractures

For the clinician who is developing a treatment plan, the functional principles and the properties of the material of the implants and instruments as well as clinical experience will be of greatest importance. Knowledge of the biologic basis of every surgical technique, however, is a further prerequisite for scientifically based medical thinking. Especially for compression osteosynthesis and the discussion about possible positive effects of axial pressure forces on bone formation, it was necessary to determine whether such pressure acting on healing bone after initial compression of the fracture ends can remain effective at all over an extended period. The analysis of this apparently simple question, however, posed considerable problems, so that it was only in 1969 that *Luhr* as well as *Perren* et al. succeeded independently in finding basic answers to these questions. For methodologic reasons, it was impossible to measure the pressure in the fracture line, as the insertion of measuring apparatus would occlude the gap and delay, if not prevent, healing. Therefore, measurement techniques were developed which made it possible to measure the forces transmitted by the compression screw plate away from the fracture line. The principle holds that the pressure forces resting on the fracture ends are in equilibrium with the tension forces arising in the plate; these forces cause a corresponding change in the length of the plate. These changes in length were observed by measurement. The pressure curves after experimental osteotomies in sheep tibia (*Perren* et al., 1969, Fig. 8.5.2-7) had a distinctly flatter course, although they were basically similar to the pressure curves after experimental fractures (*Luhr* 1969, 1972) as shown in Figure 8.5.2-8. In the curves of both groups, the initial decrease in pressure is clearly visible; this decrease is distinctly greater in experimental fractures (Fig. 8.5.2-8) than in model osteotomies (Fig. 8.5.2-7). In this connection, it is important to observe that axial pressures (and thus the principle of compression osteosynthesis) remain in force during healing of the fracture, although not completely, but at least at half of the initial values. The initial decrease in pressure, which becomes detectable within a few minutes after axial compression, is the result of a sprain of the bone substance. Due to the visco-elastic properties of bone, a permanent deformation sets in which is a function of time. As a result, the

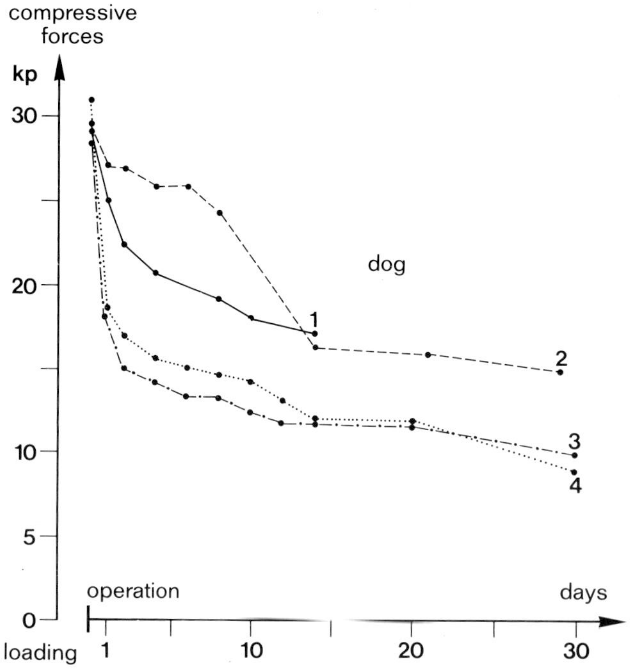

Fig. 8.5.2-8 Pressure curves for compression osteosyntheses after experimental mandibular fractures in dogs. The osteosyntheses were performed under axial compression of the fragments at about 30 kp. During the first two postoperative days, there is a relatively sharp initial decrease in pressure, primarily from permanent deformation of the bone at the contact surfaces of the fracture ends (see also Fig. 8.5.2-9). The pressure forces, however, remain at about half the initial value until fracture healing is complete (about 4 weeks).

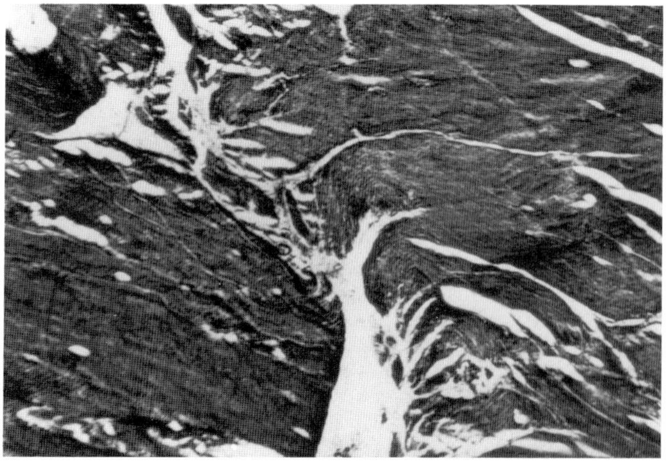

Fig. 8.5.2-9 Experimental mandibular fracture in a dog, two weeks after compression osteosynthesis at 30 kp. In the region of a pressure-bearing "supporting post", the longitudinal lamellar structure of the bone is clearly bent. The initial drop in pressure after compression osteosynthesis as shown in Fig. 8.5.2-8 is due to the morphologic deformation of the bone in the region of the contact points as illustrated here (Gomori Ag impregnation, 66x).

fragments approach each other minimally, thus causing a decrease in the plate tension and the pressure forces. The decrease in pressure is therefore not caused by possible resorption processes, as is often assumed, but is the result of morphologic deformation of the bone in the fracture line. Such pressure zones, with corresponding deformation and bending of the bone lamellae, are observed in studies of histologic serial sections (Fig. 8.5.2-9).

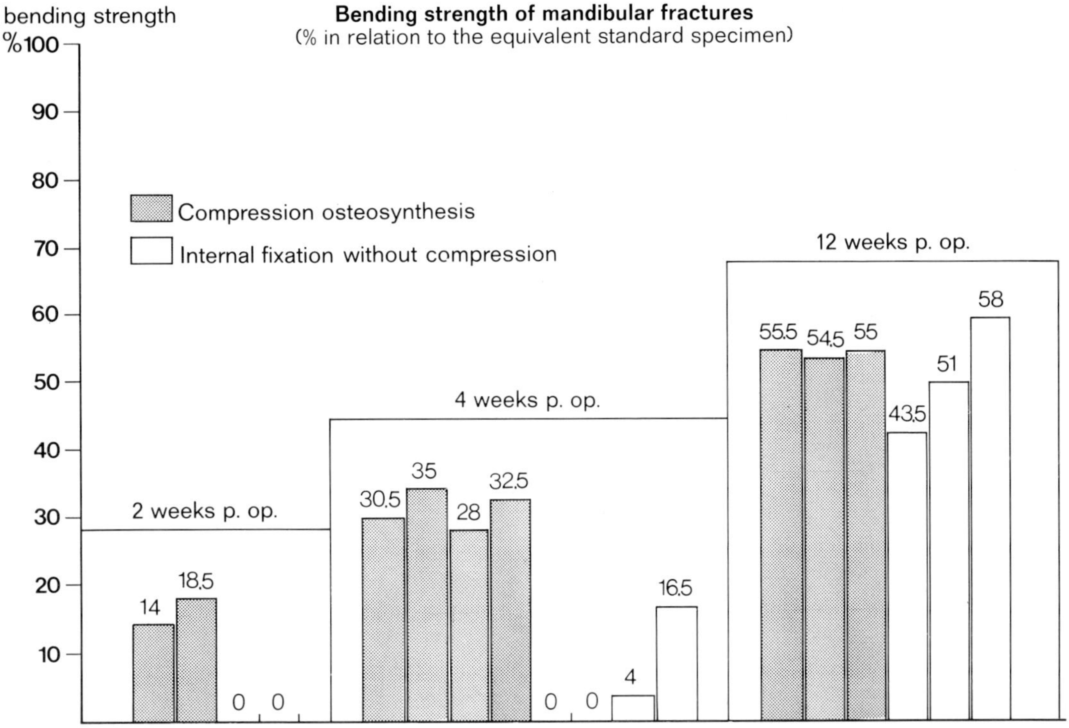

Fig. 8.5.2-10 Bending strength of fracture area correlated with the data of equivalent standard specimen of bone (100 %) 2, 4, and 12 weeks postoperatively. Fractures treated by compression screw plates (grey columns) show physical properties superior to control fragments which were reduced by simple plating without axial pressure (white columns). This demonstrates clearly the advantages of the axial compression principle in the internal fixation of fractures, as related to early weight bearing.

5.2.3.3 Resistance to Bending in Healing Bone after Compression Osteosynthesis

Rapid healing of fractures without complications is the essential criterion for the success of every treatment of a fracture. The time at which a bone becomes capable of stress is of practical clinical significance, i.e., the mechanical properties of the bone are of the greatest interest. Radiographs do not give reliable information about the mechanical stability of the healing bone (*Häbler* and *Reiss*, 1936; *Urist* and *Johnson*, 1943; *Segmüller* and *Allgöwer*, 1965; *Luhr* and *Maerker*, 1974). Therefore, a method was developed with which it is possible to measure the stability properties of experimental fractures in different stages of healing (*Luhr*, 1969, 1972). In 18 experimental mandibular fractures in dogs, such measurements on resistance to bending were carried out 2, 4, and 12 weeks after surgery in each case. Nine fractures were stabilized by compression osteosynthesis with the CSP; 9 other fractures were stabilized with the same type of plate, but without pressure on the fracture ends. The results of the measurements are shown in Figure 8.5.2-10. It is apparent that, in the first 4 weeks—and this is undoubtedly the most important phase of fracture healing—bone healing takes place more rapidly under application of axial pressure than in osteosyntheses without pressure. Thus, the investigations definitively show the advantages of compression plates compared to the simple rigid bone plates in common use previously.

5.2.3.4 Histologic Findings after Compression Osteosynthesis

Danis (1956) as well as *Müller* et al. (1963) observed that under the conditions of a stable osteosynthesis by means of axial compression of the fracture ends, the mode of healing was characterized in radiographs by the absence of a distinct endosteal and periosteal fracture callus. Analogous to wound healing, this mode of healing was designated as so-called "primary fracture healing." *Schenk* and *Willenegger* (1963, 1964, 1965) were the first to describe the histologic equivalent of such primary bone healing, but under the special experimental conditions of very delicate saw-cut **osteotomies** with stable osteosynthesis immediately following, on tubular bones of sheep and dogs. Under these special experimental conditions of what was in part an optimal adaptation of the fragments even microscopically, the authors observed in addition to the so-called gap healing on the side lying opposite the compression plate—a primary penetration of the osteotomy line by an ossification process which originated predominantly or exclusively in the cells and vessels within the Haversian canals. After such experimental osteotomies, in the course of the third week, the gradual replacement of the necrotic bone portions began, originating in the portions of the Haversian canals which had remained vital. Osteoblasts began to enlarge the canal and pushed forward new resorption channels in the direction toward the osteotomy. Six weeks after the operation, the osteotomy line was traversed by numerous osteons regenerating in the longitudinal direction of the bone (*Schenk* and *Willenegger* 1963, 1964, 1965).

In our opinion, however, osteotomies should be used with reservations as experimental models for studies on healing of fractures. This view was confirmed by our own studies (*Luhr* 1969a, 1969b, 1972) as well as those of *Luhr* et al. (1975) on **experimental fractures.** In such fracture models, we did not observe a direct transverse bone formation through the fracture gap in the compact bone during the early stage of fracture healing. We refer to the first 4 weeks as the early stage of fracture healing , for after this time, as a rule, a mandibular fracture is clinically firmly consolidated. On such clinically comparable experimental fractures, we were able, under the conditions of compression osteosynthesis, to observe only so-called **gap healing,** which we consider to be the critical mode of "primary healing of fractures." In the smallest spaces which remain even after what appears clinically to be an optimally successful reduction in many portions of the fracture site (Fig. 8.5.2-11), primary lamellar bone formation occurs in the environment of vessels which have erupted from the periosteal side and from the marrow space; this bone joins the devitalized fracture ends (Fig. 8.5.2-12). Primary fracture healing in the narrow gap segments between the "supporting pillars of the fracture vault" (Fig. 8.5.2-13) is thus directly dependent on vessels coming from the inner (marrow space) and outer (periosteal-soft tissue coat) surroundings of the fracture line. Bone regeneration from the marrow space is the more important, according to our observations of the mandible. We have never been able to observe direct transverse bone formation through the gap by regenerating material from the compact bone, as described by *Schenk* and *Willenegger* (1963, 1964, 1965) after osteotomies, after experimental fractures during the most important phase of fracture healing, i.e., the first 4 weeks.

Our histologic findings are also of interest, because they provide information about the repeatedly discussed effect of mechanical forces on bone formation. Whereas *Danis* (1949), *Eggers* et al. (1949), *Greifensteiner* (1953), and *Petrokov* (1962) consider pressure forces to be a specific irritant which directly stimulates bone formation, according to other studies by *Friedenberg* and *French* (1952), *Reynolds* and *Key* (1954), *Willenegger* et al. (1962), as well as *Müller* et al. (1963), such a possible specific action of pressure forces has not yet been explained.

By use of lamination in experimental mandibular fractures which had been treated with compression osteosynthesis, we have designed a model of a fracture site, which is represented schematically in Figure 8.5.2-14. Even with minimal displacement of the fracture ends, which cannot be perceived by the surgeon with the naked eye—i.e., even with clinically optimal

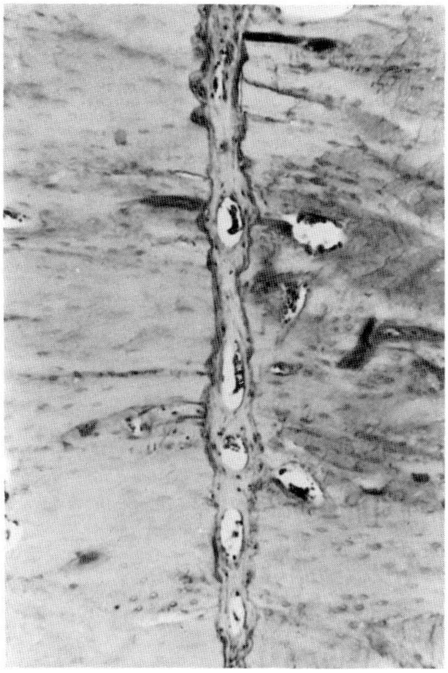

Fig. 8.5.2-11 Detail of a fracture region with a relatively narrow fracture gap (running vertically), which is filled with primary lamellar bone. Condition 4 weeks after compression osteosynthesis for an experimental mandibular fracture in the dog (Hematoxylin-eosin stain, 74 x).

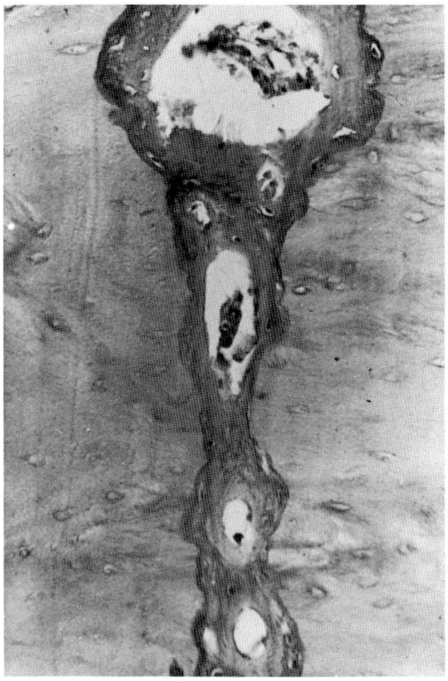

Fig. 8.5.2-12 In the vicinity of blood vessels (shown here in transverse section), direct formation of lamellar bone occurs; this bone joins together the devitalized fragment ends (left and right in the figure). Condition 4 weeks after compression osteosynthesis (PAS stain, 150 x).

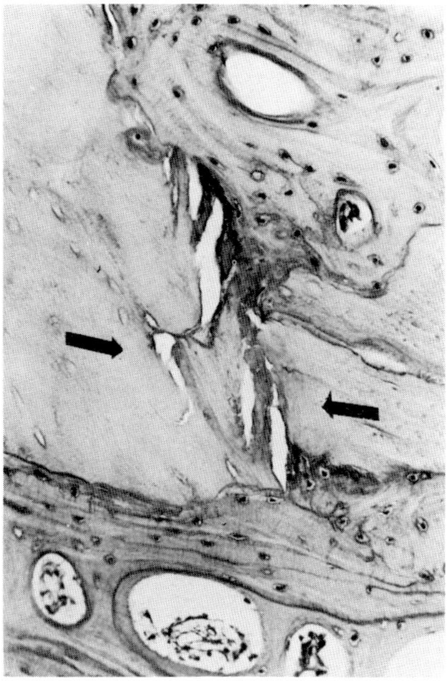

Fig. 8.5.2-13 So-called "supporting posts of the fracture vault" after compression osteosynthesis of a mandibular fracture in a dog. 12 weeks postoperatively. At the center of the picture, arrows mark the contact site of two devitalized bone edges with the typical empty bone cavities. New bone has formed only at the lateral surfaces of the supporting posts (top and bottom in the picture; Hematoxylin-eosin, 160 x).

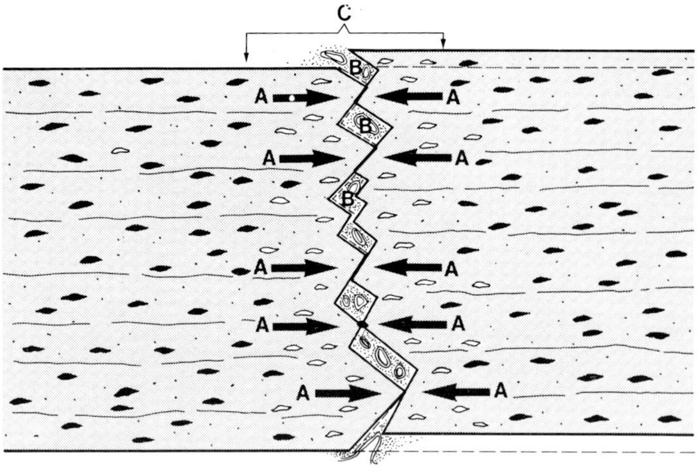

Fig. 8.5.2-14 Schematic diagram of a fracture site at the microscopic level under compression osteosynthesis. Even a minimal displacement of the fragments during reduction—hardly visible to the surgeon's naked eye—leads to microscopically distinct displacement in the region of the fracture site. Only a small number of bone protuberances (A-A) is making contact. We have called these contact areas "pressure posts of the fracture vault" (*Luhr* 1969, 1972), since only these regions support any axial pressure forces. Regeneration of bone, however, always proceeds only in the hollow segments—that is, in the vault spaces—in zones (B) which are completely neutral mechanically. Here, in the vicinity of blood vessels which have spread from the endosteal cavity and the periosteal space, primary lamellar bone is formed.
C = devitalized marginal zone (with empty bone cavities), which occurs with every fracture, independent of the type of therapy.

anatomic reduction—this ideal meshing is no longer assured in the microscopic range. Series of sections show that in fractures, with their multiple jagged fracture lines, only a small number of contact planes in present. It is only at these contact planes, which we have described as "pressure posts of the fracture vault, that pressure forces exert their effect. But as it has been known from the time of the investigations by *Bonome* (1885) that extensive segments of the fracture ends are devitalized by interruption of the blood circulation, the pressure forces are borne exclusively by the nonvital bone portions. On such contact sites of devitalized bone prominences (the so-called supporting posts of the microscopic fracture vaults), we have never been able to observe new bone formation during the first 4 weeks of fracture healing. Bone healing, however—including primary deposition of lamellar bone—always took place on the lateral surfaces of the supporting posts and in the upper segments of the fracture vault in zones of mechanical rest. This appears to have provided proof that pressure forces have no specific effect on osteogenesis during fracture healing. Our own experiments also confirm completely, for the special conditions of surgical treatment of fractures, the theories of *Pauwels* (1940, 1960, 1965), who long ago rejected the specific osteogenic effect of pressure forces. The acceleration of fracture healing under axial compression (Fig. 8.5.2-10) is based on an indirect effect, i.e., on optimal adaptation and maximal stability (mechanical rest) in the fracture region.

5.2.4 Clinical Aspects of Compression Osteosynthesis

Since we have accumulated more than 10 years of clinical experience with the compression plate system (*Luhr*, 1968), we will describe the applications, the surgical technique, as well as the results obtained with this method, which has now been adopted as a routine procedure.

5.2.4.1 Indications for Compression Osteosynthesis

With regard to indications for compression osteosynthesis, we long ago required differential indications for its use (*Luhr*, 1969a and b, 1972a and b). For fractures of the completely dentulous mandible, we still prefer (for special exceptions, see table of indications) conservative treatment with splints applied to the teeth. We use the wire-acrylic arch bar described by *Schuchardt* (1956), which can be applied by hand, i.e., independent of the laboratory, does not damage the periodontium, provides sufficient stability, and, in addition, can be corrected easily even after being inserted in the mouth. The conservative treatment of mandibular fractures is rapid, low in risk, and, in many instances, can be done on an outpatient basis. Besides, unlike almost any other procedure, it permits accurate adjustment of the occlusion. The disadvantage of dental splints consists of the rigid intermaxillary immobilization, for at least 4 weeks, which we always carry out and which we regard as necessary for biomechanical reasons.

In edentulous or insufficiently dentulous jaws and, under special circumstances, also in fully dentulous jaws (see table of indications), however, we consider compression osteosynthesis to be the method of choice today. It has almost completely replaced the formerly customary wire sutures and simple plate osteosynthesis. These were found to be insufficiently stable for the mandible when it is under bending stress (*Schwenzer*, 1967; *Luhr*, 1969a and b, 1972a and b; *Becker* et al., 1976). The second surgical procedure for removal of the osteosynthesis plates, regarded by some authors as a disadvantage (*Schüle*, 1976), can be eliminated if the highly corrosion-resistant Vitallium alloy is used, as it can remain in the organism indefinitely (*Venable* and *Stuck*, 1947). In addition, the danger of infection, said to be greater in compression osteosynthesis than in conservative treatment of fractures (*Schüle*, 1976), is not applicable, as *Höltje* et al. (1975), *Claudi* and *Spiessl* (1975), as well as *Luhr* et al. (1975) were able to show, in a review of a series of patients treated conservatively and surgically, about equal rates of infection for both treatment methods (Table 8.5.2.-I). The extraoral approach regarded by some authors as a disadvantage in compression osteosynthesis can be avoided in many instances by use of an intraoral procedure (*Schroll*, 1973; *Schilli* and *Härle*, 1976).

In basic agreement with many other authors, such as *Schilli* 1975, *Lentrodt* and *Höltje* 1975, *Schmitz* et al. 1975, *Becker* et al. 1976, *Schüle* 1976, *Freitag* and *Manderscheid* 1976, we consider compression osteosynthesis of the mandible to be indicated in the following conditions (*Luhr* 1969a and b, 1972a and b):

1. Fractures of edentulous or insufficiently dentulous mandibles. We treat fractures of a mandible with sufficient dentition by surgery also if the patient's maxilla is edentulous and thus intermaxillary fixation is difficult.
2. In the fully dentulous mandible in the following special instances:
   a) Displaced fractures outside the dental arch (fractures of the angle of the mandible, which cannot be reduced by conservative measures).
   b) Fractures of the body of the mandible combined with fractures of the mandibular joint, which require early functional therapy.
   c) Comminuted mandibular fractures.
   d) Mandibular fractures in patients with multiple trauma.
   e) Special indications: diseases involving seizures; travel by sea or air.
   f) Delayed healing of bone fractures or pseudoarthrosis.
   g) Fixation of bone grafts in continuity defects.

By using the scheme of indications given above, we now treat about 35% of all mandibular fractures by compression osteosynthesis. Fractures to which the above indications do not apply, however, are still treated conservatively by splints applied to the teeth . A wider range of indications for surgical treatment of essentially all mandibular fractures is quite possible technically (*Spiessl* and *Schroll*, 1972; *Spiessl*, 1975; *Prein* et al., 1976). But it appears to us, especially in view of the difficulties of establishing the occlusion, to be too problematic and too costly to be used routinely.

Table 8.5.2-I: **Inflammatory complications after surgical or conservative treatment of 2242 mandibular fractures**

Treatment	**Complications** Infiltration, cellulitis	Abscess	Osteo-myelitis	Late inflammatory complications	Total	%
Conservative treatment 1614 cases	19	30	11	0	60	3.8
Interosseous wiring 170 cases	2	5	4	1	12	7.1
Pin fixation 5 cases		1				
Compression plate osteosynthesis 453 cases	0	7	2	7	16	3.5

After compression osteosynthesis, the number of inflammatory complications, at 3.5 %, is not greater than after conservative treatment (3.8 %) with dental splints. After surgical treatment with interosseous wiring, however, the frequency of complications is considerably higher (7.1 %). We explain this by the inadequate stability of the wire osteosynthesis, which, despite added immobilization of the mandible with prosthetic splints and intra-extraoral devices (head cap chin shield, extraoral bars), cannot guarantee the mechanical rest in the fracture region that is necessary for undisturbed healing of the bone.

5.2.4.2 Types of Plates and Instruments for the Mandibular Compression Screw Plate System

All plates and screws of the system consist of the highly corrosion-resistant Vitallium alloy and are manufactured as precision implants with strict quality control. For various types of fractures and anatomic regions of the mandible, different types of plates are available. Plates with a basal groove (Figs. 8.5.2-15 A to G) require an extraoral approach. Because of the shape of their profile, they are distinguished by extremely great stability. Specifically for the intraoral approach, straight plates without a basal groove are appropriate (Figs. 8.5.2-16 A to D). They can be adapted easily to the bone surface even if there are considerable anatomic variants. For this purpose, bending pliers are available, the jaws of which are Vitallium-plated. The compression screws used are self-threading screws 3.6 mm in diameter and 10, 13, 16, or 19 mm long (recommended drill: 3.0 mm diameter).

The smaller retention screws have a diameter of 2.6 mm and are also 10, 13, 16, or 19 mm long (recommended drill: 2.4 mm diameter). Also needed are a measuring device for measurement of the screw length needed in each case, screwdriver with interchangeable handle, surgical drills, protective casings for transbuccal work in the intraoral approach, and two bone forceps for reduction of the fragments. All implants and instruments are stored within clear view in a sterilizable box* (Fig. 8.5.2-17).

5.2.4.3 Surgical Technique

Extraoral Approach

The fracture site is visualized as described above (5.1.3.1). The fracture ends are repositioned with two sharp bone forceps, and the compression screw plate is adapted. With appropriate pliers, the plate can be bent and adapted

* Manufacturer Howmedica International, Inc. 78.

Figs. 8.5.2-15 A to G Compression screw plates with basal rim.

Fig. 8.5.2-15 A CSP 28 mm long, for simple vertical fractures in the horizontal ramus.

Fig. 8.5.2-15 B CSP 38 mm, for oblique fractures in the horizontal ramus. A larger space between the eccentric plate holes is recommended for oblique fractures which require the longer, 38 mm type of plate.

Fig. 8.5.2-15 C CSP 48 mm, for extreme oblique sagittal fractures as well as comminuted fractures. Usually a bone fragment will be embraced by means of the grooved plate and compressed between the outer fracture ends. Additional fixation may be attained by means of a small screw inserted into one of the 7 central holes.

Fig. 8.5.2-15 D CSP 28 mm, curved, for fractures of the mandibular angle. The plate can be adapted easily to the anatomical variations of that region by bending the 2 lingual clamps.

Fig. 8.5.2-15 E CSP 48 mm, curved, for oblique and comminuted fractures of the mandibular angle.

Fig. 8.5.2-15 F CSP 38 mm, curved, for fractures of the lateral and central regions of the mandible.

Fig. 8.5.2-15 G CSP 48 mm, curved, for oblique or comminuted fractures of the lateral and central regions of the chin.

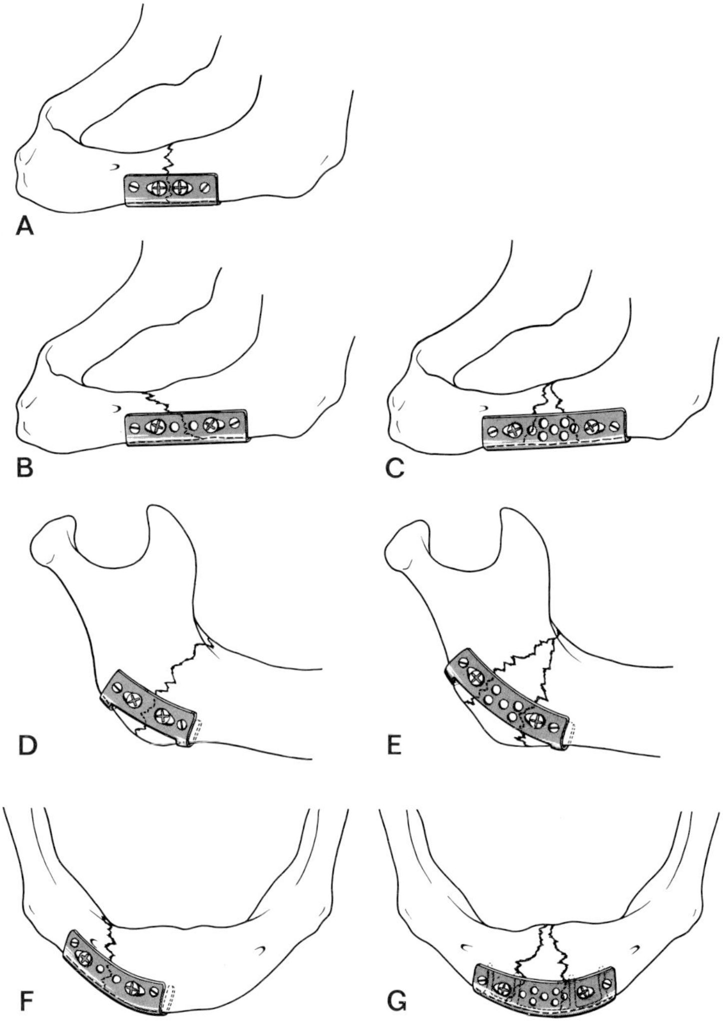

satisfactorily to the bone. For various anatomic regions, different plates with basal grooves are available. The lingual brackets should be clamped around the mandible. The periosteum and soft tissues on the interior side of the mandible are not detached. It is not necessary for the groove-shaped plate to adhere completely congruently to the bone, especially in the basal portion. Only the flat portion of the plate with the screw holes should correspond to the shape of the bone surface. After fitting of the plate, the position of the drill holes within the small diameter of the eccentric splint holes is punched (marking of the position of the drill holes either with a special instrument or with a small dental drill). After the position of the drill holes has been established, the mandibular bone is completely perforated by the drill with constant cooling by a physiologic salt solution. In addition to cooling, a low rotational velocity

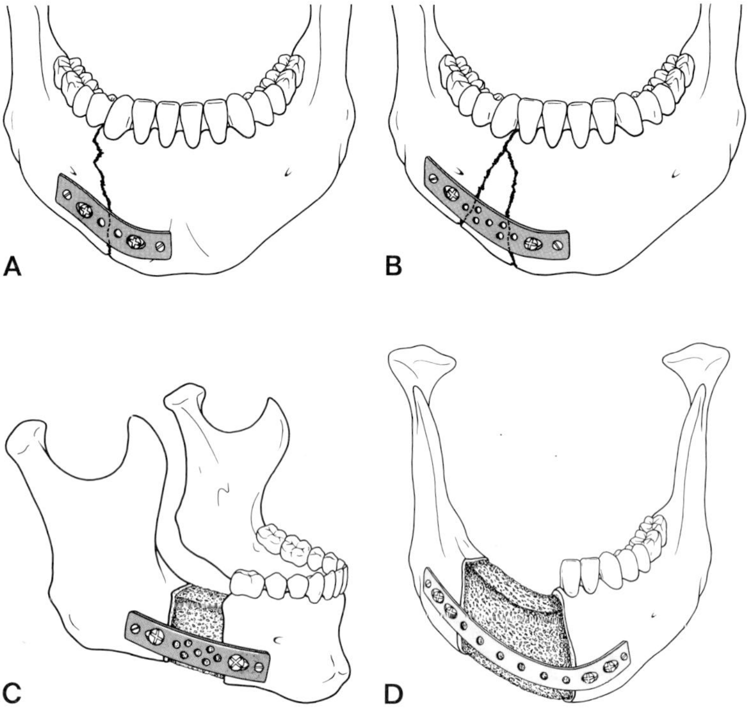

Figs. 8.5.2-16 A to D Compression screw plates without basal rim, especially for the intraoral approach.

Fig. 8.5.2.16 A 38 mm straight plate, for all fractures of the body of the mandible when adaptation of a plate with rim is difficult to achieve. Recommended for the intraoral approach.

Figs. 8.5.2-16 B and C 48 mm straight plate, for extreme oblique fractures as well as comminuted fractures and fixation of bone grafts by axial compression.

Fig. 8.5.2-16 D 130 mm straight plate, for reconstruction of larger mandibular defects with or without simultaneous bone grafting.

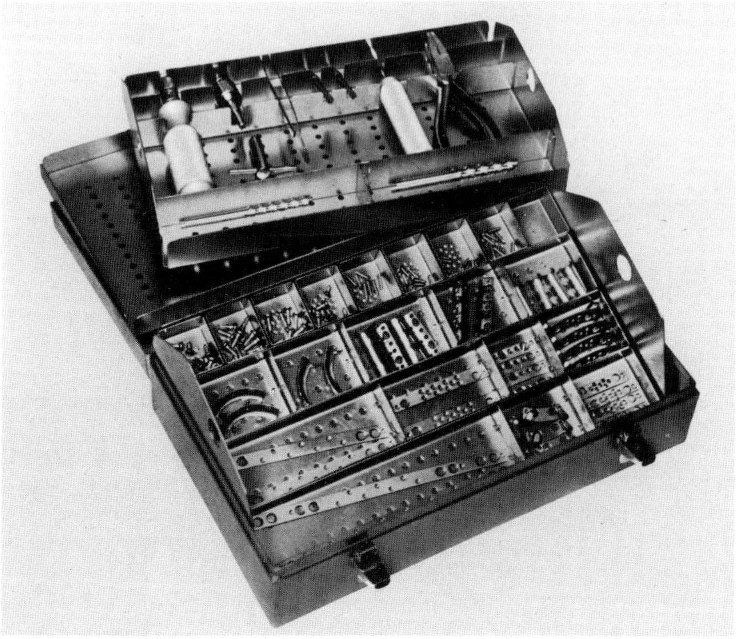

Fig. 8.5.2-17 Plates, screws, and instruments are stored in clear view in a sterilizable box with several removable inserts.

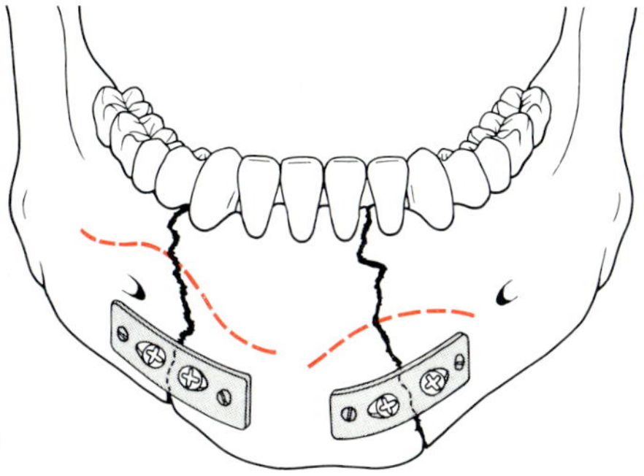

Fig. 8.5.2-18 For fractures in the premolar region, an incision curving convex upward must be used so that the mental nerve is protected. In the incisor region, however, the mucosal incision should lie deep in the vestibule.

(100 to 200 rpm) is of great importance if heat necrosis is to be avoided. With today's drills operated electrically or by compressed air, we always use a reduction drive. A special screwdriver made of Vitallium is used for insertion of the so-called compression screws (CS; see Fig. 8.5.2-1 D) of appropriate length. The screws should always emerge on the lingual side. In the last phase of screw insertion—after the screws have fully taken hold of the inner cortical bone layer—the cone-shaped screw heads are drawn into the largest diameter of the eccentric plate holes, carry along the fracture stumps, and press them together under great pressure (see Fig. 8.5.2-2). Here axial forces of 30 to 40 kp become effective. In addition, the plate is immobilized by two small retaining screws (see Fig. 8.5.2-1 E). Next, the soft-tissue flap of the periosteum is folded back and attached with resorbable suture material. A vacuum drain is applied in the immediate vicinity, above the periosteal-soft tissue suture. Then the wound is closed in layers. We use atraumatic monofilament thread, 6 x 0 or 8 x 0, for the skin sutures.

Intraoral Approach

Based on experience with our own patients, extraoral scars usually can be made quite inconspicuous if the proper technique is used. However, because younger female patients may consider them undesirable, an intraoral approach should be chosen in most instances (*Schroll*, 1974; *Schilli* and *Härle*, 1976). In frontal fractures a straight, 4 cm incision is made deep in the vestibule, which severs the mucosa and submucosa; for fractures in the premolar region, the incision is arched and convex upward (Fig. 8.5.2-18). Only after separation of these layers does the scalpel advance almost horizontally and perpendicularly to the mandibular bone and sever the muscles and the periosteum. This shape of the incision seems to us to be important, since it permits safe closure of the wound through a relatively thick layer of mucosa and muscle (Fig. 8.5.2-19). After separation of the periosteum, in the fracture region the periosteal muscle-mucosa flap located in the direction of the alveolar process is mobilized somewhat in the cranial direction, and the muscles are pushed away caudally from the mandibular border. Next, two Langenbeck or, preferably, prognathism hooks are inserted, so that the buccal soft tissues are retracted sufficiently. Corresponding to the shape of the fracture, a plate without basal rim is selected—for transverse fractures, we choose a plate 38 mm long, and for very oblique fracture lines, a 48 mm CSP—and it is shaped to the bone surface by bending with special pliers. With a special clamp, the plate is now applied to the bone surface in the fracture region. The anticipated drill holes are marked in the small diameter of the eccentric holes of the plate and placed with the appropriate surgical drill. Next, pressure screws

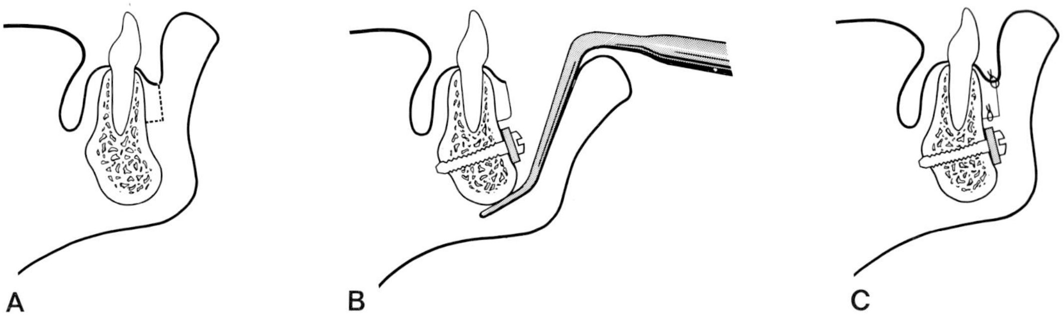

Figs. 8.5.2-19 A to C Intraoral appoach for application of the compression screw plate in the mandibular incisor region.

Fig. 8.5.2-19 A Vertical incision deep in the vestibule, with severing of mucosa and submucosa. The incision is then continued at right angles, with severing of muscles and periosteum.

Fig. 8.5.2-19 B The periosteal muscle layer is pushed aside in the caudal direction from the mandibular border and a retractor is inserted which retracts the outer soft tissues. The surgical field is now clearly visible, and the CSP can be applied without difficulty.

Fig. 8.5.2-19 C The muscles in the region of the horizontal incision are joined with catgut sutures. The mucosal margins are densely sutured with 3 x 0 synthetic sutures. The thick soft-tissue covering above the plate can help prevent dehiscence of sutures.

of appropriate length are inserted, until the fracture ends are adapted to each other under axial compression. For the proper amount of force, it is advisable, during screwing in of the pressure screws in the last phase, to grasp the screw driver only with the thumb, index finger, and middle finger and not with the whole hand, for if too strong a force is exerted, the screw threads may be torn from the bone. The application of the smaller retention screws follows next; these are centered and inserted in the small outer holes of the plate. (See also technique for extraoral approach.) We regard the insertion of vacuum drainage—here with a very thin perforated tube—as extremely important with the intraoral approach, too.

If the fracture is located more distally, e.g., in the premolar region, application of the drills and insertion of the screws can become difficult, even if the corner of the mouth is pulled far to the side. In this situation, we prefer a transbuccal approach through a small puncture incision, 3 to 4 mm in length, in the skin (Figs. 8.5.2-20 B and C), about in the middle of the planned position of the plate. Through the puncture incision, a guiding sheath is advanced with a mandrel from the extraoral site up to the intraoral incision. Then the mandrel is removed, and the proper drill is inserted through the guiding sheath (Fig. 8.5.2-20 D). Now, by displacement of the sheath mesially or distally, drill holes can be placed transbuccally in the appropriate places. The necessary screws are now inserted with a special screw holder from the intraoral incision and are held in place. The screw driver is advanced through the already existing transbuccal soft-tissue canal up to the intraoral incision, so that each screw now can be placed easily in the axial direction with the screw driver (Figs. 8.5.2-20 E and F). With this transbuccal procedure, we have not yet observed any problems with regard to any facial nerve damage, or any troublesome car formation.

If the fracture is located in the premolar region, attention must be paid to the mental nerve when the incision is made. In the premolar region, we recommended an arched incision which is convex upward (see Fig. 8.5.2-18); after

Figs. 8.5.2-20 A to F Intraoral approach for compression osteosynthesis of an oblique fracture in the region of the mental foramen.

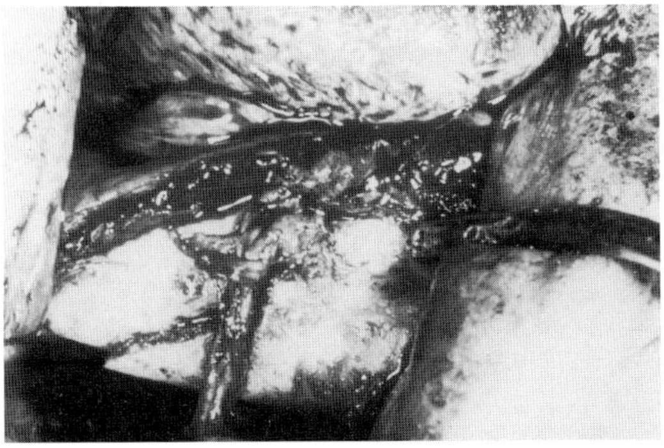

Fig. 8.5.2-20 A By means of an arched, convex-upward mucosal-periosteal incision, the fracture region was visualized and the mental nerve prepared.

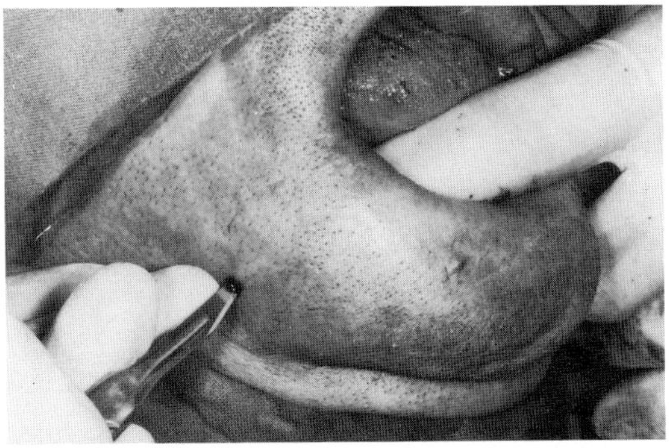

Fig. 8.5.2-20 B Puncture incision in the skin lying opposite the fracture region. For the transbuccal application of the 4 screws, one incision is sufficient.

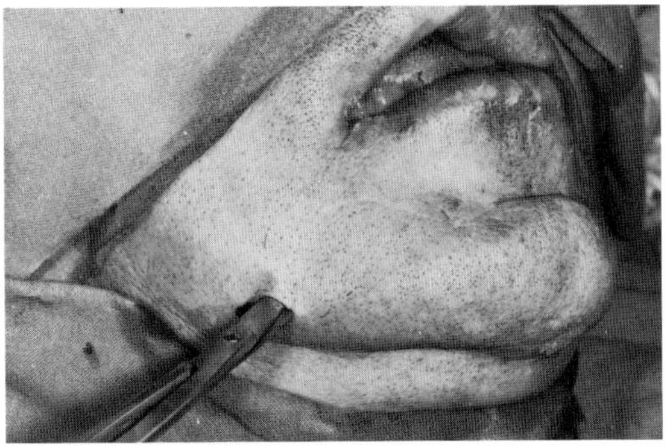

Fig. 8.5.2-20 C By spreading of the preparative scissors, the connection with the intraoral incision is established.

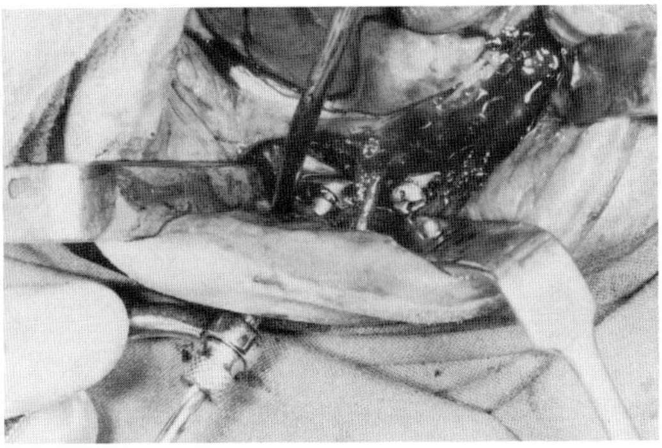

Fig. 8.5.2-20 D When the wound canal has been prepared, a protective sheath is introduced which shields the soft tissues from the surgical drill.

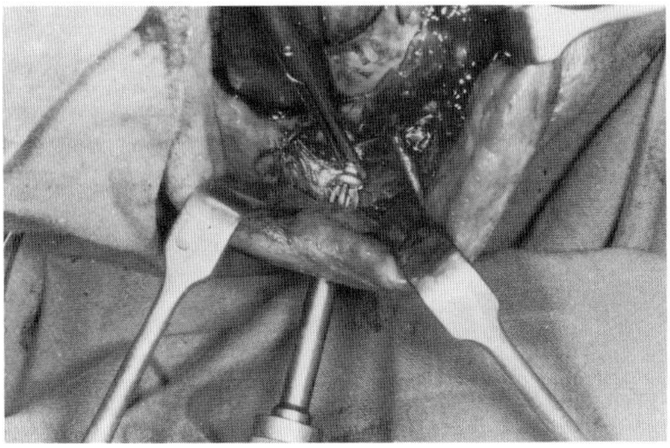

Fig. 8.5.2-20 E After placement of the drill holes, each corresponding screw is grasped with a forceps and inserted intraorally. The screw driver is introduced through the transbuccal puncture incision, and the screw is applied.

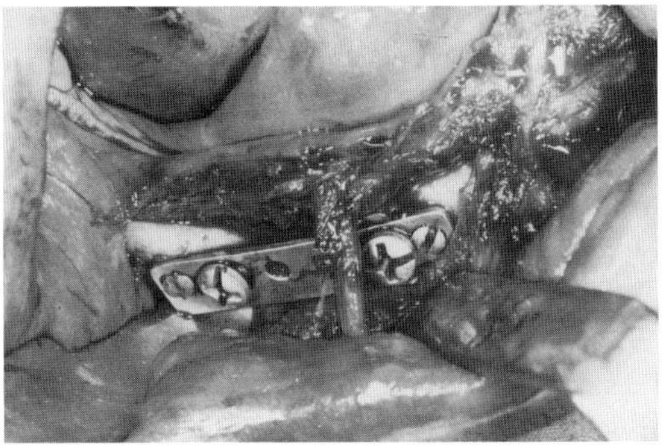

Fig. 8.5.2-20 F Position of the CSP after all 4 screws have been applied. Now the mucosal-periosteal wound is carefully sutured. This concludes the technically relatively simple procedure. The sutures are removed on about the 8th postoperative day. The CSP does not need to be removed.

severing of the mucosa and submucosa by sharp-blunt dissection, the mental nerve is visualized best by spreading the scissors perpendicular to the bone surface. The nerve must be mobilized sufficiently by this procedure at its entrance into the buccal musculature. After the muscles and the periosteum have been moved away from the bone surface, the procedure continues as described above. If the nerve is retracted with a small nerve hook, the treatment of fractures in this region also involves no difficult technical problems (Fig. 8.5.2-20). It is obvious that the plate is applied below the mental foramen.

The intraoral approach is possible also with fractures farther distal from the premolar region, up to the angle of the mandible, by means of a combined intraoral-transbuccal procedure. We prefer the intraoral approach for the management of fractures of the molar region and of the angle of the mandible too even though this procedure is more difficult technically in the distal portion. However, with the help of special instruments, i. e., drill bits and drill sleeves extra long, it is possible to overcome this interference.

After stabilization of the fracture ends by the CS plate and insertion of thin plastic tubing, the periosteal-muscle tube is adapted above the plate by 2 or 3 single sutures with resorbable suture material, and then the intraoral wound is closed with deep single sutures. For an osteosynthesis that was performed intraorally, it is advisable to provide nourishment via a stomach tube during the first 5 to 6 days, so that impregnation of the wound area with food remnants is avoided.

The compression osteosynthesis should always be carried out with administration of antibiotics—preferably beginning one day before surgery—over 5 to 6 days.

5.2.4.4 Clinical Results and Case Histories

Since 1967, more than 500 fractures have been treated successfully with the mandibular compression screw system at the Nordwestdeutsche Kieferklinik in Hamburg. Severe complications in the form of osteomyelitis occurred extremely rarely, and the overall rate of infection was no greater than for strictly conservative treatment of fractures (see also Table 8.5.2-I). It seems especially remarkable that more than 30 different operators participated in the treatment of the total number of patients. Long-term results after compression osteosynthesis have been reported for large groups of patients by *Schmitz* et al. (1975) as well as *Freitag* and *Manderscheid* (1976) among others.

In accordance with the scheme of indications for compression osteosynthesis, some typical examples below will show the clinical application of this procedure. One of the important areas of application is that of fractures of the edentulous or partially dentulous mandible.

Fig. 8.5.2-21 A shows an oblique fracture anterior to the left angle of the mandible, with cranial displacement of the central fragment, in a 42-year-old female patient. Under intubation anesthesia, the fracture was exposed by means of a submandibular incision; it was reduced and stabilized with a 38 mm CSP under axial compression (Fig. 8.5.2-21 B). The patient was discharged from the hospital on the seventh postoperative day. Already one week later, her dentures, with a lining, were reinserted, and the patient was permitted to chew soft foods. Healing proceeded without complications, and the final condition of the delicate scar below the angle of the mandible was quite inconspicuous.

Figs. 8.5.2-22 A and B, photographs taken during surgery, show the position of a 38 mm CSP inserted with an extraoral approach.

Nowadays, we prefer the intraoral approach with the exception of compound mandibular fractures with an extraoral wound involving the fracture site.

Fig. 8.5.2-23 A shows a displaced transverse fracture in the lateral chin region, which was stabilized from an intraoral approach after reduction with a 38-mm straight CSP under axial compression (Fig. 8.5.2-23 B). The patient was discharged from the hospital 5 days after the procedure. Healing proceeded without complications. New dentures were inserted 2 weeks after discharge.

Multiple fractures of the edentulous or partly dentulous mandible can also be treated effectively with the CSP (Fig. 8.5.2-24). As in all other cases, it is not necessary, in multiple fracture patients, to provide additional immobilization of the mandible by prosthetic means; instead, free movement of the mandible and ingestion of a soft diet are possible immediately after the operation.

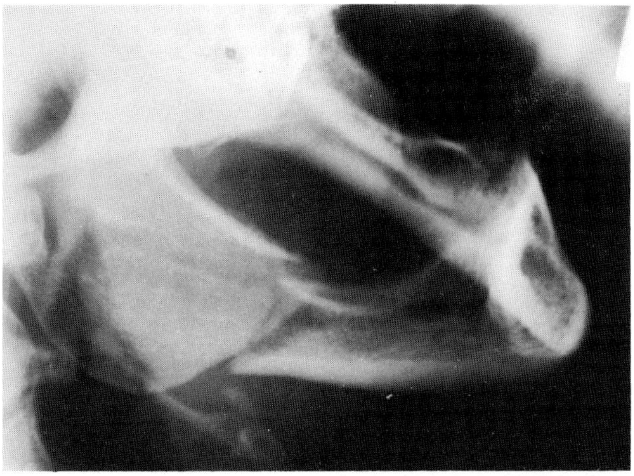

Fig. 8.5.2-21 A Displaced oblique fracture anterior to the left mandibular angle.

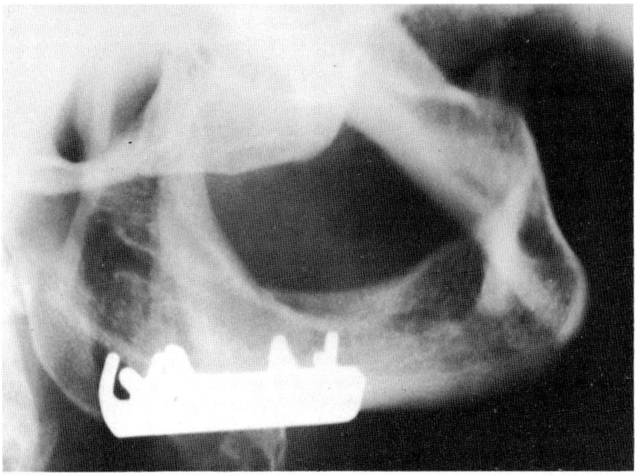

Fig. 8.5.2-21 B Postoperative follow-up radiograph after compression osteosynthesis with a 38 mm long CSP. Ideal reduction of fragments.

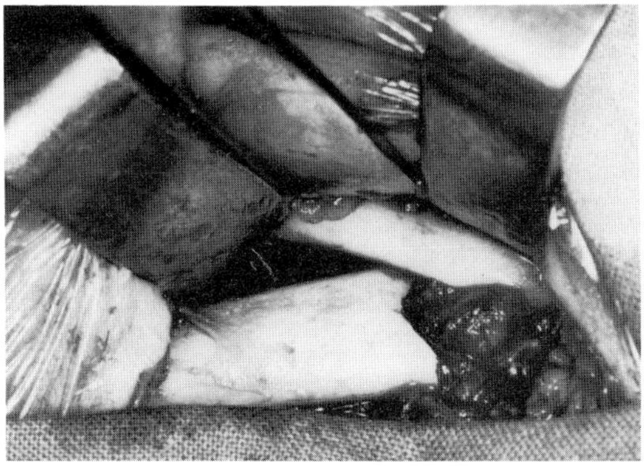

Fig. 8.5.2-22 A Displaced transverse fracture of the mandibular body, exposed by means of a submandibular incision.

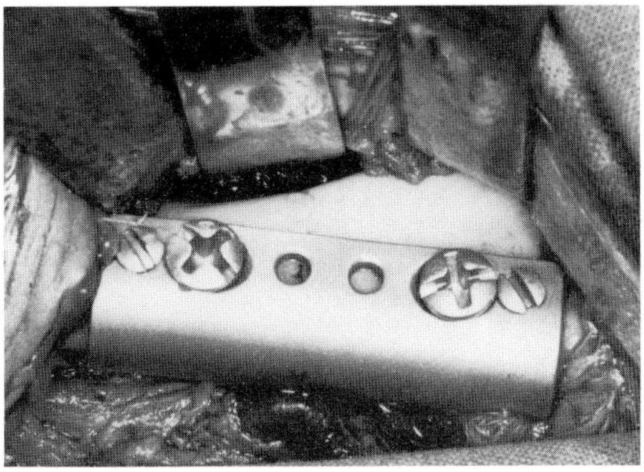

Fig. 8.5.2-22 B Anatomically exact reduction and stabilization with a 38 mm CSP.

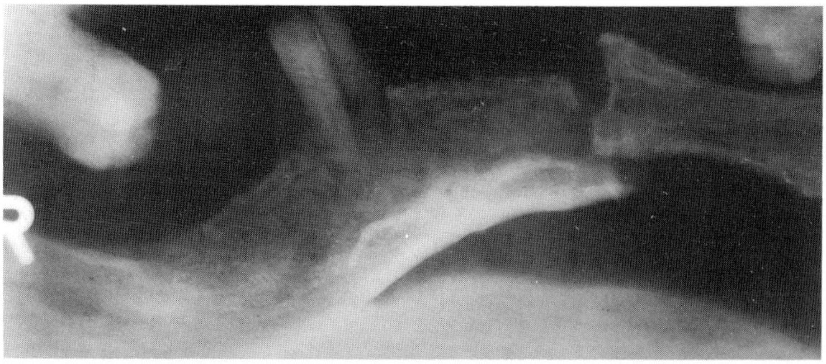

Fig. 8.5.2-23 A Displaced transverse fracture in the region of the left mental foramen.

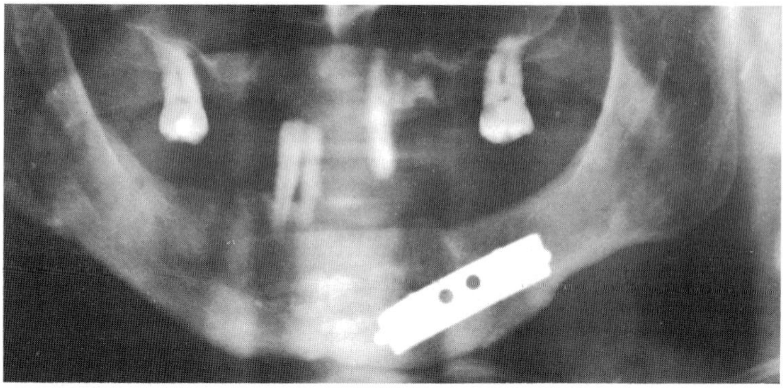

Fig. 8.5.2-23 B After application of a CSP (38 mm, without basal rim) with intraoral approach.

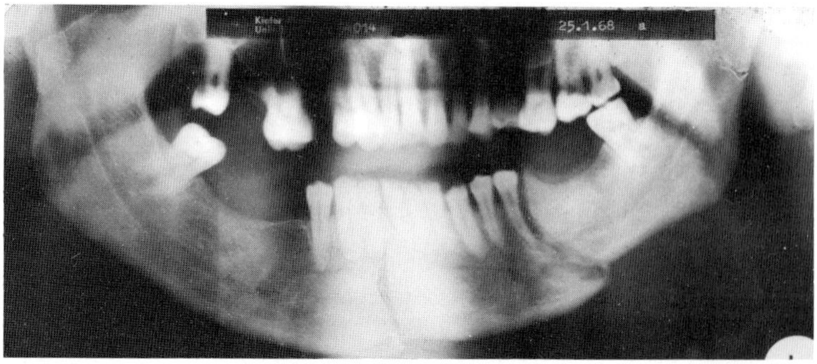

Fig. 8.5.2.-24 A Multiple mandibular fracture (chin region, body of the left mandible and bilateral fracture of the condyle) in a partly dentulous mandible.

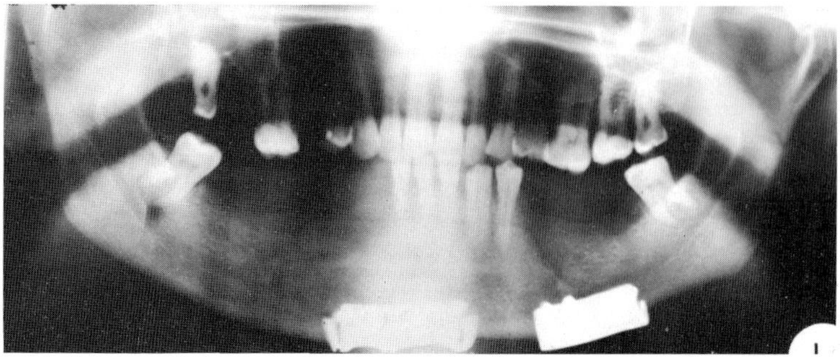

Fig. 8.5.2-24 B Condition after compression osteosynthesis with plates. No intermaxillary immobilization postoperatively.

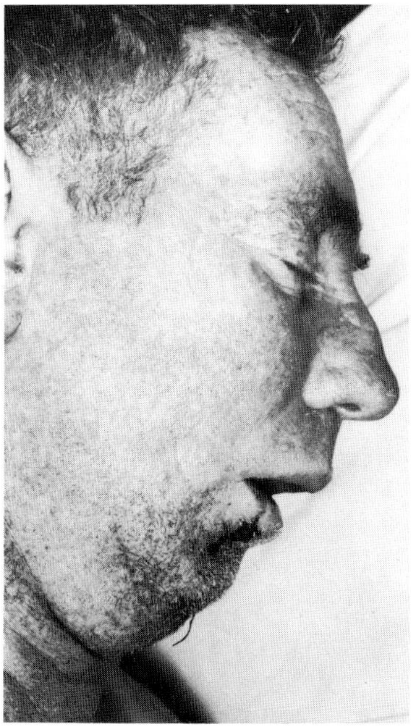

Fig. 8.5.2-24 C Before treatment, the patient has an anterior open bite and considerable posterior displacement of the mandible.

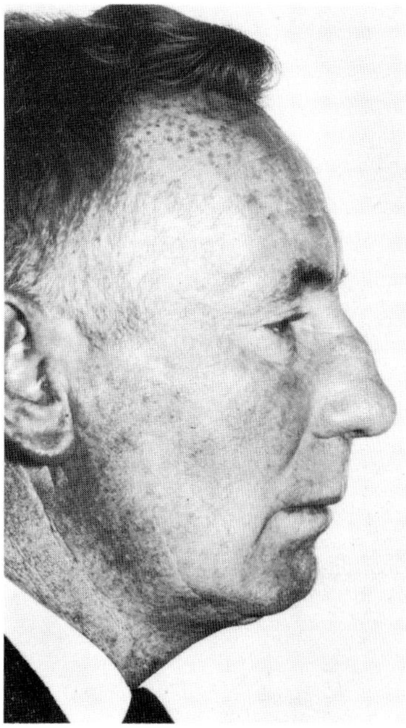

Fig. 8.5.2-24 D and E After conclusion of treatment and insertion of dentures, the facial profile and the occlusion are restored.

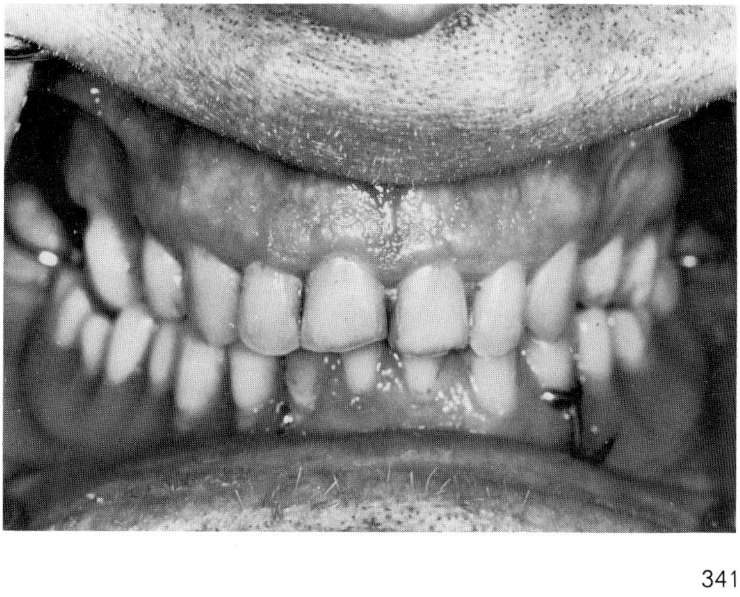

Fig. 8.5.2-24 E

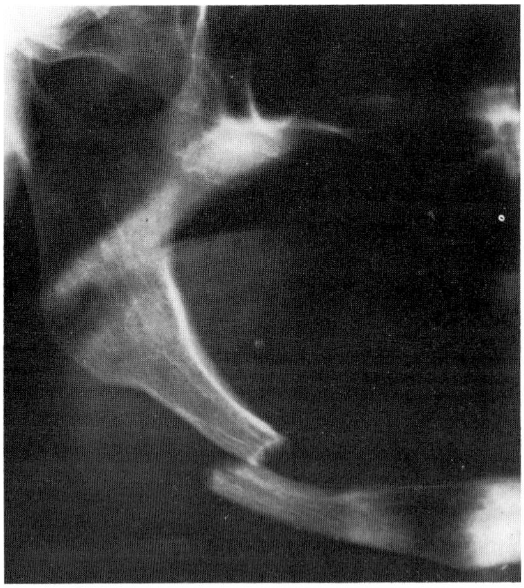

Fig. 8.5.2-25 A Displaced fracture of a markedly atrophic mandible.

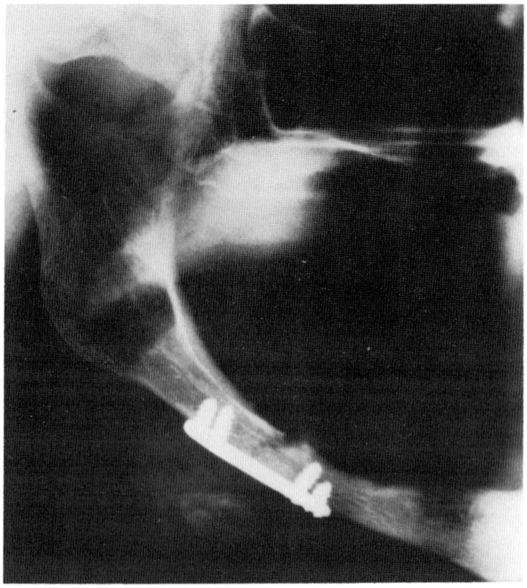

Fig. 8.5.2-25 B Compression osteosynthesis with mini-CSP which is screwed to the lower edge of the mandible in the region of the basal cortical bone.

Figs. 8.5.2-26 A and B Compression osteosynthesis of a displaced fracture of the mandibular angle, with complete dentition.

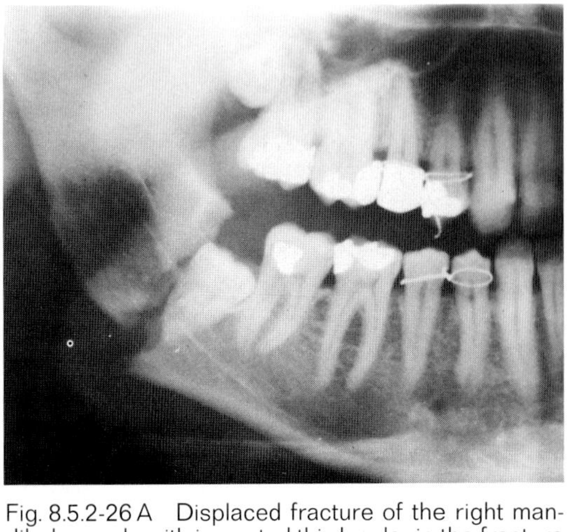

Fig. 8.5.2-26 A Displaced fracture of the right mandibular angle with impacted third molar in the fracture gap.

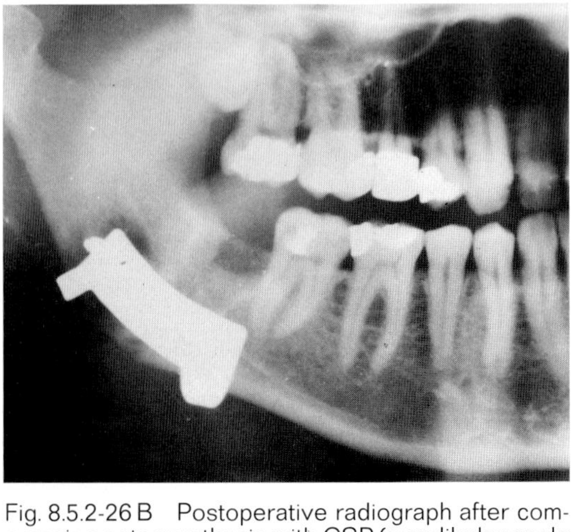

Fig. 8.5.2-26 B Postoperative radiograph after compression osteosynthesis with CSP (mandibular-angle type) and extraction of third molar. No intermaxillary immobilization was used postoperatively.

A severly atrophied mandible sometimes can make the application of the normal CS plate difficult. For such cases, extremely short screws and small plates are available which serve as mini-compression screw plates (Fig. 8.5.2-25), and which likewise provide axial compression of the fracture ends by means of eccentric holes in the plate.

Although, in principle, compression osteosynthesis is possible in each individual case, even for fractures in a mandible with complete dentition, we use this method only in special instances of this type. If subsequent occlusal disorders are to be avoided, however, the occlusion must be established during surgery by means of intermaxillary fixation.

One of the important indications for compression osteosynthesis under these circumstances is a displaced fracture in the region of the mandibular angle, which cannot be managed with dental splints alone.

Fig. 8.5.2-26 A shows such a displaced fracture of the angle of the mandible in a 26-year-old male patient, with a third molar impacted in the fracture line. Arch bars were applied prior to surgery. Under general anesthesia with nasal intubation, the impacted third molar was removed surgically from the fracture line with an intraoral approach; the occlusion was immobilized in the correct position with intermaxillary wire ligatures, and then, with a submandibular incision, the displaced fracture at the right angle of the mandible was exposed. After reduction of the central fragment which was displaced in the cranial direction, the fracture was stabilized with a CS plate at the mandibular angle and, after insertion of a Redon tube, the layers of the extraoral wound were closed. It is only after absolute stabilization of the fracture region that the intraoral wound is sutured tightly and carefully above the alveolus of the third molar. The arch bars can be removed postoperatively, so that the mandible can move freely (Fig. 8.5.2-26 B).

We see another important application of compression osteosynthesis for fractures in the completely dentulous mandible if a uni- or bilateral fracture of the temporomandibular joint is also present which requires early functional treatment. Those fractures are treated primarily with functional methods, i.e., they require early physical therapy, whereas fractures of the body of the mandible require absolute immobilization of the fragments. Such immobilization of the fracture ends in the body of the mandible is made possible in an ideal way with compression osteosynthesis, which is stable under exercise within wide limits and is stable under stress, so that even considerable traction and bending forces such as those which occur during treatment of fractures of the condyle are tolerated without interfering with healing of the fracture.

Fig. 8.5.2-27 A shows a dislocated, deep, oblique fracture of the right condylar neck, in which a fracture of the left mandibular angle was present in addition. The fracture of the mandibular angle was stabilized by means of a compression screw plate, so that after a few days, functional treatment of the TMJ fracture could begin by means of arch bars as well as a fulcrum (hypomochlion) on the involved side, with use of loose elastic bands. The follow-up radiograph taken 3 years later shows the straightening of the condylar process and the functional transformation to an almost inconspicuous condyle. One recognizes the compression plate in situ in the region of the left mandibular angle in Fig. 8.5.2-27 B.

Often—especially in dislocated fractures in the joint region—these do not heal in an anatomically ideal position. Nevertheless, early functional treatment has yielded good results, even for combined fractures which had been a problem, up to now, in most cases with regard to functioning of the joint and the absence of subjective complaints (*Schmidt-Hoberg* and *Luhr*, 1976).

We regard comminuted fractures as an indication for compression osteosynthesis even if the jaw has complete dentition. Experience has shown that such fractures often cannot be reduced accurately and immobilized with dental splints alone. By placement of a compression screw plate of appropriate length, the fragments can be joined in a stable fashion according to the individual situation (direction of the fracture, size and shape of bone fragments which might have been avulsed). For such comminuted fractures, we recommend the use of plates without a basal groove, as these are more easily adapted.

Fig. 8.5.2-28 A shows such a comminuted fracture in the left premolar region, as well as a concurrent fracture in the right mandibular angle. The result of treatment of the fracture is shown in Fig. 8.5.2-28 B.

During surgery, in every patient, it is necessary to establish the occlusion by means of inter-

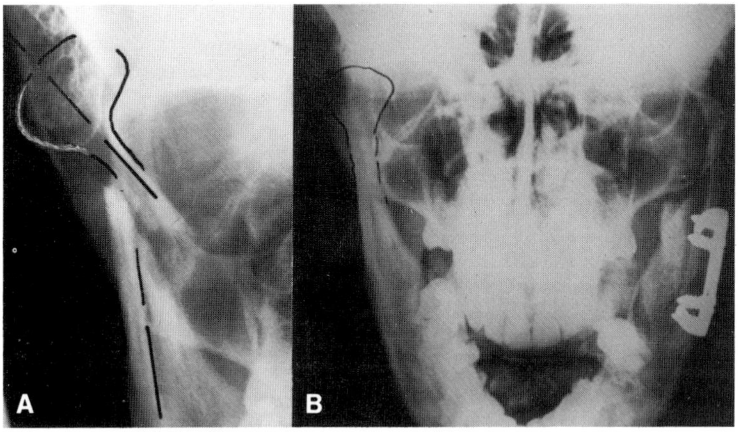

Figs. 8.5.2-27 A and B Application of compression osteosynthesis to a fracture of the completely dentulous mandible, when a concomitant dislocated fracture of the condyle is present which requires early functional therapy.

Fig. 8.5.2-27 A Dislocated deep oblique fracture of the right condylar neck.

Fig. 8.5.2-27 B Fracture in left mandibular angle, stabilized by CSP.

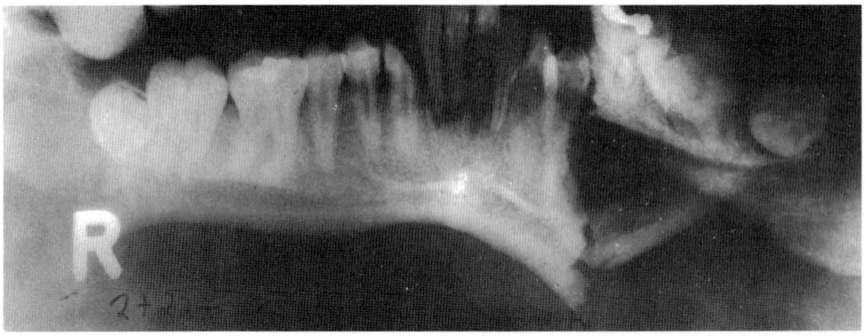

Fig. 8.5.2-28 A Bilateral fracture of the left body and the right angle of the mandible, with impacted 4 8 in the fracture line.

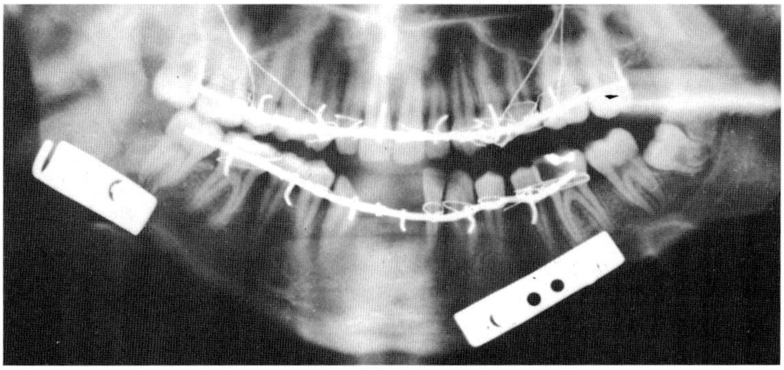

Fig. 8.5.2-28 B Condition after compression plate osteosynthesis, left, with 48 mm plate without basal groove; right, with 38 mm plate with basal groove. In addition, a maxillary fracture was present which was stabilized by internal wiring. Intermaxillary immobilization was not necessary, so that here, also, the patient was able to move the mandible freely after surgery.

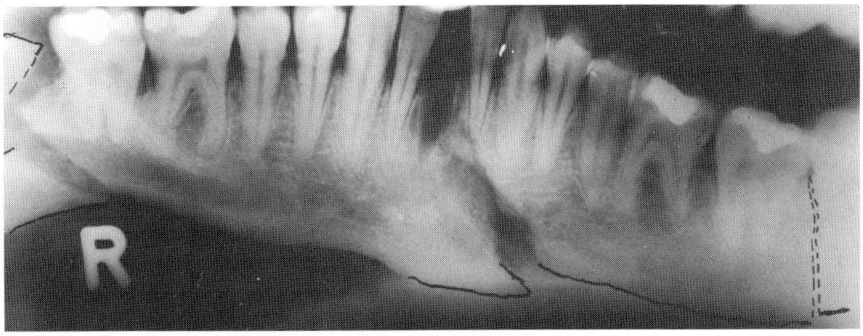

Fig. 8.5.2-29 A Triple mandibular fracture in a 35-year-old patient with multiple trauma, with additional multiple fractures of the extremities.

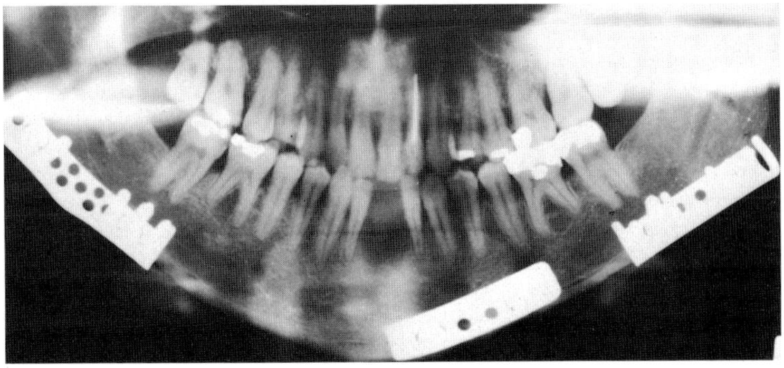

Fig. 8.5.2-29 B Condition after compression plate osteosynthesis with 3 plates. (Surgery for the fractures of the extremities was performed in the same session by the traumatology surgeon.)

maxillary fixation which, however, can be removed immediately after the operation, The splint in the mandible, however, is left in place in such cases for 4 weeks as a so-called tension band, especially since this mandibular splint does not interfere with mandibular function in any way.

For polytraumatized patients, especially those with skull and brain trauma and unconsciousness, primary surgical treatment of mandibular fractures by means of compression osteosynthesis offers great advantages. Because of the unimpeded movement of the mandible, oral hygiene as well as endotracheal suctioning and the possible need for reintubation are greatly facilitated. In addition, the patient is not burdened with intermaxillary immobilization—a considerable advantage, especially in the most seriously ill patients.

Fig. 8.5.2-29 A shows a triple mandibular fracture in a 35-year-old male patient; these fractures were treated with compression screw plates (Fig. 8.5.2-29 B); during the same surgical session, fractures of the left tibia and of the femur were stabilized surgically by the general surgeon.

In summary, compression osteosynthesis with the compression screw plates has proved eminently effective in more than 500 patients during 10 years of clinical experience, in the applications described above. The mandibular compression plate system offers the following important advantages:

1. With the use of the highly corrosion-resistant cobalt-chromium-molybdenum alloy Vitallium®, the osteosynthesis material can, if necessary, remain *in situ*, so that a second operation is avoided.
2. With plates of different shapes and lengths, which are arranged within easy view in a sterilizable box, all conceivable types and combinations of fractures in the mandibular region can be treated.

3. The surgical technique is simple and is easily performed by surgeons engaged in mandibular surgery. Furthermore, the procedure is not costly since, for example, preparation of screw threads is made unnecessary by the use of self-threading screws (in practical use, we have never observed loosening of screws with this procedure).
4. Complications from infection are no more frequent than in purely conservative treatment of fractures.
5. Maximal stability of the osteosynthesis and optimal adaptation of the fracture ends by means of axial compression guarantee rapid healing of the fracture.
6. Additional immobilization of the mandible is not needed in any case.

References

Allgöwer, M. (1969)
A dynamic compression plate. Acta Orthop. Scand. 125: 29

Beal, G., and J. Levignac (1955)
Ostéosynthèse mandibulaire (Mandibular osteosynthesis.) Rev. Stomat. (Paris) 56: 424

Bechtol, C. O., A. B. Ferguson, and P. G. Laing (1959)
Metals and engineering in bone and joint surgery. Baltimore, Williams and Wilkins

Becker, E. (1957)
Ein Instrumentarium zur perkutanen Osteosynthese und extrakutanen Überbrückung mit Kunststoffen. (An instrument set for percutaneous osteosynthesis and extracutaneous bridging, using synthetics.) Zbl. Vet.-Med. 4: 205

Becker, E. (1958)
Ein Instrumentarium zur extracutanen Osteosynthese bei Unterkieferfrakturen unter Verwendung plastischer Kunststoffe. (An instrument set for extracutaneous osteosynthesis in mandibular fractures, using plastic synthetics.) Chirurg 29: 63

Becker, R. (1974)
Stable compression plate fixation of mandibular fractures. Brit. J. oral Surg. 12: 13

Becker, R., D. Broxtermann, E. Esser, M. Meiners, and P. Topp (1976)
Indikationsstellung für verschiedene Osteosyntheseverfahren auf der Grundlage klinischer und experimenteller Untersuchungen. (Indications for various osteosynthesis procedures based on clinical and experimental studies.) Fortschr. Kiefer- u. Gesichtschir. 21: 296

Becker, R., and E. Machtens (1973)
Druckplattenosteosynthese zur Frakturbehandlung und bei orthopädisch-chirurgischen Massnahmen am Gesichtsschädel. (Compression plate osteosynthesis for fracture therapy and in surgical orthopedic treatment of the facial skull.) Osteo-News (Switz) 19

Bigelow, H. M. (1943)
Vitallium bone screws and appliances for treatment of fracture of the mandible. J. oral Surg. 1: 131

Bonome, A. (1885)
Zur Histogenese der Knochenregeneration. (The histogenesis of bone regeneration.) Virchow's Arch. path. Anat. 100: 293

Brand, D. (1937)
Verzögerte Knochenbruchheilung und Pseudarthrosenbildung. (Delayed bone fracture healing and formation of pseudoarthroses.) Leipzig

Claudi, B., and B. Spiessl (1975)
Ergebnisse bei konservativer und operativer Behandlung von Unterkieferfrakturen (ohne Kollumfrakturen). (Results of conservative and surgical treatment of mandibular fractures, except condylar fractures.) Fortschr. Kiefer- u. Gesichtschir. 19: 73

Cohen, J. (1962)
Corrosion testing of orthopaedic implants. J. Bone Jt. Surg. 44 A: 307

Danis, R. (1949)
Théorie et pratique de l'ostéosynthèse. (Theory and practice of osteosynthesis.) Paris, Masson

Danis, R. (1959)
Le vrai but et les dangers de l'ostéosynthèse. (The real purpose and dangers of osteosynthesis.) Lyon Chir. 51: 740

Eggers, G. W. N., W. H. Ainsworth, T. O. Shindler, and C. M. Pomerat (1951)
Clinical significance of the contact-compression factor in bone surgery. Arch. Surg. 62: 467

Eggers, G.W.N., T. O. Shindler, and C. M. Pomerat (1949)
The influence of the contact-compression factor on osteogenesis in surgical fractures. J. Bone Jt. Surg 31 A: 693

Freitag, V., and G. Manderscheid (1976)
Ergebnisse der Druckplattenosteosynthese nach Luhr. (Results of compression plate osteosynthesis of Luhr.) Fortschr. Kiefer- u. Gesichtschir. 21: 301

Friedenberg, Z.B., and G. French (1952)
The effect of known compression forces on fracture healing. Surg. Gynec. Obstet. 94: 743

Greifensteiner, H. (1953)
Die operative Behandlung der Unterschenkelbrüche mit verzögerter Kallusbildung unter Berücksichtigung der Kompressions-Osteosynthese. (The surgical care of leg fractures with delayed callus formation with special reference to compression osteosynthesis.) Bruns' Beitr. klin. Chir. 187: 219

Häbler, C., and O. Reiss (1936)
Experimentelle Untersuchungen über die Festigkeit des Knochens im normalen und im Zustand der Bruchheilung. (Experimental investigations of the rigidity of bone in normal conditions and during fracture healing.) Dtsch. Z. Chir. 246: 586, 760

Hayward, J. R. (1962)
Treatment methods for jaw fractures. J. oral Surg. 20: 273

Heiss, J., and H. Grasser (1968)
Stabile Osteosynthese mit Platten. (Stable osteosynthesis with plates.) Dtsch. zahnärztl. Z. 23: 1085

Hoffer, O. and P. Ariotta (1961)
Behandlung von Unterkieferbrüchen mit Metallplättchen. (Treatment of mandibular fractures with small metal plates.) Dtsch. zahnärztl. Z. 16: 807

Höltje, W. J., H.-G. Luhr and M. Holtfreter (1975)
Untersuchungen über infektionsbedingte Komplikationen nach konservativer oder operativer Versorgung von Unterkieferfrakturen. (Studies of infection-induced complications following conservative or surgical care of mandibular fractures.) Fortschr. Kiefer- u. Gesichtschir. 19: 122

Lentrodt, J., and W. J. Höltje (1975)
Indikation zur operativen bzw. konservativen Versorgung von Unterkieferfrakturen. (Indications for conservative and surgical care of mandibular fractures.) Fortschr. Kiefer- u. Gesichtschir. 19: 65

Luhr, H. G. (1968)
Zur stabilen Osteosynthese bei Unterkieferfrakturen. (Stable osteosynthesis in mandibular fractures.) Dtsch. zahnärzt. Z. 23: 754

Luhr, H.-G. (1969 a)
Die operative Behandlung von Unterkieferfrakturen unter besonderer Berücksichtigung der Kompressionsosteosynthese. (The surgical care of mandibular fractures with special reference to compression osteosynthesis.) Rep. 102nd meeting of the Vereinigung Nordwestdeutscher Chirurgen, Hamburg, 1968. Zentralbl. Chir. 94: 819

Luhr, H.-G. (1969 b)
The compression osteosynthesis of mandibular fractures in dogs. A histologic contribution to "primary bone healing". Europ. surg. Res. 1: 3

Luhr, H.-G. (1971)
Treatment of mandibular fractures and pseudoarthrosis by compression osteosynthesis. In: Trans. 5th Int. Congr. Plast. Reconstr. Surg., p. 109. Melbourne, Butterworths

Luhr, H.-G. (1972 a)
Die Kompressions-Osteosynthese bei Unterkieferfrakturen. (Compression osteosynthesis in mandibular fractures.) Munich, C. Hanser

Luhr, H.-G. (1972 b)
Die Kompressions-Osteosynthese zur Behandlung von Unterkieferfrakturen–Experimentelle Grundlagen und klinische Erfahrungen. (Compression osteosynthesis for the treatment of mandibular fractures: Experimental basis and clinical experience.) Dtsch. zahnärztl. Z. 27: 29

Luhr, H.-G., and R. Maerker (1974)
Zur Problematik der röntgenologischen Beurteilung der Frakturheilung am Unterkiefer. (Problems of radiographic evaluation of healing of mandibular fractures.) Dtsch. zahnärztl. Z. 29: 351

Luhr, H.-G., W. Busch, and R. Maerker (1975)
Histologische Untersuchungen zur Frage der primären Knochenheilung nach Kompressionsosteosynthese. (Histological investigation of primary bone healing following compression osteosynthesis.) Fortschr. Kiefer- u. Gesichtschir. 19: 13

Luhr, H.-G., W. J. Höltje, and R. Schmitz (1975)
Indikation, Technik und Ergebnisse der Kompressionsosteosynthese bei Unterkieferfrakturen. (Erfahrungen bei 400 Osteosynthesen). (Indications, technique and results of compression osteosynthesis in mandibular fracturen: Experience in 400 cases.) Paper, 4th Symp. Internal. Assn. Maxillofac. Surg., Budapest

Mittelmeyer, H. (1968)
Druckosteosynthese mit selbstspannenden Platten (Technik und Erfahrungsbericht). (Compression osteosynthesis with self-tightening compression plates: Technique and report of experience.) Saarl. Westpfälz. Orthopädentreffen, Hamburg

Müller, M. E., M. Allgöwer, and H. Willenegger (1963)
Technik der operativen Frakturbehandlung, (Technique of surgical fracture therapy.) Berlin, Springer

Niederdellmann, H. (1974)
Experimentelle Untersuchungen und klinische Beispiele zur Druckplattenosteosynthese am Unterkiefer. (Experimental investigations and clinical examples of compression plate osteosynthesis in the mandible.) Thesis (Med. Habil.), Freiburg

Niederdellmann, H. (1975)
Elekronische Messungen zur Biomechanik bei Osteosynthese am Unterkiefer. (Electronic measurements of biomechanics of mandibular osteosynthesis.) Fortschr. Kiefer- u. Gesichtschir. 19: 43

Niederdellmann, H., and W. Schilli (1972)
Funktionsstabile Osteosynthese im Unterkiefer. (Functionally stable osteosynthesis in the mandible.) Dtsch. zahnärztl. Z. 27: 138

Palfer-Sollier, M. (1956)
L'ostéosynthèse par gouttières vissées en durallium dans les fractures mandibulaires (avec ou sans perte de substance). Osteosynthesis with Durallium screw splints in mandibular fractures with or without loss of hard tissue.) Rev. Franç. Odonto-Stomat. 3: 587

Pauwels, F. (1940)
Grundriss einer Biomechanik der Frakturheilung. (Outline of a system of biomechanics of fracture healing.) Verh. Dtsch. orthop. Ges. 34: 62

Pauwels, D. (1960)
Eine neue Theorie über den Einfluss mechanischer Reize auf die Differenzierung der Stützgewebe. (A new theory of the effect of mechanical irritants on the differentiation of supporting tissue.) Z. Anat. Entwickl. – Gesch. 121: 478

Pauwels, F. (1965)
Gesammelte Abhandlungen zur funktionellen Anatomie des Bewegungsapparates. (Collected discussions on the functional anatomy of the apparatus of motion.) Berlin, Springer

Perren, S. M., M. Russenberger, S. Steinemann, M. E. Müller, and M. Allgöwer (1969)
A dynamic compression plate. Acta Orthop. Scand. 125 (Suppl.): 31

Petrokov, V. (1962)
Die Biomechanik der Kallusbildung und experimentelle Bewertung der Druckosteosynthese. (The biomechanics of callus formation and experimental evaluation of compression osteosynthesis.) Bruns' Beitr. klin. Chir. 205: 265

Pini, C. E. (1959)
Le osteosintesi mediante placchette metalliche nelle fratture della mandibola. (Metal plate mediated osteosynthesis in fractures of the mandible.) Minerva stomat. 8: 105

Prein, J., A. Eschmann, and B. Spiessl (1976)
Ergebnisse der Nachuntersuchungen bei 81 Patienten mit funktionsstabiler Unterkieferosteosynthese. (Results of follow-up studies in 81 patients with functionally stable mandibular osteosyntheses.) Fortschr. Kiefer- u. Gesichtschir. 21: 304

Reynolds, F. C., and J. A. Key (1954)
Fracture healing after fixation with standard plates, contact splints and medullary nails. J. Bone Jt. Surg. 36 A: 577

Robinson, M., and C. Yoon (1957)
New onlay-inlay metal splint for immobilization of displaced condylar fractures. J. oral Surg. 15: 164

Robinson, M., and C. Yoon (1963)
The 'L' splint for the fractured mandible: a new principle of plating. J. oral Surg. 21: 395

Schenk, R., and H. Willenegger (1963)
Zum histologischen Bild der sogenannten Primärheilung der Knochenkompakta nach experimentellen Osteotomien am Hund. (The histological appearance of so-called primary healing of the compact bone after experimental osteotomy in the dog.) Experientia (Basel) 19: 593

Schenk, R., and H. Willenegger (1964)
Zur Histologie der primären Knochenheilung. (Histology of primary bone healing.) Langenbeck's Arch. klin. Chir. 308: 440

Schenk, R., and H. Willenegger (1965)
Fluoreszenzmikroskopische Untersuchungen zur Heilung von Schaftfrakturen nach stabiler Osteosynthese am Hund. (Fluorescence microscopic studies of the healing of shaft fractures after stable osteosynthesis in the dog.) In: Richelle, L. J., and H. D. Dallemagne: Calcified Tissues. Liège, pp. 125-133

Schilli, W. (1969)
Behandlungsmöglichkeiten bei Unterkieferfrakturen. (Treatment possibilities in mandibular fractures.) Therapiewoche 41: 2005

Schilli, W. (1975)
Indikation und Technik der stabilen Osteosynthese im Unterkiefer. (Indications and techniques of stable osteosynthesis in the mandible.) Fortschr. Kiefer- u. Gesichtschir. 19: 79

Schilli, W., H. Niederdellmann, and R. Ewers (1973)
Probleme der funktionsstabilen Osteosynthese am Unterkiefer. (Problems of functionally stable osteosynthesis in the mandible.) Acta traumatol. 3: 173

Schilli, W., and F. Härle (1976)
Die funktionsstabile Osteosynthese – ein Problem des operativen Zugangs. (The functionally stable osteosynthesis: A problem of the surgical approach.) Fortschr. Kiefer- u. Gesichtschir. 21: 300

Schmidt-Hoberg, W., and H.-G. Luhr (1976)
Technik und Ergebnisse der funktionellen Frühbehandlung von Kollumfrakturen bei gleichzeitigem Vorliegen von Unterkieferfrakturen. (Technique and results of early functional treatment of condylar fractures with simultaneous mandibular fractures.) Fortschr. Kiefer- u. Gesichtschir. 21: 317

Schmitz, R., H.-G. Luhr, and H. Schubert (1975)
Indikation, Technik und klinische Ergebnisse der Kompressionsosteosynthese bei Unterkieferfrakturen. (Indications, technique and clinical results of compression osteosynthesis in mandibular fractures.) Fortschr. Kiefer- u. Gesichtschir. 19: 74

Schroll, K. (1973)
Plattenosteosynthese bei Frakturen des zahnlosen Unterkiefers. (Plate osteosynthesis in fractures of the edentulous mandible.) Öst. Z. Stomat. 70: 394, 444

Schroll, K. (1974)
Experimentelle Untersuchungen und klinische Erfahrungen mit der Plattenosteosynthese von enoral bei Frakturen des zahnlosen Unterkiefers. (Experimental investigations and clinical results of endoral plate osteosynthesis in fractures of the edentulous mandible.) Zahnärztl. Welt 83: 650, 742, 835, 934, 1042

Schuchardt, K. (1956)
Ein Vorschlag zur Verbesserung der Drahtschienenverbände. (A proposal for improving the wire arch bar.) Dtsch. Zahn-, Mund- u. Kieferheilk. 24: 39

Schüle, H. (1976)
Fortschritte und Schwerpunkte der Behandlung von Mund-, Kiefer-, Gesichtsverletzungen. (Advances and focal points in the treatment of oral and maxillofacial injuries.) Fortschr. Kiefer- u. Gesichtschir. 21: 272

Schwenzer, N. (1967)
Zur Osteosynthese bei Frakturen des Gesichtsskelets. (Osteosynthesis in fractures of the facial skeleton.) Stuttgart, Thieme

Segmüller, G., and M. Allgöwer (1965)
Realität und Relativität der primären Knochenbildung. (Reality and relativity of primary bone healing.) Chirurg 36: 504

Shira, R. B. (1954)
Open reduction of mandibular fractures. J. oral Surg. 12: 95

Smith, A. E., and M. Robinson (1954)
Individually constructed stainless steal bone onlay splint for immobilization of proximal fragment in fractures of the angle of the mandible. J. oral Surg. 12: 170

Spiessl, B. (1969)
Erfahrungen mit dem AO-Besteck bei Kieferbehandlungen. (Experience with the ASIF instrument set in treatment of mandibular fractures.) Schweiz. Mschr. Zahnheilk. 79: 112

Spiessl, B. (1975)
Funktionsstabile Osteosynthese bei Unterkieferfrakturen – Problematik und Technik. (Functionally stable osteosynthesis in mandibular fractures: Problems and techniques.) Fortschr. Kiefer- u. Gesichtschir. 19: 68

Spiessl, B., G. Schaugus, and K. Schroll (1971)
Die stabile Osteosynthese bei Frakturen des unbezahnten Kiefers. (Stable osteosynthesis in fractures of the edentulous jaw.) Schweiz. Mschr. Zahnheilk. 81: 39

Spiessl, B., and K. Schroll (1972)
Gesichtsschädel (Facial skull.) In: Igst, H., ed. Spezielle Frakturen- und Luxationslehre. (Textbook of Fractures and Luxations.) Vol. 1/1. Stuttgart, Thieme

Thoma, K. H. (1948)
Methods of fixation of jaw fractures and their indications. J. oral Surg. 6: 125

Thoma, K. H. (1952)
Methods of fixation of jaw fractures and their indications. In: Oral Surgery. Ed. 2; Ed. 3 (1958). St. Louis, C. V. Mosby Co.

Urist, M. R., and R. W. Johnson (1943)
The healing of fractures in man under clinical conditions. J. Bone Jt. Surg. 25: 375

Venable, C. S., and W. G. Stuck (1947)
The internal fixation of fractures. Springfield, Charles C. Thomas

Willenegger, H., R. Schenk, F. Straumann, M. Müller, M. Allgöwer, and H. Krüger (1962)
Methodik und vorläufige Ergebnisse experimenteller Untersuchungen über die Heilvorgänge bei stabiler Osteosynthese. (Methods and preliminary results of experimental investigations of healing events in stable osteosynthesis.) Langenbeck's Arch. klin. Chir. 301: 846

5.3 Compression Plate Osteosynthesis through the ASIF System

Wilfried Schilli

5.3.1 The ASIF System

The Association for the Study of Internal Fixation, founded in Switzerland, is now an international group of surgeons, orthopedists, anatomists, metallurgists, and technicians who devote themselves to the problems of indications for internal fixation and optimization of osteosynthesis technology. The standardization of indications, operating technique, and instrumentarium has improved the prognosis for success. Naturally, the members of the Association attempt to eliminate individual and systematic mistakes through clear, complete documentation. These efforts have resulted in specific operating instructions with a standardized instrumentarium. Principles and techniques have been set down in the **Manual der Osteosynthese** (Manual of Osteosynthesis), by *Müller* et al. (1969).

The rudiments and principles of the ASIF techniques in treatment of extremity fractures have been adapted to the maxillofacial region and put into practice in the Departments of Maxillofacial Surgery of the Universities of Basel and Freiburg. The result has been an instrumentarium assembled especially for jaw fracture treatment, with individual instruments that are compatible with the rest of the ASIF system (Fig. 8.5.3-1). The ordinary instruments of the ASIF system, especially the ones for small fragments, also can be used in the jaw. For circumstances unique to the jaw a few additional instruments were specially devised, e.g., for reduction of fragments and for transbuccal drilling and screwing. The screws used are 2 mm and 2.7 mm cortex screws. All plates are Dynamic Compression Plates (DCP), that follow the spherical gliding principle developed by *Perren* et al. (1969) and which allow axial compression (Fig. 8.5.3-2). Although designated **dynamic** compression plates (DCP), there is static compression involved when the interfragmentary pressure is built up with the help of the gliding holes. After the hemispherical screw head has been applied in the distal end of the hole, it glides in the gliding hole towards the fracture when tightened further. The bone fragment is forced along with it, and thus produces interfragmentary pressure. The position of the drilled hole is determined precisely by an eccentric drill guide (Fig. 8.5.3-3). When reverse drilling is performed (with the drill-hole on the end of the gliding hole near the fracture), the plate can be used as a neutral fixation plate without a pressure effect.

The instruments necessary for surgical treatment of jaw fractures according to the ASIF system are contained in a special basic surgical case (Fig. 8.5.3-1). We recommend a small autoclavable drill powered by compressed air. Because its rotational speed is limited, no thermal damage can occur to the bone during drilling. In principle, however, any slow-running drill can be used. Drilling and cutting of screw-threads in the vicinity of the soft tissue should be performed with a protective tap sleeve (Fig. 8.5.3-4). The hole drilled should extend through both cortical layers and its depth should be measured with a depth gauge after drilling. The fine hook of the depth gauge is hooked to the inner end of the cortex and the necessary screw length can be read on the scale after the inserted probe has made contact with the bone (Fig. 8.5.3-5). After determining the length of the screw, a thread is cut with a manual tap (Fig. 8.5.3-6) and the resulting chips are rinsed away carefully.

If care is exercised, the screw can be screwed in and out of the carved bone threads without destroying the thread and thus the grip in the bone. The screw and the bone have a large surface of contact that allows intense pressures to be transmitted through the screw to the bone. The difference between these and interosseous wires here is manifest: with the wire, there is only a small contact surface between the wire's metal and the bone in the drilled hole. Thus, the

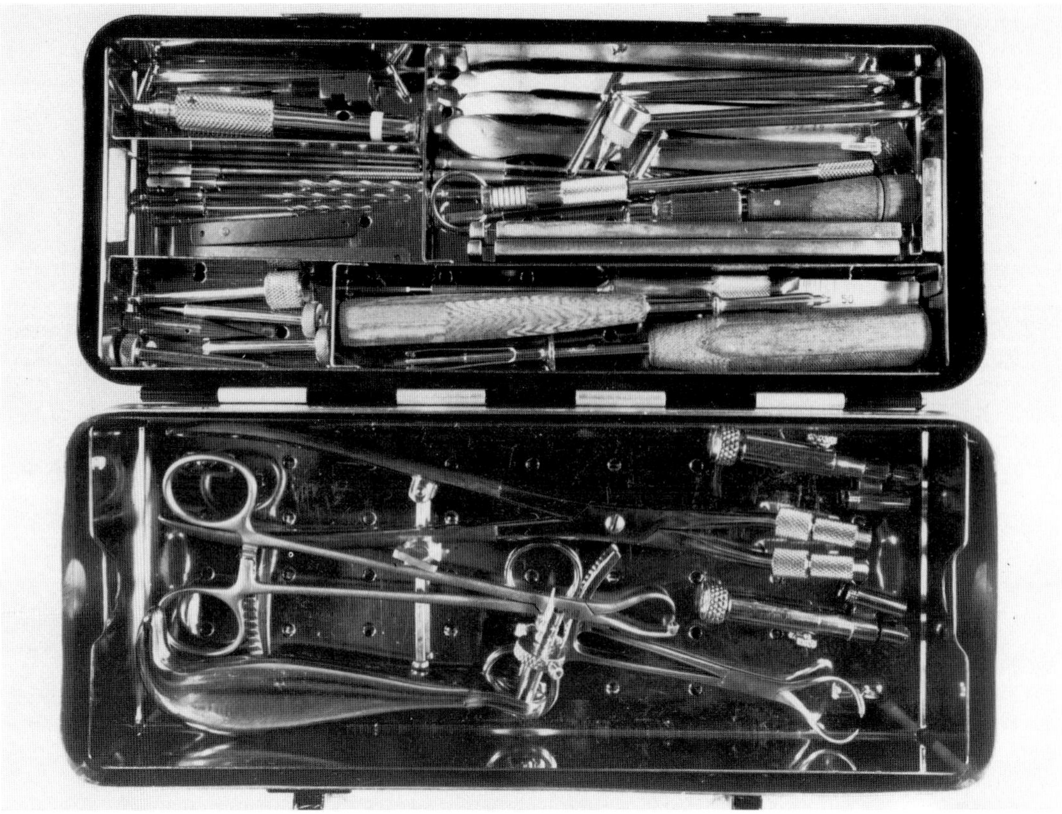

Fig. 8.5.3-1 The instrumentarium assembled by the ASIF (Association for the Study of Internal Fixation) for oral and maxillofacial surgery. All the instruments necessary for a rigid internal fixation according to the rules of the ASIF are included in the set. The only exception is the drill. The implants (plates and screws) are housed in a second case.

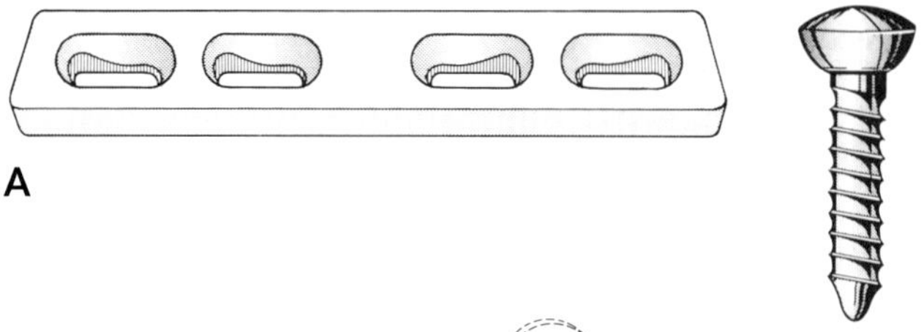

A

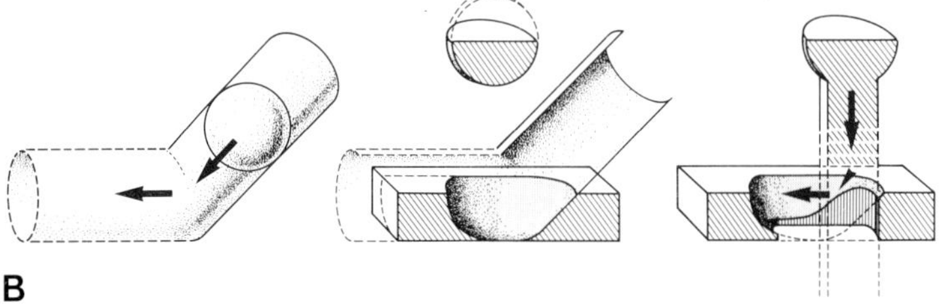

B

Figs. 8.5.3-2 A to I The principle of compression osteosynthesis with the ASIF Dynamic Compression Plate (DCP).

Fig. 8.5.3-2 A The four-hole DCP and a screw with a hemispherical screw head.

Fig. 8.5.3-2 B The spherical gliding principle of the DCP. The screw holes' gliding surface is a sector composed of two cylinders with a bend in it. A ball gliding down in the oblique cylinder is led further horizontally in the intersection plane of the two cylinders. Downward movement is transformed into horizontal movement.

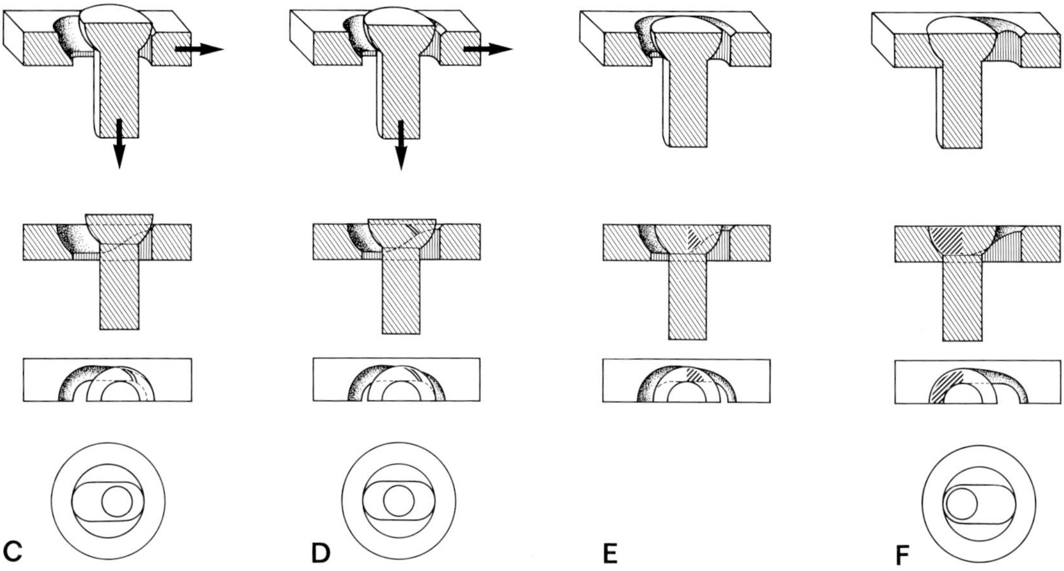

Fig. 8.5.3-2 C to E The screw is eccentrically screwed into the end of the oval screw hole which is furthest from the fracture. As soon as the hemispherical screw head touches the gliding surface, the screw begins shifting with the bone fragment toward the fracture gap.

Fig. 8.5.3-2 F The completely seated screw.

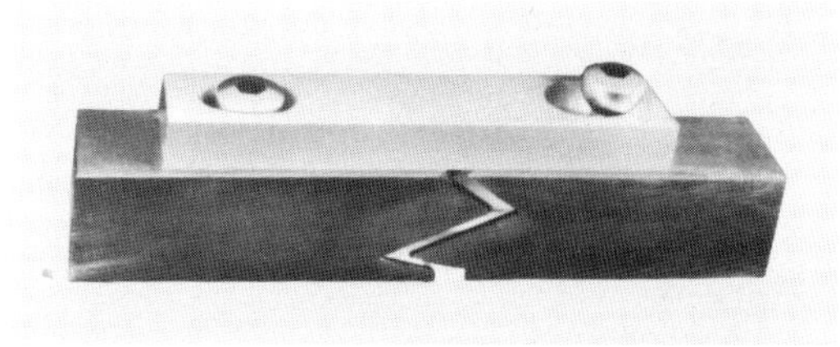

Fig. 8.5.3-2 G Left screw seated. Right screw partially screwed into the part of the DC hole furthest away from the fracture, before the screw head has entered the hole. The fracture is gaping.

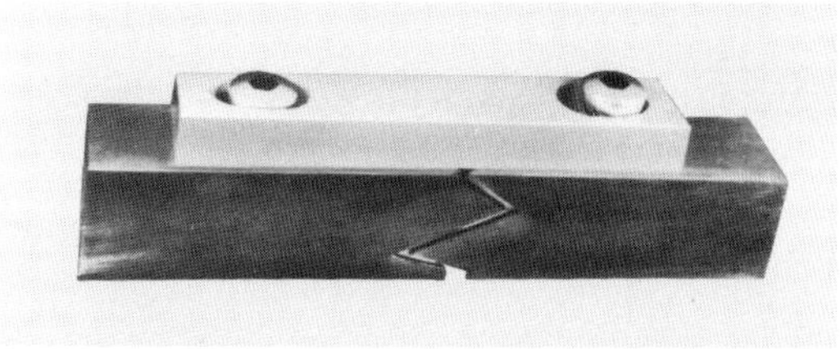

Fig. 8.5.3-2 H After the screw head has entered the DC hole, the bone fragment and the screw move against the fracture.

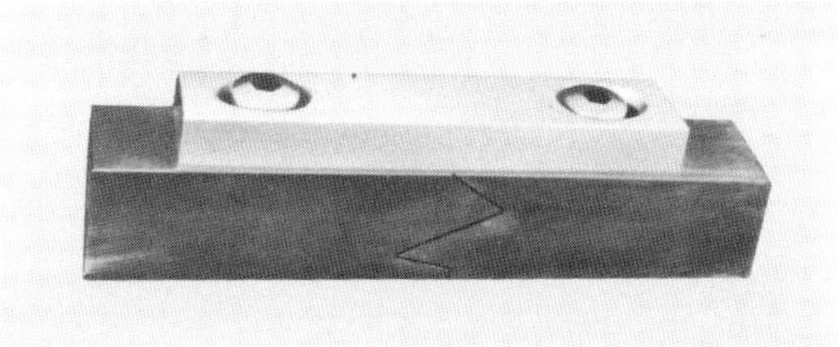

Fig. 8.5.3-2 I When the screw is firmly tightened, there is initially adaptation and finally compression of the fracture ends.
(Figs. 8.5.3-2 G to I are adaptations of those of *Müller* et al., 1969).

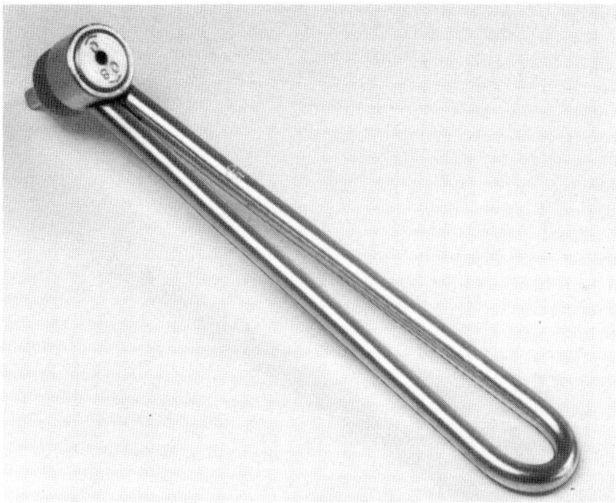

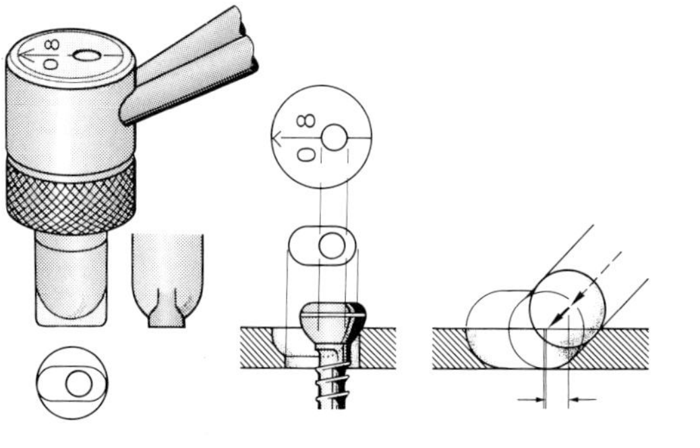

Fig. 8.5.3-3 Eccentric drill guide. The eccentric position of the drill-hole inside the oval DC hole is determined by the drill sleeve.

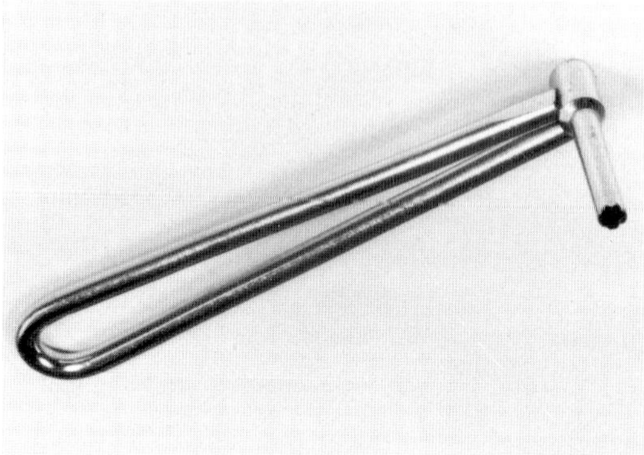

Fig. 8.5.3-4 Protective drill and tap sleeve. The grooved end provides a firm seat on the bone.

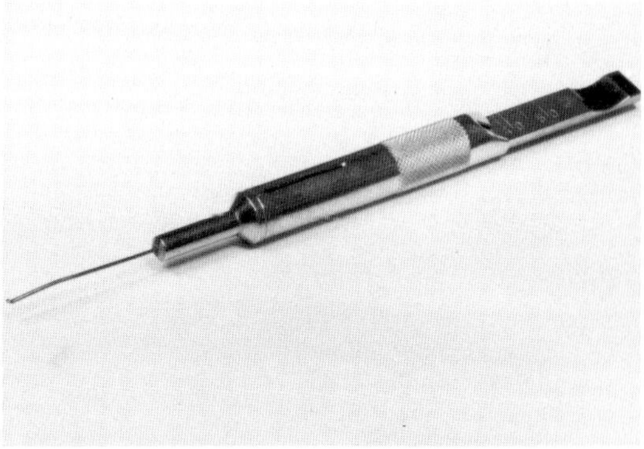

Fig. 8.5.3-5 Depth gauge. The small hook is inserted through the drilled hole. When it is pulled back, its angular end hooks to the inner bone edge of the drilled hole. The length of the screw then can be read from the scale. The instrument is laid out in such a fashion that it takes into account the thickness of the plate. The length of the hole therefore must be measured with the plate in position.

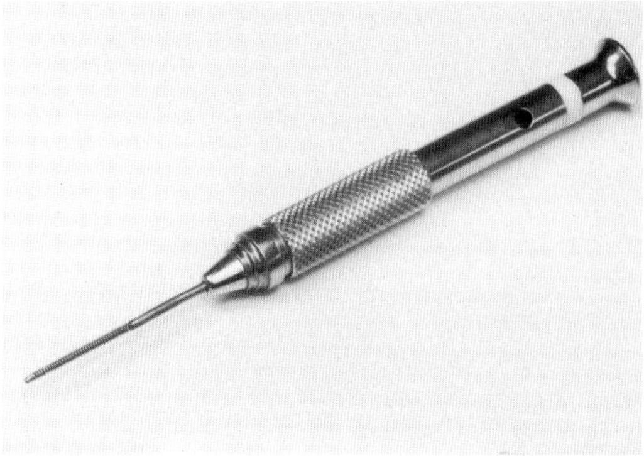

Fig. 8.5.3-6 Interchangeable manual tap with handle. Because the tap must be made from extremely hard steel, there is the danger of breakage.

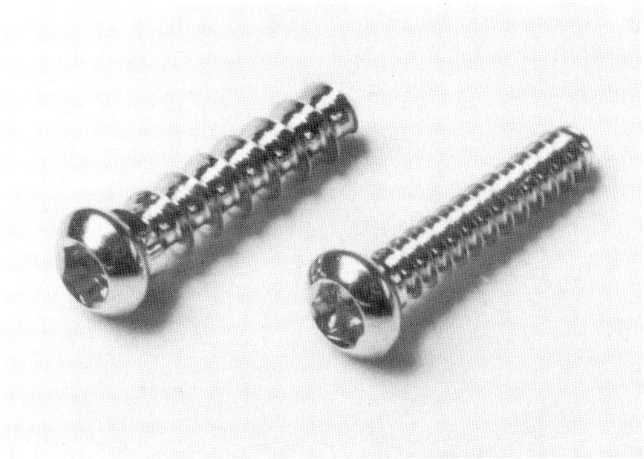

Fig. 8.5.3-7 A normal screw on the right, and an emergency screw on the left, with the same size head but with a thicker core. It is used when the thread is destroyed. It can only be screwed in once, without any prior thread-cutting.

forces which arise and stress the bone are many times greater; consequently, wire ligatures in thin bones often tear loose when they are tightened. In contrast, photoelastic studies have shown that a thread can be cut to fit a screw exactly even when the bone plate is only 2 mm thick. This is because the forces produced by the osteosynthesis screws are distributed; thus, even when a bone is thin or not particularly resistant to pressure because of a pathological change, a functional load is possible without local disturbance of, or tearing loose from, the bone. The smallest ASIF screw, with a core 2 mm thick, has a surface of application on the bone 7 times greater than the 0.5 mm wire ligature. Thus, the stress on a fracture fixed with a precise screw osteosynthesis can be 7 times greater than that on a wire ligature. An additional source of greater uncertainty with the wire ligature is that of the force developed when it is tightened. This is completely uncontrollable; with forceps, extremely high forces are produced through twisting, so that the drilled hole frequently tears when the wire is tightened.

A prerequisite for the effectiveness of the screw is a completely intact inner thread surface in the bone. In rare cases, unfavorable circumstances can make cutting a clean thread impossible, or can cause an already cut thread to be destroyed during the course of the operation. It is then frequently impossible to drill a new hole with an intact thread, as the new hole would mean shifting the DCP. The limited area afforded by the mandible often makes this, too, an impossibility.

A loose screw must not be ignored, however, because at least four firm screws are necessary to immobilize a fracture with plates and screws. When a thread tears out, a longer plate may be necessary. A second possibility is the use of a screw with a thicker core. This emergency screw (Fig. 8.5.3-7) has a core of 3 mm. It has the same screw head as the 2.7 mm screw and just fits through the DC hole of the plate. It is screwed into the hole with the stripped 2.7 mm thread without a new thread being cut. It functions in a self-cutting manner and clamps itself firmly into the hole by virtue of its greater diameter. It must not be unscrewed again for any reason during the operation.

5.3.2 The Various ASIF Plates

In terms of dimensions, in principle the ASIF plates used for the small extremities (fingers) also can be applied to the jaw, i.e., easily adaptable plates 2 mm thick with neutral round holes, and 2.5 mm thick plates with horizontally aligned DC holes. The finger plates alone, however, are not sufficient for rigid internal fixation of the mandible. When a horizontal DC plate is used, a tension band also must be implemented. In order to avoid this, DC holes can be positioned obliquely or at right angles. In the Freiburg 4-hole plate, the slope of the outer DC holes is 45°, which effects a slight rotation upwards and a central compression. The gaping in the tension zone thus can be avoided Fig. 8.5.3-8; *Niederdellmann* and *Schilli*,

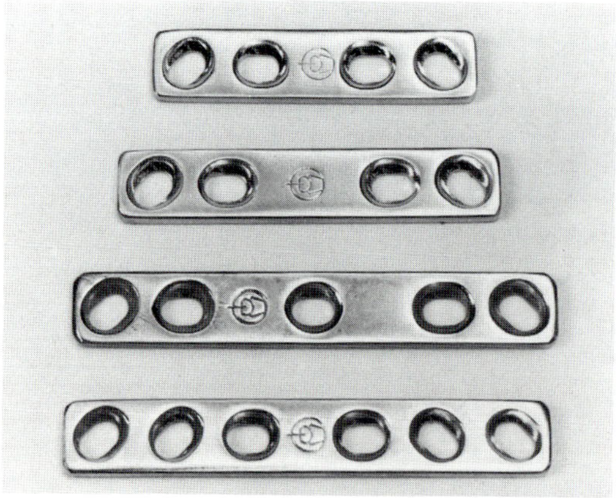

Figs. 8.5.3-8 A to E The mode of action of the Freiburg tension band plate with the 45° outer holes.

Fig. 8.5.3-8 A Freiburg tension band plates of different sizes.

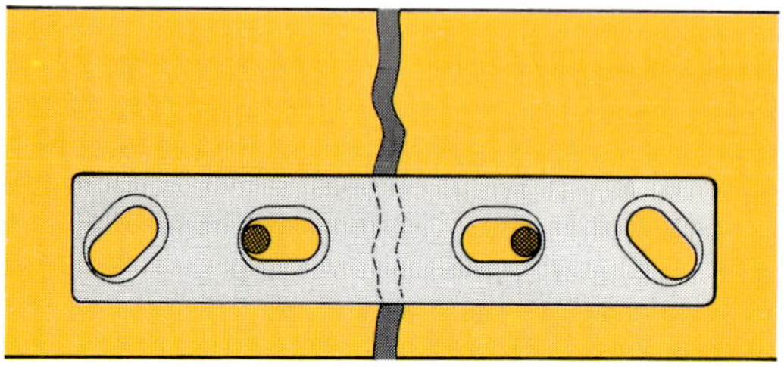

Fig. 8.5.3.8 B Initially, both inner holes are drilled. The holes are situated with the eccentric drill guide away from the fracture.

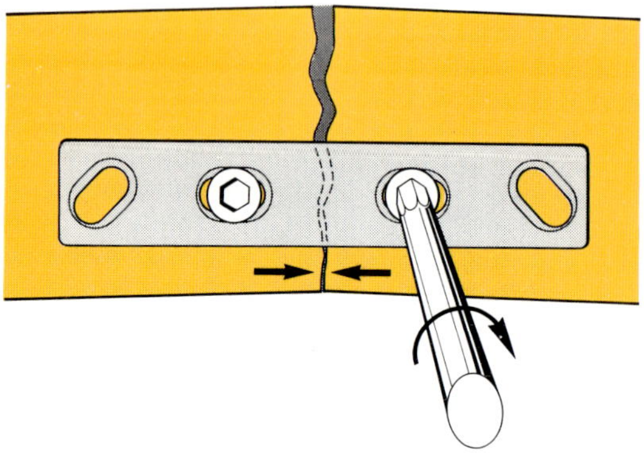

Fig. 8.5.3-8 C The fragments are brought closer to each other and pressed together in the lower region through tightening of the screws in the two horizontal DC holes. In the upper region, however, which corresponds to the alveolar process, a gap remains.

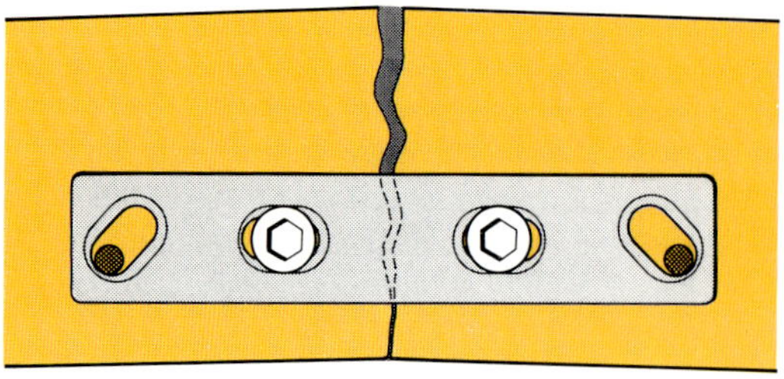

Fig. 8.5.3-8 D Holes placed in the obliquely arranged DC holes.

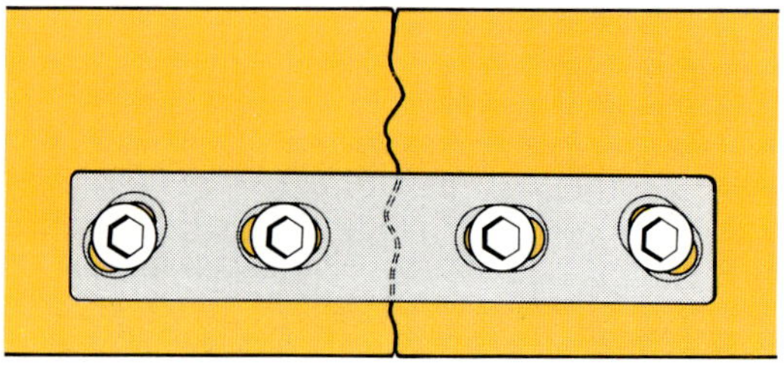

Fig. 8.5.3-8 E The plate is stressed through tightening of the two outer screws in the obliquely arranged holes in such a fashion that both fragments rotate upwards; thus, the fracture is closed and compressed in the alveolar process region.

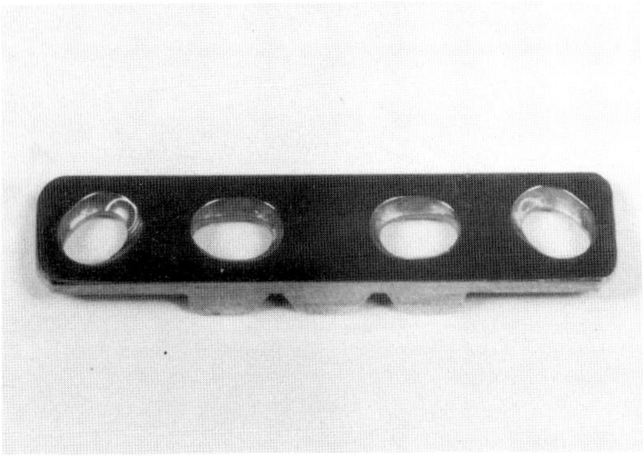

Fig. 8.5.3-9 A Inlay plate. The notched inlay part is recessed into a slit drilled in the bone.

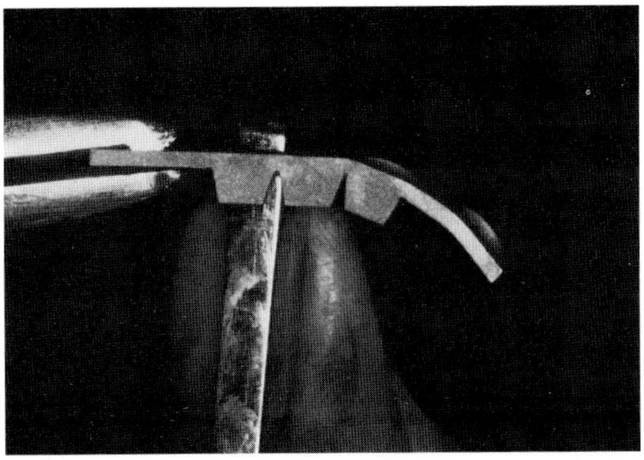

Fig. 8.5.3-9 B The notches in the inlay part allow the plate to be bent in this area as well.

1973). For extreme cases, *Spiessl* (1974) recommends plates with vertically situated inner or outer DC holes (eccentric dynamic compression plate, EDCP). Within the vertically positioned DC holes the central compression is completely eliminated and only the rotation components, located in the part of the tension zone away from the plate, are used to produce pressure.

For extreme cases with especially high mechanical stress, there is also a Freiburg DC plate equipped with an inlay section. The inlay section has grooves that make the plate adaptable (Fig. 8.5.3-9). This plate is indicated either where smooth oblique fractures allow the ends of the bone to slip along each other despite perfect plate adaptation or where massive torsion stresses arise, as in the case of very strong patients—particularly those with median or paramedian fractures. Also, if additional fracture of the alveolar process makes producing interfragmentary pressure with the help of the oblique DC holes impossible, the inlay plate offers the only possibility of achieving reliable stability. Use of this plate is further indicated with free bone grafts; the inlay part provides stabilization through a third dimension. This is important especially with bone grafts, because there is no large surface of interfragmentary contact to be expected. The adaptation of the plates occurs with plate bending pliers and bending irons (Fig. 8.5.3-10).

In comminuted as well as in discontinuity defect fractures, a long distance has to be bridged by the plate. Interfragmentary compression cannot be achieved under these circumstances since the contact of the fragments is insufficient. In these cases a reconstruction plate, as it is used for fixation of bone grafts (see Chapter 18), is recommended. For sufficient fixation, as a rule, at least three screws are necessary within each fragment.

For the repositioning of the fragments, reduction forceps (Fig. 8.5.3-11) are used. In the intraoral approach, *Homann*'s bone elevator with the short tip has proven particularly useful. In the extraoral approach and for difficult repositioning, the mandibular reduction forceps (Fig. 8.5.3-12) is helpful. This instrument is fixed with two additional cortex screws in the lower border of the mandible, which are screwed to a depth of 5 to 8 mm. These reduction forceps permit exact repositioning and the build-up of interfragmentary pressure through the forceps while the drilling and plate placement ensue. The screw heads function here as ball joints (Fig. 8.5.3-13).

Plate-holding forceps (Fig. 8.5.3-11)—especially in the extraoral approach—provide for temporary fixation of the plate adapted by the bending pliers and bending irons. The pointed end spans the mandible lingually, and the blunt end is inserted into a hole in the plate. When the forceps is closed, the plate is pressed against the surface

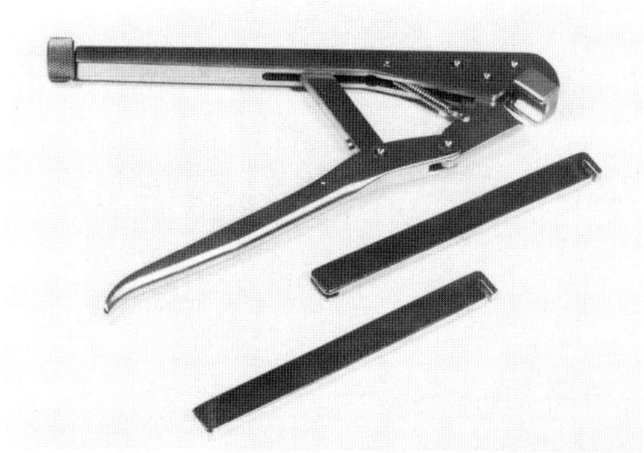

Fig. 8.5.3-10 Plate bending pliers and bending irons.

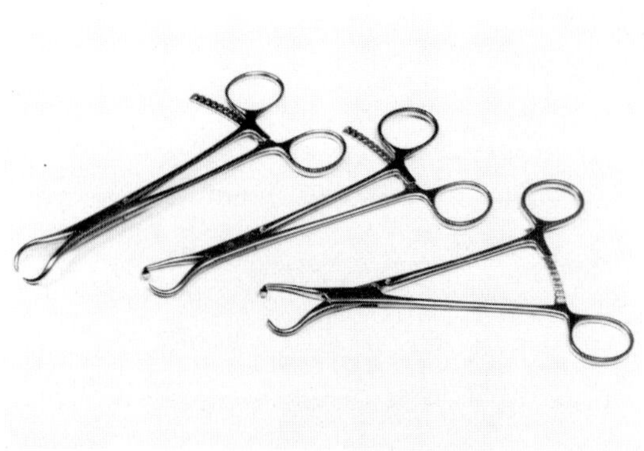

Fig. 8.5.3-11 Reduction forceps (left) and plate-holding forceps (right).

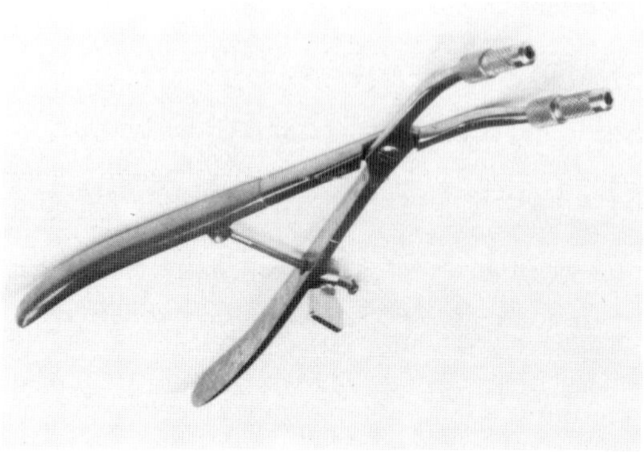

Fig. 8.5.3-12 Reduction forceps for repositioning both fragments. The ends of the forceps grip two screws into the mandibular border on both sides of the fracture. These forceps allow both fragments to be reduced and held in the correct position until the DCP has been applied.

of the bone. A well-adapted plate can be affixed to the bone with two plate-holding forceps until the first two screws have been inserted.
Setting the holes and determining the drilling angle require a certain amount of experience. For a rigid internal fixation, at least four firmly seated screws are necessary. Sometimes one of the plate screws is also used as a lag screw (see section 6, pp. 372 f.).

5.3.3 Prerequisites and Indications for Compression Plate Osteosynthesis

A *conditio sine qua non* in the dentulous jaw is an occlusal reconstruction which is exact to the millimeter. To this end, continuous interdental wires are almost always applied before the beginning of the operation to provide intermaxillary fixation of the fragments in the correct occlusion. We have found elastic connections with rubber bands to be effective. With small rubber rings, an exceptionally strong continuously effective reduction force can be developed. At the same time, the elastic fixation nevertheless permits small corrective movements after the fracture site has been exposed.
In the completely dentulous jaw, continuous interdental wiring is not necessary when the occlusion can be easily established—e.g., for fractures in the angle of the mandible. Here, the occlusion is sufficiently fixated by the application of some eyelet wires or Ernstian

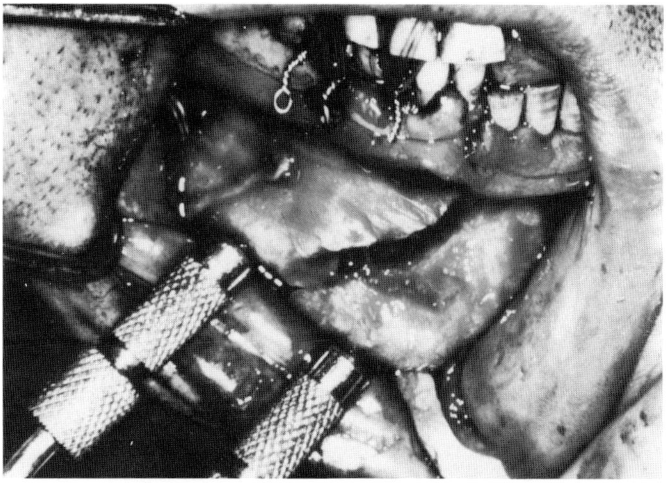

Fig. 8.5.3-13 A Reduction forceps *in situ* with a gaping fracture.

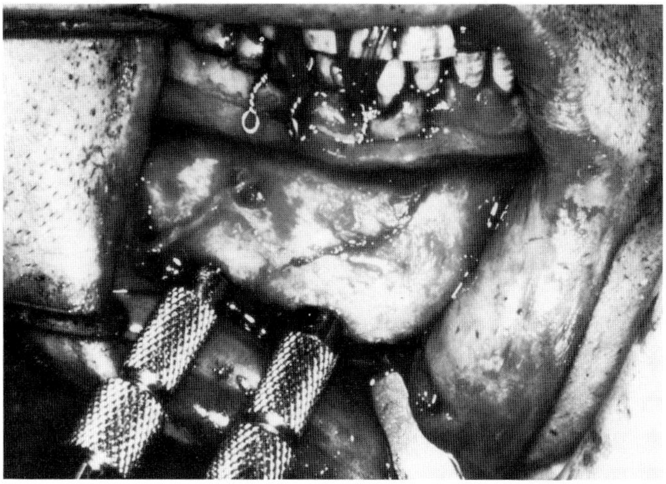

Fig. 8.5.3-13 B Appearance after reduction of the fragments.

ligatures, juxtaposed in each case. These ligatures then must be rigidly secured with intermaxillary wires and additionally with cold-curing acrylic.

In contrast to the conservative treatment of fractures, rigid internal fixation requires not only an occlusal reconstruction exact to the millimeter but also a most exact reduction in the vicinity of the fracture. Only if the fragments fit together exactly can interfragmentary pressure achieve sufficient rigidity. In the case of intermaxillary fixation, the difficulty arises from having control over the occlusion only in the vestibular region When the fracture lines are within the dental arch, the fragments can turn toward the outside when the tie wires are tightened (Fig. 8.5.3-14). giving rise to lingual malocclusion which is not readily noted.

With the use of compression plates on the outside of the mandible, there is the additional danger of lingual gaping of the fracture line. This must be prevented by a compensation bend (Fig. 8.5.3-15). The danger of displacement as a result of the rigid DCP is not as great

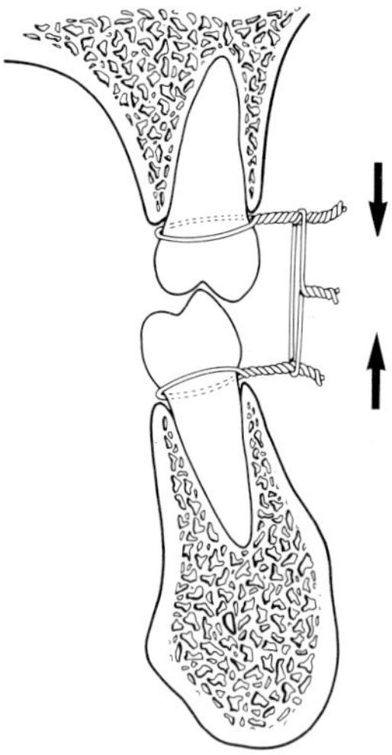

Fig. 8.5.3-14 Interdental ligatures, which are drawn together in the oral vestibule, give rise to the danger of lingual gaping of the occlusion because of the mobility of the parts of the jaw. This cannot be controlled. After rigid fixation with wire ligatures this cannot be corrected.

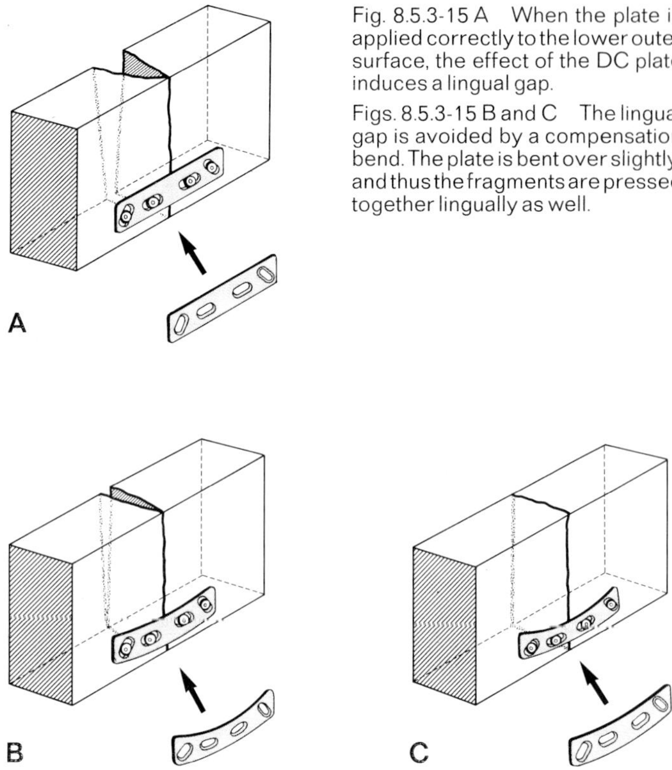

Fig. 8.5.3-15 A When the plate is applied correctly to the lower outer surface, the effect of the DC plate induces a lingual gap.

Figs. 8.5.3-15 B and C The lingual gap is avoided by a compensation bend. The plate is bent over slightly, and thus the fragments are pressed together lingually as well.

when one of the plate fixation screws functions simultaneously as a lag screw.

Fractures in the anterior portion of the mandibular arch are very distinct. Usually they can be reduced manually, especially in completely dentulous jaws. After intraoral exposure of the fracture site, the fragments can be held in the correct occlusion with a Homann hook. In such cases, intermaxillary ligatures are superfluous. Keeping this in mind always allows an exact reduction of simple fractures with the devices mentioned, and thus permits the correct occlusion to be re-established through internal fixation. The prerequisite is that the osteosynthesis be absolutely stable. After completion of the operation, function can be resumed immediately.

In principle, the masticatory part of function need never be considered. Any patient can derive sufficient nourishment for weeks or even months from a liquid diet. The possibility of moving the jaw and opening the mouth is, however, often of vital necessity for patients suffering from systemic diseases; if intermaxillary fixation makes opening the mouth impossible, indications for tracheotomy might well arise sooner. Early resumption of function is also desirable after additional injuries of the TMJ. Disregarding borderline cases in which personal situations influence the decision, we find rigid internal fixation indicated if rapid resumption of mouth opening function is necessary or desirable, or if the impossibility of reduction by conservative means necessitates surgical exposure of the fracture. Specifically, rigid internal fixation of the mandible is indicated in the following conditions:

1. Fractures in the non-dentulous or sparsely dentulous jaw, where a sufficient tooth-borne fixation cannot be achieved.
2. Fractures in the dentulous jaw with:
   a) Simultaneous fractures of the TMJ requiring functional treatment;
   b) Displaced mandibular fractures which cannot be reduced by conservative methods;
   c) Already existing soft tissue infections (if an infection is already present, the danger of the infection spreading to the bone and the development of fracture osteomyelitis is exceptionally great if the fragments are not fixed rigidly);
   d) Patients for whom an intermaxillary immobilization is contraindicated because of some other condition, e.g.
      - susceptibility to seizures,
      - diseases of the respiratory tract,
      - extensive multiple injuries (bronchial toilet),
      - necessity of transportation over long distances after the procedure (for better supervision of the breathing passages and avoidance of the danger of aspiration of vomitus).

In determining whether the indication exists for rigid internal fixation, with the advantages of rapid resumption of function and the less severe and shorter overall incapacitation to the patient which result from the intermaxillary fixation, we must always weigh the disadvantages of a surgical procedure, with all its possible complications and consequences. Osteosynthesis is easier to select if the threat of extraoral scar formation is not present, i.e., if the fracture can be exposed easily via an intraoral approach. Additionally, existing soft tissue injury, through which the fracture area is already more or less exposed, gives preference to osteosynthesis. The surgeon's personal preference and experience also play a significant role. A maxillofacial surgeon in a trauma center is frequently called to treat patients who are already intubated and for whom there are no adequate radiographs. In such a case, he must rely on the clinical examination. With an experienced team, surgical treatment of a jaw fracture sometimes can be performed simultaneously with extremity treatment. Because accident victims are primarily young, extended anesthetic exposure may be justified. It is always surprising how quickly polytraumatized patients recover from extended osteosynthesis operations. Immediate treatment with a precise reduction of the fragments and rigid internal fixation has the advantage of assuring the surgeon that his work was not performed in an infected region. Thus, the chances of healing are greater, the danger of complications is less, and the entire postoperative treatment time is shortened. For these reasons, the experienced maxillofacial surgeon will find internal fixation indicated with relative frequency.

5.3.4. Technique of the ASIF Compression Plate Osteosynthesis, explained through Typical Examples

Case 1:
22-year-old patient with a displaced mandibular fracture on the right side between 42 and 43 brought in during the night shift on the weekend moped accident). Fully conscious, with slight bleeding from a gaping mucosal wound. The fragments can be moved against each other but not brought into the proper position. There is clearly interference at the fracture surfaces. Nasal intubation, application of a few continuous wires in all four quadrants to facilitate reduction. Incision in the oral vestibule from 46 to 33 (Fig. 8.5.3.-16 A). Mental nerve dissected free and mobilized (Fig. 8.5.3.-16 B). Subsequently, the mucoperiosteal flap is shifted aside in the vicinity of the fracture site down to the mandibular border; then the fracture site can be correctly aligned with a periosteal elevator

Figs. 8.5.3-16 A to J Surgical treatment of a fracture in the anterior mandibular region by means of the Freiburg tension band plate.

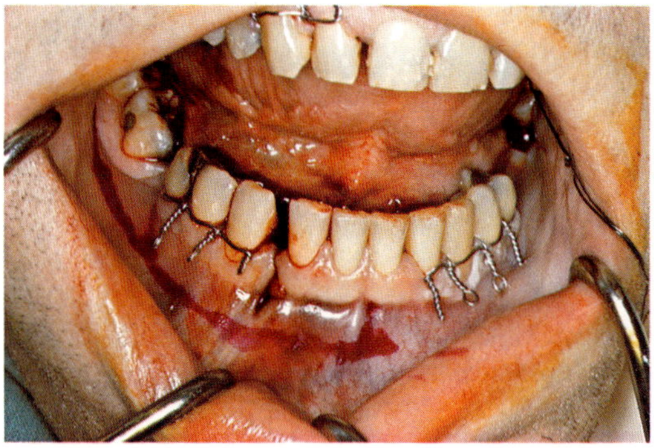

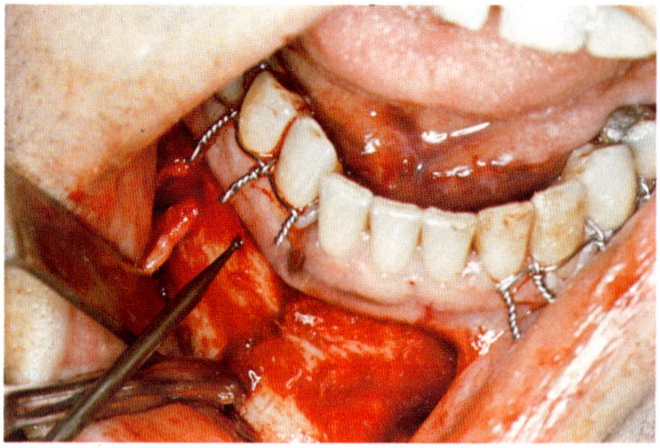

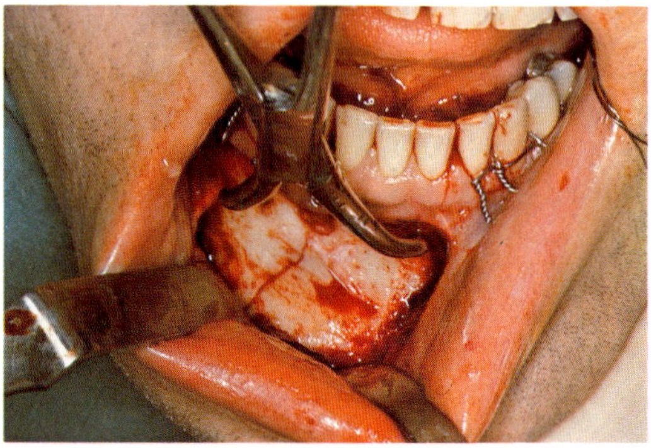

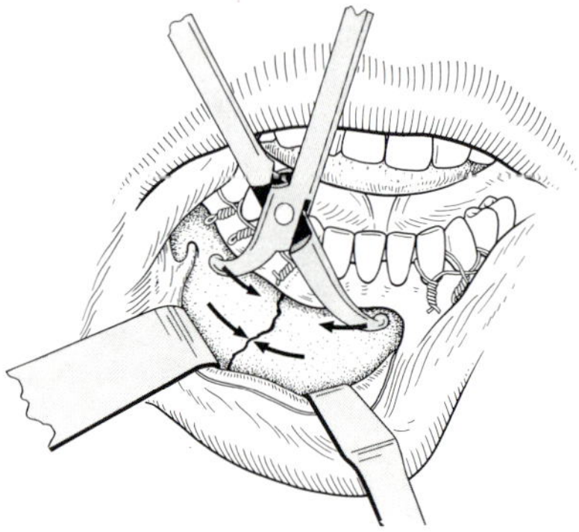

Figs. 8.5.3-16 A to C Incision in the oral vestibule; as a safety measure, several wire ligatures were placed before the surgical exposure. They were not needed, however, because the fragments were easily reduced with a bone forceps and two Homann hooks on the mandibular border.

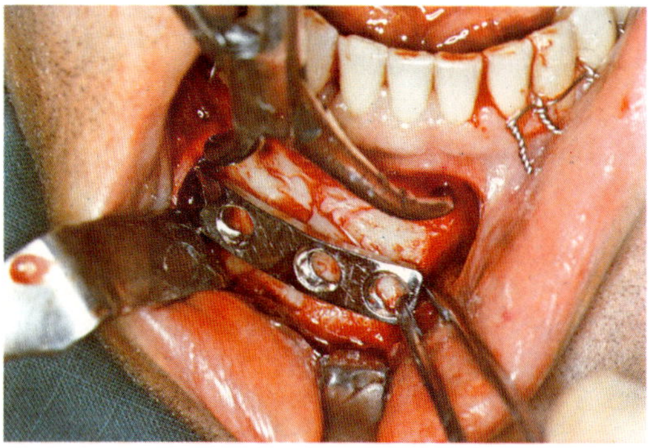

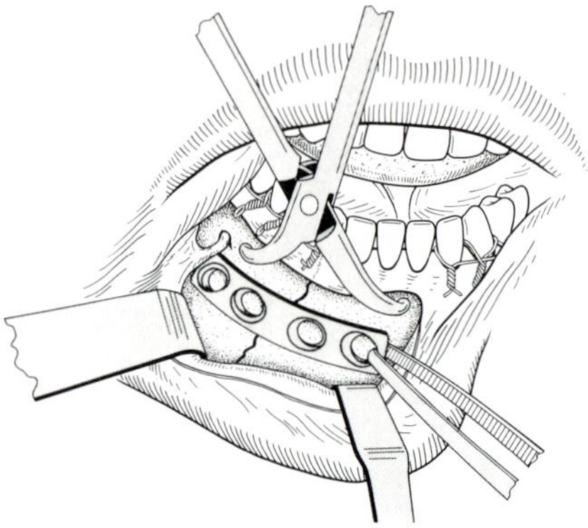

Figs. 8.5.3-16 D The plate is adapted on the fracture site. It is situated under the mental nerve, which has been dissected free. After adaptation, the plate is given a slight compensation bend so that it is somewhat hollow in the middle.

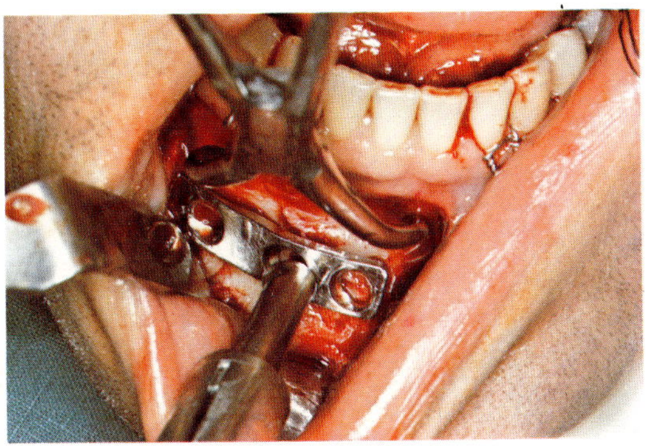
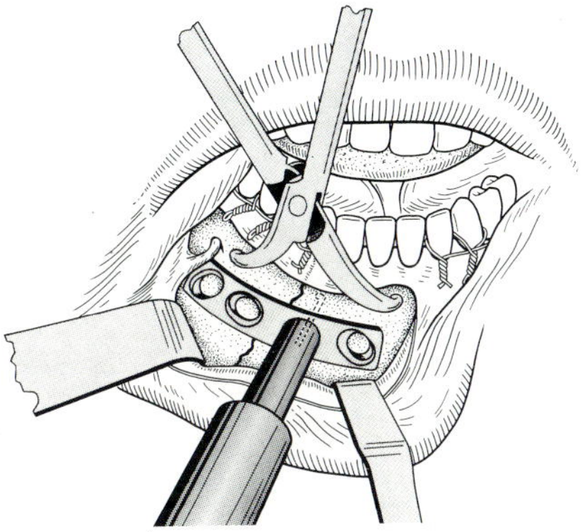

Figs. 8.5.3-16 E After the first holes near the fracture have been drilled, the necessary screw length is determined with the depth gauge.

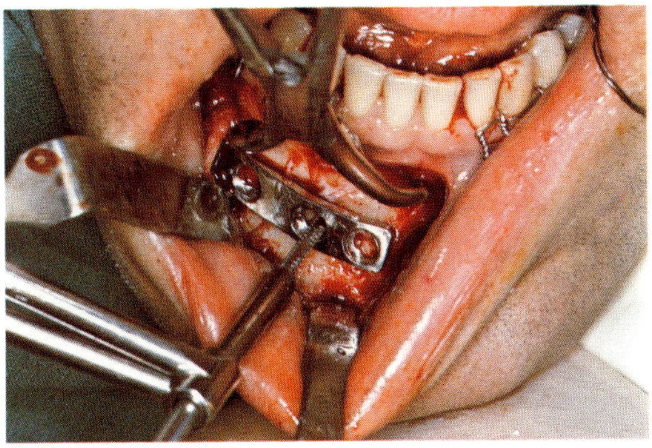
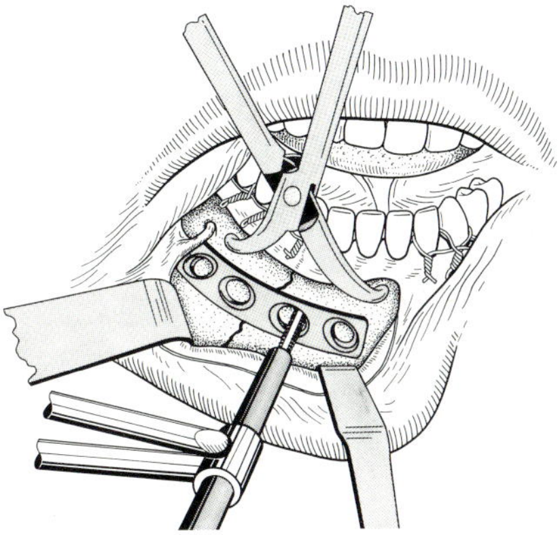

Figs. 8.5.3-16 F The thread is cut. The tap is extremely sharp and should be used only in conjunction with the tap sleeve.

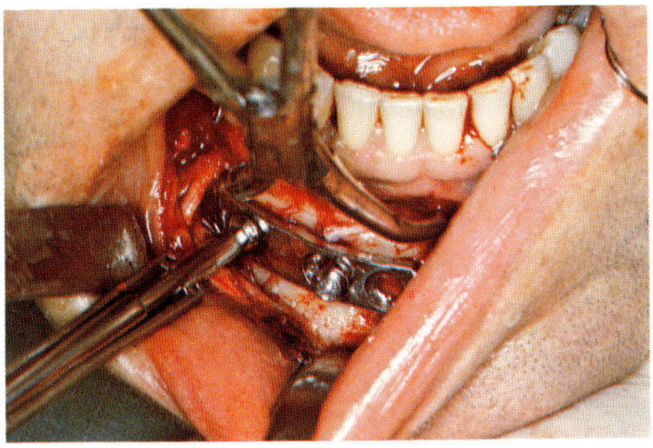
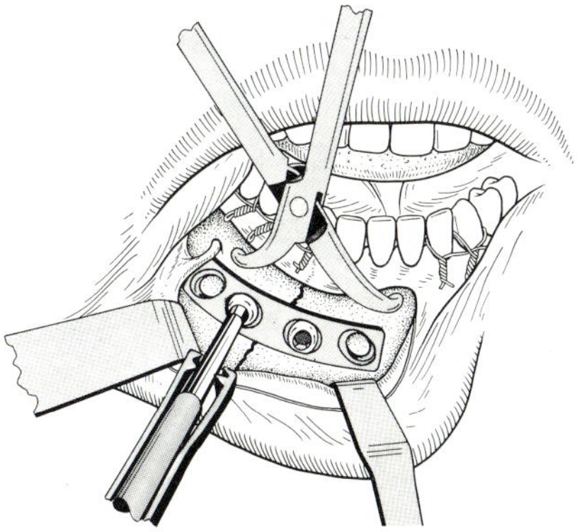

Figs. 8.5.3-16 G The fracture ends are fixated through tightening of the two middle screws. The screw heads have not yet completely entered the DC holes.

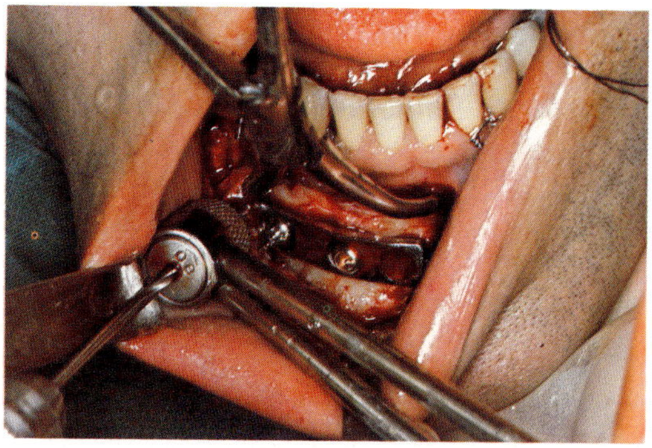
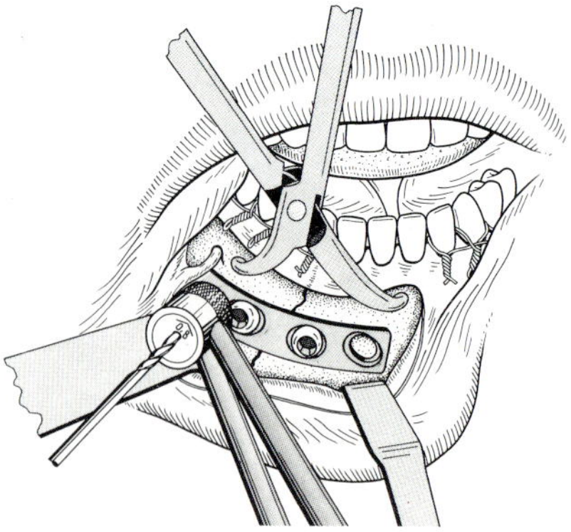

Figs. 8.5.3-16 H Drilling of the holes within the oblique DC holes with the help of the eccentric drill guide.

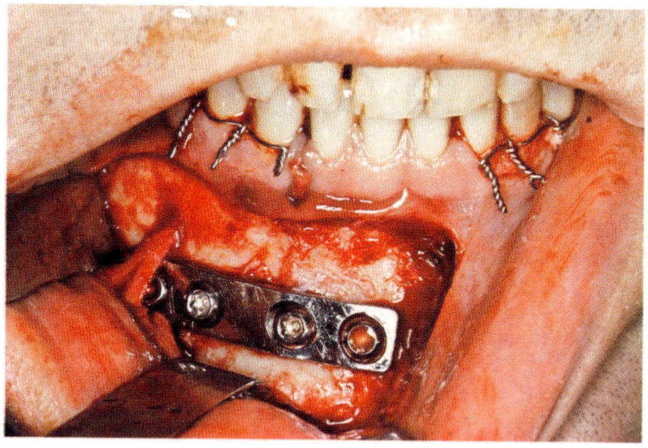
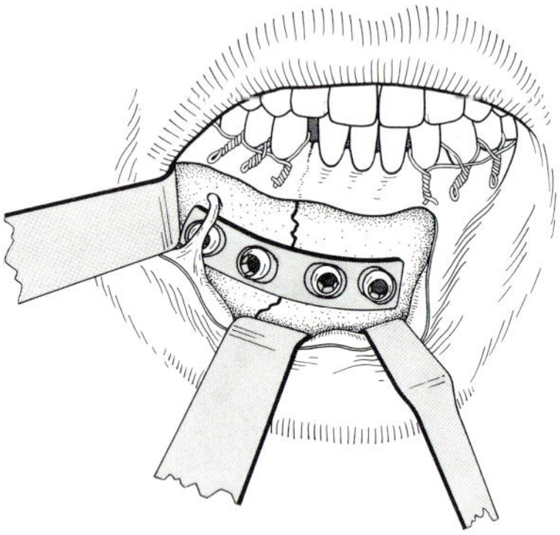

Figs. 8.5.3-16 I All screws are tightened again at the end. The occlusion is tested. The screw heads are deep in the DC holes.

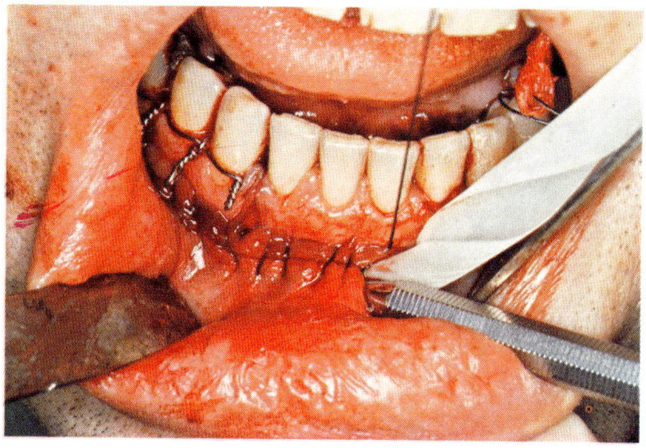

Fig. 8.5.3-16 J The oral vestibular wound in closed with a continuous suture; drainage ensues with a small rubber drain or a Monovac catheter.

Figs. 8.5.3-17 A to C Surgical treatment of a fracture in the lateral mandibular region with a Freiburg tension band plate.

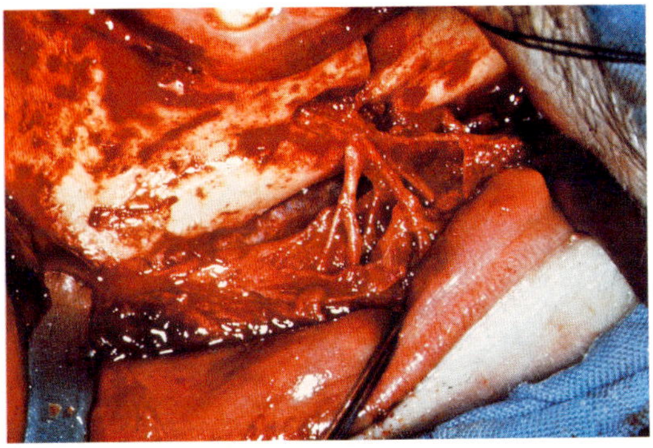

Fig. 8.5.3-17 A Appearance after exposure of the fracture site and dissection of the mental nerve.

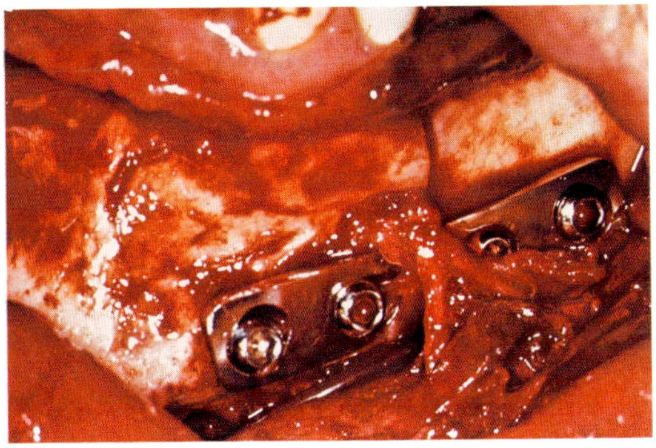

Fig. 8.5.3-17 B The plate *in situ*. The mental nerve is located above the plate.

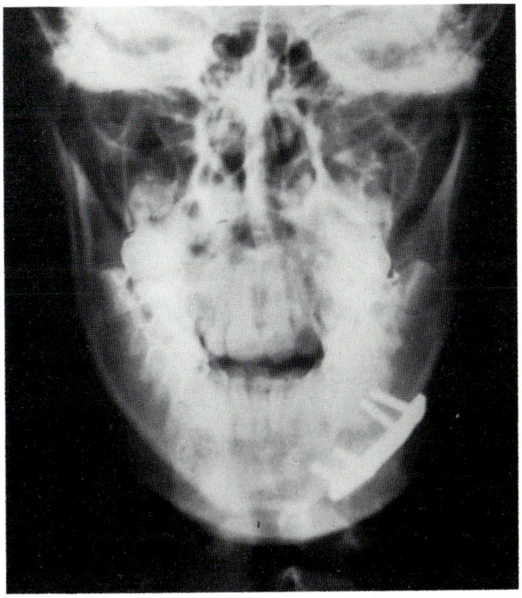

Fig. 8.5.3-17 C Radiograph after osteosynthesis. A second fracture in the right condylar process is treated functionally.

and a Homann hook. The fragments are held with pointed bone forceps (Fig. 8.5.3.-16 C), and a four-hole plate is bent to fit it (Fig. 8.5.3.-16 D). The inner holes are drilled and the lengths are measured (Fig. 8.5.3-16 E), the threads are cut (Fig. 8.5.3-16 F), and the inner screws are inserted (Fig. 8.5.3-16 G). The outer holes are drilled (Fig. 8.5.3-16 H), the threads are cut, and the screws placed (Fig. 8.5.3-16). Primary suture closure (Fig. 8.5.3-16 J). Length of operation: 1 hour.

Case 2:
18-year-old student at examination time, with a fracture only slightly displaced in the horizontal ramus at 35, and fracture of the right condylar process. The patient wishes to be able to speak again in four days, in order to continue his exams.
Nasal intubation, exposure of the fracture through an incision in the oral vestibule, dissection of the mental nerve (Fig. 8.5.3-17 A), adaptation of the plate. Drilling of and thread-cut-

Figs. 8.5.3-18 A to D Surgical treatment of a double fracture of the mandible, at 4 3 and in the left angle, by means of Freiburg tension band plates.

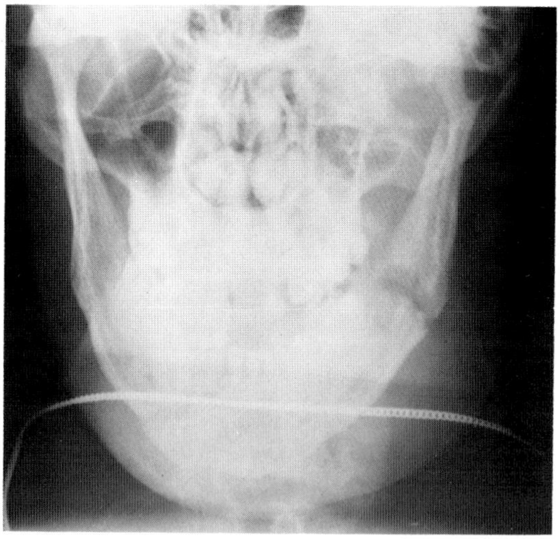

Fig. 8.5.3-18 A Radiograph (from the referring hospital) shows displaced fractures at 4 3 and in the left angle of the mandible.

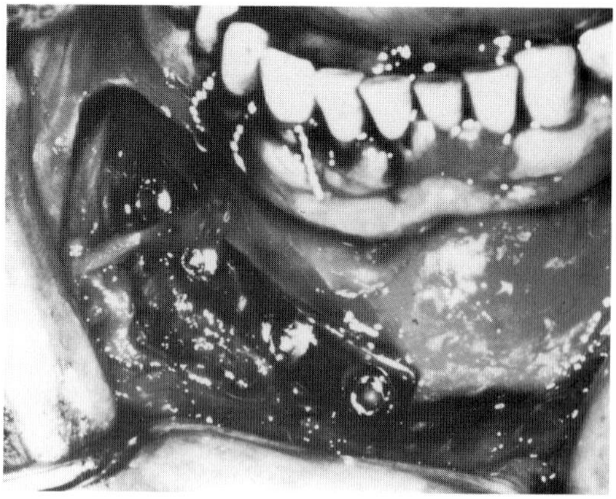

Fig. 8.5.3-18 B The Freiburg tension band plate *in situ* below the mental nerve.

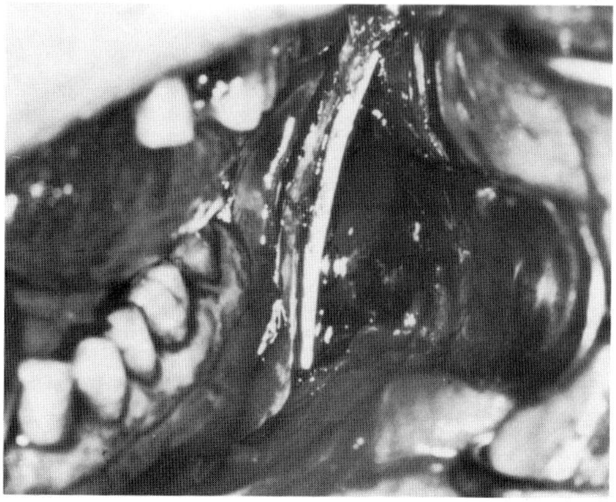

Fig. 8.5.3-18 C The plate in the angle of the mandible, placed intraorally.

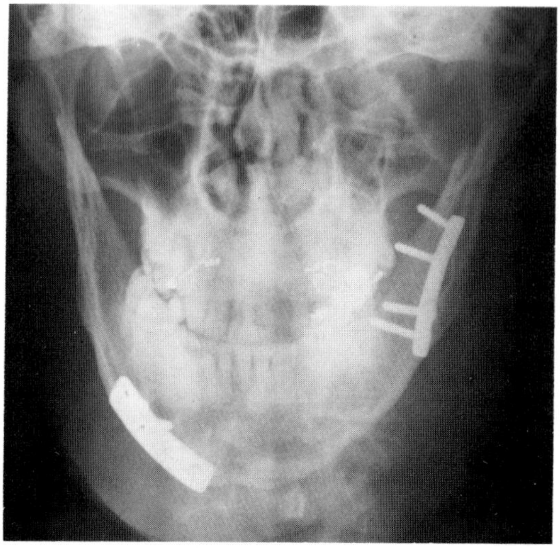

Fig. 8.5.3-18 D Radiograph after treatment.

ting in the distal holes had to be performed transbuccally through a puncture incision (see Fig. 8.5.1-10, section 5.1.1.2). The suction drainage was led off through this puncture incision for two days (see Fig. 8.5.1-11, section 5.1.1.2). The plate is situated under the mental nerve (Figs. 8.5.3-17 B and C).

Case 3:
28-year-old patient after a traffic accident. Thoracic contusion, fracture of the femur, displaced mandibular fractures in the vicinity of the right canine and in the left angle of the mandible (Fig. 8.5.3-18 A). The patient had to be intubated for treatment of the compound femur fracture, and for this reason an immediate simultaneous surgical treatment of the jaw fracture was chosen.
Nasal intubation and re-establishment of the occlusion through the placement of interdental ligatures in maxilla and mandible and institution of intermaxillary fixation. Intraoral exposure of the fracture site in the right canine region. Discovery of a widely gaping fracture (see Fig. 8.5.3-13 A) which could not immediately be manually reduced; therefore, reduction forceps were used (see Fig. 8.5.3-13 B). Fixation of the fracture with the help of a Freiburg tension band plate (Fig. 8.5.3-18 B). Intraoral exposure of the fracture site on the left angle of the mandible and adaptation of the plate (Fig. 8.5.3-18 C). Drilling and screwing ensued transcutaneously with the help of a drill sleeve. Good reduction of the fragments (Fig. 8.5.3-18 D). The intermaxillary fixation was removed after closure of the wound.

Case 4:
32-year-old patient with a compound mandibular fracture in the vicinity of the right mandibular first molar combined with an external wound involving the fracture line. After intermaxillary fixation and trimming of the wound edges, the fracture site is exposed via the external wound. At the lower border of the mandible, holes are drilled on both sides of the fracture (Fig. 8.5.3-19 A). Screws are inserted for fixation of the reduction forceps, and with the aid of these forceps the fragments are reduced and held in the correct position (Fig. 8.5.3-19 B). A Freiburg tension band plate is adapted, given a slight compensation bend and fixed by means of two plate-holding forceps (Fig. 8.5.3-19 C). Thereafter the holes are drilled, the lengths are measured, the threads are cut, and the screws are placed as described in case 1 (Figs. 8.5.3-19 D to G). After insertion of the inner screws, plate-holding and reduction forceps are removed. Insertion of a suction tube for Redon drainage. Wound closure.

Case 5:
17-year-old patient with displaced mandibular fractures in the vicinity of the left canine and in both angles. The third molars are involved in the fracture lines (Fig. 8.5.3-20 A). Wire-acrylic arch bars are applied in the maxilla and the mandible. The mandibular arch bar is separated between 32 and 33. After surgical removal of both mandibular third molars, the occlusion is adjusted for each fragment separately and fixed by application of intermaxillary tie wires. After open reduction, two Freiburg tension band plates are placed in the vicinity of the left canine and in the left angle of the mandible as described above. In the right angle, a more oblique running and wide gaping fracture is found. For better fixation, a plate with 6 holes is inserted. Intermaxillary fixation is left for 8 days (Fig. 8.5.3-20 B).

5.3.5 Results of ASIF Compression Plate Osteosynthesis

The large number of methods available for the treatment of mandibular fractures suggests that there is no single ideal technique for all cases. The variety of methods, and therefore the determination of indications for each, is particularly dependent on results in borderline situations for which several methods have proven effective. Results must consider the outcome of fracture treatment from the perspective not only of re-establishing form and function, but also of the injury which could stem from the particular method.
The most important criterion for judging results of restorative therapy after jaw fractures is the inspection of the **occlusion**. Modern dentistry has found that occlusal deviations of fractions of a millimeter can cause far-reaching late sequelae. In evaluating the occlusion, therefore,

Figs. 8.5.3-19 A to G Extraoral approach for treatment of a fracture of the right horizontal ramus, by means of a Freiburg tension band plate.

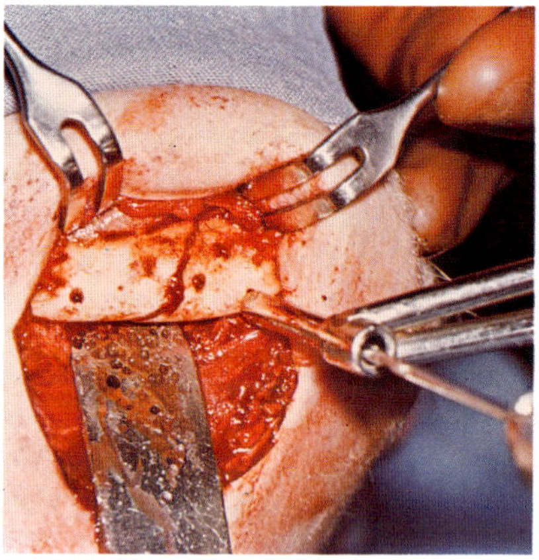

Fig. 8.5.3-19 A Exposed fracture site. Drilling the holes for cortex screws provided for fixation of the reduction forceps.

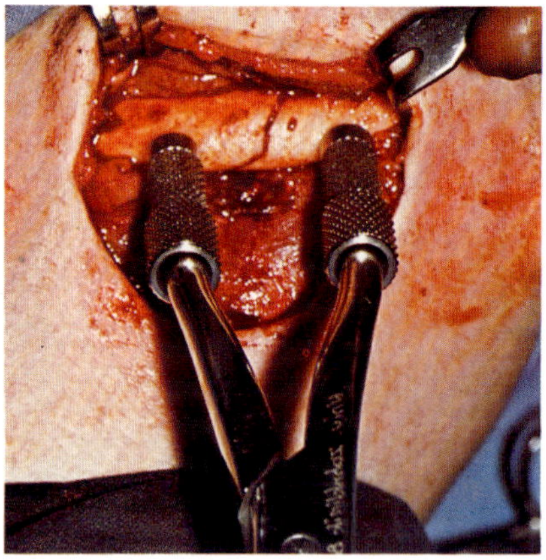

Fig. 8.5.3-19 B Reduction forceps *in situ* after reduction of the fragments.

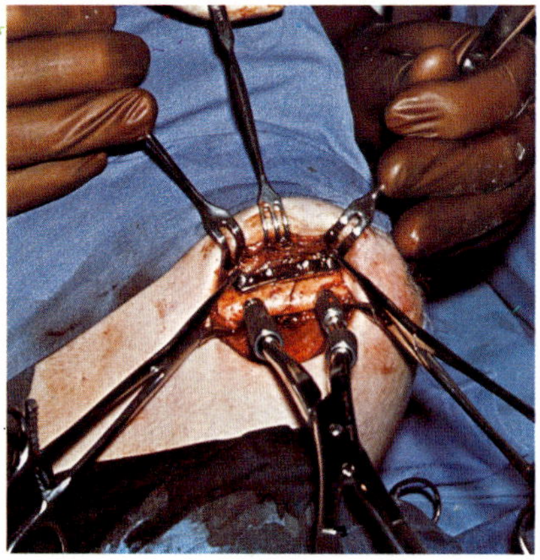

Fig. 8.5.3-19 C DCP adapted on the fracture site and fixed by means of two plate-holding forceps.

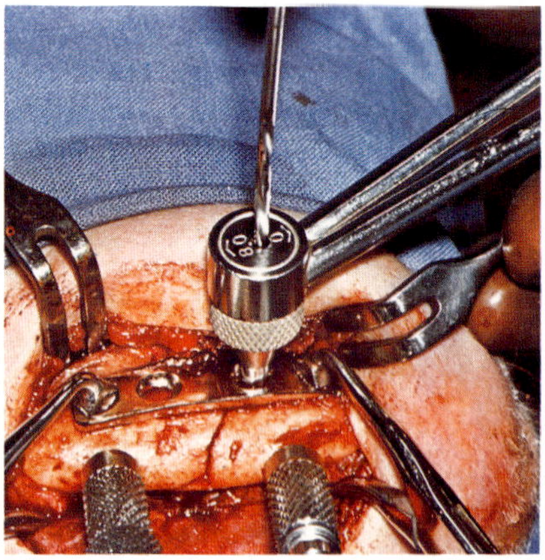

Fig. 8.5.3-19 D The first hole is drilled with the aid of the eccentric drill guide.

simple oral inspection is not enough; at the very least, an inspection with occlusal indicator wax in the dorsal contact position (centric relation) should be undertaken in addition to this oral clinical inspection. An investigation of this sort was carried out at the Freiburg Clinic by *Reuter* and *Scharf* (1976) on patients who had been treated either by conservative measures, i.e., tooth-borne splints, and by compression plate osteosynthesis according to the ASIF principles. In evaluating the results, it must be borne in mind that the greater the displacement of the fractures, the more frequently an indication for surgical treatment through osteosynthesis was found. The group of patients who were treated conservatively with tooth-supported splints and

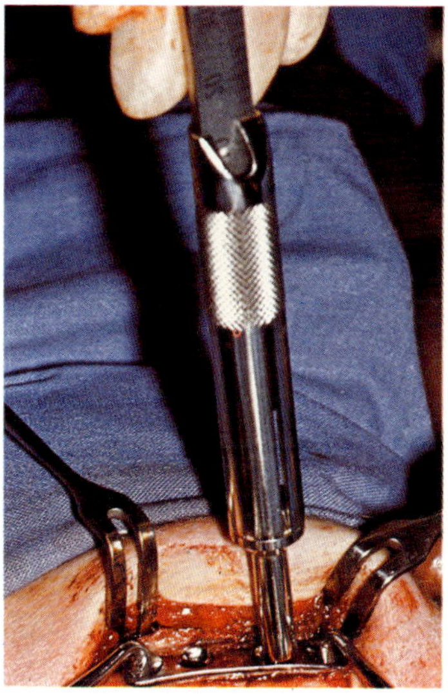

Fig. 8.5.3-19 E The length of the screw is determined with a depth gauge.

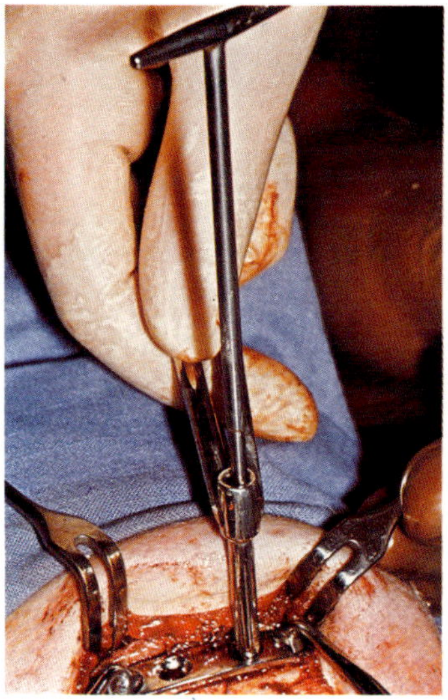

Fig. 8.5.3-19 F The thread is cut.

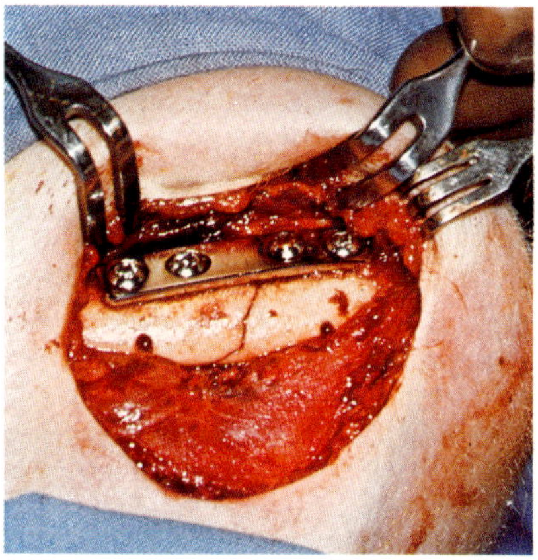

Fig. 8.5.3-19 G All screws are tightened. The fracture ends are exactly reduced and under compression.

intermaxillary immobilization had, therefore, the more favorable prerequisites for *restitutio ad integrum.* Thus, a significantly lower percentage of permanent damage was to be expected with them. This makes it all the more surprising that a normal occlusion was found in 94 % of all cases treated by compression plate osteosynthesis, in contrast to 72 % of the cases treated with conservative methods. Grinding to correct finer occlusal deviations had to be performed in 18 % of the osteosynthesis subjects and in 43 % of the patients treated by conservative measures. The completion of the fracture treatment dated back more than one year for all patients.

Pape and his collaborators came to similar con-

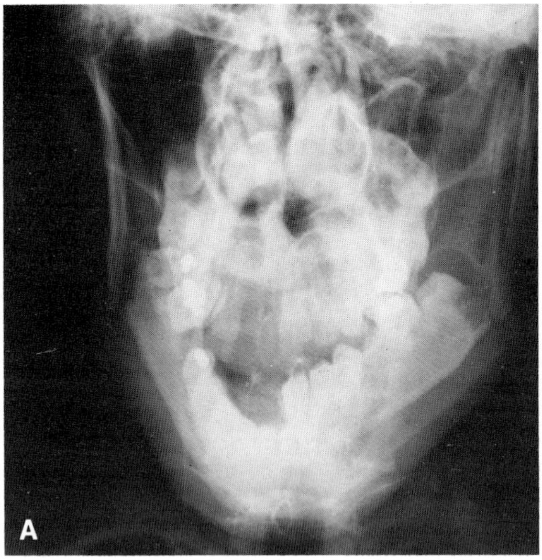

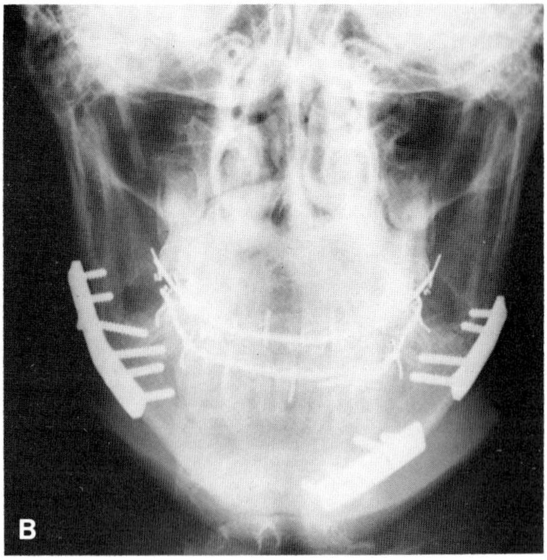

Figs. 8.5.3-20 A and B Surgical treatment of a triple fracture of the mandible, at 3 3 and in both angles, by means of three Freiburg tension band plates.

Fig. 8.5.3-20 A Radiograph before treatment.

Fig. 8.5.3-20 B Radiograph after rigid internal fixation by means of two Freiburg tension band plates with four holes at 3 3 and 3 8 and a Freiburg tension band plate with six holes at 4 8. Both third molars have been removed.

clusions when they retrospectively investigated fracture patients treated in the Cologne Clinic. The superiority of the surgical fracture treatment was particularly evident with patients who were also suffering from fractures of the temporomandibular joint. They showed an occlusal deviation rate of only 6% after surgical fracture treatment, while 17% of the conservatively treated patients exhibited such deviations. The favorable results after rigid internal fixation are probably the result of anatomical reduction. The rate of TMJ problems after jaw fractures with and without TMJ fractures was the same in both groups.

A second possible permanent injury after the loss af mandibular continuity is permanent **damage to the mandibular nerve**, with perception disorder in the vicinity of the lower lip. The declared losses of sensitivity range in the literature between 1.4% and 8.9% (*Müller*, 1967; *Fuchs*, 1967; *Schmieg* and *Niemcyzk*, 1975). A comparison here of the two Freiburg groups investigated is especially difficult in this respect, because it is only natural that the possibility of traumatic damage to the mandibular nerve is disproportionately greater in the cases with greater displacement of the fragments, which was the determining factor for the osteosynthesis indication, than in the barely displaced fractures which were all treated conservatively. The initial findings before the reduction and immobilization cannot be taken into consideration for evaluation. First of all, transient post-traumatic edema can lead to neural function disturbance, and second, the reduced general condition of many patients before either conservative or surgical treatment often precluded a definitive test of nerve function.

In the neurological examination of the Freiburg patient groups, the sensitivity of the lower lip—sensitivity to contact, tactile acuity, and sensitivity to pain—was tested. In contact sensitivity, in comparison to symmetrical sites a weaker sensitivity was categorized as hypoesthesia and abnormal sensitivity as paresthesia. The maximum tactile acuity found in the vicinity of the lower lip, with simultaneous touching at two points, is 4 mm. Inability to separate distances smaller than 11 mm between the test points was categorized as hypoesthesia. Using this neurological standard, normal sensitivity was found in 96 % of conservatively treated patients, as opposed to 87 % of those treated by osteosynthesis. Hypoesthesia was found in 4 % of the conservatively treated patients and in 13 % of the osteosynthesis subjects; total anesthesia was not observed in either of these groups (*Reuter* and *Scharf*, 1976).

In evaluating the disruption of sensitivity after compression plate osteosynthesis in the mandible, it must be taken into account that part of the damage resulted from the trauma. Similarly, danger of damage to the nerve exists during the surgical exposure and reduction. The danger, however, is very great when the drilled holes and screws within them, which are necessary for the fixation, penetrate and thus damage the contents of the canal. The Freiburg cases were all inspected radiologically for this reason, to ascertain the relationship between the hole, the screw, and the mandibular canal. This revealed that in 53 % of the patients at least one screw was partly or completely situated in the canal. Despite this, there was no greater incidence of hypoesthesia in these patients than in those with no connection between the holes and canals. It can be assumed, therefore, that in more than half the cases with lasting damage to neural function, the cause lay not with the operating technique, but rather with the trauma. Follow-up examinations ensued one year or more after the treatment was completed; in general, predictable post-traumatic improvement in sensitivity has appeared. In individual instances, however, it can take even longer than two years for a demonstrable amount of neural function improvement (*Fries*, 1969).

A particular disadvantage of surgical fracture treatment is the inevitable appearance of an operation scar. In the extraoral approach, we observed this in 14 % of the cases (*Schilli* and *Härle*, 1976). This corresponds roughly with the investigations by *Prein* et al. (1976). This danger of a visible extraoral scar is a great disadvantage of internal fixation. It prevents many patients, particularly women and younger subjects, from agreeing to surgery after having the procedure explained to them. In any case, the intraoral approach method seems to us to limit greatly the necessity of extraoral fracture exposure for a stable osteosynthesis. In our department, the fracture is exposed extraorally only in extremely rare cases, when there are extensive comminuted fractures of the angle of the mandible and of the ascending ramus. The intraoral approach, however, also involves a certain amount of scar formation. Even if this scar is not outwardly visible, there is still the danger of a broad cicatricial adhesion to the gingival margin. In all these instances, we then deepen the vestibule as a preventive periodontal operation when the metal removal is performed. The possibility of late periodontal damage thus can be largely avoided.

Deciding on an intraoral approach also eliminates the danger of damaging the mandibular branch of the facial nerve. This possibility of damage, which can be reduced significantly through careful operating technique and the use of an electric nerve probe, is nonetheless still present with this approach. Its frequency is given as between 1 and 30 % (*Freytag* and *Manderscheid*, 1976; *Prein* et al., 1976). This possibility of motor nerve damage further convinced us to prefer the intraoral approach whenever possible.

References

Freitag, V., and G. Manderscheid (1976)
Ergebnisse der Druckplattenosteosynthese nach Luhr. (Results of compression plate osteosynthesis by the Luhr method.) Fortschr. Kiefer u.Gesichtschir. 21: 301

Fries, R. (1969)
Die stabile Osteosynthese von Unterkieferfrakturen unter besonderer Berücksichtigung der offenen axialen Markdrahtung. (Stable osteosynthesis of mandibular fractures with special attention to open axial medullary wiring.) Öst. Z. Stomat. 66: 265 and 298

Fuchs, P. (1967)
Zur Behandlung posttraumatischer Neutritiden und Neuralgien im Kieferbereich. (Treatment of post-traumatic neutritis and neuralgia in the maxillofacial region.) Fortschr. Kiefer- u. Gesichtschir. 12: 41

Krüger, E. (1976)
Lehrbuch der chirurgischen Zahn-, Mund- und Kieferheilkunde. (Textbook of oral and maxillofacial surgery.) Vol. II., 2nd ed. Berlin, Buch- und Zeitschriften-Verlag "Die Quintessenz", 3rd ed. 1981

Müller, W. (1967)
Häufigkeit und Art der Spätfolgen bei 2733 Frakturen des Gesichtsschädels. (Frequency and type of late consequences in 2733 fractures of the facial skeleton.) Fortschr. Kiefer- u. Gesichtschir. 12: 220

Müller, M. E., M. Allgöwer, and W. Willenegger (1969)
Manual der Osteosynthese. (Manual of osteosynthesis.) Berlin, Springer.

Niederdellmann, H., and W. Schilli (1973)
Zur Plattenosteosynthese bei Unterkieferfrakturen. (Rigid internal fixation of mandibular fractures by means of compression plates.) Dtsch. zahnärztl. Z. 28: 638

Pape, D.
Personal communication

Perren, S. M., J. Russenberger, S. Steinemann, M. E. Müller, and M. Allgöwer (1969)
A dynamic compression plate. Acta orthop. scand. (Suppl.) 125: 29

Prein, J., A. Eschmann, and B. Spiessl (1976)
Ergebnisse der Nachuntersuchungen bei 81 Patienten mit funktionsstabiler Unterkieferosteosynthese. (Results of follow-up studies in 81 patients with functionally stable mandibular osteosyntheses.) Fortschr. Kiefer- u. Gesichtschir. 21: 304

Reuter, E., and F. Scharf (1976)
Spätfolgen nach Unterkieferfrakturen unter Berücksichtigung von Frakturverlauf, Dislokation und Behandlungsmethode. (Late sequelae of mandibular fractures with special attention to course of fracture, displacement, and treatment methods.) Fortschr. Kiefer- u. Gesichtschir. 21: 307

Schilli, W., and F. Härle (1976)
Die funktionsstabile Osteosynthese – ein Problem des operativen Zugangs. (The functionally stable osteosynthesis: A problem of the surgical approach.) Fortschr. Kiefer- u. Gesichtschir. 21: 300

Schmieg, E., and H. M. Niemczyk (1975)
Intraorale Drahtosteosynthese bei Kieferwinkelfrakturen. (Intraoral wire osteosynthesis in fractures of the angle of the mandible.) Fortschr. Kiefer- u. Gesichtschir. 19: 107

Spiessl, B. (1975)
Funktionsstabile Osteosynthese bei Unterkieferfrakturen – Probleme und Technik. (Functionally stable osteosynthesis in fractures of the mandible: Problems and techniques.) Fortschr. Kiefer- u. Gesichtschir. 19: 68

Spiessl, B., and K. Schroll (1972)
Gesichtsschädel. (Facial skeleton.) In Nigst, H.: Spezielle Frakturen- und Luxationslehre. (Textbook of fractures and dislocations).) Vol. I/1, Stuttgart, G. Thieme

6. Rigid Internal Fixation by Means of Lag Screws

Herbert Niederdellmann

In osteosynthesis, the requirement of a minimum of implant material with maximum stability always should be considered. This goal is particularly appropriate for lag screw osteosynthesis. Therefore, one should examine, in planning any operation on traumatized patients, whether a lag screw osteosynthesis is feasible.

Surgical treatment of fractures requires analysis of radiographs which show many of the details of the fracture in advance of surgery. During surgical visualization of the fracture site, further details become apparent which, together with the preoperative interpretation of the radiographs, determine the choice of the osteosynthesis material.

6.1 Definition and Action of the Lag Screw

The concept of lag screw osteosynthesis is defined as the stable union of two bone fragments under pressure with the aid of screws which, in turn, are under tension. These screws can be used alone or in combination with a compression plate for stabilization of a fracture. Any osteosynthesis screw can be used for lag screw osteosynthesis, however, screws which have a constant thread diameter along their entire length are the best. It is essential for the bone fragments to be subjected to pressure by the action of the lag screws.

The concept of the lag screw at first appears paradoxical in terms of joining bone fragments under pressure by means of screws. In fact, however, the lag screw acts to draw one fragment to the other, so that, finally, pressure forces exist between the fragments. This is possible because the threads of the screws are firmly anchored only in one of the fragments (the fragment furthest from the screw head). In the other fragment, the screw encounters only little resistance initially—before the final firm screw connection—in a so-called gliding hole, which has a larger diameter. Only at the instant when the fracture surfaces approach one another with further turns of the screws does the low-resistance bed become a firm means of retention for the screw head. When the screw is in its firm final position, the screw head lies in complete congruence on the bone surface, which has been prepared to fit properly. During this process, the fracture surfaces are pressed on one another.

For a better understanding of this principle, it is useful to know diameters of the screws (Fig. 8.6-1). In the ASIF cortical screw, one distinguishes between the spherical head of the screw, the diameter of the core, and the diameter of the threads. The core diameter of a screw corresponds to the drilled diameter of the thread hole. The thread diameter determines the size of the drilled gliding hole, through which the screw threads can slide, so that the screw cannot move sideways, but the threads do not hold. For the screw head, it is necessary to create a corresponding depression at the end of the gliding hole in the outer cortical bone. This bed forms a wide-surface area for the spherical screw head and prevents the occurrence of pressure points which could rupture the cortical bone during the final screw union of the fracture. It is important for the proper function of a lag screw osteosynthesis that the gliding hole corresponds to the diameter of the thread and the thread hole to the core diameter of the screw, and that a cavity corresponding to the screw head is created in the cortical bone (Fig. 8.6-2 A).

If the gliding hole is drilled with a smaller diameter than that of the thread of the lag screw (Fig. 8.6-2 B), the screw already takes hold in the gliding hole itself. Until the screw takes hold in the threaded hole of the other fragment, the fragments will separate from one another and not follow the principle of lag screw osteosynthesis. In such a misinterpreted lag screw osteosynthesis, at best, the fragments may remain anatomically reduced without compression.

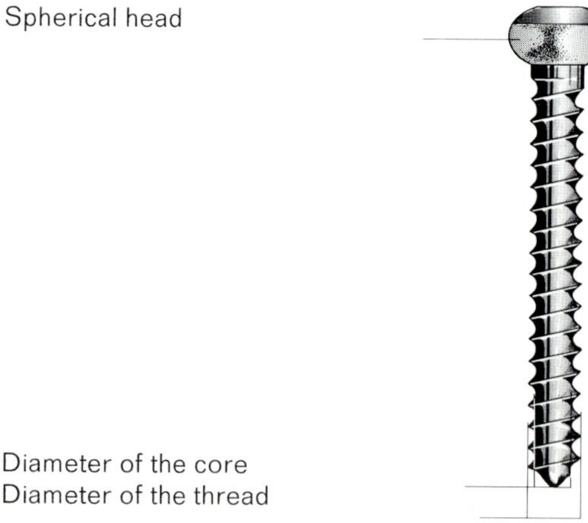

Fig. 8.6-1 Osteosynthesis screw with spherical head.

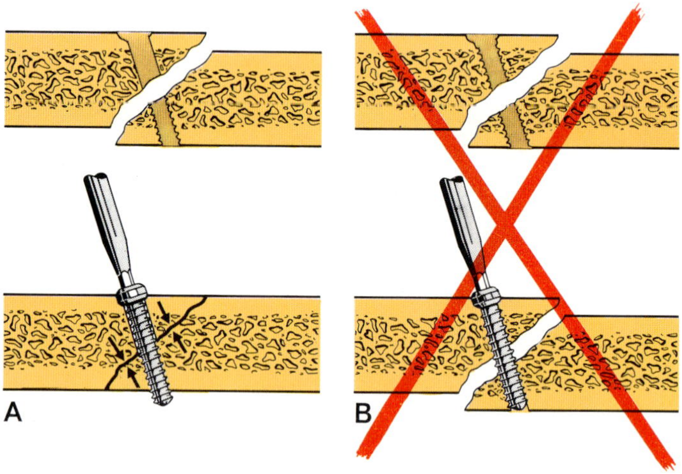

Figs. 8.6-2 The principle of lag screws: (A) correct: gliding hole and thread hole. (B) incorrect: thread holes in both fragments. (After *Müller*, *Allgöwer*, and *Willenegger*, 1969).

6.2 Indications for Lag Screw Osteosynthesis

Lag screw osteosyntheses generally are applied in the treatment of lamellar fractures. Lag screws can be used in conjunction with a dynamic compression plate (DCP) or they can serve exclusively as screw osteosyntheses for stabilization of a fracture.

Short lamellae are stabilized in addition by a dynamic compression plate (Fig. 8.6-3). In wide lamellar fractures, one can dispense with the DCP because, by means of the pressure forces of several screws, sufficient friction between the lamellae and thus sufficient stability of the fragments can be achieved (Fig. 8.6-4).

In comminuted fractures, lag screw osteosynthesis is used primarily to simplify the fracture situation. With the aid of lag screws, several fragments can be transformed into a simple fracture. Additional stabilization is achieved with a neutralization plate which protects the previously applied lag screws effectively (Fig. 8.6-5).

In fractures of the angle of the mandible, lag screws can be applied at the site of the tension

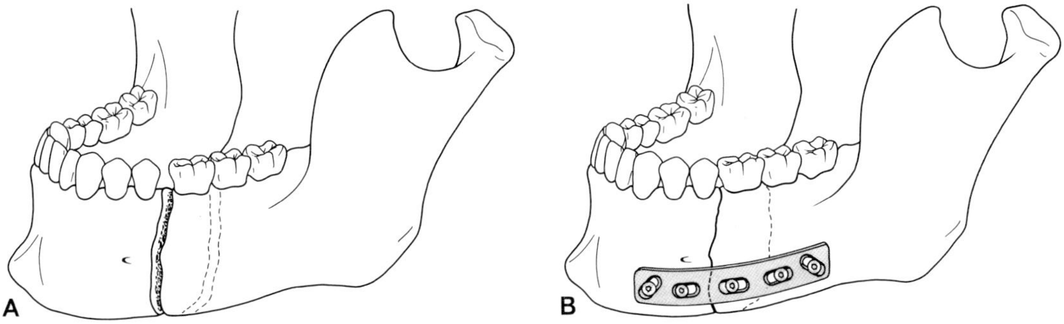

Figs. 8.6-3 A and B Lag screw osteosynthesis in a short lamellar mandibular fracture, in combination with a neutralization plate.

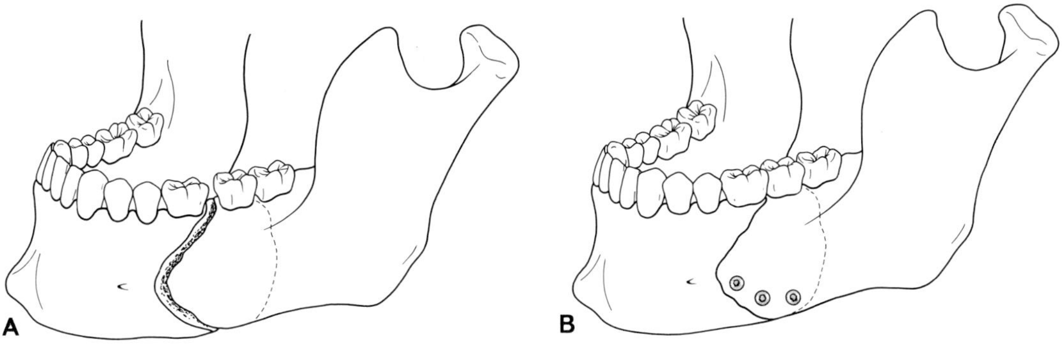

Figs. 8.6-4 A and B Lag screw osteosynthesis in a wide lamellar fracture.

forces. These fractures can be stabilized by means of a single lag screw as a tension band osteosynthesis (Fig. 8.6-6).
In mandibular fractures, as a rule the available space is limited, therefore, one should always begin with a screw of small dimensions.

6.3 Technique of Lag Screw Osteosynthesis

For lag screw osteosynthesis, when the usual cortical bone screw is used, a gliding hole is drilled in the outer cortical bone with a spiral drill. The gliding hole must have a diameter that corresponds at least to the diameter of the screw thread. The inner cortical bone contains the thread hole. To avoid shearing of the fragments, care must be taken during drilling that the axis of the screw bisects the angle between the perpendicular to the fracture line and the perpendicular to the bone surface (*Danis*, 1947; *Müller* et al., 1969; Fig. 8.6-7).
For the systematic screw union of fractures with the aid of lag screws, special ASIF instruments are recommended (Fig. 8.6-8):

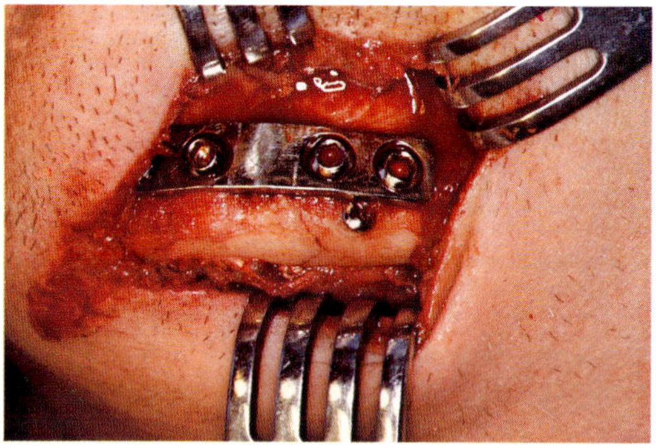

Fig. 8.6-5 Clinical picture of a multiple fracture in which, by means of lag screw osteosynthesis, the number of fragments which had to be fixed by means of a neutralization plate could be reduced to two.

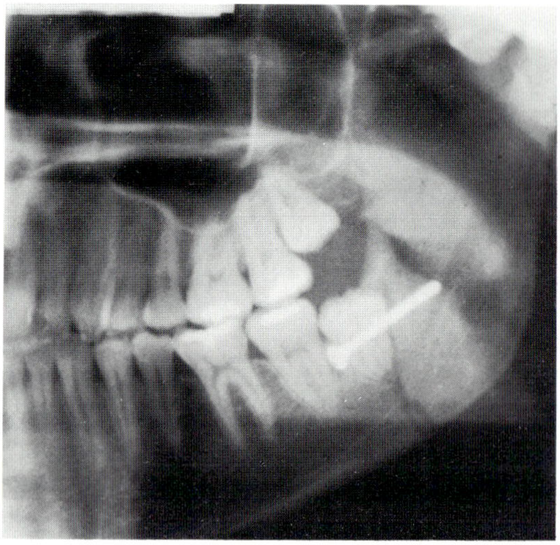

Fig. 8.6-6 Lag screw osteosynthesis for fracture of mandibular angle.

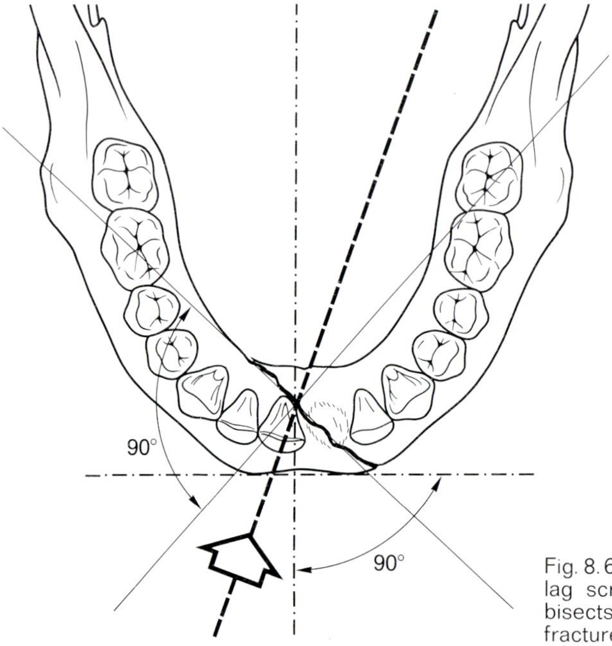

Fig. 8.6-7 Schematic diagram of screw axis for a lag screw osteosynthesis. The axis of the screw bisects the angle between the perpendiculars to the fracture line and the bone surface.

Fig. 8.6-8 Recommended ASIF intruments for a lag screw osteosynthesis (from top to bottom):
drill guide, useful for transcutaneous drilling,
drill bit (extra long) within a drill sleeve,
drill bit (short),
ASIF universal air drill with drill bit (extra long) within a drill sleeve,
drill bit (extra long),
depth gauge,
countersink for manual work,
tap (short) for manual work,
tap (extra long),
screw driver with screw.

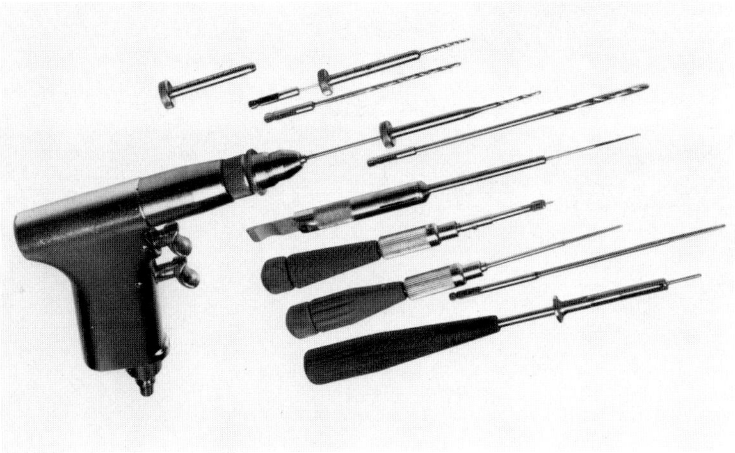

1. Drill bits, extra long, 1.5 mm diameter, 2.0 mm diameter, 2.7 mm diameter.
2. Taps, extra long, 2.0 mm diameter, 2.7 mm diameter.
3. Drill sleeve for transcutaneous drill guide.
4. Transcutaneous drill guide.
5. Countersink.

For a lag screw osteosynthesis with 2.7 mm screws, the fracture is first reduced and then a hole is drilled through the outer cortical bone with a 2.7 mm drill bit, along the axis described above (Fig. 8.6-9 A). It is advisable initially, with the aid of a drill guide, to pit the bony surface by means of a 2.0 mm drill bit in order to obtain a secure hold and a precise direction for the 2.7 mm drill bit. When the bore in the outer fragment end is finished, a sleeve with 2.7 mm outer diameter and 2.0 mm inner diameter is inserted and a hole is drilled further along this predetermined axis into the inner fragment end with a 2.0 mm drill bit (Fig. 8.6-9 B). It is obvious that in this procedure the fragments must remain exactly reduced. After drilling is completed, the length of the screw is measured with the depth gauge (Fig. 8.6-9 C). With the 2.7 mm tap, the thread hole is cut into the inner fragment. For the spherical screw head, a corresponding bed must be created in the outer cortical bone over the gliding hole (Fig. 8.6-9 D). Besides the countersink of the ASIF instrumentarium 5mm spherical burs that fit the dental handpiece can also be used to make this depression. The 2.7 mm cortical bone screw can now slide through the hole in the outer fragment end and obtain its firm hold in the thread of the inner cortical bone (Figs. 8.6-9 E and F). By firmly tightening the screws, the fracture surfaces are stabilized under pressure.

The procedure will be illustrated for a paramedial lamellar fracture. After stabilization of the occlusion with multiple-loop wiring and intermaxillary fixation with rubber bands, the incision is made in the vestibule from 35 to 45. After reflection of the mucoperiosteum and insertion of Homann hooks, the fracture site is clearly visualized. Then the fracture ends are carefully reduced. Next, one drills a gliding hole in the outer fragment end with a 2.7 mm drill bit (Fig. 8.6-10 A) and, after insertion of the drill sleeve, a thread hole is made in the inner fragment end with a 2.0 mm drill bit (Fig. 8.6-10 B). Then the screw length is determined with the depth gauge. The thread is cut with a 2.7 mm tap in the inner fragment end (Fig. 8.6-10 C). With a 5 mm spherical bur, the bed for the screw head is created on the surface of the outer cortical bone above the gliding hole (Fig. 8.6-10 D). Now the hole for the screw is completely prepared. The next step is stabilization with a 2.7 mm lag screw. It is essential that the lag screw completely penetrates the inner cortical

Figs. 8.6-9 A to F Step-by-step procedure in lag screw osteosynthesis.

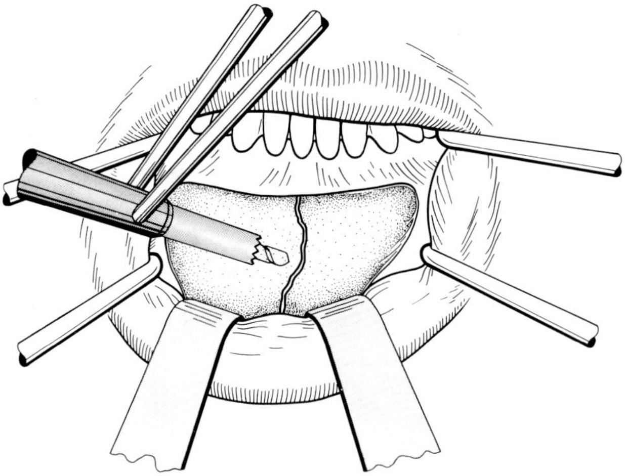

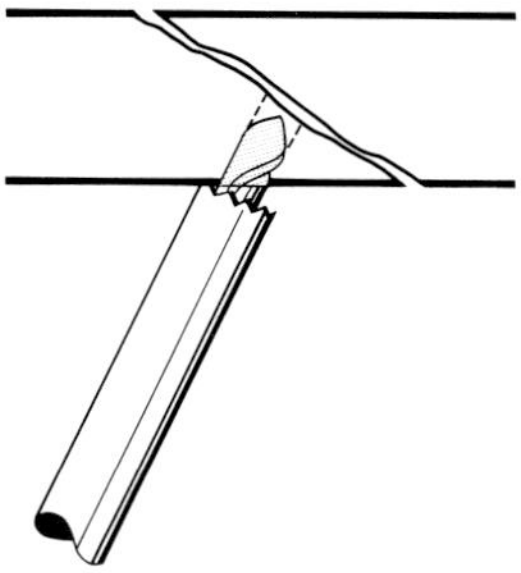

Fig. 8.6-9 A Preparation of gliding hole in the outer fragment.

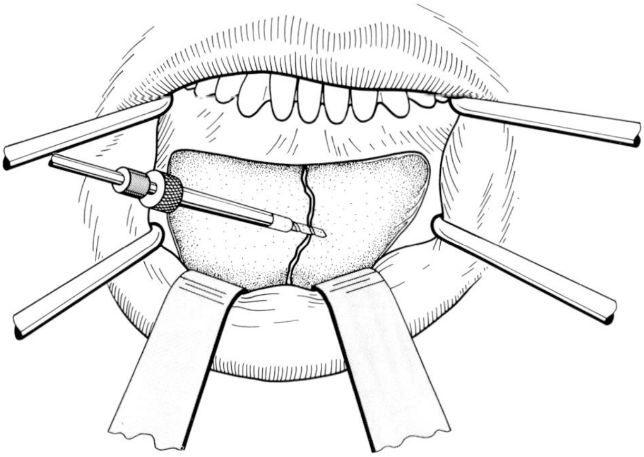

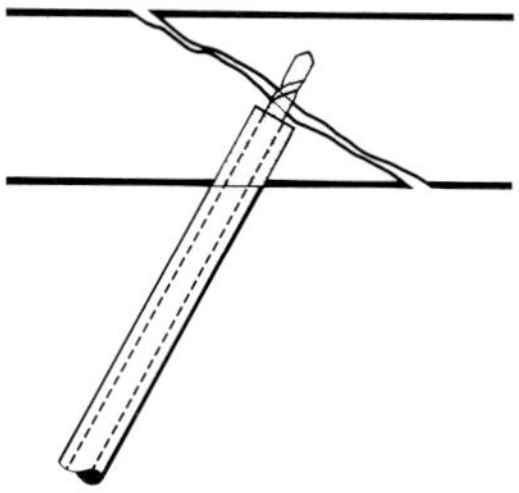

Fig. 8.6-9 B Preparation of thread hole in the inner fragment.

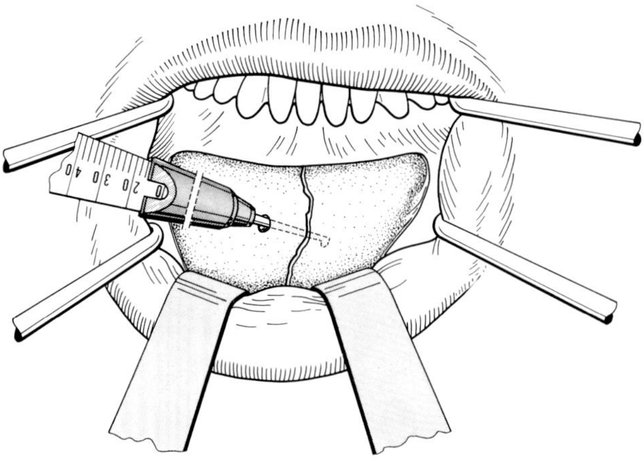

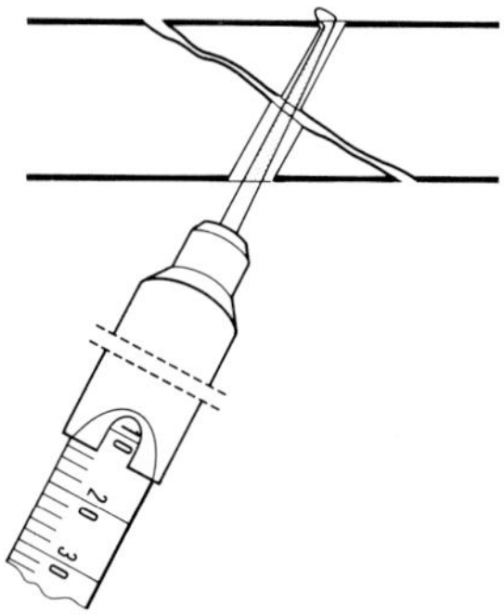

Fig. 8.6-9 C Determination of screw length with the depth gauge.

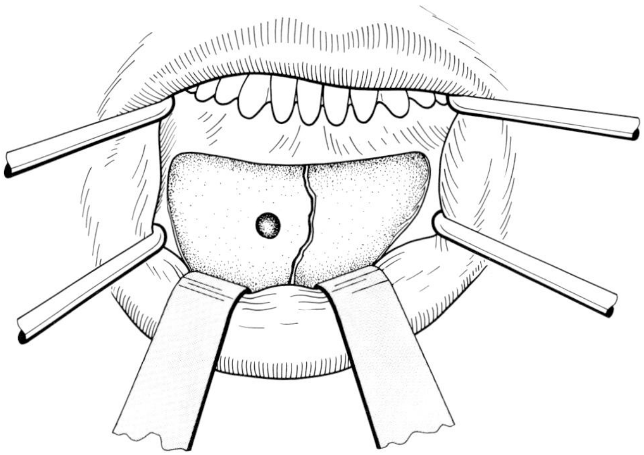

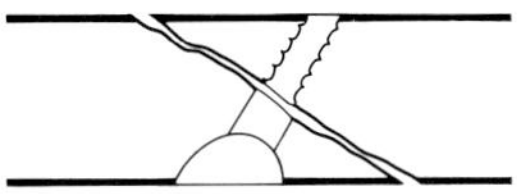

Fig. 8.6-9 D Completely prepared gliding hole and thread hole and bed for screw head.

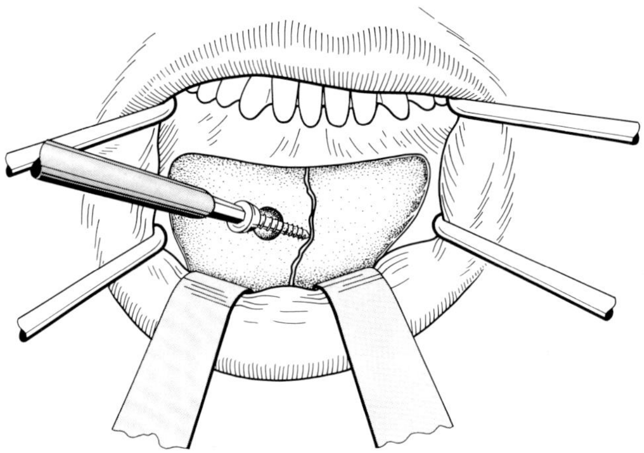

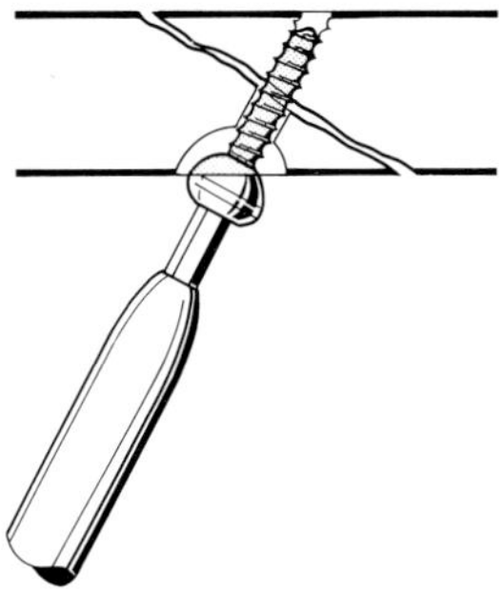

Fig. 8.6-9 E Placement of the first lag screw.

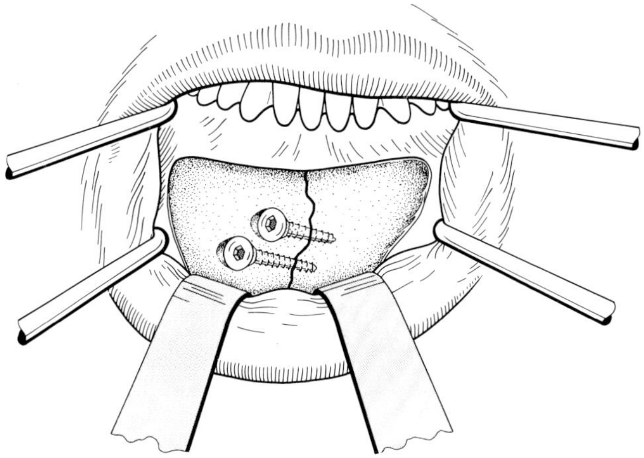

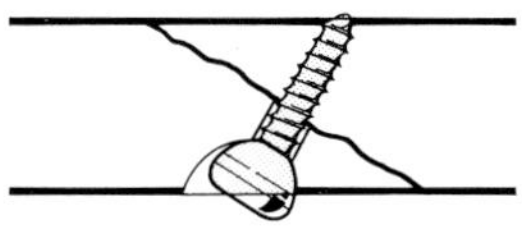

Fig. 8.6-9 F Final fixation of fracture by means of two lag screws.

Figs. 8.6-10 A to E Treatment of an anterior wide lamellar mandibular fracture by lag screw osteosynthesis.

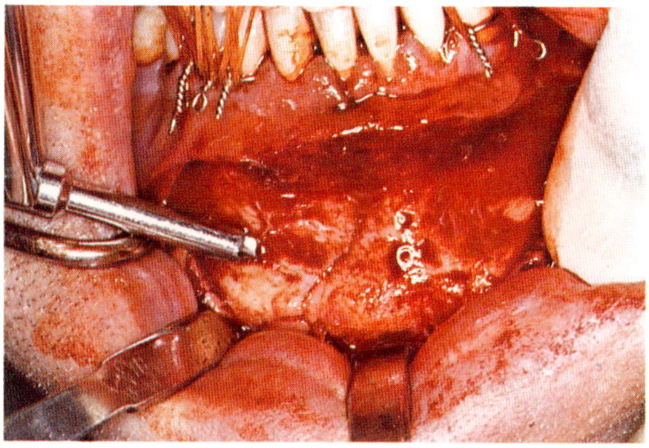

Fig. 8.6-10 A Preparation of gliding hole in the outer fragment.

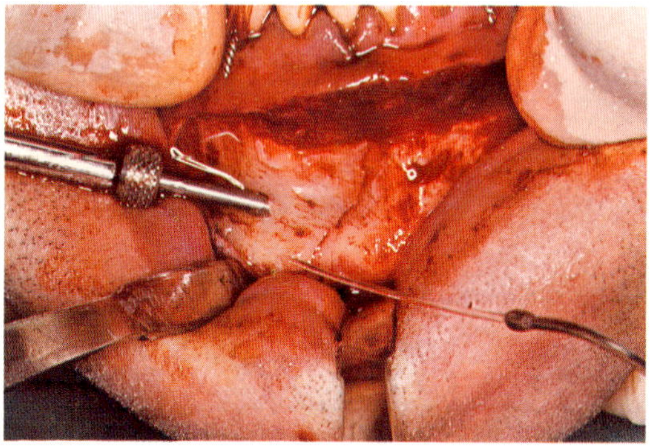

Fig. 8.6-10 B Preparation of thread hole in the inner fragment.

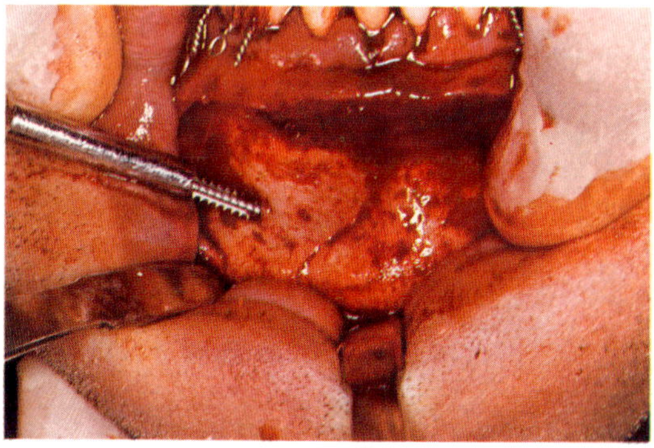

Fig. 8.6-10 C Cutting of thread in the inner fragment.

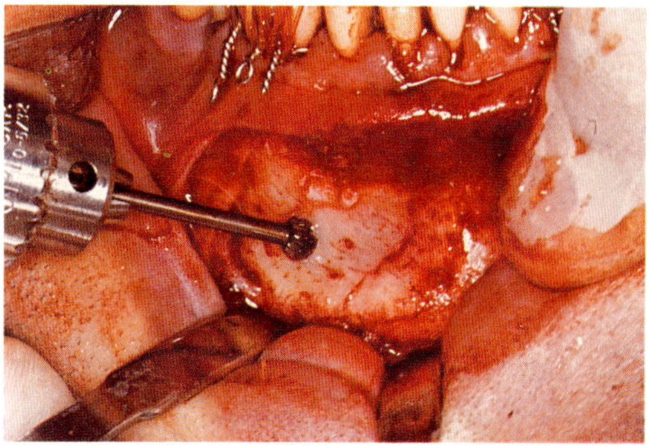

Fig. 8.6-10 D Preparation of bed for screw head in the outer cortical bone.

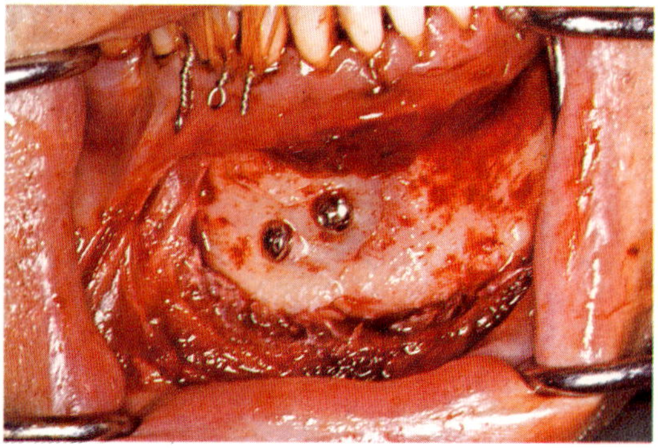

Fig. 8.6-10 E Final rigid fixation of fracture by means of two lag screws.

bone; it is allowed to extend several millimeters beyond the inner bone surface, but must never be too short, because the bony thread can be damaged during tightening of the screw if it is too short. The application of the second, and, if needed, also a third screw proceeds in the same way (Fig. 8.6-10 E). As a rule, wide lamellar fractures can attain functionally stable rigidity with two or three 2.7 mm cortical screws.
For short lamellar fractures, the dentulous jaw should be provided with a neutralization plate in addition. For such a case, one of the middle screw holes of the osteosynthesis plate is used for lag screw osteosynthesis. The formation of the corresponding head space comes about because the osteosynthesis plate itself provides this space in the form of the gliding hole. The other screw holes in the osteosynthesis plate are again provided with screws according to the usual principles.
In wide lamellar fractures, a neutralization plate is superfluous because the large-area adhesion of the interlocking fragments results in additional stabilization of the fracture after lag screw attachment of the fragments. It fractures are treated exclusively with lag screws, however, it is essential to assure that a sufficient bed is present in the outer cortical bone for the spherical screw head.
In comminuted fractures, the fracture situation is simplified initially by means of lag screw osteosyntheses and, in addition, a neutralization plate is applied in the usual way for protection of these lag screws.
Here too, one proceeds entirely according to the principle of the lag screw osteosynthesis described above. If the fragments are very small, it is advisable to use miniscrews. The procedure is completely identical to that for 2.7 mm cortical bone lag screw osteosynthesis:
In place of the 2.7 mm spiral drills, one uses 2.0 mm spiral drills, and in place of the 2.0 mm spiral drills, 1.5 mm spiral drills are used. The sleeve which, in turn, is used to guarantee that one drills along the axis, has an outer diameter of 2.0 mm. With miniscrews, small fragments can be attached to larger ones. The number of fragments which must be stabilized with plate osteosynthesis can thus be decreased with this method.
Experience has shown that lag screw osteosynthesis in the anterior portion of the mandible can be carried out by means of an intraoral approach. Fractures located farther distally require an additional transcutaneous stab incision after an intraoral approach under direct vision. The only exception is that of fractures with a primary external opening.
For lag screw osteosynthesis in the angle of the mandible, the technique is basically the same as has been described. If the screws are to be inserted from caudo-lateral to cranio-lingual, the above-mentioned extraoral stab incision is made at the level of the premolars and the border of the mandible. After manual reduction of the fracture—preferably with centric occlusion—one performs the individual steps already described for lag screw osteosynthesis, by way of the transbuccal channel with the aid of a drill guide and extra-long drills (Figs. 8.6-11 A and B).
It is important in this procedure that drilling be done at a very acute angle to the bone surface and, in the outer cortical bone, at a sufficient distance from the fracture line, at the level of the *linea obliqua*. The creation of a sufficient bed for the spherical screw head (Fig. 8.6-11 C) is again accomplished most readily with a spherical bur in the dental handpiece, with an intraoral approach. This is of considerable importance for the success of the operation. The bed for the screw head must be formed in such a way that the sphere does not make contact prematurely with the bone surface. If these two points are considered sufficiently, tearing of the cortical bone above the gliding hole of the screw can be avoided. The screws required for the treatment of such fractures are between 26 and 32 mm in length.

6.4 Results and Typical Examples

Some clinical cases will illustrate clearly the procedure of osteosynthesis with lag screws:

Case 1:
A 32-year-old patient suffered a broad lamellar fracture of the right mandible and a bilateral fracture of the condyle. These fractures had been immobilized at another hospital with arch bars and intermaxillary rubber bands

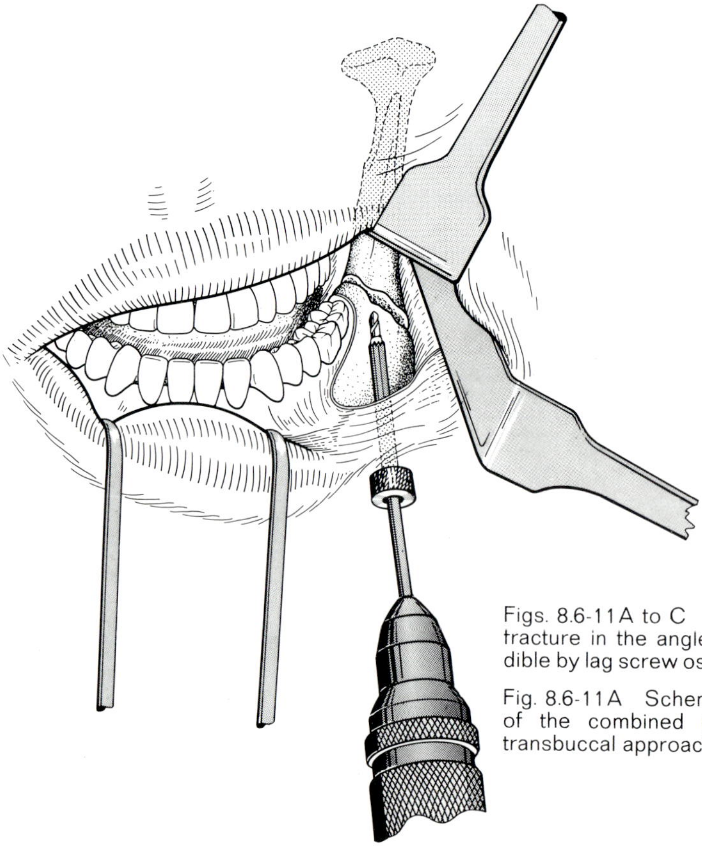

Figs. 8.6-11 A to C Treatment of fracture in the angle of the mandible by lag screw osteosynthesis.

Fig. 8.6-11 A Schematic drawing of the combined intraoral and transbuccal approach.

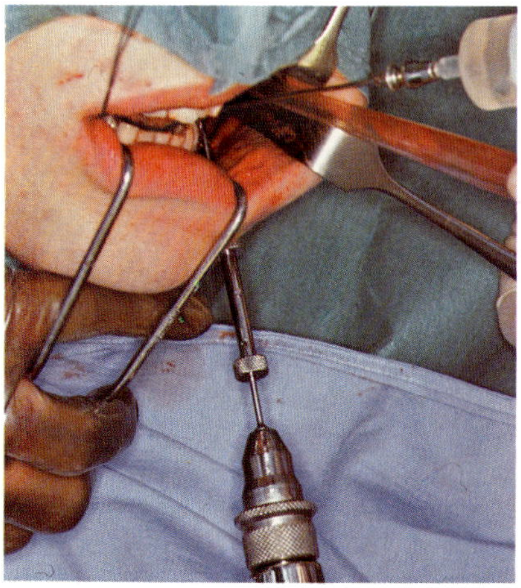

Fig. 8.6-11 B Transbuccal use of instruments for intraoral surgery with direct vision.

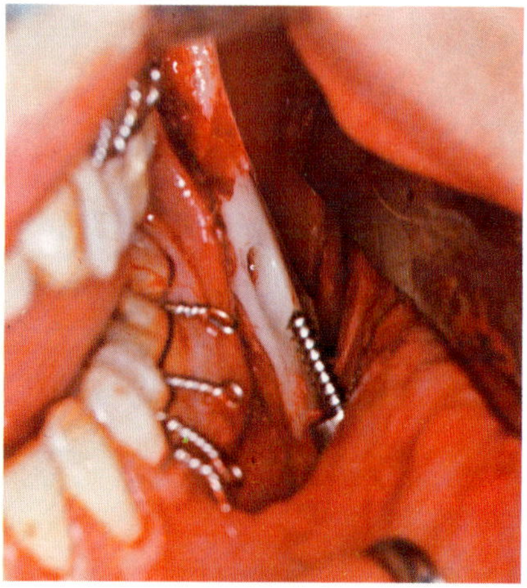

Fig. 8.6-11 C Condition after preparation of the gliding hole and drill hole; application of the lag screw from transbuccal direction for stabilization of the fracture of the mandibular angle.

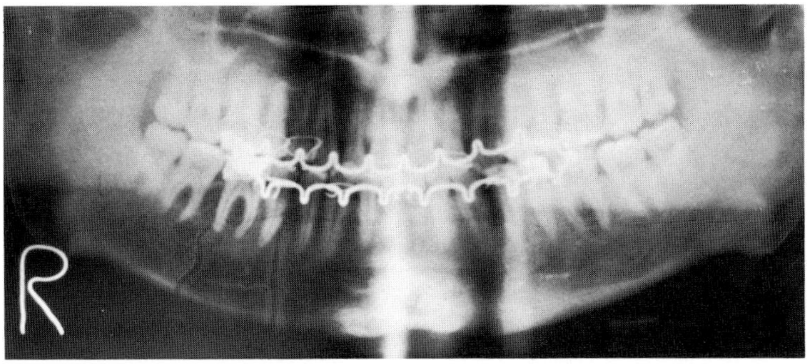

Fig. 8.6-12 A Wide lamellar fracture in the right body of the mandible with accompanying bilateral condyle fractures, after intermaxillary fixation applied elsewhere.

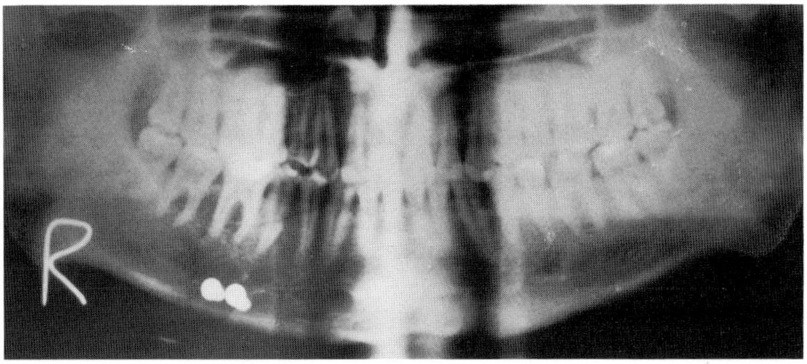

Fig. 8.6-12 B Condition after lag screw osteosynthesis for early functional treatment of the condyle fractures.

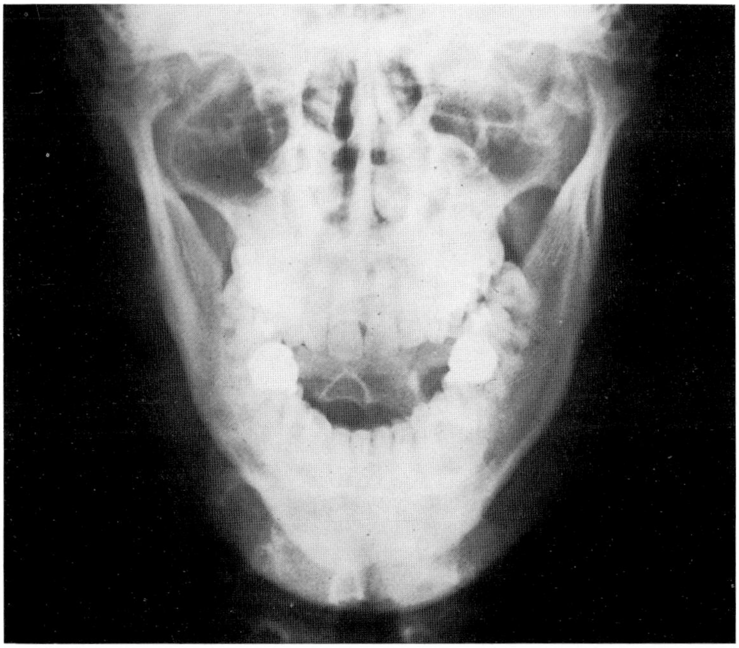

Fig. 8.6-12 C Condition after removal of metal, three months later. The condyle fractures are still visible. The functional result was excellent.

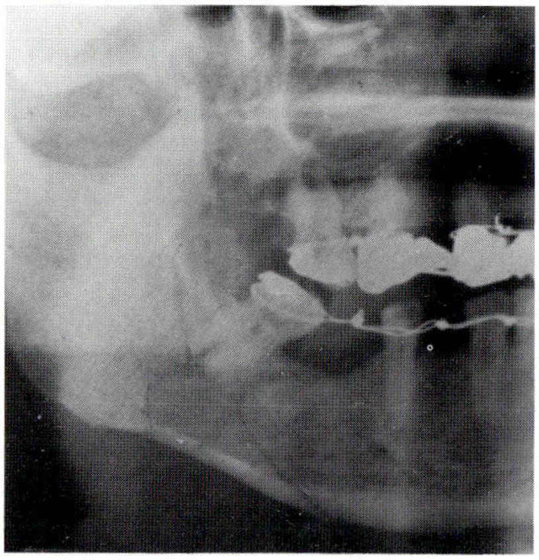

Fig. 8.6-13 A Intermaxillary fixation of a comminuted fracture in the right mandibular angle.

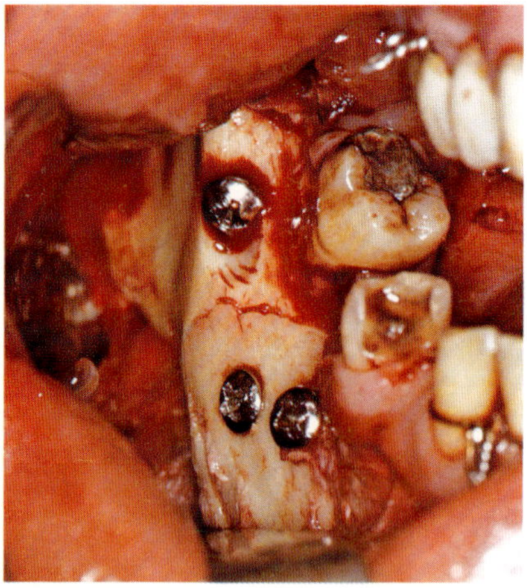

Fig. 8.6-13 B Lag screw osteosynthesis for stabilization.

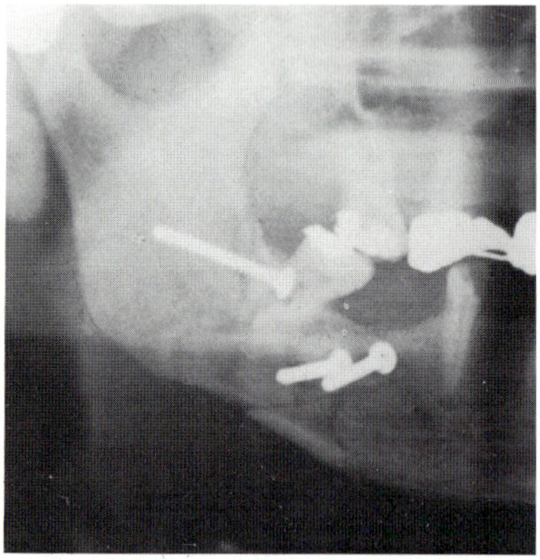

Fig. 8.6-13 C Position of the lag screws.

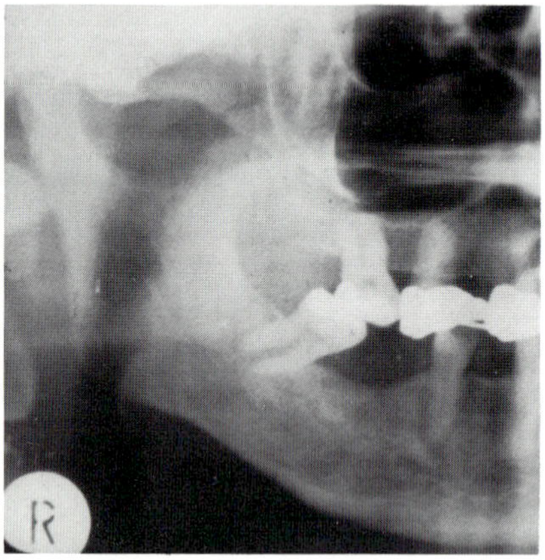

Fig. 8.6-13 D Condition after removal of metal.

(Fig. 8.6-12 A). Two weeks after the primary treatment, a combined transbuccal-intraoral approach was used for stabilization of the lamellar mandibular fracture with two lag screws. The arch bars were subsequently removed. In this way, it was possible to provide functional treatment relatively early for the condyle fractures (Fig. 8.6-12 B). After removal of the metal, three months later, the radiograph still shows the condyle fractures (Fig. 8.6-12 C); the functional result was excellent.

Case 2:
A 43-year-old patient was admitted to the hospital as a night-time emergency patient with a comminuted fracture in the region of the mandibular angle. After application of multiple-loop wires and intermaxillary fixation, radiographs recording the patient's status were obtained (Fig. 8.6-13 A). Long-term intermaxillary fixation was not appropriate here because the patient, for occupational reasons, refused this. Therefore, a lag screw osteosynthesis was under-

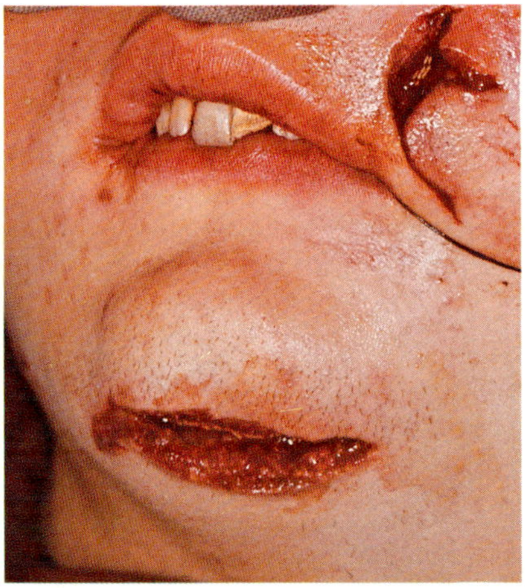

Fig. 8.6-14 A Paramedial multiple fracture of mandible, with extraoral opening; closed fracture of the mandibular angle on the right.

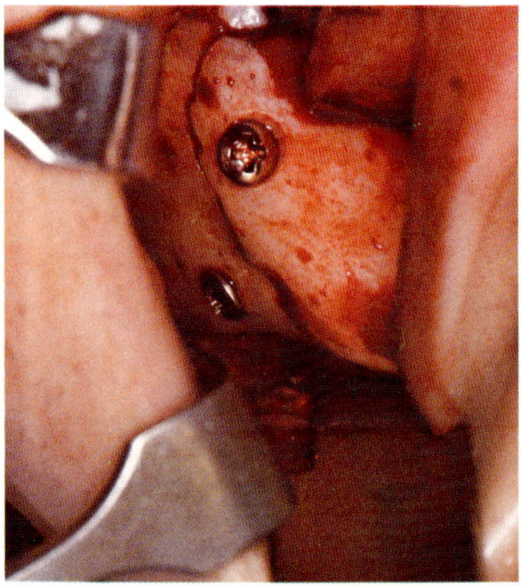

Fig. 8.6-14 B Condition after lag screw osteosynthesis of the mandibular angle fracture.

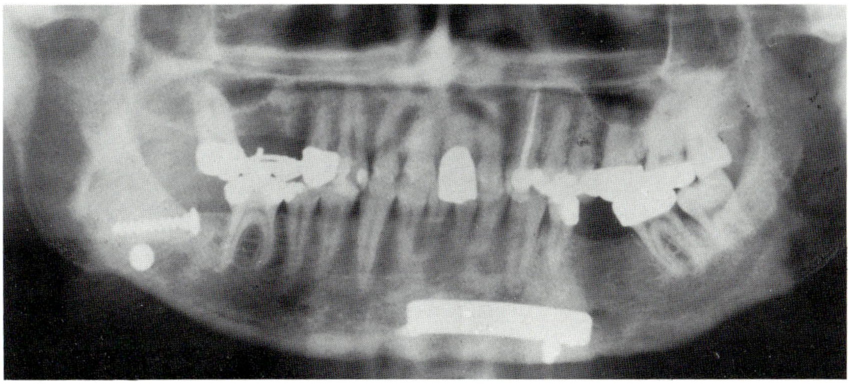

Fig. 8.6-14 C Radiographic control. The paramedial fracture had been treated by means of lag screw osteosynthesis and neutralization plate (see Fig. 8.6-5).

taken (Figs. 8.6-13 B and C). This treatment resulted in healing of the fracture without complications. One year later, the screws were removed under local anesthesia via an intraoral approach (Fig. 8.6-13 D).

Case 3:
A 24-year-old patient was admitted with soft-tissue injuries and a chin fracture with an external opening as well as an externally closed fracture of the mandibular angle (Fig. 8.6-14 A). A rigid internal fixation with plates and screws was performed. The clinical photographs show the mandibular angle fracture after intraoral stabilization with two lag screws (Fig. 8.6-14 B) and the comminuted fracture in the anterior region after treatment with a lag screw and an osteosynthesis plate (see Fig. 8.6-5). A final radiograph shows the treatment result after bony consolidation of the fractures before the metal was removed (Fig. 8.6-14 C).

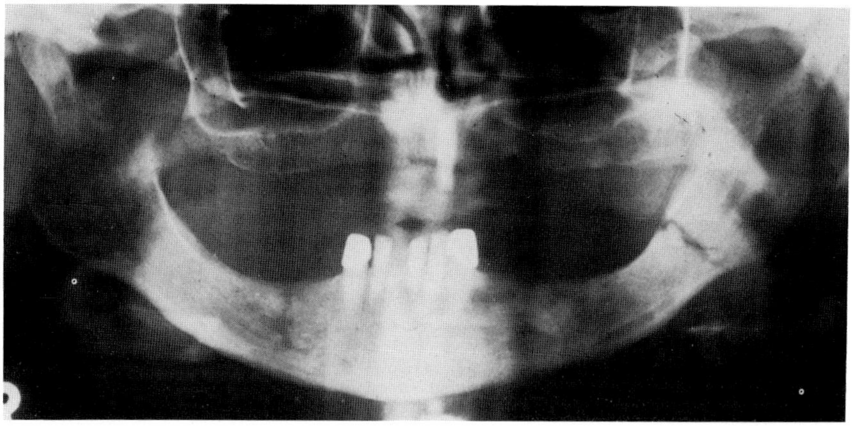

Fig. 8.6-15 A Moderately displaced fractures of mandibular angle and the right condylar process.

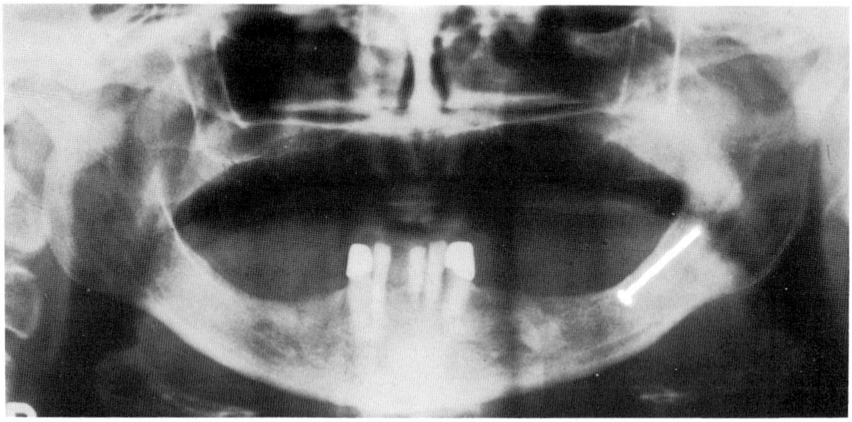

Fig. 8.6-15 B Bony consolidation after lag screw osteosynthesis.

Case 4:
A 45-year-old woman was admitted with displaced fractures of the left mandibular angle and the right condylar process. Her remaining dentition was exclusively in the anterior part of the mandible, and her teeth were in desolate condition. The radiographs show the displaced fractures (Fig. 8.6-15 A) and bony consolidation after lag screw osteosynthesis at the left angle of the mandible (Fig. 8.6-15 B).

In many instances we have obtained excellent results with lag screw osteosynthesis, as did *Brons* and *Boering* (1970), who also used ASIF implants.

Lag screw osteosynthesis represents a valuable complement to compression plate osteosynthesis. It is especially suitable for stabilization of short lamellar fractures and comminuted fractures in combination with a neutralization plate. Functionally stable fixation of wide lamellar fractures can be achieved with two or three lag screws only.

References

Brons, R., and G. Boering (1970)
Fractures of the mandibular body treated by stable internal fixation. J. oral Surg. 28: 407

Danis, R. (1949)
Théorie et pratique de l'ostéosynthèse. (Principles and technique of osteosynthesis.) Paris, Masson & Cie.

Müller, M. E., M. Allgöwer, and H. Willenegger (1969)
Manual der Osteosynthese. (Handbook of osteosynthesis.) Berlin – Heidelberg – New-York, Springer

7. Intramedullary Wire Fixation

Rudolf Fries

7.1 Introduction and Definition

Hey-Groves as early as 1913 introduced rods with a resilient cross-section into the marrow space of tubular bones for stabilization of fractures. This type of intramedullary splinting was refined by *Küntscher* (1962) and became the accepted form of pinning of the marrow. In mandibular fractures, marrow pinning can be applied only rarely, for anatomical reasons such as the absence of a straight marrow canal, the neurovascular bundle in the mandibular canal, and the danger to the roots of the teeth, and for technical reasons, including the rigidity and dimensions of the pin. Only *Lukjanenkow* (1957, 1958) has reported on pinning of the mandible in which, after surgical exposure of the fracture site from a submandibular approach, he prepares a drilled bone channel—at some distance from the fracture line—starting from the mandibular border and at a shallow angle with it and, after reduction of the fragments, uses a jeweler's mallet to insert a pin (rectangular cross-section) which crosses the fracture line.

In traumatology, *Kirschner* wires originally were used for treatment by extension. Later, *Kirschner* wires of very small size also were used for intramedullary fixation of bone fractures in the form of covered or open wiring of the marrow in cases of clavicular fractures (*Knöfler*, 1949; *Stratter*, 1957; *Labes*, 1957; *Küntschner*, 1962; *Bodrogi* and *Hangos*, 1966) and fractures of the forearm (*Knight* et al., 1949; *Aichner* and *Rupp*, 1960). On the basis of this experience, the method of *"open axial marrow wiring"* was developed for mandibular fractures, and thus a functionally stable intramedullary osteosynthesis was made possible (*Fries*, 1966, 1968).

Definition: "Axial" means the insertion, by drilling, of Kirschner wires from the fracture line parallel to the mandibular border. The term intramedullary wiring was adopted from general traumatology as a common concept, even though the mandible does not contain marrow spaces as such, but the *Kirschner* wire is inserted by drilling in the spongiosa region (see Fig. 8.7-3).

7.2 Experimental Investigations

In experiments on dogs (*Fries*, 1969), although the marrow wire was introduced into the mandibular canal, no lesions were observed in the soft tissue.

Bone sections stained with hematoxylin-eosin showed irregular formation of new bone in the mandibular canal, extending about 3 cm distally and proximally from the fracture line. The periosteal formation of new bone occurred in a cuff shape and also was not limited to the fracture site, but was observed to have the same extent as the endosteal formation, even in zones distant from the fracture site.

When the rate of new bone formation was evaluated with the aid of tetracycline marking, the rate of new bone formation at the fracture site was found to be increased 8-fold compared to that in the nonfractured other half of the mandible. The rate of new bone formation was increased, however, not only in the fracture region, but in the entire mandible on the fractured side, decreasing with distance from the fracture line; it was considerably higher postoperatively than when bone healing had ended.

7.3 Indications for Open Axial Intramedullary Wiring

All fractures of the edentulous or partly edentulous body of the mandibule in which conservative treatment is not successful can be considered for intramedullary wiring. Experience has shown that the posterior fracture fragment should be at least 2 cm long. Therefore, fractures of the angle of the mandible cannot be

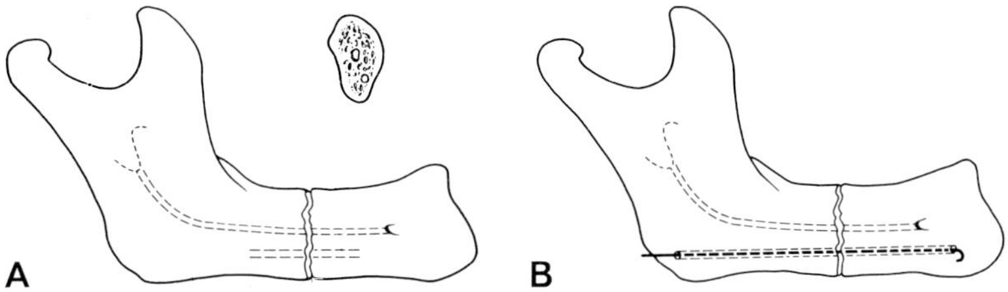

Figs. 8. 7-1 A and B Schematic diagram of axial marrow wiring.

Fig. 8. 7-1 A The guidance channels are prepared in advance with a drill within the spongiosa, starting from the fracture line and proceeding latero-caudally from the mandibular canal.

Fig. 8. 7-1 B Condition after intramedullary wiring has been carried out. It should be noted that the proximal end of the *Kirschner* wire penetrates the compact bone of the mandible; the anterior end of the wire is bent at a sharp angle, shortened, and lowered beneath the skin.

treated with intramedullary wiring. We have no direct experience with the surgical treatment of extracapsulary fractures of the condylar process with the use of wiring, as described by *Rausch* and *Stanischeff* (1952).

Open axial intramedullary wiring is indicated for the following:

- Fractures of the body of the mandible in cases of deficient dentition.
- Fractures posterior to the dental arch.
- Fractures healed in a displaced position.
- Pseudoarthroses.
- Temporary mandibular osteotomy in tumor surgery.
- Fixation and retention of bone transplants in connection with reconstruction of the mandible.

Broader indications:

- Fractures in an edentulous, atrophied mandible. In such cases, burdening the patient with long-term immobilization of the jaws can be avoided.
- Fractures in mandibles with adequate dentition, in which open reduction is unavoidable. In such cases (see below), it is recommended that additional intermaxillary immobilization be used intraoperatively and for one to two weeks postoperatively.

7.4 Methods of Open Axial Intramedullary Wiring

"Covered" intramedullary wiring, in which the *Kirschner* wire is inserted by drilling, from an anterior approach, into the mandible, traversing the fracture line, has not proved practical, since it is difficult to insert the marrow wire without control, without damage to the roots and to the contents of the mandibular canal.

In **open axial intramedullary wiring**, the fracture site is exposed from the submandibular approach. Starting from the fracture line, one prepares, in each of the fragments latero-caudally from the mandibular canal in the spongiosa region, a 1.5 cm long guiding channel by drilling (Fig. 8.7-1). Now a *Kirschner* wire (1.6 to 1.8 mm diameter), sharpened at both ends into a lancet shape, is inserted in the guiding channel and drilled into the anterior fragment with the aid of a pistol-like instrument which can be connected to any dental unit (Fig. 8.7-2) until the wire emerges through the skin of the chin (Fig. 8.7-3 A). Now the drilling engine is applied to the anterior end of the *Kirschner* wire, the posterior tip of the wire is inserted in the guiding channel of the proximal fragment, and the *Kirschner* wire is drilled through the posterior fragment (Fig. 8.7-3 B). It is important to be certain that the tip of the wire pierces the compact bone layer of the posterior

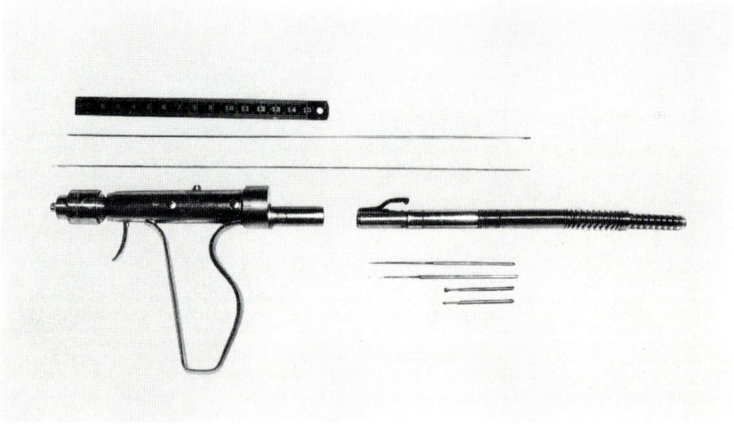

Fig. 8.7-2 A Instruments used for intramedullary wiring.
Top: *Kirschner* wires (1.8 or 1.6 mm diameter) pointed in lancet shape at both ends.
Bottom: "Pistol handle" (left) which can be connected to the cable (right) of any dental unit with a chuck to which working appliances of various dimensions (*Kirschner* wire, drill, dental burs) can be attached (B. Braun, D-3508 Melsungen, Germany).

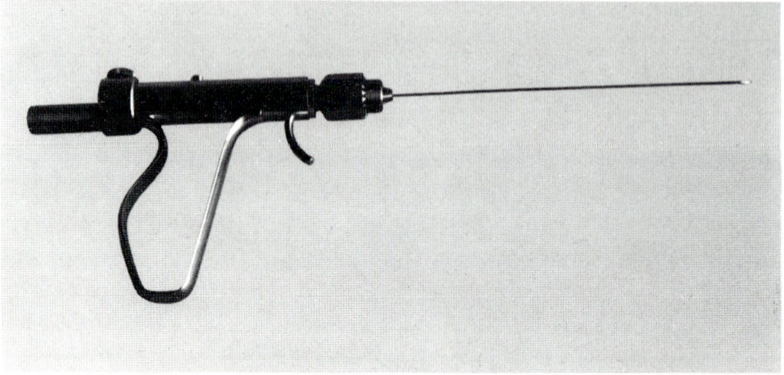

Fig. 8.7-2 B Pistol handle with attached *Kirschner* wire.

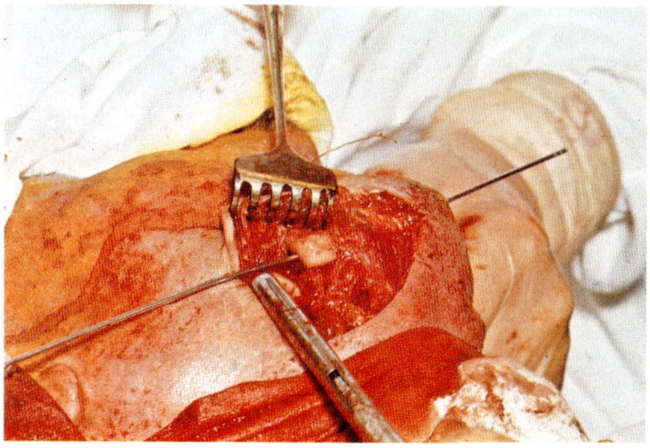

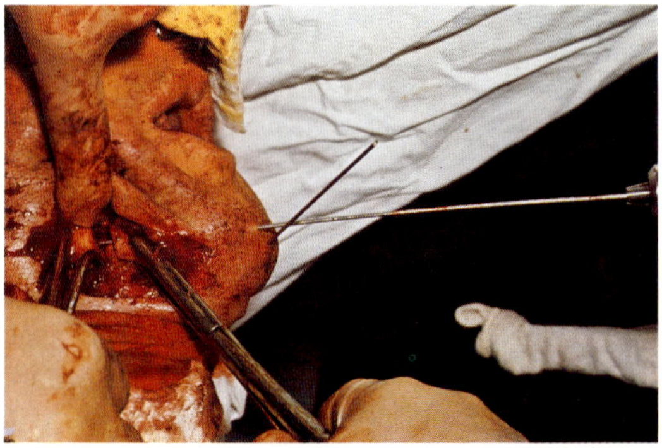

Figs. 8.7-3 A and B View at operation.

Fig. 8.7-3 A The tip of the *Kirschner* wire is introduced into the guidance channel of the anterior fragment, and the mandible is drilled in the anterior direction until the tip of the wire emerges from the skin of the chin.

Fig. 8.7-3 B Now the drill is applied to the anterior wire end, the posterior wire tip is introduced into the guidance channel of the proximal fragment, and the latter is perforated by the drill in the dorsal direction. It is important that the posterior tip of the marrow wire penetrate the compact bone dorsally.

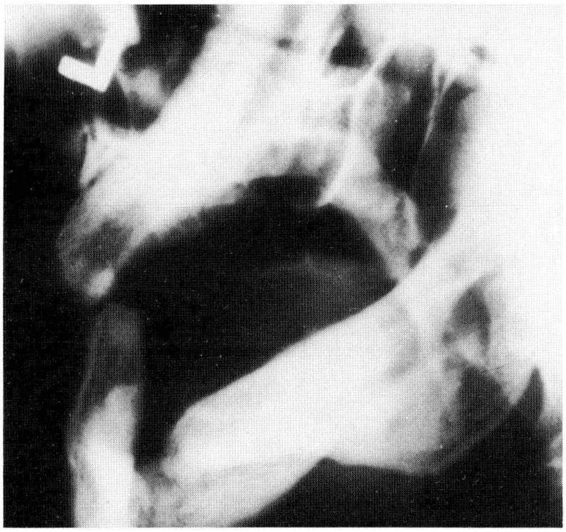

Fig. 8.7-4 A Large midsection fracture of the mandible, which healed in a displaced position. Fracture lines in the premolar region bilaterally.

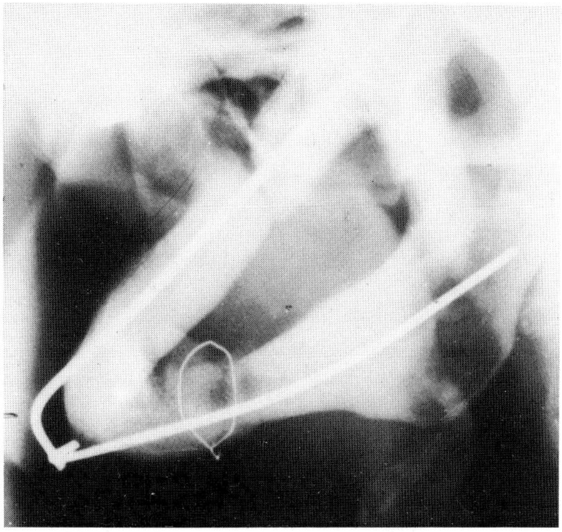

Fig. 8.7-4 B Condition several weeks after intramedullary wiring bilaterally. An ejected bone wedge was fixed in position by means of circumferential wiring.

fragment. Next, the anterior end of the wire is bent at an angle of about 60° at the site of its emergence from the bone, shortened to 1 cm, and submerged beneath the skin.

After 12 weeks at the earliest, if the fracture has consolidated, the anterior end of the *Kirschner* wire is visualized by means of a small skin incision and the wire is removed.

Suggestions: During passage of the *Kirschner* wire through the compact bone, **frictional heat** is formed. *Pallan* (1960) has shown experimentally that rotating speeds of 500 rpm cause least damage. More heat is developed, in our experience, if the wire is passed too close to the compact bone layer over a long distance, or if the *Kirschner* wire is guided at a sharp angle instead of parallel to the mandibular border. In such cases, a radiograph will show small, circumscribed bone necroses. Bone healing, however, is not affected.

Patients can open their mouths immediately after the operation, and take a soft diet. Additional intermaxillary immobilization is necessary only in the dentulous mandible during osteotomy when the posterior fragment is drilled; it remains in place for about 10 days.

The **timing of open intramedullary wiring**, for noninfected fractures, should not be before the seventh day, so that the fracture hematoma, which possesses regenerative potential, is not drained off. If the fracture gap is abscessed, however, it is necessary to wait at least 3 weeks. Early osteitis or osteomyelitis must be excluded as a possibility.

Type of fracture: Transverse and oblique fractures do not differ with respect to healing. For open comminuted fractures exposed to the oral cavity, removal of very small bone fragments is recommended.

Teeth in the fracture line which show no evidence of severe loosening or inflammatory changes can be left in place.

Infections at the site of fracture were seen twice among 52 of our follow-up patients with intramedullary wiring. In one case, the operation was carried out too soon after healing of a fracture abscess. Four weeks after the operation, the patient had clear signs of osteomyelitis along the intramedullary wire on both sides of the fracture line.

In another case, during surgical treatment of an iatrogenic fracture of the angle of the mandible after surgical removal of a third molar, a small root remnant was overlooked, and the result was a circumscribed osteomyelitis.

In another patient, osteitis was controlled by extraction of the tooth located in the fracture line and by antibiotic therapy. Intramedullary wiring, performed two weeks later, resulted in an oral fistula from which a small sequestrum was removed after 8 weeks. This did not delay the healing of the fracture.

In two additional fracture abscesses, osteosynthesis was performed about 6 weeks after the start of the infection. In both cases, the fractures healed without complications.

Radiographic findings: The course of healing of a fracture cannot easily be evaluated radiographically because of the precise adaptation of the fracture ends (Fig. 8.7-4). Periosteal calluses were present after 10 to 12 weeks only in a few patients. Radiographic evaluation of pathologic changes in the bone is of greater importance. Following healing of fracture abscesses, one must look for changes due to osteitis. In addition, the determination of the relationships of teeth to the fracture line is important.

Lesions of the mandibular nerve caused by surgery were not observed, even in animal experiments.

On the other hand, it was shown that, compared to the investigations of *Ditchfield* (1960), regeneration of the mandibular nerve in the presence of lesions is decidedly better when intramedullary wiring is used than if damage is caused by wire sutures in the bone. We ascribe this result to the precise reduction and to the accurate postoperative immobilization of the mandibular fragments by means of a functionally stable osteosynthesis.

In tumor surgery, intramedullary wiring has been found to be very satisfactory for temporary osteotomies of the mandibular bone. In contrast to the wire osteosyntheses in use previously, we observed almost no interference with wound healing in the osteotomy region.

Advantages of open axial intramedullary wiring:
- Stability of the osteosynthesis.
- No need for additional splints in edentulous mandibles.
- Short period of immobilization in dentulous mandibles.
- Rapid restoration of function.
- Protection of the mandibular canal and of the dental roots.
- Precise determination of the position of the *Kirschner* wire.
- Possibility for fixation of larger ejected bone fragments after establishment of continuity of the mandibular arch with supplemental circumferential wiring.
- Avoidance of the disadvantages of blind, covered intramedullary wiring.

7.5 Results

Fifty-two wirings (5 covered and 47 open) were studied during follow up, and 3 failures were observed.
- In one covered intramedullary wiring, the proximal fragment could not be located. Intramedullary wiring was replaced by interosseous wire fixation.
- In one patient, intramedullary wiring was done too early (10 days) after the inflammatory infiltrate subsided following an abscess of the fracture gap. Five weeks later, the patient was hospitalized because of osteomyelitis. After removal of the *Kirschner* wire and high doses of antibiotics, the condition improved rapidly. The patient was not bedridden; nevertheless, a massive pulmonary embolism which developed 12 days later caused the patient's death.
- In one female patient, a small root fragment of the third molar was overlooked in the fracture line; osteitis resulted. The *Kirschner* wire was removed and, after the inflammatory symptoms had subsided, interosseous wiring and intermaxillary immobilization were carried out. Thereafter, the fracture healed without complications.

As more experience has been gathered, it has thus far been possible to avoid further mishaps.

References

Aichner, H., and G. Rupp (1960)
Die gedeckte Markdrahtung unstabiler, geschlossener Schaftbrüche des Vorderarms. (The closed intramedullary wiring of unstable, closed shaft fractures of the forearm. Chir. Prax. 55: 60

Bodgrogi, I., and G. Hangos (1966)
Zur operativen Behandlung der Clavicularfrakturen. (The surgical treatment of clavicular fractures.) Zbl. Chir. 86: 856

Ditchfield, A. (1960/61)
Interosseous wiring of mandibular fractures. A follow-up of fifty cases. Brit. J. plast. Surg. 13: 146

Fries, R. (1966)
Markdrahtung bei Unterkieferfrakturen. (Intramedullary wiring in mandibular fractures.) Fortschr. Kiefer- u. Gesichtschir. 11: 225

Fries, R. (1968)
Die axiale Markdrahtung bei Unterkieferfrakturen. Erfahrungen und Ergebnisse. (Axial intramedullary wiring for mandibular fractures.) Öst. Z. Stomat. 65: 170

Fries, R. (1964)
Methoden der Frakturbehandlung. (Methods of fracture care.) Proc. 14th Biennial Int. Cong. Int. Coll. Surg.

Fries, R. (1969)
Die stabile Osteosynthese von Unterkieferfrakturen unter besonderer Berücksichtigung der offenen axialen Markdrahtung. (Stable osteosynthesis of mandibular fractures with special emphasis on open intramedullary wiring.) Öst. Z. Stomat. 66: 265, 319

Hey-Groves, E. W. (1913)
An experimental study of the operative treatment of fractures. Brit. J. Surg. 438-513

Knight, R. A., and G. D. Purvis (1949)
Fractures of bones of the forearm in adults. J. Bone Jt. Surg. 31 A: 755

Knöfler, H. (1949)
Ein Beitrag zur optimalen Behandlung der Clavicularfrakturen. (Optimal treatment of clavicular fractures.) Chirurg 33: 308

Küntscher, G. (1962)
Die Marknagelung. (Intramedullary wiring.) Berlin, Springer

Labes, H. (1957)
Zur Spiessung der Clavicular- und Unterarmfrakturen. (Intermedullary wiring of fractures of the clavicle and forearm.) Zbl. Chir. 82: 1156

Luklanenko, W. J. (1957)
Clinical observations in the use of intraosseous osteosynthesis in the healing of mandibular fractures. (Translated title). Stomatologiya (Moskva) 36: 31

Lukjanenko, W. J. (1958)
Comparative observations of various methods of intraosseous osteosynthesis and their indications for use. (Translated title). Stomatologiya (Moskva) 37: 15

Pallan, F. G. (1960)
Histological changes in bone after insertion of skeletal fixation pins. J. oral Surg. 18: 400

Rausch and Stanischeff
Cited by Wackerbauer, R. (1952):
Zur operativen Behandlung von Kiefergelenkköpfchenfrakturen. (Surgical treatment of fractures of the mandibular condyle.) Dissertation, Munich

Stratter, P. (1957)
Über Verletzungen der Clavicula und ihre Behandlung. (Clavicular injuries and their treatment.) Chirurg 28: 373

Index

Krüger/Worthington

Oral Surgery in Dental Practice

A textbook of oral surgery for dentists must above all be directed to the special needs of general dental practice.
The practitioner needs a description of surgical techniques and a review of pain control methods, but equally important are the descriptions of aftercare and those complications which may arise in practice. To this end the dentist needs some background knowledge of general surgery if he wishes to successfully use his specialized dentoalveolar surgery.
This book contains the essential information for a course in oral surgery for dentists, including dental implantology and periodontal surgery – as well as those basic elements of general surgery which are particularly significant for the dentist. It results from years of accumulated experience in the practical teaching of dental students and in designing continuing education courses for dentists in practice. It is intended to help the student through the oral surgery course and to serve as a reference work for the dentist in his daily practice.

Foreign editions: German, Italian, Greek, Japanese.
392 pp; 330 single-color illustrations; 17.5 × 24.5 cm format; cloth bound, dust cover.

quintessence books

Richard W. Chaikin

Elements of Surgical Treatment in the Delivery of Periodontal Therapy

The concept of this book is to provide complete and detailed step by step photographs of various current soft tissue periodontal surgical techniques. An attempt has been made to describe the procedures in very specific detail. Pictures were taken during the course of each phase of the procedure as well as afterwards. The detail of the technique of obtaining each particular step is thus vividly portrayed. This monograph, then, is a manual of technique with a minimum of text. By following the abundant and minutely detailed photographs, the postdoctoral student, whether in General Practice, or in a school program, may commence to refine his particular surgical technique.
Included is a fine introductory chapter on philosophy of periodontal therapy, as well as chapters on Electrosurgery and Implantology from a periodontist's point of view. No restorative procedure will be of value unless the supporting structures are first placed in adequate health.
It, therefore, becomes the obligation of every dentist to recognize periodontal pathosis and to have it corrected for adequate biomaintainability. Since this text discusses many soft tissue problems and their corrections, it should be in the library of every dentist.

Foreign editions: German, Spanish, Japanese.
176 pp; 129 single-color and 137 multi-color illustrations;
17.5 × 24.5 cm format; cloth bound, dust cover.